DISEASES OF THE HAIR AND SCALP

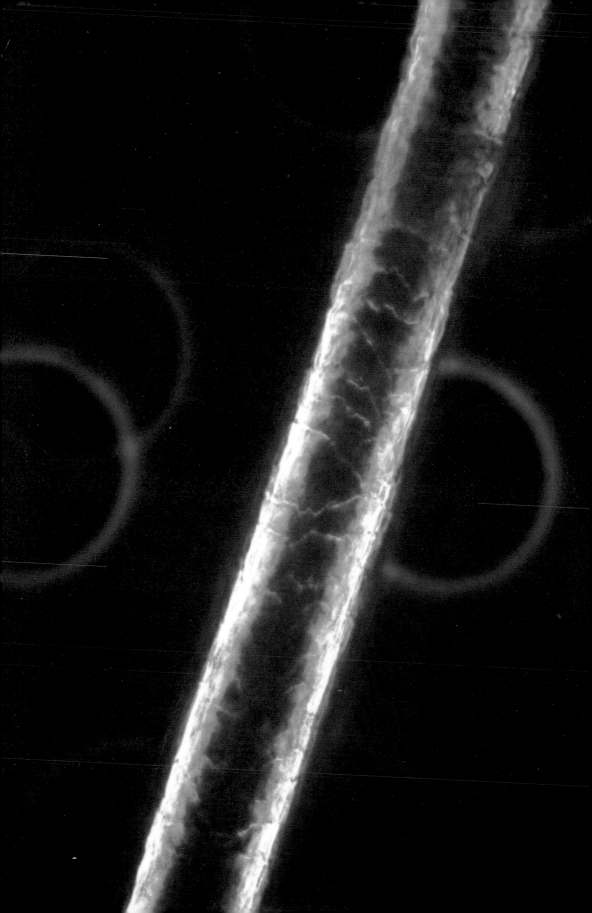

Diseases of the Hair and Scalp

ARTHUR ROOK

MA, MD, FRCP

Consultant Dermatologist
Addenbrooke's Hospital, Cambridge

RODNEY DAWBER

MA, MB, ChB, FRCP

Consultant Dermatologist
John Radcliffe Hospital, Oxford

BLACKWELL SCIENTIFIC PUBLICATIONS

OXFORD LONDON EDINBURGH

BOSTON MELBOURNE

First published 1982

Printed in Great Britain at
the Alden Press, Oxford
and bound at
Kemp Hall Bindery, Oxford

DISTRIBUTORS

USA
    Blackwell Mosby Book Distributors
    11830 Westline Industrial Drive
    St Louis, Missouri 63141

Canada
    Blackwell Mosby Book Distributors
    120 Melford Drive, Scarborough
    Ontario, M1B 2X4

Australia
    Blackwell Scientific Book Distributors
    214 Berkeley Street, Carlton
    Victoria 3053

British Library
Cataloguing in Publication Data

Rook, Arthur
    Diseases of the hair and scalp.
    1. Hair—Diseases
    2. Scalp—Diseases
    I. Title   II. Dawber, Rodney
    616.5'46   RL151

ISBN 0-632-008229

Contents

Preface

With a few notable exceptions most physicians, including most dermatologists, took little interest in disorders of the hair, apart from ringworm and alopecia areata and certain rare hereditary disorders of the hair shaft, until the development of scientific endocrinology in the present century provided some understanding of the mechanisms underlying certain common disturbances of hair growth. Recent research has greatly increased our knowledge of the complex endocrine influences on the hair, and has also established that a wide range of other metabolic and nutritional disturbances, and some psychiatric states, may first be clinically manifest as, or be accompanied by, changes in the density, pattern, colour or texture of the hair. Apart from those abnormalities of the hair which result from direct external infection, or from chemical or physical trauma, almost all are caused by or are related to systemic processes. The patient who complains of loss of hair, or of the growth of hair which she considers abnormal or excessive, is presenting her physician with a symptom which is as worthy of careful study and investigation as is abdominal pain or cough or any other symptom.

Research by anthropologists and zoologists has thrown much light on the origin and significance of certain common changes in hair pattern, which have in the past wrongly been regarded as abnormal. They have also made it clear that there is no scientific justification for the study of the scalp hair in isolation from the reduced but far from vestigial hair coat in other regions of the body.

This book attempts to present a practical clinical account of the hair and its disorders. It is hoped that it will be of value not only to the dermatologist, but also to other physicians who wish to understand the significance of changes in their patients' hair. The comparative physiology of hair growth is described because it throws light on clinical situations in man. The history of each disorder is discussed briefly, where it explains international inconsistencies in nomenclature, and at greater length where it explains how discredited 'scientific' theories of the past have taken a prominent and sometimes a misleading place in contemporary folk-lore.

Diseases of the scalp are included because they are so often associated with some disturbance of hair growth.

Addenbrooke's Hospital, Cambridge   Arthur Rook
Slade Hospital, Oxford   Rodney Dawber

Acknowledgements

We would like to express our gratitude to the many colleagues who have supplied us with clinical photographs of their patients. The source of each illustration is acknowledged in the legend which accompanies it.

We greatly appreciate the assistance of Mr C.Gummer, Scientific Officer, Slade Hospital, Oxford, for drawing many figures and for offering constructive criticisms.

Schering Chemicals Limited have kindly paid the cost of the colour frontispiece.

Chapter 1
The Comparative Physiology, Embryology and Physiology of Human Hair

Comparative aspects of the physiology of hair growth
  Endocrine influences on follicular activity
The embryology of hair
The growth cycle of the human hair follicle

Comparative aspects of the physiology of hair growth
(References p. 4)

Hair is a characteristic feature of the mammals. The factors which control hair growth and replacement in some mammals other than man have been extensively studied for a variety of motives. Economic pressures have certainly provided a stimulus for research into hair growth in the sheep and in other species which directly or indirectly serve man's needs. In addition very numerous experimental investigations have been carried out on the common laboratory mammals.

These studies in mammals other than man are of great importance to the physician in clinical practice for they throw much light on the origin and significance of the complex mechanisms by which the growth and replacement of human hair are regulated.

Although a striking feature of hair in man is its relative sparsity, where it is present it is often long and plentiful and by no means vestigial (Goodhart 1960). Man has largely lost the general covering of body hair which protects the skin of other primates. Ashley Montagu (1964) suggests that this reduction in body hair may have followed the adoption of a hunting way of life which necessitated the development of a mechanism for the rapid loss of body heat. The eccrine sweat glands were evolved, and selection pressures then favoured the partial loss of the covering of hair which impaired their function.

The head hair and the beard are adornments directly concerned with sexual display. Pubic hair is in general much better developed in man than in other species and axillary hair is an almost exclusively human characteristic. It is probable that the hair in both sites is concerned with the wider dissemination of the odour of the apocrine glands, which become functional at the age at which this hair develops.

The general covering of body hair in many mammals has an important function in conserving heat, and in some the colour or pattern of colours serves as camouflage. In mammals living in geographical regions in which there are

I

marked seasonal changes in temperature, a heavy coat which made survival possible throughout the cold winter could well be a handicap in warmer weather. Moulting evolved under such climatic conditions to allow the necessary seasonal adjustment of the weight (and in some species also of the colour) of the coat. However, moulting is not necessarily seasonal; it may correlate with age or with reproduction cycles (Ebling 1965).

Wave moulting
The pattern of moulting varies greatly from species to species and even in successive cycles in a single species (Ebling 1965). Moulting may be related to age, the texture, density and colour of successive coats adapting the young animal to the changed circumstances of each stage of development. Synchronous shedding of hair is a pathological event except in the very young. In many species spontaneous moults start in one region and progress in a wave across the body. Age-related moulting in rats and mice starts on the belly and moves over the flanks to the back. In the adult rabbit these waves of hair shedding and replacement start in the anterior dorsal region and move posteriorly and ventrally.

Seasonal moulting occurs in many species in the spring and autumn; in others there are three moults each year. For example in the stoat, *Mustela erminea* (Rothschild 1942, 1944), moults occur in the autumn, winter and spring. The winter moult starts on the belly and moves towards the back. In the spring the wave passes in the opposite direction. Aquatic rodents such as the beaver and the muskrat undergo almost continuous coat replacement, but suspend moulting at the peak of the breeding season (Ling 1972). Aquatic mammals, such as seals, moult usually after the breeding season.

Many other mammals have seasonal moults. Ebling (1965) makes the important point that all the follicles in any particular region of the body do not necessarily behave in the same fashion. For example in a wild sheep, the mouflon, the moult is complete only in the outer coat; the shorter wool fibres continue to grow (Ryder 1960).

Mosaic moulting
In the species so far mentioned, with the exception of the mouflon, with the two distinct populations of follicles, the follicles in each region of the body are synchronized in more or less the same stage of the moulting cycle. In the human scalp, on the contrary, the activity of each follicle appears to be independent of that of its neighbours. This so-called mosaic pattern of moulting has been said to occur in the guinea-pig which, on this account, has been regarded as a particularly valuable species for laboratory studies on hair growth (Bosse 1965). Subsequent studies in the guinea-pig (Jackson & Ebling 1970, 1971, 1972) on the effects of oestradiol on the hair cycles suggest that there is a wave pattern of

follicular activity in this animal, which is partially obscured by the lack of synchrony between different types of follicle, although there is a marked degree of synchrony within each type. Waves of hair growth appear to move from anterior to posterior (Tejima *et al.* 1968). A number of observations (reviewed by Jackson 1972) suggest that moulting in the human scalp too, may not be strictly of the mosaic pattern, because more than one type of follicle may be concerned.

The significance of moulting
Moulting is in general a mechanism of adaptation to changing environmental temperatures and conditions but in some species it shows also some correlation with the sexual cycle. In the rabbit (Farooq *et al.* 1963) hair loosening occurs towards the end of pregnancy and the doe plucks the loosened hair to line her nest. Postpartum shedding of hair occurs also in women, but its practical significance is questionable.

The regulation of moulting
The photoperiod—the duration of daylight—has been shown to have a strong influence on the moulting cycle as well as on the sexual cycle in a number of animals (Ebling 1965). Temperature itself appears to have little direct influence on the cycles. It is postulated that the increase in the photoperiod in the spring and its decrease in the autumn influence the moulting cycle through the eyes, the hypothalamus and the hypophysis, which then directly modifies follicular activity through the thyroid and adrenal and indirectly through the gonads.

Both the sexual cycle and the hair cycle are intrinsic rhythms, which may in some species be adjusted by environmental factors acting through the endocrine system. In man the sexual cycle and the hair cycle have become largely disengaged from environmental influences, but the hormones of environmental adaptation and the sex hormones still influence follicular activity under physiological as well as pathological conditions. Hormonal influences on the hair follicle in species other than man can throw much light on the phenomena observed in man, and will therefore be reviewed in some detail.

Endocrine influences on follicular activity

The investigation of the mechanisms by which follicular activity is regulated has been greatly advanced by grafting experiments carried out in rats (Johnson 1965, 1977). The transplantation of dorsal and ventral skin flaps in rats, in a two-stage operation to avoid interference with the blood supply of the flaps, showed that the wave of hair replacement developed in each graft at the same time as on the donor and several grafts showed the direction of passage of the wave in the graft to be the opposite to that in the surrounding skin. If grafts are exchanged between rats of different ages so that the waves of hair replacement are out of phase, the timing of the waves on the graft is that of the donor for at least two cycles when the donor is the younger rat. If the donor is the older rat the timing of the first and subsequent cycles is that of the host. The implication of these studies, and of others in rats joined in parabiosis, is that each follicle has an inherent rhythm of cyclical activity, but that the timing of the events of that cycle can be influenced by systemic factors.

The donor dominance in grafted skin is of great practical importance in plastic surgery, and provides the basis for the treatment of common baldness by grafting from the occipital to the frontovertical regions of the scalp.

The influence of the nervous system on hair growth is uncertain. Hair follicles have a well-developed nerve supply (Heyden 1969; Giacometti & Montague 1969), mediating their sensory function. It has been claimed that after denervation of the skin in mice, the hair grew more slowly after plucking and remained shorter (Omard 1970). Other work in various species showed increased hair growth after sympathectomy, but this seems likely to be a result of increased blood flow. Moreover, in the normal hair cycle the cyclical increase in blood flow in anagen is a consequence of increased metabolic activity and not its cause.

The effects of hormones on the hair cycles in laboratory rodents have been extensively studied. Cortisol inhibits the initiation of anagen in the resting follicle, and gonadectomy and adrenalectomy accelerate it. Oestradiol in the albino rat also delays the initiation of follicular activity and reduces the rate of hair growth and the loss of club hairs. Thyroid stimulates follicular activity. Thyroidectomy in rats and mice slightly reduces the rate of growth of hair and retards the initiation of anagen in resting follicles (Houssay *et al.* 1965). Thyroidectomy in sheep reduces wool growth by 25–45% but has no effect on the shaft diameter of the wool fibres (Rougeot 1965).

In the rat the covering of hair in adult life is probably brought about by prolactin. Thyroxin increases hair length in female rats (Rensels & Callahan 1959).

References

Bosse K. (1965) Growth and replacement of hair in the guinea-pig. In *Comparative Physiology and Pathology of the Skin*, eds. A.J. Rook & G.S. Walton. Oxford, Blackwell Scientific Publications, p. 151.

Ebling F.J. (1965) Comparative and evolutionary aspects of hair replacement. In *Comparative Physiology and Pathology of the Skin*, eds. A.J. Rook & G.S. Walton. Oxford, Blackwell Scientific Publications, p. 87.

Farooq, A., Denenberg V.H., Ross S., Savin P.B. & Zarrow M.X. (1963) Maternal behaviour in the rabbit: endocrine factors involved in hair loosening. *American Journal of Physiology*, **204**, 271.

Giacometti L. & Montagna W. (1969) The innervation of human hair follicles. In *Advances in Biology of Skin*, vol. IX, *Hair Growth*, eds. W. Montagna & R.L. Dobson. Oxford, Pergamon Press, p. 393.

Goodhart C.B. (1960) The evolutionary significance of human hair patterns and skin colouring. *Advances in Science*, **17**, 53.

Heyden B. (1969) Uber die Innervation des behaarten Haut des Menschen. *Acta anatomica*, **74**, 20.

Houssay A.B., Epper C.E. & Pazo J.H. (1965) Neurohormonal regulation of the hair cycles in rats and mice. In *Biology of the Skin and Hair Growth*, eds. A.G. Lyne & B.F. Short. Sydney, Angus & Robertson, p. 641.

Jackson D. (1972) Hair replacement in the guinea-pig and in man. *British Journal of Dermatology*, **87**, 509.

Jackson D. & Ebling F.J. (1970) The effect of oestradiol on moulting in the guinea pig, *Cavia porcellus*, L. *Journal of Endocrinology* **48**, lv.

Jackson D. & Ebling F.J. (1971) The guinea-pig hair follicle as an object for experimental observation. *Journal of the Society of Cosmetic Chemists*, **22**, 701.

Jackson D. & Ebling F.J. (1972) The activity of hair follicles and their response to oestradiol in the guinea-pig, *Cavia porcellus*, L. *Journal of Anatomy*, **111**, 303.

Johnson E. (1965) Growth and replacement of hair in rodents. In *Comparative Physiology and Pathology of the Skin*, eds. A.J. Rook & G.S. Walton. Oxford, Blackwell Scientific Publications, p. 137.

Johnson E. (1977) The control of hair growth. In *The Physiology and Pathology of the Skin*, vol. 4, *The Hair Follicle*, ed. A. Jarrett. London, Academic Press, p. 1351.

Ling T.K. (1972) Adaptive function of vertebrate molting cycles. *American Zoologist*, **12**, 77.

Montagu A. (1964) Natural selection and man's relative hairlessness. *Journal of the American Medical Association*, **187**, 357.

Omard E. (1970) Regeneration of hair: a neural effect. *American Zoologist*, **10**, 323.

Rensels E.G. & Callahan W.P. (1952) The hormonal basis for pubertal maturation of hair in the albino rat. *Anatomical Record*, **135**, 21.

Rothschild M. (1942) Change of pelage in the stoat, *Mustela erminea*, L. *Nature (London)*, **149**, 78.

Rothschild M. (1944) Pelage change of the stoat, *Mustela erminea*, L. *Nature (London)*, **154**, 180.

Rougeot J. (1965) Thyroid hormones and the wool cuticle. In *Biology of the Skin and Hair Growth*, eds. A.G. Lyne & B.F. Short. Sydney, Angus & Robertson, p. 625.

Ryder M.L. (1960) A study of the coat of the mouflon, *Ovis musimon*, with special reference to seasonal change. *Proceedings of the Zoological Society of London*, **135**, 387.

Tejima Y., Okada Y., Kanno F., Kikuchi K. & Isobe G. (1968) Studies on hair cycle in the guinea-pig. *5th Congress of the International Federation of Societies of Cosmetic Chemists*, Tokyo, p. 40.

The embryology of hair
(References p. 8)

A knowledge of the embryology of the hair follicle is essential for the dermatologist, not only because it may eventually lead to an understanding of many of the structural defects of the hair shaft, but also because the sequence of events by which the hair follicle is formed in fetal life is partially recapitulated in each cycle of follicular activity. It is surprising therefore that, as Pinkus (1958) has pointed out, the subject attracted until relatively recently little interest among either clinicians or anatomists except in Germany. Albert von Kölliker (1817–1905), Swiss by birth, became Professor of Anatomy in Würzburg in 1847, and was a pioneer in the application of the cell theory in comparative anatomy and embryology. In 1850 he published an important article on the embryology of the skin in the journal of which he was co-founder (Kölliker 1850). P.G. Unna (1850–1929) of Hamburg was the first dermatologist to give serious attention to this subject (Unna 1876). It is, however, not discussed in the influential English translation by Norman Walker of Unna's *Histopathology of the Diseases of the Skin* (Unna 1896). The few English-language texts that did not ignore completely the embryology of the hair quoted Stöhr's *Histology*, which also appeared in English translation in 1896. The German work became still more widely known with the publication in 1910 of the *Manual of Human Embryology*, edited by Keith and Moll, to which F. Pinkus contributed an important chapter.

The scientific approach in the United States to diseases of the hair, based on studies of the embryology and physiology of the hair follicle, was given great impetus by Martin Engman, Professor of Dermatology, Washington University, St Louis, who had worked for a year in Unna's clinic. Engman initiated a long-term research programme, in which C.H. Danforth, Mildred Trotter, L.D. Cady and others took part. The publications of this group (Danforth 1925) laid the foundations for much subsequent work on the hair.

This account of the embryology of the hair follicle is based largely on the writings of Pinkus (1958), Sengel (1976) and Spearman (1977).

The primitive hair germs, seen as focal crowding of the nuclei of basal cells in fetal epidermis, form at the end of the second or the beginning of the third month, in the eyebrow region and on the upper lip and the chin. These are the sites in which vibrissae are present in mammals other than man. In the electron microscope (Breathnach & Smith 1968) the initial crowding of the cells in the primitive or pregerm stage is not at first associated with other significant changes in the cells concerned. The factors determining the sites of individual hair formations are unknown. During the fourth month primary hair germs begin to form over the general body surface. As the fetus grows, new primary germs form between the existing ones, and secondary germs develop in relation to the primary germs, so that the follicles are in groups of three.

As the hair germ enlarges it becomes asymmetrical and grows obliquely downwards (Fig. 1.1). This solid column of cells, now known as the hair peg, the broad tip of which becomes slightly concave, carries before it the aggregation of mesodermal cells which will form the papilla.

As the follicle elongates its lower end becomes bulbous, and the concavity at the tip deepens to enclose the dermal papilla. Two swellings appear at the posterior edge of the follicle; the upper swelling is the germ of the sebaceous gland (Fig. 1.2).

The layer of cells immediately surrounding the enclosed papilla constitutes the matrix. Between the epithelial cells melanocytes can be seen, and at first are scattered throughout the lower part of the bulb and in the outer root sheath. The

Fetal development of the hair follicle

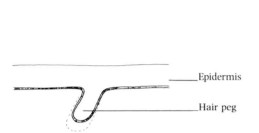

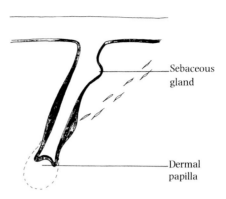

Fig. 1.1. Formation of the epidermal hair peg.

Fig. 1.2. Oblique growth of the peg. The tip of the peg has become concave and encloses the dermal papilla. The upper bulge represents the future sebaceous gland, the lower bulge the site of attachment of the arrector muscles.

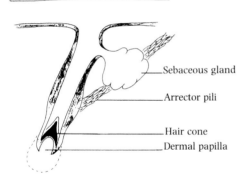

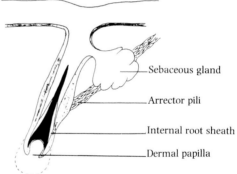

Fig. 1.3. The sebaceous gland has formed. The cone of the internal root sheath is evident.

Fig. 1.4. The tip of the hair emerges from the protection of the internal root sheath.

mesodermal cells surrounding the bulb begin to form the connective tissue sheath (Fig. 1.3).

Above the bulb a cone of cells differentiates from the matrix; these will form the hair. A second concentric cone of cells surrounding the first is the future inner root sheath. The outer of the three components of the inner root sheath differentiates first as Henle's layer, which keratinizes just above the bulb of the follicle. Inside it is the thicker Huxley's layer which keratinizes slightly higher in the follicle, and inside this again is the cuticle of the internal root sheath, the overlapping tile-like cells of which project downwards towards the base of the follicle. The differentiation of Henle's and Huxley's layers reaches an advanced stage before presumptive cuticular or corneal cells can be detected (Robins & Breathnach 1970). The inner cone gives rise to the cortex and the hair cuticle; there is no medulla in fetal hair. The cone of the internal root sheath pushes upwards and protects the tip of the hair as it grows up into the hair canal (Fig. 1.4). In subsequent hair cycles the internal root sheath disintegrates below the level of the sebaceous duct.

The first hair coat of long fine lanugo is shed in utero about one month before birth at full term (Kligman 1961). The second coat of shorter lanugo, in all areas except the scalp where the hair may be both longer and of larger calibre, is shed during the first three or four months of life, almost imperceptibly, or as a wave terminating in almost complete alopecia. The more or less unsynchronized mosaic pattern of hair growth then becomes established.

References

Breathnach A.S. & Smith J. (1968) Fine structure of the early hair germ and dermal papilla in the human foetus. *Journal of Anatomy*, **102**, 511.

Danforth C.H. (1925) Hair with special reference to hypertrichosis. *A.M.A. Archives of Dermatology and Syphilology*, **11**, 494, 637 and 804.

Kligman A.M. (1961) Pathologic dynamics of hair loss. *Archives of Dermatology*, **83**, 175.

Kölliker A. (1850) Zur Entwicklungsgeschichte der äussern Haut. *Zeitschrift für wissenschaftlicher Zoologie*, **2**, 67.

Pinkus F. (1910) The development of the integument. In *Manual of Human Embryology*, vol. 1, eds. H. Kübel & F. Mall. Philadelphia, Lippincott, p. 243.

Pinkus H. (1958) Embryology of hair. In *The Biology of Hair Growth*, eds. W. Montagna & R.A. Ellis. New York, Academic Press, p. 1.

Robins E.J. & Breathnach A.S. (1970) Fine structure of bulbar end of human foetal hair follicle at stage of differentiation of inner root sheath. *Journal of Anatomy*, **107**, 131.

Sengel P. (1976) *Morphogenesis of Skin*. Cambridge, Cambridge University Press.

Spearman R.I.C. (1977) Hair follicle development, cyclical changes and hair form. In *The Hair Follicle*, ed. A. Jarrett. London, Academic Press, p. 1268.

Unna P.G. (1876) Beiträge zur Histologie und Entwicklengsgeschichte der menschlichen Oberhaut und ihrer Anhangsgebilde. *Archiv für microscopisch Anatomie und Entwicklungsmach*, **12**, 665.

Unna P.G. (1896) *The Histopathology of the Diseases of the Skin*, trans. N. Walker. Edinburgh, Clay.

The growth cycle of the human hair follicle
(References p. 16)

From the time it is first formed each hair follicle undergoes repeated cycles of active growth and of rest. The relative duration of phases of the cycle varies with the age of the individual and the region of the body, and can be modified by a variety of factors, physiological and pathological.

The events of the follicular cycle (Kligman 1959) are most readily understood if a follicle is first examined in the final stage of its full development and active growth—metanagen (Fig. 1.5).

Catagen
Mitosis in the matrix decreases and then stops and the follicle enters catagen (Parakkal 1970) which is complete within a few days. The melanocytes in the tip of the papilla resorb their dendrites and as keratinization of hair and inner root sheath continues, the terminal portion of the hair which has become club-

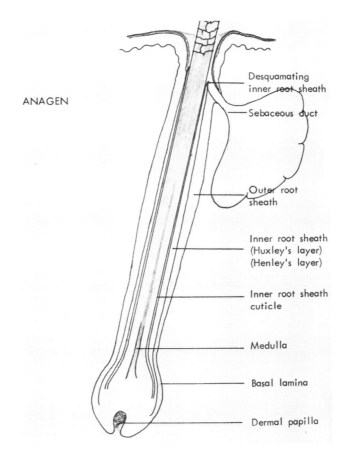

ANAGEN

Desquamating inner root sheath

Sebaceous duct

Outer root sheath

Inner root sheath (Huxley's layer) (Henley's layer)

Inner root sheath cuticle

Medulla

Basal lamina

Dermal papilla

Fig. 1.5. A follicle in metanagen.

shaped lacks pigment, and keratinized fibres extend from it to between epithelial cells. Since mitosis has ceased the lower part of the follicle becomes shortened and the connective tissue sheath, particularly the vitreous membrane, becomes thickened and corrugated. The inner root sheath disintegrates and disappears. The cells of the external root sheath form a sac in the base of which are the germ cells of the follicle. Beneath the sac lies the dermal papilla, which moves upwards as the follicle shortens. The club is surrounded by a capsule of partially keratinized cells and becomes bound to the unkeratinized cells in the base of the sac. The follicle is now in telogen. It is still not clear what initiates spontaneous catagen; the reduction in blood supply is not a primary change; the destruction of the lower two thirds of the follicle is already underway before the capillary loops are affected (Ellis & Moretti 1957) (Fig. 1.6).

Telogen
Telogen is the resting phase of the hair cycle. The club hair with its relatively

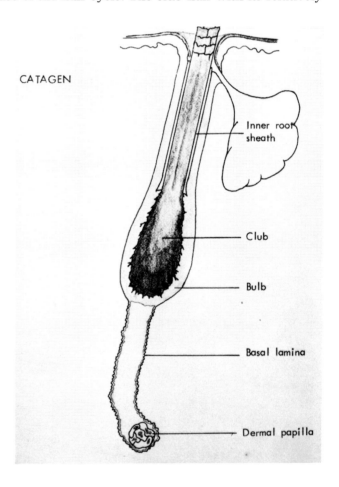

Fig. 1.6. Catagen.

unpigmented bulb is held in the sac by the intercellular junctions and may be retained in the follicle until metanagen is well established in the next cycle or for more than one subsequent hair generation (Fig. 1.7). The follicle re-enters anagen spontaneously at the end of telogen, or may be induced to do so prematurely if the resting club hair is plucked.

Anagen (Chase 1954)

The sequence of events in anagen to some extent recapitulates those of the original morphogenesis of the follicle in fetal skin. In stage I of anagen the cells of the dermal papilla increase in size and show increased RNA synthesis; simultaneously the germinal cells at the base of the sac show vigorous mitotic activity. In stage II the lower part of the follicle grows down, partially enclosing the dermal papilla. As the follicle reaches its maximum length the proliferation of the matrix cells gives rise to the cone of the internal root sheath, a distinctive feature of stage III. In stage IV the melanocytes lining the papilla develop dendrites and begin to form melanin; the hair has formed but is still within the cone of the internal root sheath. The keratogenous zone becomes established just below the level of the sebaceous duct. In stage V the tip of the hair has emerged from the cone of internal root sheath (Fig. 1.8). Stage VI, also known as metanagen, begins as soon as the hair emerges at the skin surface and it continues until the onset of catagen. Stages I to V of anagen are known collectively as proanagen.

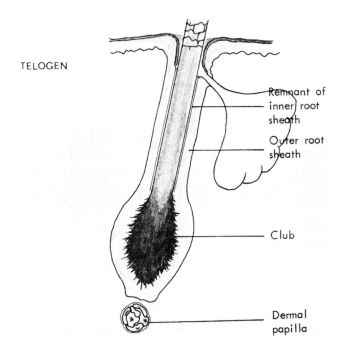

TELOGEN

Remnant of inner root sheath

Outer root sheath

Club

Dermal papilla

Fig. 1.7. A club hair in a telogen follicle.

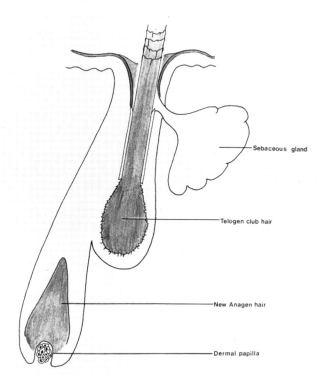

Fig. 1.8. Early anagen. The new hair will grow up beside the club hair.

The dynamics of the follicular cycle in the human scalp
The normal duration of anagen in any individual scalp follicle is genetically determined and ranges from two to over five years. The approximate average duration of anagen is easily remembered as 1000 days (Orentreich 1969). Telogen lasts approximately 100 days. The ratio of anagen to telogen hairs is therefore approximately 90 to 10 since under normal conditions the percentage of hairs in catagen at any given moment is small.

The population of follicles in the human scalp is approximately 100,000—blondes have more and redheads fewer. The average number of hairs shed daily is therefore 100.

The average density of hair follicles in the newborn is 1135/cm². Dilution by growth in surface area has reduced this to 795 towards the end of the first year and to 615 by the third decade. Between the ages of 30 and 50 the destruction of some follicles has reduced the number to 485 after which there is only slight further reduction in old age. In a clinically bald scalp many follicles are reduced in size but the total count is less drastically reduced. Average figures for bald scalp (age 45–70 years) were 330 and (70–85 years) 280 (Giacometti 1965).

The role of the photoperiod in adjusting moulting cycles in some species of mammal (p. 3) has suggested that similar effects might occur in man. Most observers have failed to record any consistent relation between moulting in man and the seasons. However, Orentreich (1969) recorded short-term variations superimposed on a long-term seasonal variation with maximum loss in November in the northern temperate regions.

The trichogram
Studies of the dynamics of the follicular cycle depend largely on the trichogram, the ratio of anagen to telogen hairs, as established by the microscopic examination of plucked hairs (Fig. 1.9) (Braun-Falco 1966; Meiers 1967). This technique gives reliable results, provided that certain precautions are taken; over 50 hairs must be plucked as the standard deviation is unacceptably high if the sample is too small (Bosse 1967); the hair should not have been washed during the week before the examination, as washing the hair extracts hairs nearing the end of telogen and thus artificially reduces the percentage in this phase recorded in the trichogram (Braun-Falco & Fischer 1966). The hair root is less damaged by a sharp quick pluck than by slow traction.

Important differences in the trichogram are recorded with age and with the region of the scalp. The highest A/T ratio—over 90%—is found in children. In adult men, even in those not clinically bald, the proportion of hairs in telogen is highest in the frontovertical region. No marked regional variations were found in

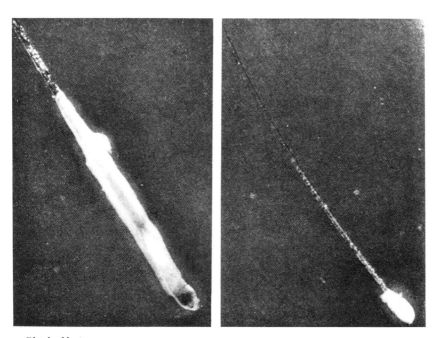

Fig. 1.9. Plucked hairs:
(a) left, anagen
(b) right, telogen.

non-bald women (Braun-Falco 1966), but differences are present in women with androgenetic alopecia. Witzel & Braun-Falco (1963) examined scalp hairs from 146 clinically normal subjects; they found an average in all sites in women of 85% in anagen and 11% in telogen, and in men 83% and 15% respectively. Catagen hairs accounted for 2.1% of the trichogram in women and 2.9% in men but were demonstrable in only 19% of women and 31% of men. Dystrophic anagen hairs made up 2.5% of the total in women and 3.2% in men but were demonstrable in only 48% of women and 46% of men.

Racial variation in follicular density is well illustrated by studies of the predominantly dark-haired population of the Argentine (Barman *et al.* 1965). The follicular density in adults ranged from 175–300 per cm² with an average of 223. The density of follicles decreased with age in all regions and the hair became finer, but the diameter was not related to the total population. The proportion of telogen hairs increased with age and was greatest in the frontovertical region in both sexes.

In regions of the body other than the scalp anagen is relatively short and telogen relatively long. There is some disagreement between the figures given by different authors, most of whom reported wide variations in each site. Saitoh *et al.* (1970) made their observations by time-lapse photography and also reviewed the findings of some earlier observers.

	Anagen	*Telogen*
Moustache	16	6
Finger	12	9
Arms	13	13
Leg	21	19

Pinkus (1947) observed a single follicle on the dorsum of one hand daily for six years, during which 12 hairs were formed. The average life span of each hair was 180 days (107–195). The hairless intervals lasted, in six instances, 27–52 days, and in the other six 76–92 days.

The rate of hair growth
Several different techniques have been employed to measure the rate of hair growth in man. Myers & Hamilton (1951) observed the length of time required for the regrowth of the hair in 90% of follicles after plucking. The time interval ranged from 129 days on the vertex of the scalp and 117 days on the temples, to 92 days on the chin. Plucking the hair damages the follicle, and observations based on regrowth after plucking are not necessarily applicable to spontaneous regrowth (Silver *et al.* 1969). Observations of individual uninjured follicles (Saitoh *et al.* 1970) showed that new hairs took 3 weeks to reach the scalp surface. By direct measurement of the regenerated hairs, Myers & Hamilton (1951) found the daily growth rate to be 0.35 mm/day on the vertex and on the

temple and slightly greater in these sites in women than in men. Barman *et al.* (1964) measured daily shavings and obtained essentially similar figures. Using the intradermal injection of sulphur 35L cystine to measure linear growth of scalp hair gave a daily average of 0.37 mm (range 0.31–0.41) (Munro 1966). Saitoh and his colleagues in Japan (Saitoh *et al.* 1969) used a capillary tube technique for measuring the rate of hair growth. They recorded an average growth rate of 0.44 mm on the vertex and on the chest, 0.29 mm at the temples and 0.27 mm in the beard. Time-lapse photography showed a constant growth rate in each follicle and no significant diurnal variation.

Pecoraro *et al.* (1970) studied, in 126 subjects aged 10–74, the density and rate of growth of axillary hair. The axilla was divided into three subregions, central, brachial and thoracic. There were no significant sex differences in hair density. Hair density and growth rate were highest in the central area. The hairs in the three subregions showed different quantitative responses to pregnancy. In all three subregions the hair density decreased with age. In contrast the pubic hair (Astore *et al.* 1979) showed a trichogram little influenced by ageing or by pregnancy.

The mitotic activity at a given level of the germinative matrix of a follicle is inversely proportional to the distance from the base of the dermal papilla (Van Scott *et al.* 1963). There is a consistent proportional relationship between the volume of the hair matrix and the size of the papilla; the latter depending on the size of the population of germinative cells and hence the size of the hair (Epstein & Maibach 1969).

The length of the hair
The length of each hair is genetically determined. It depends obviously on the duration of anagen and the rate of growth (Fig. 1.10).

Systemic influences on the hair cycle
Androgens increase the growth rate as well as the calibre of the shaft in androgen-dependent sites such as the beard. Androgen-blocking agents reduce the growth rate in such sites (p. 112). In the scalp genetically predisposed to androgenetic alopecia, however, androgen reduces the shaft diameter and the rate of growth and the duration of anagen.

Oestrogen retards the rate of growth during anagen but prolongs the duration of anagen. Thyroxin advances the onset of anagen in resting follicles and cortisone retard it.

Local influences on hair growth
Anything causing epithelial hyperplasia will initiate a new anagen in resting follicles, e.g. wounds cause hair growth beyond the edges of the wound (Chase 1969).

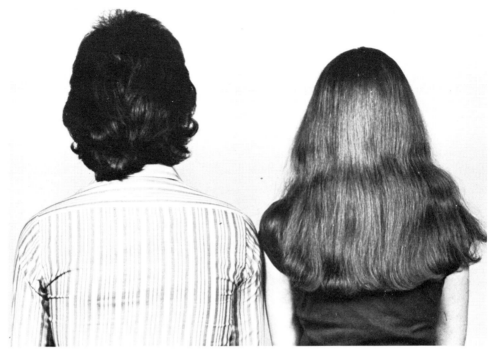

Fig. 1.10. Differences in hair length depend on the duration of anagen, a genetically determined characteristic. Neither of these subjects had had a haircut for over 18 months.

Inflammatory changes, as in ringworm infections, cause telogen to synchronize in the area of scalp surrounding the lesion, thus limiting the extension of the lesion (Bosse 1967).

The widespread belief that shaving increases the rate of growth and shaft diameter of hair is difficult to destroy. Trotter in 1923 showed that neither shaving nor exposure to sunlight had any effect on hair growth. In a further paper in 1928 she repeated that shaving did not have any effect on the growth of the beard. Over 40 years later, Lynfield & Macwilliams (1970) reported that five young men had shaved one leg only for several months, leaving the other leg as a control. There was no difference between the two sides in the weight of hair produced or in the shaft diameter or in the rate of growth.

References
Astore I.P.L., Pecoraro V. & Pecoraro E.G. (1979) The normal trichogram of pubic hair. *British Journal of Dermatology*, **101**, 441.
Barman J.M., Pecoraro V. & Astore I. (1964) Method, technic and competence in the study of the trophic state of the human scalp hair. *Journal of Investigative Dermatology*, **42**, 421.
Barman J.M., Astore I. & Pecoraro V. (1965) The normal trichogram of the adult. *Journal of Investigative Dermatology*, **44**, 233.

Bosse K. (1967a) Der Einfluss der Entzündigung auf das Haarwachstum. *Hautarzt*, **18**, 218.

Bosse K. (1967b) Vergleichende Untersuchungen zur Physiologie und Pathologie des Haarwechsels unter besonderer Berücksichtigung seiner Synchronisation. II. Methodische Untersuchungen zur Haarwechselstatusbestimmung und ihre Anwendung an Mensch und Meerschweinchen. *Hautarzt*, **18**, 35.

Braun-Falco O. (1966) Dynamik des normalen und pathologischen Haarwachstum. *Archiv für klinische und experimentelle Dermatologie*, **227**, 419.

Braun-Falco O. & Fischer C. (1966) Uber den Einfluss des Haarwaschens auf das Haarwurzelmuster. *Archiv für klinische und experimentelle Dermatologie*, **226**, 136.

Chase H.B. (1954) Growth of the hair. *Psysiological Reviews*, **34**, 113.

Chase H.B. (1969) Physical factors which influence the growth of hair. In *Advances in Biology of Skin*, vol IX, *Hair Growth*, eds. W. Montagna & R.L. Dobson. Oxford, Pergamon Press, p. 435.

Ellis R.A. & Moretti G. (1957) Vascular pattern associated with catagen hair follicles in the human scalp. *Anals of the New York Academy of Science*, **53**, 448.

Epstein E.L. & Maibach H.I. (1969) Cell proliferation and movement in human hair bulbs. In *Advances in Biology of Skin*, vol. IX, *Hair Growth*, eds. W. Montagna & R.L. Dobson. Oxford, Pergamon Press, p. 83.

Giacometti, L. (1965) The Anatomy of the human scalp. In *Advances in Biology of Skin*, vol. IX, *Hair Growth*, eds. W. Montagna & R.L. Dobson, Oxford, Pergamon Press, p. 97.

Kligman A.M. (1959) The human hair cycle. *Journal of Investigative Dermatology*, **33**, 307.

Lynfield Y.L. & Macwilliams P. (1970) Shaving and hair growth. *Journal of Investigative Dermatology*, **55**, 170.

Meiers H.G. (1967) Die Methode des Trichogrammes. *Artzsliche Kosmetologie*, **6**, 22.

Munro D.D. (1966) Hair growth measurement using intradermal sulphur 35L-cystine. *Archives of Dermatology*, **93**, 119.

Myers R.J. & Hamilton J.B. (1951) Regeneration and rate of growth of hair in Man. *Annals of the New York Academy of Science*, **53**, 862.

Orentreich N. (1969) Scalp hair regeneration in man. In *Advances in Biology of Skin*, vol. IX, *Hair Growth*, eds W. Montagna & R.L. Dobson. Oxford, Pergamon Press, p. 99.

Parakkal P.F. (1970) Morphogenesis of the hair follicle during catagen. *Zeitschrift für Zellforschung*, **104**, 174.

Pecoraro V., Astore I. & Barman J.N. (1970) Growth rate and hair density of the human axillae. *Journal of Investigative Dermatology*, **56**, 362.

Pinkus F. (1947) The story of a hair root. *Journal of Investigative Dermatology*, **9**, 91.

Saitoh M., Uzuka M., Sakamoto M. & Kobori M. (1969) Rate of hair growth. In *Advances in Biology of Skin*, vol. IX, *Hair Growth*, eds. W. Montagna & R.L. Dobson. Oxford, Pergamon Press, p. 183.

Saitoh M., Uzuka M. & Sakamoto M. (1970) Human hair cycle. *Journal of Investigative Dermatology*, **54**, 65.

Silver A.F., Chase H.B. & Arsenault C.T. (1969) Early anagen initiated by plucking compared with early spontaneous anagen. In *Advances in Biology of Skin*, vol. IX, *Hair Growth*, eds. W. Montagna & R.L. Dobson. Oxford, Pergamon Press, p. 265.

Trotter M. (1923) The resistance of hair to certain supposed growth stimulants. *Archives of Dermatology and Syphilology*, **7**, 93.

Trotter, M. (1928) Hair growth and shaving. *Anatomical Record*, **37**, 373.

Van Scott E.J., Ekel T.M. & Auerbach R. (1963) Determinants of rate and kinetics of cell division in scalp hair. *Journal of Investigative Dermatology*, **41**, 269.

Witzel M. & Braun-Falco O. (1963) Über den Haarwurzelstatus am menschlichen Capillitium unter physiologischen Bedingungen. *Archiv für klinische und experimentelle Dermatologie*, **216**, 221.

Chapter 2
Hair Follicle Structure, Keratinization and the Physical Properties of Hair

Physiology and biochemistry
(References p. 38)

All the cell layers within the outer root sheath are products of the hair matrix in the bulb (Fig. 2.1a and b). The area of active cell division is in the lower bulb and in the upper bulb adjacent to the dermal papilla. From the upper bulb to the zone of complete keratinization cells stream upwards and undergo successively the phases of orientation into layers, hardening and keratinization.

The outer root sheath is not a product of the hair matrix but consists of a sleeve of cells continuous with, and similar in structure to, the surface epidermis. It is, however, an intimate part of the hair follicle.

Hair bulb

The hair matrix is made up of rapidly dividing cells in the lower bulb and the upper bulb surrounding the dermal papilla. These cells are several layers deep and have a very rapid turnover; it has been suggested that each matrix cell divides every 23–72 hours (Van Scott *et al.* 1963). Unlike the epidermal basal layer, there appears to be no diurnal variation in mitotic rate or chalone inhibition in the matrix (Bullough & Lawrence 1958; Kligman 1959; Epstein & Maibach 1969). At the end of the anagen phase of the follicular cycle, continuous cell division slows down and finally ceases in catagen (p. 9).

Matrix cells possess a characteristic ultrastructure (Fig. 2.2). Most of the cell is occupied by the large spherical nucleus; within the scanty cytoplasm are many ribosomes and some mitochondria. Rough surface endoplastic reticulum, a compact Golgi zone adjacent to the nucleus and arrays of cisternae and vesicles

Fig. 2.1. A mature anagen hair follicle: (a) a scanning electron micrograph; (b) line diagram with parts labelled.

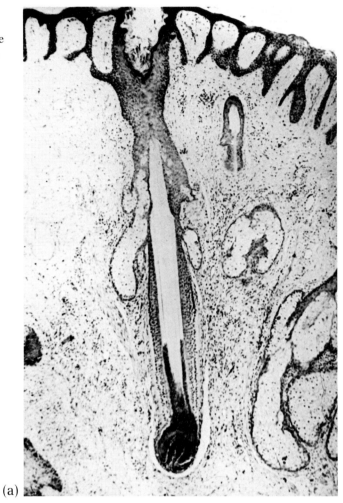

(a)

(b)

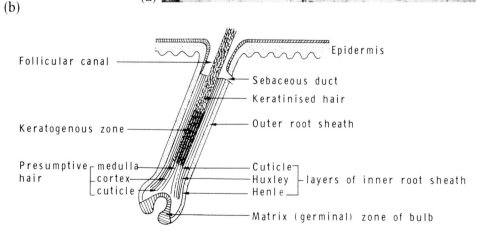

Follicular canal

Keratogenous zone

Presumptive hair — medulla
— cortex
— cuticle

Epidermis

Sebaceous duct

Keratinised hair

Outer root sheath

Cuticle ⌉
Huxley ⌡ layers of inner root sheath
Henle ⌋

Matrix (germinal) zone of bulb

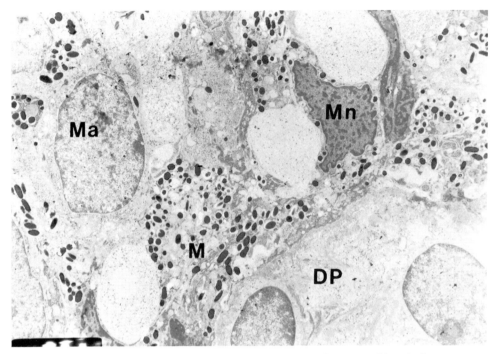

Fig. 2.2. Electron micrograph at the junction of the dermal papilla (DP) and hair bulb. A melanocyte (Mn) containing mature melanosomes (M) is seen adjacent to a hair bulb matrix cell (Ma).

compose the rest of the cytoplasm. The cells are rich in RNA (Fraser *et al.* 1972). Desmosomal attachments and gap junctions are present between adjacent cells and, as in epidermal keratinocytes, filaments extend from the desmosomes into the cell cytoplasm. There are considerably fewer cell attachment sites between matrix cells than are found in the epidermal basal layer; this may facilitate easier movement of cells from the matrix to the upper bulb and suprabulbar area. The cells surrounding the dermal papilla are precursors of the hair fibre and the more peripheral matrix cells give rise to the inner root sheath. In the suprabulbar part of the follicle these cells become relatively long and thin, with distinct cell boundaries (Auber 1952). The overall size of the cells and the relative amount of cytoplasm noticeably increase (Montagna & Van Scott 1958). These changes may relate to greater water content and protein synthesis. Ribosomes are mostly strung together as polysomes and a few bound ribosomes are evident. Golgi bodies are poorly developed in this region and consist of a few vesicles adjacent to the nucleus; the endoplastic reticulum is poorly developed (Parakkal & Maltoltsy 1964). Both nuclei and nucleoli remain prominent in suprabulbar cells.

The various layers ascending the follicle (Fig. 2.3a and b) first become

Fig. 2.3. (a) Concentric layers of the hair follicle (resin embedded section). Within the cortex (Co) only occasional medullary cells are present (M). Within the outer root sheath (ORS), all layers show keratinization, which in the Huxley layer (Hu) is only evident in the upper area. (b) Concentric cell layers of suprabulbar portion of an anagen hair follicle.

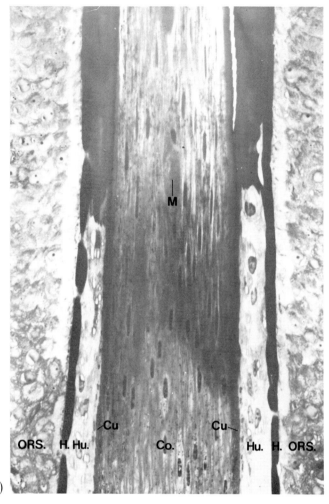

(a)

(b)

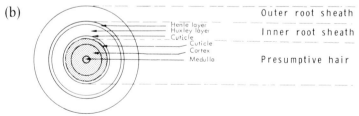

noticeable as cells of different shapes. Medullary cells remain relatively large and spherical whilst presumptive hair cortex cells become spindle-shaped. The structure of each layer will be considered separately, from its development from the appropriate bulbar matrix cells, through differentiation and cell death associated with keratinization higher up the follicle.

Medullary cells
These differentiate from matrix cells adjacent to the apex of the dermal papilla. Distinctive microscopic changes can be observed before other cell layers are distinguishable. Irregular dense granules develop from the Golgi apparatus (Auber 1952) and these enlarge by coalescing. By cytological and histochemical methods the granules can be differentiated from epidermal keratohyalin, though as will be seen later, the granules have some biochemical similarities to the inner root sheath protein (Harding & Rogers 1971). Medullary cells do not produce these proteins in significant amounts and harden by a different biochemical process than the keratin-forming cells of the cortex and cuticle. The function of medullary granules in man is not known. Medullary cells produce some filaments which are aggregated into bundles and are randomly distributed in the cytoplasm. As differentiation proceeds, glycogen granules become evident particularly near the nucleus. In the final stages of differentiation, the nucleus and other cytoplasmic organelles begin to disintegrate. Mitochondria begin to swell, the cristae lose orientation and the density of the matrix decreases. Finally the mitochondria become vacuolated like empty vesicles. Fully formed medullary cells are wedged between projections of cortical cells and in the fully developed hair, mature cells are arranged along the core of the hair with spaces between them.

In vellus and lanugo hair no medullary cells form and even terminal hair follicles may reveal complete absence or only infrequent medullary cells (Fig. 2.3a).

Cortical cells
These become visible microscopically at a higher level in the follicle than presumptive medullary cells as spindle-shaped cells which produce increasing amounts of cytoplasmic filaments parallel both to the long axis of the cell and the hair follicle (Figs. 2.4 and 2.5) the filaments grade into dense α-keratin fibrils but have no clear connection with tonofibrils. This zone of keratinization shows evidence of intense protein synthesis (Parakkal 1969), many polysomes being seen together with strong nucleolar and cytoplasmic staining for RNA. The higher keratogenous zone shows increasing evidence of cytolysis—hydrolases are released from lysosomes (acid phosphatase stain) and the phospholipid reaction increases (Braun-Falco 1958a); at the same stage, nuclear degradation occurs. Ribosomes are the final organelle to disappear. Stable sulphydryl groups (cysteine reaction) are increasingly found towards the upper keratogenous zone. The fully keratinized 'dead' cortical cells retain a membranous nuclear outline (nuclear 'ghost') which persists into the hair shaft.

Cuticle cells
Presumptive cuticular cells elongate in the suprabulbar region and become

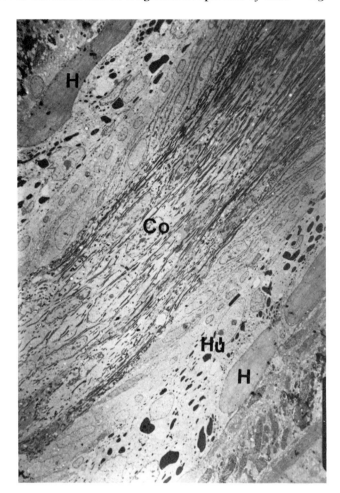

Fig. 2.4. Hair follicle (longitudinal section), showing the central cortex (Co) surrounded by the root sheaths. The Henle layer (at H) is keratinized.

flattened; during differentiation the cells increasingly overlap (Fig. 2.5). Tonofibrils and desmosomes are present but no α-keratin fibrils are produced. Increasing protein synthesis occurs during hardening and keratinization and dense cytoplasmic granules are visible. Reactive phospholipids and cysteine sulphydryl groups are detectable, contributing to the formation of a matrix rather than fibrillar, protein structure (Birkbeck & Mercer 1957).

Hardening (keratin bonding) zone (Fig. 2.1b)
During this phase before complete cell death and keratinization, the hair first acquires its strength and flexibility in the cuticle and cortex (Auber 1952). The hair fibre decreases in diameter by about 25% probably due to a combination of water loss due to plasma membrane permeability changes, and contraction of keratin complexes from cytoplasmic water loss. In the final stages of keratin-

Chapter 2

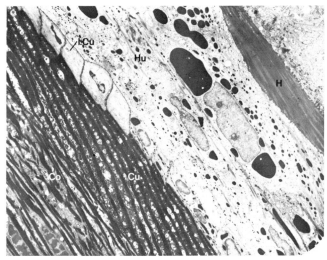

Fig. 2.5. Hair follicle (electron micrograph). The inner root sheath cuticle (I.Cu) is visible adjacent to the hair cuticle (Cu). The Huxley layer (Hu) shows numerous (black) trichohyalin granules.

bonding, bound sulphydryl is oxidized to cystine and the cysteine reaction of the keratinized area decreases to negligible amounts.

Inner root sheath (Figs. 2.3b, 2.5)

The inner root sheath consists of three layers, from within outwards, the cuticle, Huxley's and Henle's layers; the cuticle is one cell thick whilst Huxley's layer is several cells deep. The cuticle interlocks with the cells of the hair cuticle and is intimately associated with it. All three layers are formed from the peripheral mass of matrix cells in the hair bulb. There is no evidence in man to support the idea that the basal cells of the outer root sheath cells overlying the hair bulb contribute to the formation of the Henle layer.

All three layers undergo differentiation in the same sequence but at different rates—firstly, the Henle layer, then the Huxley layer and finally the cuticle. The late stages of hardening and cell death further up the follicle begin in the Henle layer (Fig. 2.4), then the cuticle and finally Huxley's layer. It is important to note that complete hardening and differentiation of the inner root sheath occurs before the layers of the developing hair within it. Keratinization proceeds by the secretion of increasing amounts of trichohyalin and flattening of the cells. The trichohyalin granules (Fig. 2.5) are mostly attached to tonafilaments. The final stage of differentiation involves the disintegration of the nucleus, other organelles and the trichohyalin which become diffusely visible as electron-dense material between keratin filaments. This is particularly evident in the inner root sheath cuticle. In the lower follicle the junction between the outer root sheath and the Henle layer is maintained by desmosomes and gap junctions; higher up the follicle, after inner root sheath differentiation is complete, the relation with the outer root sheath is maintained by intercellular cement and by interdigitation between cells. The Huxley and Henle layers possess similar intimate methods of contact. With maturation, inner root sheath cells demonstrate thickening of plasma membranes and the deposition of amorphous intercellular material; cells shrink during keratinization, the mature inner root sheath thus becoming a rigid cylindrical tube surrounding the softer ascending hair structures within it (Fig. 2.3a). The fully formed inner root sheath shows detectable amounts of cystine, RNA and phospholipid probably released from the degradation of hydrolysed organelle membranes and trichohyalin (Jarrett 1958). At the level of the follicular canal, desmosomal contacts between adjacent cells begin to be broken down and the cells, singly or in groups, are shed into the follicular canal. This desquamation is probably facilitated by hydrolases of lysosomal origin. The exact source of these enzymes is not known but they may be from the inner or outer root sheath (Straile 1962) or from sebaceous secretion.

The prime function of the inner root sheath is to mould the hair within it. It effects this by hardening in advance of the hair; since the cuticles of the hair and inner root sheath are closely apposed, in health, the fully keratinized fibre takes the shape of the root sheath (Straile 1962; Swift 1977).

Outer root sheath (Figs. 2.3a, 2.6)
This layer surrounds the hair follicle as a sleeve of cells several layers thick that is continuous with the epidermis. It is divisible into two parts: a short lower part surrounding the outer part of the bulb and the upper part from the neck of the bulb to the level of the sebaceous duct. The area surrounding the follicular opening has the same structure and biochemical characteristics as the surface epidermis and will not be considered further.

The part surrounding the hair bulb is one or two cells thick, the outer layer

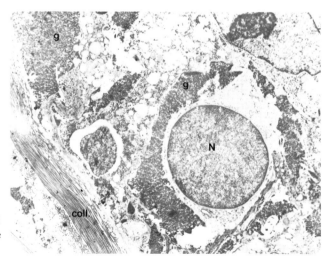

Fig. 2.6. Outer root sheath. The nucleus (N) is surrounded by cytoplasmic glycogen (g). Adjacent to the cell is the perifollicular connective tissue membrane (coll.).

being elongated and the inner layer markedly flattened. In the suprabulbar area it is usually three cells thick and only becomes multilayered approximately half way along the follicle. The outer cell layer is the germinative layer continuous with the epidermal basal cells (Parakkal 1969); differentiation occurs in a centripetal direction towards the inner root sheath, the cells enlarging, flattening and becoming vacuolated. The exact fate of the cells adjacent to the Henle layer is not known though it seems likely that movement towards the surface occurs; this certainly occurs in some sheep and mice in which keratinized cells from the upper part of the outer root sheath are shed into the follicular canal along with the inner root sheath. It is possible that some keratinization occurs in the differentiating cells next to the inner root sheath (Jarrett 1958).

The outer root sheath differs from the follicular canal in containing prominent Golgi vesicles associated with well-developed rough endoplasmic reticulum; the amorphous cytoplasmic granules produced during differentiation probably develop from this organelle. The granules are not membrane bound. Membrane-limited vesicles are also present together with glycogen particles (Parakkal 1969). The outer root sheath does not produce keratohyalin. The epidermis of the follicular canal differs from the surface epidermis only in degree. Ribosomes are arranged as polysomes lying free in the cytoplasm with only small Golgi vesicles and very little endoplasmic reticulum. The keratohyalin granules are smaller and rounder and more membrane-coating granules are seen than in the surface epidermis. Towards the sebaceous duct the membrane-coating granules decrease both in size and number (Knutson 1974). The exact function of the outer root sheath is not known. During the early stages of the anagen phase of the hair cycle it elongates rapidly because of a high rate of mitotic activity which ceases when the follicle reaches its full length; subsequent mitotic activity only continues at a rate equal to cell death or cytoplasmic obliteration (Bullough & Lawrence 1958; Montagna & Van Scott 1958) though some investigators have detected higher rates than this (Straile 1962). In general, the outer root sheath is considered a relatively static region displaying little indication of cell movement. However, the observation that partial keratinization occurs in the innermost cells adjacent to the Henle layer suggests that the moving cylinder of inner root sheath plus hair may pull along the inner cells of the outer root sheath; these cells may also have a role in the differentiation and breakdown of the Henle layer. The outward migration of outer root sheath cells in facilitating the movement of the cell layers within it during metanagen, may account for the final outward movement of the terminal part of the hair during the last half of catagen after hair growth has ceased (Straile *et al.* 1961).

Histochemistry (Swift 1977)

Knowledge of the chemical nature of the various morphological components of the hair follicle has accumulated by three major methods—histochemistry and electron histochemistry, autoradiography and analysis of material extracted from different parts of the follicle.

Cystine and cysteine
In the hair follicle, the presumptive cuticle and cortex contain cysteine sulphydryl groups followed by cystine disulphide cross-links (hard keratin) in the fully keratinized hair; only small amounts are to be found in root sheaths, particularly the Henle layer. Stabilization and hardening in the follicle are accompanied by an increase in birefringence of the cortical zone. An α-keratin pattern without orientation has been found in the lower bulb using X-ray diffraction studies: keratinization is associated with the development of orientated α-keratin as seen in the hair cortex. This α-pattern precedes the formation of disulphide-rich proteins and corresponds to the development of fibrillar bundles in the cortical zone which subsequently acquire cystine-rich proteins (Rudall 1945). Autoradiographic studies have suggested that α-keratin-like, low sulphur fibrils (microfibrils) are formed first and at a later stage an amorphous sulphur-rich matrix protein (interfibrillar) is deposited.

Nucleic acids
The dividing cells of the hair follicle matrix stain densely for DNA; through the suprabulbar region the intensity fades and the nuclei lose this stain during keratinization. Dermal papillary cell nuclei are strongly positive for DNA. The basal cells of the follicle show the greatest concentration of RNA. Differentiating cortical cells also contain large amounts of RNA associated with great numbers of ribosomes between cytoplasmic fibrillar bundles. As the cortical cell keratinize, RNA staining stops abruptly.

Carbohydrates
Glycogen is the main carbohydrate reserve store. Dermal papillary vascular endothelial cells contain glycogen but this is absent from follicular matrix cells; all the differentiated cell layers in the follicle contain glucogen but as cells harden the amount decreases progressively. Glycogen staining disappears as catagen succeeds the various phases of anagen.

   Acids mucopolysaccharides are detectable in the follicular connective tissue sheath and the dermal papilla; metachromatic stains are also positive in the peripheral layers of the outer root sheath. Very little acid mucopolysaccharide is detectable in the presumptive hair. Using electron histochemical methods a polysaccharide-rich layer is detectable around matrix cells of the hair bulb, particularly near desmosomes; this coat vanishes from differentiating hair cells but is retained in the inner root sheath—the retention of this coat may be important in the breakdown of the inner root sheath higher up the follicle.

Lipids

Very little histochemical work has been carried out to detect lipids in hair follicles. Typically only undifferentiated matrix cells show lipid staining and only in small amounts. Prior to trichohyalin deposition, early inner root sheath cells contain lipid granules. Phospholipid is evident in matrix cells and in the inner root sheath; these decrease as hardening proceeds.

Arginine and citrulline

Intense staining for arginine is found in association with trichohyalin droplets in the developing medulla and inner root sheath. This decreases as cells undergo hardening. The structure of trichohyalin has been investigated extensively (Rogers 1964a, b; Fraser *et al.* 1972). Both the inner root sheath and medullary proteins are rich in acidic and basic aminoacids, contain citrulline and are virtually devoid of cystine. Rogers (1964a, b) proposes that the medullary and inner root sheath trichohyalin globules contain arginine-rich protein (arginine trichohyalin) which by desimidation of the arginine is transferred into citrulline-rich, insoluble, hardened proteins which ultimately fill the cells (citrulline trichohyalin). The establishment of isopeptide cross-links in these proteins takes place either before or during the conversion of arginine into citrulline. In biological terms, it seems likely that this method of inner root sheath and medullary hardening has evolved to limit the use of disulphide bond keratinization, which requires considerable amounts of sulphur-containing amino-acids, to the cuticle and cortex. This is of great importance in coat formation in animals but whether it is of significance in man is not known.

Enzymes (Braun-Falco 1958b)

Optical histochemical techniques have demonstrated the presence of many enzymes within the hair follicle, in particular phosphorylase, aldolase, succinic dehydrogenase, cytochrome oxidase, alkaline phosphatase, acid phosphatase, glucose-6-phosphatase, esterases, carbonic anhydrase, aminopeptidase, β-glucuronidase, and arginase. Alkaline phosphatase activity is present along the basement membrane and around the periphery of dermal papillary cells. Acid phosphatase activity is associated with premelanosomes, Golgi apparatus and endoplasmic reticulum of melanocytes.

Dermal papilla (Fig. 2.7)

The connective tissue contained within the hair bulb is the dermal papilla. The size of the papilla and surrounding bulb are directly related to the size of the hair produced (Durward & Rudall 1958; Schinckel 1961). In anagen follicles the dermal papilla is attached to a basal plate of connective tissue by a narrow stalk. In small follicles there may be no visible vasculature but terminal hair follicles show variable numbers of papillary blood vessels. Papillary cells in the anagen

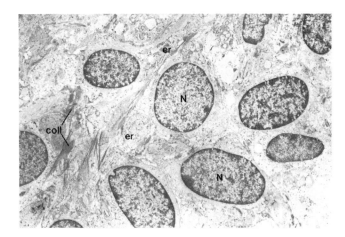

Fig. 2.7. Dermal papillary cells. The cytoplasm shows endoplasmic reticulum (er). Collagen fibres (coll) are present between the cells.

follicle (Fig. 2.7) have prominent Golgi complexes and rough endoplasmic reticulum with bound ribosomes; even in the telogen phase appreciable cytoplasmic volume is still evident. At the beginning of anagen, papillary cells show a marked increase in RNA content (Roth 1965). There is a close relationship between the cytogical activity of dermal papillary cells and hair bulb matrix cells (Straile 1965). The fact that papillary cell activity does not predate that in matrix cells is against the idea of the papilla initiating the anagen phase, but it seems probable that the dermal papilla determines the cyclical rhythm of the follicle (Cohen 1965). Papillary capillary endothelial cells undergo mitotic activity during anagen (Helwig 1958) but these changes occur secondary to those in bulb matrix cells. In human anagen follicles the ratio of papillary cells to matrix cells is approximately 1:9.

Hair structure
(References p. 38)

The main part of the fully keratinized hair fibre is the cortex, which is made up of closely packed, interdigitating spindle-shaped cells whose axis is parallel to the hair axis. Covering this is the cuticle, composed of six to eight layers of flattened cells which overlap each other from root to tip (Fig. 2.8). In man, a third component may be present in terminal hairs, the central medulla (Fig. 2.9). It consists of specialized cells which contain air spaces (Fig. 2.10).

Surface structure
Mammalian hairs are covered with a thin layer termed the epicuticle (Fraser *et al.* 1972) which is approximately 2.5 nm thick. It has been suggested in the past that the epicuticle covers the entire surface of the hair but more recently it has been localized as part of the cell membrane complex (Robbins 1979), perhaps

chemically associated with the intercelular binding material. The epicuticle is not morphologically evident on microscopy. It is probably best to consider the epicuticle to be a lipid-containing surface membrane made up of the cytoplasmic membrane and/or the A-layer to which remnants of protein from the exocuticle are attached (Swift & Holmes 1965; Swift 1977).

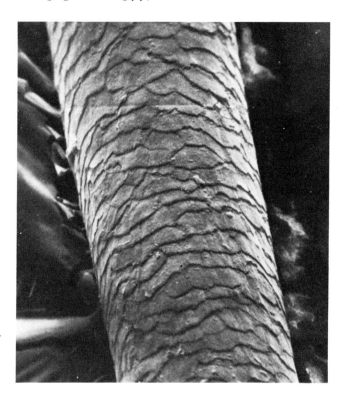

Fig. 2.8. Surface structure of scalp hair at root end, showing overlapping cuticular cells closely apposed to underlying cells. The lower margin points towards the tip (scanning electron micrograph).

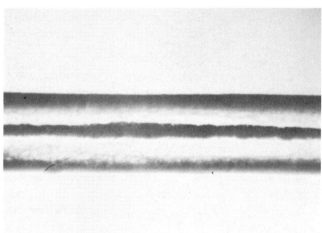

Fig. 2.9. Medullated terminal hair showing continuous (dark) central medulla.

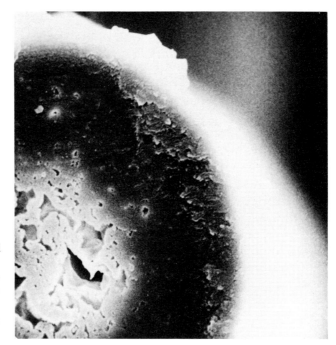

Fig. 2.10. Normal medullated terminal scalp hair (transverse section). Scanning electron micrograph showing air spaces in the medulla (lower left) and darker compact surrounding cortex.

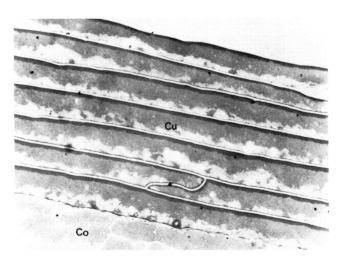

Fig. 2.11. Hair cuticle layers (Cu) surrounding the central cortex (Co) (electron micrograph).

Cuticle (Wolfram & Lindemann 1971) (Fig. 2.11)
Human hair is surrounded by six to ten layers of cuticle cells, each being approximately 0.2–0.5 μm thick; at the proximal end the hair is therefore encased by a 1 μm thick layer of cuticular material. The number of layers varies but little from coarse to fine hairs and thus in the latter the cuticle may account for up to 10% of the fibre by weight. Cuticular cells overlap and on surface

examination of the fibre they are seen to be imbricated (like roof tiles). The free margin of the cells points towards the tip. The free length of each fibre visible at the surface is mainly dependent on the overall diameter of the hair, i.e. in vellus hair three-quarters of the surface cuticle cell is visible with a relatively large distance between the free margin of successive scales of terminal hair in which scale margins appear closer. The cell junctions between adjacent cuticle cells and the cuticle and underlying cortex are usually flat, and folds are infrequently but regularly seen, which may contribute to the mechanical strength of the cuticle.

Each cuticle cell is composed of lamellar components (Fig. 2.12). The outer cell membrane complex is from 5 to 25 nm thick. Within each cell are three major layers—the cystine-rich A-layer, the exocuticle and the endocuticle. The cuticle cell contents generally lack fine structure, though Orfanos & Ruska (1968a) have observed fine structure in the exocuticle made up of interwoven thread-like osmophilic units approximately 3 nm in diameter; other authors have interpreted these results cautiously (Swift 1977) suggesting that the units could be the product of the high magnification methods used.

The outer exocuticle is approximately 0.2 μm thick and the inner endocuticle 0.1 μm thick in human scalp hair; the junction between the two layers is generally irregular. The A-layer is of constant thickness in each cell and

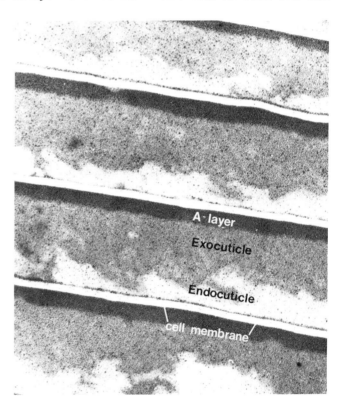

Fig. 2.12. Hair cuticle (electron micrograph—silver methenamine stain).

approximately 40 nm thick. The endocuticle has an irregular substructure of membrane-like elements which are probably the remnants of cytoplasmic structures.

Cortex (Orfanos & Ruska 1968b)

This component constitutes the main bulk of the hair and is the part contributing most to the mechanical properties of the fibres. Cortical cells are closely packed and orientated to the axis of the hair; they are approximately 3–6 μm in diameter and up to 100 μm long. Each cell contains a nuclear remnant (nuclear 'ghost') which is stellate in transverse section. The major structures within cortical cell are the closely packed macrofibrils (Fig. 2.13).

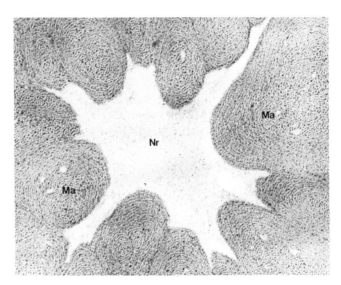

Fig. 2.13. Hair cortex. The central nuclear remnant (Nr) is surrounded by macrofibrils (Ma) (electron micrograph—silver methenamine stain).

Each macrofibril is a solid cylindrical unit 0.1 to 0.4 μm in diameter and of variable length but often the whole cell length. Between the macrofibrils is a variable amount of intermacrofibrillar matrix and melanin granules; this matrix is analogous in structure to the cuticular endocuticle and contains the remnants of cytoplasmic organelles. In some cells macrofibrils are so densely packed that individual units are difficult to see on electron microscopy (paracortical cell), whilst others are less densely aggregated (orthocortical cells). Human hair cortex is generally considered to be of the paracortical cell type throughout the cortical thickness, though Swift (1977) has described Mongolian (straight) hair as paracortical, Caucasian (curly) as mainly paracortical and Negro (woolly) as segmented into two zones—the outer side of the crimp curl being ortho-, and the inner parcortical.

Macrofibrils are composed of rod-like microfibrils approximately 7 nm in diameter, arranged in whorls (pseudo-hexagons), and embedded in a structure-less intermicrofibrillar matrix (Fig. 2.14). Routine transmission electron microscopic studies suggest that these microfibrils are parallel and are longitudinally orientated within the macrofibril, but Johnson & Sikorski (1965) have described a spiral arrangement of macrofibrils.

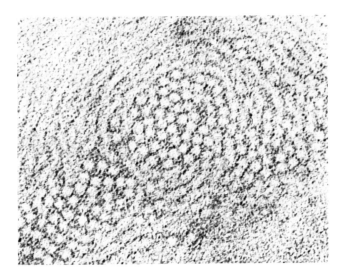

Fig. 2.14. Details of the structure of a hair cortex macrofibril. The dark staining matrix protein surrounds densely packed circular microfibrils (silver methenamine stain).

Medulla (Marhle & Orfanos 1971)
In many lower animals, e.g. the porcupine quill, the medulla constitutes a continuous central part of the fibre. However, in human hair the medulla is typically only found in terminal hair and may be continuous (Fig. 2.9), discontinuous or even absent. Wildman (1954) has subdivided medullary types into a 'latticed' and 'simple' pattern for continuous medulla, and a 'fragmented' and 'ladder' pattern for discontinuous medulla.

The medulla in all keratin fibres consists of a cortex-like framework of spongy keratin supporting thin shells of amorphous material bounding air spaces of variable size.

Chemical composition of hair (Montagna 1974; Robbins 1979)
Human hair is a very complex fibre made up of various morphological components and several different chemical species. For convenience and simplicity the different chemical components are described separately in most texts and in relating the chemical basis of hair function and physical properties. However, it is very important to note that human hair is an integrated system with the chemical components acting together. The chemical composition of hair varies somewhat with its water content. The main component is protein which is 65–95% of the hair by weight; the protein is a condensation polymer of

amino acids. Other constituents include water, lipids, pigment and trace elements.

Protein

Most of the keratinous protein is contained within cortical cells. It is characteristically insoluble and resistant to proteolytic enzymes. Because of solubility problems it is difficult to compare quantitative results from different laboratories. Solubility may vary from 10 to 70%. Solubilization involves breaking disulphide bonds by either reduction or oxidation. The proteins produced by reduction are kerateins; those from oxidation are keratoses, S-carboxymethyl kerateins (SCMK proteins). SCMK proteins produced by reduction separate into a low sulphur group (SCMKA proteins, mol. wt. 45,000) and a high sulphur group (SCMKB proteins, mol. wt. 20,000)—these compose 60% and 30% respectively of the total protein of hair (Fraser *et al.* 1972). After oxidation, the keratoses can be separated into α-keratose and γ-keratose; in relation to sulphur content and amino-acid content α and γ keratoses are similar to SCMKA and SCMKB proteins respectively. As well as these two protein groups, 2–3% of the protein consists of low-sulphur heterogeneous protein that is rich in glycine and tyrosine (Zahn & Biela 1968).

To summarize, hair contains perhaps up to fifty proteins extracted by a variety of methods but it is quite likely that these are the technical products of much fewer proteins present in vivo. It has been shown by electron histochemical methods that in the hair cortex, the high-sulphur proteins are predominantly in the matrix and the low-sulphur in the filamentous protein.

During the last 20 years many investigators have analysed the constituent amino acids of whole hair specimens; such analysis is often quoted for genetically diseased hair. The results are of limited use since they only provide average values for the amino-acid contents of average proteinaceous substances of the hair; also some amino acids undergo hydrolytic decomposition (Bloch & Weiss 1956). 5–6 N Hydrochloric acid is most commonly used for keratin fibre analysis and using this method the following amino acids have been shown to undergo partial decomposition—cystine, threonine, tyrosine, phenylalanine, arginine and tryptophan.

The amino acids isolated from normal hair are shown in Table 2.1 together with average relative amounts found by quantitative analysis (Dawber 1978). The figures are gross and in health and disease cannot be compared unless a large number of varying factors are taken into consideration; these include genetic variation, weathering, diet, cosmetic treatment and the extraction and analytical methods used. In general, male scalp hair contains more cystine than female hair, whilst dark hair is said to contain more cystine than light shades. The tip of scalp hair contains significantly less cystine and cysteine than the root end; the converse applies for cysteic acid. For details of these and other studies of

Table 2.1. Amino acid composition of normal hair expressed as residues per 100 residues extracted

Amino acid	Amount	Amino acid	Amount
Lysine	2.8	Alanine	4.8
Histidine	0.8	$\frac{1}{2}$ Cystine	17.5
Arginine	5.6	Valine	5.9
Aspartic acid	5.0	Methionine	0.5
Threonine	6.9	Isoleucine	2.7
Serine	11.7	Leucine	6.1
Glutamic acid	11.1	Tyrosine	1.9
Proline	3.6	Phenylalanine	1.4
Glycine	6.5		

factors varying amino-acid composition, the reader is referred to more comprehensive texts (Asquith 1977; Robbins 1979).

Human hair cuticle is said to contain more cystine, cysteic acid, proline, threonine, isoleucine, methionine, leucine, tyrosine, phenylalanine and arginine than whole hair (Bradbury 1973); using different methods, other workers obtained broadly similar results (Blout *et al.* 1960). In general cuticular cells contain a higher proportion of amino acids not usually found in α-helical polypeptides than whole hair. The chemical composition of the A-layer and exocuticle are considerably different from the endocuticle in that they are highly cross-linked by cystine, giving a tough and resilient layer. The endocuticle contains very little cystine.

Since both by weight and volume the cortex makes up the main part of the hair fibre, whole fibre analytical studies relate closely to cortical chemistry. The greatest error will be in those amino acids present in smallest quantities.

Medullary protein is notoriously insoluble and difficult to isolate; consequently complete analytic studies have not so far been possible; much of the known information has come from analysis of porcupine quill proteins (Rogers 1964a). Medulla has a very low cystine and sulphur content and contains relatively large quantities of acidic and basic amino acids and hydroxyamino acids.

Water content

Water content of hair is important in relation to its physical and cosmetic properties. The density of dry hair is 1.09 on the basis of geometrical weight measurements and 1.37 from pycnometric measurements. Consequently the porosity is about 20% and hence is hygroscopic. When impregnated with water its weight increases by 12–18%. The process of absorption is very rapid; 75% of the maximum possible amount of water is absorbed within 4 minutes (Ryabukhin 1980). The water binding of amino and guanidino groups are responsible for the large percentage of water absorption capacity of keratin, particularly at low humidities; peptide bonds are preferential sites for hydration. It is thought that at low relative humidities ($< 25\%$), water molecules are bonded to hydrophilic sites by hydrogen bonds. With increasing humidity more water is absorbed producing a decrease in the energy binding of water already associated with the protein. At greater than 80% relative humidity water on water absorption becomes more and more important.

Hair lipids
Much of our knowledge of hair lipids comes from 'fat solvent' studies. Depending on the solvent used, different results are obtainable; ethanol removes more lipid from hair than do solvents such as benzene, ether or chloroform. The values obtained represent mainly sebum and the chromatographic fractions obtained consist primarily of free fatty acids and neutral fats—esters, glyceryl, wax, hydrocarbons and alcohols.

   The lipids of human hair are often thought of as of minor importance. It has been shown that hair lipid increases after puberty in both sexes. This declines with age in women but not to the same extent in men. Negroid hair produces more lipid than Caucasian hair. Squalene content in children is approximately one-quarter that of adults, whilst cholesterol exists in similar proportions. In relation to age or sex there is no difference with regard to fatty alcohol content of human hair lipid.

Trace elements (Brown & Crounse 1980)
It is not known to which chemical group in hair structure trace elements are attached; however, the principal metal content of human hair probably exists as an integral part of fibre structure i.e. as salt linkages or coordinated complexes with the side chains of pigment or proteins.

   Trace elements may be incorporated into hair from several sources, both exogenous and endogenous (Hopps 1971). Of endogenous sources, the matrix, connective tissue papilla, the sebaceous, eccrine and apocrine glands and the surface epidermis are important. The environment also contributes greatly, particularly by pollution, e.g. from industry and hair cosmetics; scalp hair has been used in many studies as a sensitive index of environmental pollution. Until recently the most frequently investigated elements in hair have been As, Cd, Cr, Cu, Hg, Pb and Zn (Chatt *et al.* 1980). Techniques such as nuclear activation, X-ray fluorescence, and emission, and atomic absorption and emission have enabled submicrogram quantities to be determined. An international coordinated programme on activation analysis of trace element pollutants in human hair has been set up by the International Atomic Energy Agency based in Vienna (Ryabukhin 1980). It is hoped to standardize methods used so that different studies around the world can be coordinated and correlated. With standardization of methods it is possible that the method of photon activation analysis may give a unique measurement of trace elements present along hair shafts—a complete profile may prove to be unique for each individual as fingerprints. This method enables elements such as C, N, O, F, Cr, Y, Zn, Mo, Cd, Sn, I, Sr, Pb, Tl and Bi to be analysed that are difficult by other methods.

The total ash content of human hair varies from 0.26% to 0.94% of dry weight. The number of elements reported in human hair depends on the method used but the following have been detected—Ca, Mg, Sr, B, Al, Si, Na, K, Zn, Cu, Mn, Fe, Ag, Au, Hg, As, Pb, Sb, Ti, W, Mo, I, P and Se. The vast majority are from extraneous sources but substances such as As and thallium used as poisons are sensitively localized in hair after ingestion.

Hair shape

The shape of hair varies with body site and with race (Swift 1977).

Mongoloid hair is typically straight and of round bore, whilst Caucasoid hair is curly and tends to be oval in cross-section; Negroid hair is woolly and distinctly oval. Caucasoid and Negroid hair tends to have a smaller diameter than Mongoloid hair.

Pubic, beard and eyelash hairs are generally oval in all racial types. There is no detectable difference in hair shape between men and women with respect to race or body site.

References

Asquith R.S. (1977) *Chemistry of Natural Protein Fibers.* London, Wiley.

Auber L. (1952) The anatomy of follicles producing wool fibres with special reference to keratinisation. *Transactions of the Royal Society of Edinburgh,* **62,** 191.

Birkbeck M.S.C. & Mercer E.H. (1957) The electron microscopy of the human hair follicle. II. The hair cuticle. *Journal of Biophysical and Biochemical Cytology,* **3,** 215.

Blout E.R., de Loye D., Bloom S.M. & Forman G.D. (1960) *Journal of the American Chemical Society,* **82,** 3787.

Bradbury J.H. (1973) The structure and chemistry of keratin fibres. *Advances in Protein Chemistry,* **27,** 111.

Braun-Falco O. (1958a) The fine structure of the anagen hair follicle of the mouse. In *Advances in the Biology of the Skin,* vol. IX, *Hair Growth,* eds. W. Montagna & R.L. Dobson. Oxford, Pergamon Press, ch. 29.

Braun-Falco O. (1958b) Histochemistry of the hair follicle. In *The Biology of Hair Growth,* eds. W. Montagna & R.A. Ellis. New York, Academic Press, ch. 4.

Brown A.C. & Crounse R.G. (1980) *Hair, Trace Elements and Human Illness,* part I. New York, Praeger.

Bullough W.S. & Lawrence E.B. (1958) The mitotic activity of the follicles. In *The Biology of Hair Growth,* eds. W. Montagna & R.A. Ellis. New York, Academic Press, p. 171.

Chatt A., Secord C.A., Tiefenbach B. & Jervis R.E. (1980) Scalp hair as a monitor of community exposure to environmental pollutants. In *Hair Trace Elements and Human Illness.* Eds. A.C. Brown & R.G. Crounse. New York, Praeger, ch. 3.

Cohen J. (1965) The dermal papilla. In *Biology of the Skin and Hair Growth,* eds. A.G. Lyne & B.F. Short. Sydney, Angus & Robertson, ch. 12.

Dawber R.P.R. (1978) Unpublished results.

Durward A. & Rudall K.M. (1958) The vascularity and patterns of growth of hair follicles. In *The Biology of Hair Growth*, eds. W. Montagna & R.A. Ellis. New York, Academic Press, p. 189.

Epstein W.L. & Maibach H.L. (1969) Cell proliferation and movement in human hair bulbs. In *Advances in Biology of Skin*, vol. IX, *Hair Growth*, eds. W. Montagna & R.L. Dobson. Oxford, Pergamon Press, p. 89.

Fraser R.D.B., MacRae T.P. & Rogers G.E. (1972) *Keratins: Their Composition, Structure and Biosynthesis*. Springfield, Thomas.

Harding H.W.J. & Rogers G.E. (1971) The E-lysine cross-linkage in citrulline-containing protein fractions from hair. *Biochemistry*, **10**, 624.

Helwig E.B. (1958) Pathology of psoriasis. *Annals of the New York Academy of Sciences*, **73**, 924.

Hopps H.C. (1971) The biological basis of using hair and nail for analysis of trace elements. *Proceedings of the Symposium on Trace Substances in Environmental Health*, VIII, ed. Hemphill, D.D. Columbia, University of Missouri.

Jarrett A. (1958) The chemistry of inner root sheath and keratins. *British Journal of Dermatology*, **70**, 271.

Johnson D.J. & Sikorski J. (1965) *Proceedings of the 3rd International Wool Textile Research Conference (Paris)*, **I**, 53.

Kligman A.M. (1959) The human hair cycle. *Journal of Investigative Dermatology*, **33**, 307.

Knutson D.D. (1974) Ultrastructural observations in acne. *Journal of Investigative Dermatology*, **62**, 288.

Marhle G. & Orfanos G.E. (1971) The spongious keratin and the medullary substance of human scalp hair. *Archiv fur Dermatologische Forschung*, **241**, 305.

Montagna W. & Van Scott E.J. (1958) The anatomy of the hair follicle. In *The Biology of Hair Growth*, eds. W. Montagna & R.A. Ellis. New York, Academic Press, ch. 3.

Montagna W. & Parakkal P.K. (1974) In *The Structure and Function of Skin*. New York, Academic Press, ch. 7, p. 232.

Orfanos C. & Ruska H. (1968a) The fine structure of human hair. I. Hair cuticle. *Archiv fur klinische und experimentelle Dermatologie*, **231**, 97.

Orfanos C. & Ruska H. (1968b) The fine structure of human hair. II. The hair cortex. *Archiv fur klinische und experimentelle Dermatologie*, **231**, 264.

Parakkal P.F. & Matoltsy A.G. (1964) A study of the differentiating products of the hair follicle cells with the electron microscope. *Journal of Investigative Dermatology*, **43**, 23.

Parakkal P.F. (1969) The fine structure of the anagen hair follicle of the mouse. In *Advances in Biology of the Skin*, vol. IX, *Hair Growth*, eds. W. Montagna & R.L. Dobson. Oxford, Pergamon Press, ch. 29.

Robbins C.R. (1979) *Chemical and Physical Behaviour of Human Hair*. New York, Van Nostrand–Reinhold, p. 7.

Rogers G.E. (1964a) Structural and biochemical features of the hair follicle. In *The Epidermis*, eds. W. Montagna & W.C. Lobitz, Jr. New York, Academic Press, p. 202.

Rogers G.E. (1964b) Isolation and property of inner root sheath cells of the hair follicle. *Experimental Cell Research*, **33**, 264.

Roth S.I. (1965) The cytology of the murine resting (telogen) hair follicle. In *Biology of the Skin and Hair Growth*, eds. A.G. Lyne & B.F. Short. Sydney, Angus & Robertson, ch. 14.

Rudall K.M. (1964) The biomolecular structure of hair keratins. In: *Progress in the Biological Sciences in Relation to Dermatology*, eds. A.J. Rook & R.H. Champion. Cambridge University Press, p. 355.

Ryabukhin Y.S. (1980) International coordinated program of trace element pollutants in human hair. In *Hair, Trace Elements and Human Illnesses*, eds. A.C. Brown & R.G. Crounse. New York, Praeger, ch. 1, p. 5.

Schinckel P.G. (1961) Mitotic activity in wool follicle bulbs. *Australian Journal of Biological Sciences*, **14**, 659.

Straile W.E., Chase H.B. & Arsenault C. (1961) Growth and differentiation of hair follicles between periods of activity and quiescence. *Journal of Experimental Zoology*, **148**, 205.

Straile W.E. (1962) Possible functions of the external root sheath during growth of the hair follicle. *Journal of Experimental Zoology*, **150**, 207.

Straile W.E. (1965) Root sheath dermal papilla relationships and the control of hair growth. In *Biology of the Skin and Hair Growth*, eds. A.G. Lyne & B.F. Short. Sydney, Angus & Robertson, ch. 3.

Swift J.A. & Holmes A.W. (1965) Degradation of human hair by papain. *Textile Research Journal*, **35**, 1014.

Swift J.A. (1977) The histology of keratin fibres. In: *Chemistry of Natural Protein Fibres*, ed. R.A. Asquith. London, Wiley, ch. 3.

Van Scott E.J., Ekel T.M. & Auerback R. (1963) Determinants of rate and kinetics of cell division in scalp hair. *Journal of Investigative Dermatology*, **41**, 269.

Wildman A.B. (1954) *The Microscopy of Animal Textile Fibres*. Wool Industries Research Association, Leeds.

Wolfram L.J. & Lindemann M.K.O. (1971) Some observations on the hair cuticle. *Journal of the Society of Cosmetic Chemists*, **22**, 839.

Zahn H. & Biela M. (1968) Tyrosin reiche proteine im ameisensaureextrakt von reduzierter welle. *European Journal of Biochemistry*, **5**, 567.

Physical properties of hair
(References p. 47)

The physical properties of biological materials are a function of their geometric shape and of the intrinsic properties of the individual constituent materials. Hair keratin is the only human protein that is able to have its exact physical properties analysed. Most of the early work on keratin fibres was carried out on wool (Chapman 1969) and much of the equipment now used for assessing human hair characteristics has evolved from prototypes used in earlier wool research (Robbins 1979). A considerable amount of work has been carried out in applying basic laws of physics and engineering to hair tensile properties but it is important to state that such laws cannot exactly apply in the field of biomechanics. The 'strength' of human hair resides in the cortex which has a composite structure in which discontinuous fibres—keratin fibrils within longitudinal orientated cell envelopes—are embedded in a sulphur-rich matrix. In engineering terms, fibre/matrix composites are structures in which two or more components are combined to make best use of the favourable properties of the components whilst at the same time mitigating against some of their less desirable characteristics. Natural composites can sustain loads and resist loads far more efficiently than man-made composites, and hair is no exception (Fraser & Macrae 1980; Harris 1980). The cortical matrix is easily deformed by mechanical stress and energy is transmitted evenly into the fibrils, possibly by shearing forces at the fibre/matrix interface. Whatever the efficiency of the hair cortex as a composite, without an intact overlying cuticle human hair resists external mechanical stresses poorly, as in excessive weathering due to cosmetic abuse. Therefore in assessing hair for biochemical efficiency it is important to consider the cuticle, epicuticle, intercellular cement substance and the plasma membranes of both the cortex and cuticle (Spearman 1977). Since the medulla is absent from vellus hair and is frequently absent or discontinuous in terminal hair, it is not generally considered important in this context, though in lower animals this is certainly not the case.

The physical properties of hair can be divided into elastic deformations including stretching, bending, stiffness, torsion, cross-sectional area and shape, density, friction and static charge.

Elastic properties

Probably the most important mechanical property of hair is elasticity by which it resists forces tending to change its shape, volume and length and also enables it to recover its original form when the force is removed. Every deforming force of an elastic substance is balanced by a force tending to return it to its normal condition. The commonest types of strain are stretching (the ratio of increase in length to the original length), compression (the ratio of decrease in length to the original length), shear, bending and torsion (Mitchell & Feughelman 1960). Each type of stress and strain has a modulus (the ratio of stress to strain). The modulus that has received the greatest amount of attention in hair studies has been Young's modulus, a measure of elasticity to stretching. Young's modulus is defined by the equation:

$$\frac{FL}{al} \quad \text{dynes per unit area (cm}^2\text{)}$$

where F = force (dynes) applied per unit area of cross-section.

a = unit area of cross-section.
L = length of fibre before stretching
l = increase in length on stretching

In considering the response of hair to stretching, another law of physics must be considered, Hooke's Law. This states that in elastic substances, strains are proportional to the stresses producing them. Thus, when an elastic fibre is pulled, the change in length is proportional to the force applied. A typical load-elongation curve for human hair is shown in Fig. 2.15; Hooke's law only applies up to point 1 on the curve. Up to this point the fibre is able to return to its original state. Irreversible changes occur in the hair in the yield region even if the fibre returns to its normal length. In the post-yield region resistance to stress increases greatly until the breaking point is reached. When hair is stretched up to 30% of its original length in water and allowed to return to its former length, the curve of relaxation is separated from the elongation curve (Fig. 2.16). Under these circumstances, the work of elongation is greater than the work of recovery; the ratio of these two work values is known as the hysteresis (resilience) ratio. The elongation/relaxation graph is known as the hysteresis curve. When normal hairs are stretched to between 30 and 70% more than their original length above the hysteresis region, the relaxation curve is the same as for extension (Alexander, Hudson & Earland 1963). Normal scalp hair fibres break if stretched to approximately 80% of the initial length.

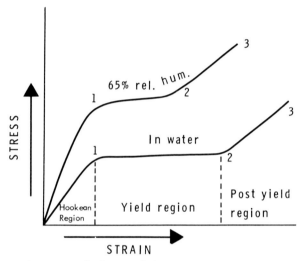

Fig. 2.15. Load/extension curves for human hair.

The effects of many different factors on the tensile properties of hair have been studied in great detail.

The moisture content of hair increases with increasing relative humidity (RH). The effect of 65% RH and 100% RH on the load-extension curve can be seen in Fig. 2.15. In general, Young's modulus falls as RH rises, whilst hair extensibility prior to breaking is directly proportional to RH (Robbins 1979).

Both the wet and dry elastic properties of hair are directly proportional to shaft diameter as assessed by investigations at fixed RH. The breaking stress decreases with increasing hair diameter.

The elastic modulus of human hair decreases with increasing temperature as do the post-yield modulus and fibre strength. Hair extensibility prior to breaking point increases directly with temperature.

Bleaching and permanent waving markedly alter the elastic properties of hair, the latter particularly so. Bleaching decreases tensile properties by up to 25% (Alexander *et al.* 1963; Robbins 1979). Permanent waving reduces disulphide cross-links and causes molecular 'shifting' on reoxidation. Both the

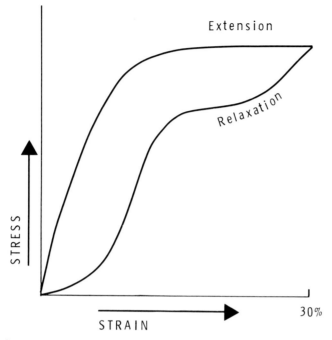

Fig. 2.16. Load/extension and recovery curves for human hair.

reduction and re-oxidation phases alter tensile properties; stress to breaking point is up to 15% less, and stress to 20% extension up to 18% less than for untreated hair. Stretching hairs in aqueous reduction solutions results in lower stresses to achieve a particular strain; re-oxidation improves this towards normal.

Dying from a light to a darker shade produces negligible change in elastic properties, whilst any impairment on lightening hair colour depends on the extent of disulphide bond oxidation (bleaching).

Sunlight and artificial ultraviolet β-radiation cause photochemical degradation of cystine to cysteic acid and thus impair elastic properties in a similar way to bleaching, but to a smaller degree since disulphide bond disruption is less following UVR exposure.

Elastic properties of hair in disease (Goldsmith & Baden 1971)
Dawber (1972) found that hair from a family with pili annulati, though not clinically fragile, always breaks through the abnormal bands; breaking stress analysis however, showed only a 2% reduction compared to normal controls.

Swanbeck *et al.* (1970) studied tensile strength, strain at breaking point and elastic modulus in male pattern baldness, alopecia areata and defluvium capillorum; no significant abnormalities were found. However, in congenital ectodermal dysplasia both tensile strength and elastic modulus were reduced whilst in congenital ichthyosiform erythroderma only elastic modulus was decreased.

Both hypothyroidism and acromegaly cause an alteration in the yield region of the stress/strain curve at low levels of RH (Korostoff *et al.* 1970).

In view of the importance of the disulphide bond with regard to tensile strength of hair, it is likely that all sulphur, cystine and high-sulphur, protein-deficient hairs will have abnormal tensile properties (Clarke & Buhrke 1954), though only occasional reports have appeared to substantiate this. Brown *et al.* (1970) studied a congenital defect of hair showing trichoschisis, alternate birefringence and low sulphur content and found that dry hair had a lower degree of extension at a lower stress than normal. Stress–strain testing of low sulphur hair in water (Baden *et al.* 1976) showed that the fibres extended more at lower tensions before breaking; these results were similar to those from hairs with chemically reduced disulphide bonds.

Most of the studies described above, investigating elastic properties of hair, are carried out at fixed rates of extension with the hair held at each end. For other methods of evaluating stretching properties of hair the reader is referred to the description by Robbins (1979); the use of techniques such as the oscillating beam method, stress relaxation, stretch rotation and the set and supercontraction method has largely been limited to the hair cosmetic and wool industries.

Hair structure following stretching
The fusiform cortical cells increase in length during stretching; this change occurs during the Hookean phase of extension (Fig. 2.15). It seems unlikely that any slip occurs between adjacent cells in view of the firm adhesion present due to plasma membrane interdigitations and strong cement substance. X-ray diffraction studies have shown that further stretching modifies intracellular keratin structure. There is an increase in the meridional spacings which are considered to correspond with distances between the coils and supercoils in the alpha helix (Fraser *et al.* 1972) which are like stretched spiral springs. This action is possible because of the weak hydrogen bonds between the keratin fibrils and the matrix protein. As strain increases in the yield and post yield zones (Fig. 1) matrix disulphide bonds are disrupted and cell membranes may fracture in advance of the breaking point (Rudall 1964). Following elastic recoil, disulphide bonds probably reform at different points in the keratin molecule as in permanent waving.

It is important to note that many of the properties of hair fibres described above may not be relevant under normal circumstances since the force required to pull hair out of its follicle (Tsuda 1957) even in the anagen phase of the hair cycle, may frequently be less than that needed to construct load-extension curves

(Figs. 2.15 and 2.16). Certainly the majority of hairs plucked for anagen–telogen analysis possess roots i.e. they are released from the scalp before the breakage point is reached.

Hair bending and stiffness

When a hair fibre is bent the arc that is formed contains three longitudinal zones within it—the outer layers of the arc are stretched, the inner layers compressed and a central zone undergoes neither stretching or compression. Stiffness of hair implies a resistance to bending. This property of hair has received very little attention from clinicians though several authors have shown that bending forces damage cuticular structure in the outer part of the bending arc in normal (Swift & Brown 1972) and knotted hair (Dawber 1974). Also the transverse fracture and breakage of monilethrix internodes is probably due to the inability of the narrowed hair to withstand bending forces (Dawber, 1980).

Several methods have been described in an attempt to quantitate bending forces (Robbins 1979) but none of the techniques can specifically measure the extension and compression forces within the bent section. It has been suggested that hair stiffness parallels the linear stretching properties and is varied by similar factors.

Density of human hair (Morton & Hearle 1962)

The absolute density of keratin fibres is difficult to measure (Hearle & Peters 1960). At RH of 60% the density is approximately 1.320, the same as wool fibres. No studies of hair density in disease have been carried out; bleaching and permanent waving have no significant effect on hair density.

Variations in hair fibre dimensions

The measurements which are most commonly used for comparative studies are length and diameter. If the hair is taken to be cylindrical, then volume, cross-sectional area, radius and surface area can easily be calculated. These measurements need to be made to enable fundamental elastic properties to be studied. Single hair cross-sectional dimensions can be measured by various methods, including linear density, light microscopy, vibrascopy, calipers and laser beam diffraction. Centrifugation can be used for multiple hair determinations (Robbins 1979).

Much of the work carried out in this field has been by physical anthropologists, anatomists, forensic scientists and cosmetic scientists. Hayashi *et al.* (1975) studied differences in hair diameter, the hair index—the ratio of the least diameter to the greatest diameter—and the area of the cuticle expressed as a percentage of the area of cross-section in 55 subjects of 18 races in Europe, Asia and America. The diameter measurements showed that hair from white races and their hybrids—German, Italian and English—are finer than hair from Latin countries, Afro-Americans and Ghanaians. The coarsest hair was found in Mongoloid races. Scalp hair diameter varies from 40 to 120 μm; Caucasoid scalp hair varies from 50 to 90 μm whilst Mongoloid scalp hair is the coarsest with a mean diameter of approximately 120 μm.

Hair length increases slightly as RH rises, whilst hair diameter increases to a much greater degree. Swelling of this type is much less than unstretched hair when the hair is under tension below 60% RH; at greater than 60% RH swelling of hair is greater than that of unstretched fibres.

Mechanical properties of hair cuticle

Linear stretching of hair fibres alters cortical structure before any cuticular damage occurs. Cuticular cells are able to move over each other, since the flat overlapping cells do not normally interdigitate like cortical cells. These overlapping scales give a rough surface to hair fibres which are thus susceptible to frictional damage.

Friction is defined as the force tending to resist motion when one body slides over another. The force (F) necessary to slide one object over another is proportional to the normal load pressing the surfaces together (W):

$$F = \mu W$$

The constant μ is the coefficient of friction; the force to start movement governs the coefficient of static friction (μ_s) and that force necessary to maintain force determines the coefficient of kinetic friction (μ_{kk}). μ_k is usually less than μ_s. The methods used to measure friction in keratin fibres have been well described (Meredith & Hearle 1959).

Hair exhibits a directional frictional effect in that it is easier to move a surface in a root to tip direction than in a tip to root direction. Wet friction is higher than dry friction for both human hair and wool fibres; friction is not dependent on hair shaft diameter or temperature. Bleaching and permanent waving increase the coefficient of kinetic friction whilst high conditioning shampoos and cream rinses decrease μ_k.

Electrical (static) charge of hair

Dry hairs are poor conductors of electricity whilst wet hairs are very good. When dry hair is rubbed and pressed during combing and brushing, under suitable conditions static electricity is produced. This is associated with 'flyaway' hair and is due to electrons or ions that are not moving. Frictional electricity is called tribo-electricity; it is more likely to develop in fibres with a high electrical resistance, for example hair or wool, than those with a lower resistance such as cotton and rayon (Morton & Hearle, 1962). Decreasing levels of RH decrease electrical resistance and lessen the propensity for tribo-electricity production. Most women know that combing and brushing in hot conditions causes greater flyaway than in cool conditions; experimental combing has confirmed this observation in showing that electrical resistance decreases as the temperature rises. Semi-quantitative experiments have shown that a useful way to minimize static build up is to reduce the effort of combing by making the hair comb easier.

The sign of the charge that develops when hairs are rubbed against each other is related to the direction of rubbing. If a single fibre in a group of hairs all orientated in the same direction is pulled out root first it becomes positively charged; if it is pulled out tip first a negative charge is produced. Hair is thus dielectrically anisotropic at its surface.

Cream rinses and certain shampoos (high cleansing or high conditioning) decrease flyaway by reducing static charge as a result of lower kinetic frictional force during combing or brushing. They also lower the electrical resistance of fibres by increasing hair moisture.

References

Alexander P., Hudson P.F. & Earland C. (1963) *Wool: Its Chemistry and Physics*, 2nd edn. London, Chapman & Hall.

Baden H.P., Jackson C.E., Weiss L., Jumbow K., Lee L., Kubilus J. & Gold R.J.M. (1976) The physicochemical properties of hair in the BIDS syndrome. *American Journal of Human Genetics*, **28**, 514.

Brown A.C., Belser R.B., Crounse R.G. & Wehr R.F. (1970) A congenital hair defect, trichoschisis, with alternating birefringence and low sulphur content. *Journal of Investigative Dermatology*, **34**, 496.

Chapman B.M. (1969) A review of the mechanical properties of keratin fibres. *Journal of the Textile Institute*, **60**, 181.

Clarke G.L. & Buhrke V.E. (1954) Effects of elemental sulphur in the diet on the load extension hysteresis in single wool fibres. *Science (New York)*, **120**, 40.

Dawber R.P.R. (1972) Investigations of a family with pili annulati associated with blue naevi. *Transactions of St John's Hospital Dermatological Society*, **58**, 51.

Dawber R.P.R. (1974) Knotting of scalp hair. *British Journal of Dermatology*, **91**, 169.

Dawber R.P.R. (1980) Weathering of hair in some genetic hair dystrophies. In *Hair, Trace Elements and Human Illness*, eds. A.C. Brown and R.G. Crounse. New York, Praeger Scientific Publishers.

Fraser R.D.B., MacRae T.P. & Rogers G.E. (1972) *Keratins: Their Composition, Structure and Biosynthesis*, 1st edn. Springfield, Thomas. p. 133.

Fraser R.D.B. & MacRae T.P. (1980) Molecular structure and mechnical properties of keratins. In *The Mechanical Properties of Biological Materials*, Cambridge, Cambridge University Press, ch. 9.

Goldsmith L.A. & Baden H.P. (1971) The mechanical properties of hair. Chemical modifications and pathological hairs. *Journal of Investigative Dermatology*, **56**, 200.

Harris B. (1980) The mechanical behaviour of composite materials. In *The Mechanical Properties of Biological Materials*. Cambridge, Cambridge University Press, ch. 3.

Korostoff E., Rawnsley H.M. & Shelley W.B. (1970) Normalised stress–strain relationships of human hair perturbations by hypothyroidism. *British Journal of Dermatology*, **83**, 27.

Meredith R. & Hearle J. (1959) *Physical Methods of Investigating Textiles*. New York, Interscience, ch. II.

Mitchell T.W. & Feughelman M. (1960) The torsional properties of single wool fibres. I. Torque–twist relationships and torsional relaxation in wet and dry fibres. *Textile Research Journal*, **30**, 662.

Morton W. & Hearle J. (1962) *Physical Properties of Textile Fibres*. London, Butterworth Scientific Publications, ch. 17.

Robbins C.R. (1979) *Chemical and Physical Behaviour of Human Hair*, 1st edn, New York, Van Nostrand–Reinhold.

Rudall K.M. (1964) The biomolecular structure of hair keratins. In *Progress in the Biological Sciences in Relation to Dermatology*, vol 2, eds. A. Rook & R.H. Champion. London, Cambridge University Press.

Spearman R.O.C. (1977) The physical properties of hair. In *The Physiology and Pathophysiology of the Skin*, vol. 4, ed. A. Jarrett. London, Academic Press, ch. 44.

Swanbeck G., Nyren J. & Juhlin L. (1970) Mechanical properties of hairs from patients with different types of hair diseases. *Journal of Investigative Dermatology*, **54**, 248.

Swift J.A. & Brown A.C. (1972) The critical determination of fine changes in the surface architecture of human hair due to cosmetic treatment. *Journal of the Society of Cosmetic Chemists*, **23**, 695.

Tsuda K. (1957) Extractive properties of human hair. *Journal of Kyoto Prefecture Medical University* **61**, 936.

Chapter 3
The Hair in Infancy
and Childhood

Physiological aspects
(References p. 51)

As described above, the number and distribution of hair germs are genetically determined and, in all but exceptional circumstances, no new follicles are formed after birth. It follows that during growth the density of hair follicles is progressively reduced. Giacometti (1965) found an average density in the newborn scalp of 1135 per cm². In infants aged 3–12 months the density had been reduced to 795 per cm² and by the age of 20–30, to 615 per cm².

The dilution of follicle density is accompanied by an increase in the diameter of individual hairs—a rapid increase for the first 3 or 4 years, a less rapid increase for the next 6, and thereafter a slow increase or none at all (Duggins & Trotter 1951). At birth very few hairs are medullated. In the first months of life the percentage of medullated hairs rises rapidly, but after 7 months appears to fall, to rise again slowly and irregularly from the second year. The variation in shaft diameter, which shows a rough correlation with medullation, is considerable in any individual subject (Wynkoop 1929). This wide variation is probably explained by the variable proportion of hairs still of vellus type (Duggins & Trotter 1951). Cuticular scale counts show significant individual differences, but no constant correlation with age (Trotter & Duggins 1960). Such physical properties as extensibility and tensile strength increase during infancy and childhood (Goldman & Mason 1948).

The refraction indices and birefringence of the cuticle were determined in hair samples from subjects ranging in age from earliest infancy to twenty years (Duggins 1954). The refraction index fluctuates widely in the first few years of life, coinciding with the transition from vellus to terminal hair. There is a sharp drop in the refraction index in girls between 8 and 16 years, and a slow drop in boys between 8 and 13 years; over the age of 16 it is the same in both sexes.

In infancy the colour of hair is commonly lighter than in later childhood, but the age at which it reaches its full depth of colour shows considerable individual variation.

The differences between the hair of children and that of adults have been reviewed by Bogaty (1969).

Hair cycles
Cyclical activity of the hair follicles begins in utero as soon as they are completely formed. During fetal life and for the first 3 weeks after birth changes in the phases of the scalp hair cycles are sudden and of short duration and are synchronized (Barman *et al.* 1967). Until about the seventh month of extrauterine life all the scalp hairs, except those of the occipital region, are in the same phase.

In the fifth month of fetal life vellus of uniform length and calibre covers both the forehead and the scalp. The follicles in the frontal and parietal regions then suddenly and simultaneously enter telogen (Pecoraro *et al.* 1964b, 1968). In the occipital region the follicles remain in anagen almost until birth. Five or six weeks before birth a new anagen wave occurs in the frontal and parietal regions, but less sudden and less complete than the earlier wave. Thus the hair is shed in utero twice from the frontal and parietal regions and once from the occipital region.

At birth and during the first 3 days after it there are regional differences in the percentage of hairs in each phase of the cycle. In the frontal region about 65% of the follicles are in anagen and about 33% in telogen. In the parietal regions over 70% are in anagen, about 20% in catagen and about 10% in telogen, whilst in the occipital region 90% are in anagen. These figures were all obtained in Rosario, Argentina. No sex differences in hair cycles were recorded, but it was noted that in dark-skinned children the percentage of anagen hairs in the frontal and parietal regions at birth was significantly higher than in fair-skinned children, implying that the onset of a further catagen leading to telogen occurs earlier in the latter. This trend towards less synchronization of cycles continues during the first months of extrauterine life. In some infants during the first 2 or 3 weeks of life all or most of the scalp follicles are in telogen (Kostanecki *et al.* 1965) and the hair is diffusely shed during the early months. Steigleder & Schultka (1963) noted that hair was shed most profusely from the sites later affected in some individuals by common baldness. Gradually the asynchronized mosaic pattern of adult life becomes established. In normal infants only about 25% of follicles are in telogen by the sixth month (Bosse & Rubisz-Brzezinska 1965), but there is much individual variation.

During childhood the mosaic pattern becomes consolidated. During the years before puberty an average of 94% of follicles are in anagen and 6% in telogen, but there are regional variations; in the frontal region 10% of follicles are in telogen and in the occipital only 3% (Pecoraro *et al.* 1964a).

References

Barman J.M., Pecoraro V., Astore I. & Ferrer J. (1967) The first stage in the natural history of the human scalp hair cycle. *Journal of Investigative Dermatology*, **48**, 138.

Bogaty H. (1969) Differences between adult and children's hair. *Journal of the Society of Cosmetic Chemists*, **20**, 159.

Bosse K. & Rubisz-Brzezinska J. (1965) Der Haarwechsel des Säuglings. *Archiv für klinische und experimentelle Dermatologie*, **221**, 166.

Duggins O.H. (1954) Refraction indices and birefringence of the cuticles of hair of children. *American Journal of Physical Anthropology*, **12**, 89.

Duggins O.H. & Trotter M. (1951) Changes in morphology of hair during childhood. *Annals of the New York Academy of Sciences*, **53**, 569.

Giacometti L. (1965) The anatomy of the human scalp. *Advances in Biology of Skin*, **6**, 97.

Goldman L. & Mason L.M. (1948) Investigational studies in some congenital and acquired defects of the hair in children. *Journal of Investigative Dermatology*, **11**, 323.

Kostanecki W., Pawlowski A. & Lozinska D. (1965) Der Haarwenzelstatus bei Neugetorenen. *Archiv für klinische und experimentelle Dermatologie*, **221**, 162.

Pecoraro V., Astore I., Barman J. & Aranjo C.I. (1964a) The normal trichogram in the child before puberty. *Journal of Investigative Dermatology*, **42**, 427.

Pecoraro V., Astore I. & Barman J.M. (1964b) Cycle of the scalp hair of the newborn child. *Journal of Investigative Dermatology*, **43**, 145.

Pecoraro V., Astore I. & Barman J.M. (1968) The prenatal and postnatal hair cycles in man. In *Biopathology of Pattern Alopecia*, eds. A. Baccaredda-Boy, G. Moretti & J.R. Frey. Basel, Karger, p. 29.

Steigleder G.K. & Schultka O. (1963) Wechsel des Kopfhaars bei Kindern im ersten Lebensjahr. *Zeitschrift für Haut und Geschlects-krankheiten*, **34**, XI.

Trotter M. & Duggins O.H. (1960) Age changes in head hair from birth to maturity. III. Cuticular scale counts of hair of children. *American Journal of Physical Anthropology*, **8**, 467.

Wynkoop E.M. (1929) A study of the age correlations of the cuticular scales, medullas and shaft diameters of human head hair. *American Journal of Physical Anthropology*, **13**, 177.

Trichoglyphics—hair slope patterns
(References p. 52)

All hair follicles grow obliquely in relation to the epidermis. The direction of slope of the follicles, varying from one region of the body to another, gives rise to the hair tracts and the study of the pattern of these tracts is known as trichoglyphics.

Hair slope patterns were the life's work of Walter Kidd (1853–1929) (Kidd 1903). He claimed that the patterns had been determined by function and this Lamarckian hypothesis aroused some controversy (Rook 1975). The true significance of hair slope patterns in general remains uncertain. The hair streams and epidermal ridge patterns probably have some homologous directional growth properties (Findlay & Harris 1977). The available evidence suggests that the directional pattern of scalp hair is determined by the growth and shape of the developing brain before or during the period of downward growth of the hair follicles from the 10th to the 16th fetal week.

Kiil (1948a) classified frontal hair slope patterns in a Norwegian population into three types. He showed complete concordance of patterns in uniovular twins. Kiil (1948b) later found the same three types in mental defectives in Connecticut USA, with some racial variation in their relative frequency. One of the three patterns failed to occur in the 66 patients with Down's syndrome included in the survey.

One distinctive feature of the hair-slope pattern is the hair whorl. It is impossible completely to cover a sphere, such as the human head, with hair without there being at least one point from which the hair-slope radiates. The hair whorl is determinable in the human fetus from the 16th to the 18th week (Wunderlich & Heerema 1975). Of 404 newborn infants examined by these authors 98.5% had single parietal whorls and 1.5% had double. In 93.8% the whorls were clockwise and in 4.7% counter clockwise. In over half the infants (57.9%) the whorls were central, in 32.4% were on the right side and only 8.3% on the left.

Aberration in the growth of the brain occurs between the 10th and 25th week of fetal development. In a number of well-defined dysmorphic syndromes (Smith & Gong 1973, 1974) the whorls are abnormal. For example, 85% of patients with primary microcephaly had abnormal patterns and 25% had no parietal whorl.

Excessive unruliness of scalp hair in infancy is seen in 2% of normal infants. It is much more frequent in microcephaly, Down's syndrome and de Lange syndrome (Smith & Greely 1978).

References

Findlay G.H. & Harris W.F. (1977) The topology of hair streams and whorls in man with an observation on their relationship to epidermal ridge patterns. *American Journal of Physical Anthropology*, **46**, 427.

Kidd W. (1903) *The Direction of Hair in Animals and Man*. London, Black.

Kiil V. (1948a) Inheritance of frontal hair direction in man. *Journal of Hereditary*, **39**, 206.

Kill V. (1948b) Frontal hair direction in mentally deficient individuals with special references to mongolism. *Journal of Hereditary*, **39**, 281.

Rook A. (1975) The clinical significance of abnormal hair-slope patterns—trichoglyphics. *British Journal of Dermatology*, **92**, 239.

Smith D.W. & Gong B.T. (1973) Scalp hair patterning as a clue to early fetal brain development. *Journal of Pediatrics*, **83**, 374.

Smith D.W. & Gong B.T. (1974) Scalp-hair patterning: its origin and significance relative to early brain and upper facial development. *Teratology*, **9**, 17.

Smith D.W. & Greely M.J. (1978) Unruly scalp hair in infancy: its nature and relevance to problems of brain morphogenesis. *Pediatrics*, **61**, 783.

Wunderlich R.C. & Heerema N.A. (1975) Hair crown patterns of human newborn. *Clinical Pediatrics*, **14**, 1045.

Abnormalities of the hair line

The hair line separates the scalp follicles which give rise to terminal hairs from those which continue to produce vellus hairs.

Displacement of the hair line occurs in a number of syndromes:

Low frontal hair line—Cornelia de Lange syndrome (p. 246); lipoatrophic diabetes (p. 246); fetal hydantoin syndrome (p. 253)

Low nuchal hair line—multiple pterygium syndrome; Turner's syndrome; Noonan's syndrome.

Circumscribed alopecia in infancy
(References p. 55)

The differential diagnosis of circumscribed alopecia present at or soon after birth depends on an accurate history and careful examination (reviewed by Dubreuilh & Petges 1908; Huriez & Desmons 1961).

Obstetric trauma at birth may be followed by scarring, or by the temporary shedding of hair over a contusion or haematoma.

Trauma is often wrongly incriminated in the presence of circumscribed areas of *aplasia* (see p. 55) but the shape and situation of these raw areas should establish the true diagnosis.

Naevi are the commonest cause of circumscribed congenital alopecias. Epidermal naevi in infancy are flat or only slightly thickened and totally or partially devoid of hair. The slightly warty texture of the surface may suggest the diagnosis, which becomes obvious as the child ages (see p. 500).

Cicatricial alopecia not preceded by inflammatory changes is rarely present at birth but may develop in early childhood in association with a number of hereditary syndromes, e.g. incontinentia pigmenti (p. 339).

Circumscribed alopecia without scarring and in the absence of a naevus is rarely reported, but is easily overlooked.

The most distinctive form of *follicular aplasia* is triangular alopecia of the temples (p. 59) but more common, though often discovered only in the course of a routine examination of the scalp, is a small circumscribed but not sharply defined area of alopecia of the vertex in which follicles are absent or are few and of vellus type. The first postnatal hair coat may be normal, in which case the defect is undetectable until a few months after birth (Friederich 1949). Similar patches are occasionally seen elsewhere in the scalp and may be multiple (Gedda et al. 1954).

Sutural alopecia is an inconstant feature of the Hallermann–Streiff syndrome but is not present in early infancy.

Alopecia areata (p. 298) has occurred in infancy, but the diagnosis should be made with caution.

Occipital alopecia of the newborn. In discussing the physiology of hair growth in fetal life it was pointed out that whilst the hair in other regions of the scalp is shed twice in utero, the occipital hair is shed only once (p. 50). The delayed onset of telogen of the follicles in that region of the scalp results in the development of occipital alopecia during the early weeks of life (Brocq 1907). Friction on the pillow has been held responsible and it is probably a factor but it is the late telogen which renders these hairs so vulnerable to friction.

There may be only some thinning of the occipital hair but in the fully developed case of occipital alopecia the bald patch is circular and it is in the upper occipital region (Fig. 3.1). Its lower margin is sharp and consists of a band of hair extending to the nape towards the mastoid regions. Laterally the patch extends to the parietal bosses. The upper margin is less definite and merges gradually with the hair on the vertex.

Complete recovery occurs spontaneously as the affected follicles have re-entered anagen.

Three infants with *subdural meningocoeles* developed alopecia (Bitz & Donalies 1970); in one it began over the lesion. The hair re-grew after surgical treatment.

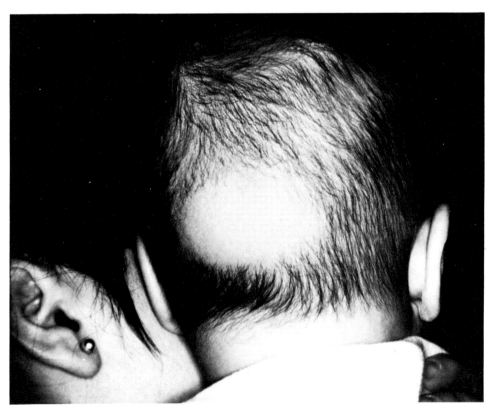

Fig. 3.1. Occipital alopecia of the newborn (Professor J.-M. Lachappelle).

References

Bitz D. & Donalies C. (1970) Alopecia partialis beim klinische progradiunten chronischen subduralen Hydrom des Säuglings. *Paediatrie und Grenzgebiete*, **9**, 101.

Brocq L. (1907) *Traité Élémentaire de Dermatologie Pratique*, vol. 1. Paris, Doin, p. 358.

Dubreuilh W. & Petges G. (1908) Des alopécies congénitales circonscrites. *Annales de Dermatologie et de Syphiligraphie*, **9**, 257.

Friederich H.C. (1949) Zur Kentnis des angeborenen umschriebenen Haarausfalls. *Dermatologische Wochenschrift*, **120**, 712.

Geda L., Testa I. & Benigni A. (1954) Trigemellanze dizigooica con Alopecia congenita, acromtrichia e linea palmare trasverse concordanti nei trigemine monozigooici. *Acta Geneticae Medicae et Gemellologiae*, **3**, 117.

Huriez C. & Desmons F. (1961) Les Alopécies circonscrites de l'enfant, leurs aspects cliniques et leur traitement. *Révue du Practicien (Paris)*, **11**, 1927.

Aplasia cutis

History and nomenclature

An early account of this developmental defect was published by William Campbell in 1826. However, it appears to have escaped the notice of dermatologists until the present century, during which very numerous case reports have appeared, using the term aplasia cutis, congenital skin defect or congenital absence of skin. Aplasia cutis is perhaps to be preferred since the aplasia varies greatly in degree.

Aetiology

Aplasia cutis is a primary failure of differentiation early in embryonic life. The role of amniotic adhesions or intrauterine pressure cannot be substantiated (Pers 1963).

Most cases are sporadic but there are many pedigrees showing autosomal dominant inheritance of strictly circumscribed defects (Markowitz 1933; Deekin & Caplan 1970, Fisher & Schneider 1973). It is not clear, however, whether only a single genotype is involved. In some families autosomal dominant inheritance of extensive aplasia has occurred (Rauschkolb & Enriquez 1962) and in one pedigree the twenty-six individuals in five generations who were affected also had bullae and absent or defective nails (Bart *et al.* 1966). It seems probable that at least the latter syndrome is genetically distinct.

The incidence of aplasia cutis in a Mexican hospital was 1.1/1,000 births (Balsa *et al.* 1974).

Pathology

The aplasia may involve only absence of the skin appendages from otherwise normal skin. For such cases the term 'aplastic naevus' has been suggested (Schoenfeld & Mehregan 1973). However, usually the epidermis is totally absent, and if the dermis is present it lacks normal elastic fibres (Gross *et al.*

1957). At times the defect extends deeply to involve subcutaneous fat, skull and dura, and even the underlying brain (Ruiz-Maldonado & Tamayo 1974).

Clinical features

Since aplasia cutis shows wide variation in extent and in depth, the resulting syndromes range from a trivial cosmetic disability to gross deformity incompatible with a normal life. Indeed extensive congenital absence of epidermis may be rapidly fatal (Fuchs *et al.* 1971).

Aplasia cutis is of course present at birth as a sharply marginated ulcer with a raw red base, simulating a wound. Over 60% of cases involve the scalp (Boureau 1961), usually near the vertex (Fig. 3.2), and although they are often round, they may be rectilinear or irregular in outline. Usually 1–2 cm in diameter, they may be much larger. On the limbs and trunk they tend to be symmetrical. The limbs are affected in about 25% of cases, most commonly the knees. The lesions are sharply angular in outline. The trunk is involved in about 12%, alone or in conjunction with other sites.

The defects may heal rapidly to leave an atrophic or, more rarely, a cheloidal scar (Moschella 1962). Sometimes recurrent crusting delays healing for months or years. Even extensive defects may heal if they are not deep, though with

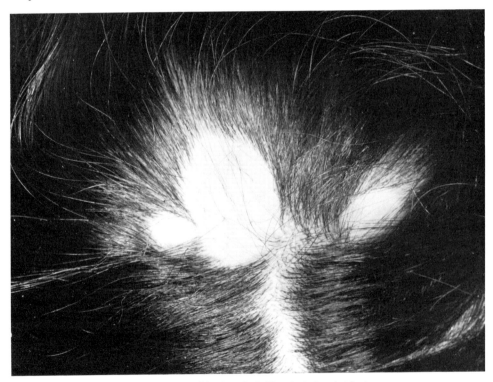

Fig. 3.2. Aplasia cutis of the vertex (Addenbrooke's Hospital, Cambridge).

considerable cosmetic disfigurement. The mortality from meningitis or haemorrhage of infants with scalp defects was about 20% (Anderson & Novy 1942): although infection is now more often controllable there is still an appreciable mortality from erosion of the sagittal sinus or respiratory failure (Peer & Van Duyn 1948; Gross *et al.* 1957).

Aplasia involving only the follicles (Meyer & Civatte 1960; Schoenfeld & Mehregan 1973) is present at birth as an area of alopecia, less sharply marginated than when other cutaneous structures also are involved.

Associated defects of many kinds may accompany aplasia cutis. There may be developmental defects in the region of the skin aplasia, for example anomalous veins (Resnik *et al.* 1965) which increase the risk of haemorrhage. Very rarely cerebral atrophy underlying the defect may result in spastic paralysis and mental retardation (Ruiz-Maldonado & Tamayo 1974).

Aplasia cutis of the scalp is a feature of the Johanson–Blizzard syndrome in which it is associated with a wide spectrum of defects (Johanson & Blizzard 1971), including aplastic alae nasi, microcephaly and mental retardation, absence of permanent teeth buds, deafness, exocrine pancreatic deficiency, leading to malabsorption, and primary hypothyroidism. Inheritance of the syndrome is probably determined by an autosomal dominant gene (Schussheim *et al.* 1976). The scalp hair is fine sparse and hypopigmented (Solomon & Keuer 1980).

In some cases the aplastic areas have presented at birth as bullae, which soon ruptured; in others bullae occur in addition to raw areas of aplasia. Some such cases have been reported as epidermolysis bullosa (Schüssler 1936). Some of the older case reports are insufficiently detailed for evaluation, but most such cases clearly differ from epidermolysis bullosa in that bullae do not continue to form after birth (Scott 1967; Bart 1970).

Finally there may be associated defects at sites remote from the area or areas of aplasia. The most frequent defects of this type are constriction bands, occasionally leading to spontaneous amputation (Pers 1963).

Diagnosis

When aplasia cutis is seen at any early stage the only diagnosis likely to need consideration is birth injury. The site and the configuration of the aplastic areas usually establish the diagnosis, which may be a matter of medicolegal importance.

Once the raw areas have healed the main differential diagnosis is an epidermal naevus. These may be flat until their sebaceous component becomes more prominent with the approach of puberty. A biopsy may be required to establish the diagnosis.

Treatment

Until healing has taken place the control of infection is the principal consideration. If the bald area is unsightly, plastic surgery may be practicable when the child is older (Walker *et al.* 1980).

References

Anderson N.P. & Novy F.G. (1942) Congenital defects of the scalp. *A.M.A. Archives of Dermatology and Syphilology*, **46**, 257.

Balsa R.E., Petruccelli M.C. & de Nichilo M.A. (1974) Aplasia cutis congenita. *Dermatologia (Mexico)*, **18**, 5.

Bart B.J. (1970) Epidermolysis bullosa and congenital localized absence of skin. *Archives of Dermatology*, **101**, 78.

Bart B.J., Gorlin R.J., Anderson V.E. & Lynch F.W. (1966) Congenital localized absence of skin and associated abnormalities resembling epidermolysis bullosa. *Archives of Dermatoloy*, **93**, 296.

Boureau M. (1961) Les aplasies cutanées congénitales du nouveau-né. *Presse Médicale*, **69**, 2175.

Campbell W. (1826) Case of congenital ulcer on the cranium of a foetus. *Edinburgh Journal of Medical Science*, **2**, 82.

Deekin J.H. & Caplan R.M. (1970) Aplasia cutis congenita. *Archives of Dermatology*, **102**, 386.

Fisher M. & Schneider R. (1973) Aplasia cutis congenita in three successive generations. *Archives of Dermatology*, **108**, 252.

Fuchs K., Lichtig C. & Peretz B.A. (1971) Extensive congenital absence of epidermis. *Dermatologica*, **142**, 219.

Gross H., Lindemayr W. & Pospisil E. (1957) Zur Kenntnis der Aplasia cutis. *Neue Österreiche Zeitschrift für Kinderheilkunde*, **2**, 94.

Johanson A. & Blizzard R. (1971) A syndrome of congenital aplasia of the alae nasi, deafness, hypothyroidism, dwarfism, absence of permanent teeth, and malabsorption. *Journal of Pediatrics*, **79**, 982.

Markowitz M. (1933) Alopecia congenitalis hereditaris verticis. *Archives of Dermatology and Syphilology*, **28**, 587.

Meyer J. & Civatte J. (1960) Alopécies congénitales du tourbillon. *Bulletin de la Société française de Dermatologie et de Syphiligraphie*, **67**, 457.

Moschella S.L. (1962) Congenital defects of scalp with keloid formation. *Archives of Dermatology*, **86**, 63.

Peer L.A. & Van Duyn J. (1948) Congenital defect of the scalp. Report of a case with fatal termination. *Plastic and Reconstructive Surgery* (Baltimore), **3**, 722.

Pers M. (1963) Congenital absence of skin: pathogenesis and relation to ring-constriction. *Acta Chirurgica Scandinavica*, **126**, 388.

Rauschkolb B.R. & Enriquez S.I. (1962) Aplasia cutis congenita. *Archives of Dermatology*, **86**, 54.

Resnik S.S., Koblenzer P.J. & Pitts F.W. (1965) Congenital absence of the scalp with associated vascular anomaly. *Clinical Pediatrics*, **4**, 722.

Ruiz-Maldonado R. & Tamayo L. (1974) Aplasia cutis congenita, spastic paralysis and mental retardation. *American Journal of Diseases of Children*, **128**, 699.

Schoenfeld R.J. & Mehregan A.H. (1973) Aplastic nevus—the 'Minus Nevus'. *Cutis*, **12**, 386.

Schussheim A., Choi S.J. & Schrebraz M. (1976) Exocrine pancreatic insufficiency with congenital anomalies. *Journal of Pediatrics*, **89**, 782.

Schüssler A. (1936) Zur Krankheit-bild die 'Kongenitaler Epidermolysis bullosa uber Hautdefek-ton'. *Zeitschrift für Kinderheilkunde*, **58**, 533.

Scott F.P. (1967) Congenital skin defects. *Dermatologica*, **135**, 84.

Solomon L.M. & Keuer E.J. (1980) The ectodermal dysplasias. *Archives of Dermatology*, **116**, 1295.

Walker J.C., Kornig J.A., Irwin L. & Meijer R. (1960) Congenital absence of skin. *Plastic and Reconstructive Surgery*, **26**, 208.

Congenital triangular alopecia

History and nomenclature
The first description and illustration of this distinctive congenital defect were given by Sabouraud (1905) in his *Manual of Topographical Dermatology*, under the term 'aire alopécique temporale congénital'. Although most of the larger textbooks have since that date referred to the condition, remarkably few actual case reports have been published, yet although it is uncommon it is not excessively rare. Kubba & Rook (1976) reported three cases.

Aetiology and pathology
The embryological basis of this circumscribed defect has not been established. Two siblings were similarly affected (Degos & Robert 1949) but no other evidence of a possible genetic factor has been recorded.

The affected area is slightly atrophic with a reduced number of follicles of vellus type (Sabouraud 1905).

Clinical features
The practically bald triangular areas are present at birth but, if the infant's hair is generally fine and sparse, may not be noticed by the parents until after the first

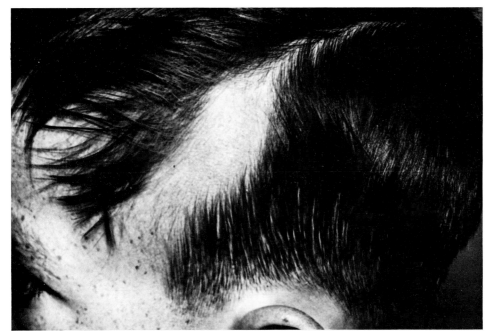

Fig. 3.3. Triangular alopecia. In this patient it was bilaterally symmetrical (Addenbrooke's Hospital, Cambridge).

year: sometimes indeed not until 2 or 3 years later. It is possible that in some cases the first hair coat is normal as in some other forms of congenital circumscribed alopecia. The base of each triangle impinges on, and may or may not involve, the temporal hair line. The triangle overlies the frontotemporal suture and measures 3–5 cm from base to apex. It is usually unilateral, but may be bilaterally symmetrical. It remains unchanged throughout life, and as far as is known is of no more than minor cosmetic significance (Canizares 1941; Minars 1974; Kubba & Rook 1976) (Fig. 3.3).

Diagnosis
The site and the shape of the area of alopecia readily establish the diagnosis.

References
Canizares O. (1941) Alopecia triangularis congenitalis. Report of a case. *Archives of Dermatology and Syphilology*, **44**, 1106.
Degos R. & Robert R. (1949) Alopécie angulaire congénitale de la tempe. *Bulletin de la Société française de Dermatologie et de Syphiligraphie*, **5**, 457.
Kubba R. & Rook A. (1976) Congenital triangular alopecia. *British Journal of Dermatlogy*, **95**, 657.
Minars N. (1974) Congenital temporal alopecia. *Archives of Dermatology*, **109**, 995.
Sabouraud A. (1905) *Manuel Elémentaire de Dermatologie Topographique Régional*. Paris, Masson, p. 197.

The scalp in infancy
(References p. 62)

Many naevi (Chapter 18) may be present in the scalp at birth or may develop during the first weeks of life.

Greasy scaling and crusting, particularly in the frontovertical regions, is characteristic of seborrhoeic dermatitis (see Fig. 3.4).

Hypertrichosis and hypotrichosis in infancy have many causes which are discussed in Chapter 8 and 6 respectively.

Abnormalities of the frontal or nuchal hair line are often of diagnostic significance. Some are listed on p. 53.

Two unusual conditions not conveniently classified elsewhere are briefly described.

Cephalhaematoma

Birth trauma resulting in subperiosteal haemorrhage is the cause of this uncommon scalp lesion which, in about 25% of cases, is associated with an underlying fracture of the skull (Kendall & Woloshin 1952). It presents as a firm but compressible swelling, often with a palpable rim of periosteum.

Most cephalhaematomas are resolved during the first 6 weeks of life, but sometimes they may calcify (Solomon & Esterly 1973).

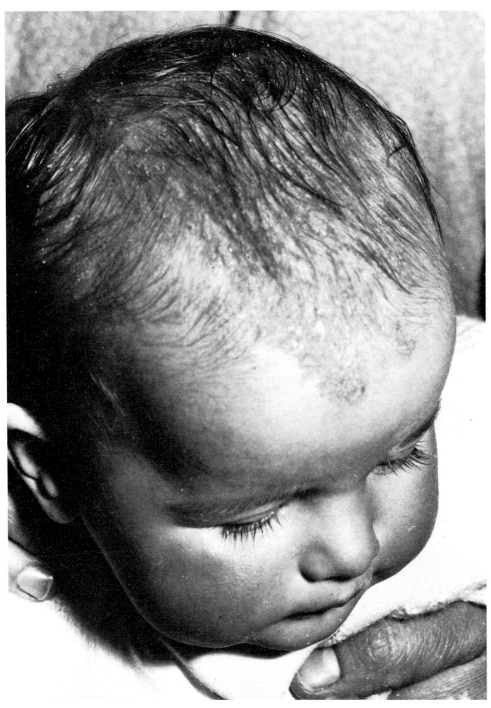

Fig. 3.4. Seborrhoeic dermatitis in the scalp of an infant (Addenbrooke's Hospital, Cambridge).

Gonococcal scalp abscess

The slight injury to the scalp which may be inflicted by the application of an electrode for monitoring the fetal heart rate may provide a portal of entry for infection. In two such infants gonococcal abscesses developed.

References
Kendall N. & Woloshin H. (1952) Cephalhematoma associated with fracture of the skull. *Journal of Paediatrics*, **41**, 125.
Reveri M. & Krishnamurthy C. (1979) Gonococcal scalp abscess. *Journal of Pediatrics*, **94**, 819.
Solomon L.A. & Esterly M.B. (1973) *Neonatal Dermatology*. Philadelphia, Saunders, p. 47.

Chapter 4
Hair Patterns:
Baldness and Hirsutism

History and nomenclature: hirsutism and hypertrichosis
(References p. 70)

Hippocrates mentioned a woman who grew a beard soon after menstruation had ceased. Medical authors and laymen alike have through the ages recorded with curiosity unusual patterns of hair growth in both sexes, and lay attitudes to those who have been the victims of such failure to conform have perhaps changed rather little.

The scientific study of abnormal patterns of hair growth may be said to have begun in 1905 when Bullock and Sequeira recognized the association of hyperplasia or adenomas of the adrenal cortex with hirsutism and virilization.

Many authors use the terms hypertrichosis and hirsutism as synonymous. There is however an increasing tendency to confine hirsutism to the growth in either sex of terminal hair in part or all of the male sexual pattern. Hirsutism will be so defined in this book. Hypertrichosis is the growth of hair in any other pattern, circumscribed or widespread, which is inappropriate to the site and to the age and sex of the patient (see p. 233). The distinction is scientifically valid, since hirsutism is invariably androgen-induced, whilst hypertrichosis is caused by a wide variety of different mechanisms.

Hair patterns
(References p. 70)

The hair pattern is determined by the length and the shaft diameter and the structure of the hair occupying each follicle at the moment of examination. The number of hair follicles is essentially the same in males and females (Szabo 1958). Differential growth of the body surface from fetal life to adulthood dilutes the originally dense population of follicles and in some regions changes their relative distribution. No new follicles are formed after fetal life, and there is no wholesale destruction of follicles: however, there is some reduction of follicle density in the scalp between the ages of 30 and 50 years. Giacometti (1965) found 615 follicles/cm^2 in the age group 20–30, but only 485 per cm^2 between 30 and 50. There was a relatively small further reduction in later decades. Quantitative studies of other regions of the body have not been reported, but clinical experience suggests that there is probably a comparable reduction of follicle density, but perhaps somewhat later in life, and with variations from region to region.

From the formation of the follicles in fetal life (see p. 5) until death, the hair pattern is never completely stable (Garn 1951). There are, admittedly, decades such as the first, in which no gross change in hair pattern is evident. Yet even in childhood vellus hair, variable in extent and length, makes its appearance on the trunk and limbs, and the terminal hair on the scalp increases progressively in shaft diameter (Atkinson *et al.* 1959).

The first conspicuous change in hair pattern occurs at puberty. Terminal hair gradually replaces vellus, first in the pubic region and then in the axillae and then in fairly regular sequence over a period of several years, on the legs, thighs, forearms, abdomen, buttocks, chest, back, arms and shoulders (Reynolds 1951). The transition from vellus to terminal hair on the face also occurs in an orderly sequence, at the corners of the upper lips, then on the chin, on the cheeks and on the rest of the beard area. The pattern of terminal hair does not reach its full extent until the fifth or even the sixth decade, nor does the hair in any site assume its ultimate diameter and length until after a number of years. In each body region the terminal hair acquires structural features characteristic of that region.

This growth of terminal hair on face, trunk and limbs is induced by androgenic hormones. Genetic factors, including those associated with racial differences, determine the ultimate extent of the hirsutism and variations in its pattern. However, changes related to ageing also modify the follicular response, as is apparent from the relatively late development of the full pattern, and from the fact that even abnormally high levels of androgenic stimulation do not necessarily induce the full pattern in the young adult. The clinical problems resulting from the presence of abnormal degrees of hirsutism in the female, or from her failure to accept normal degrees as physiological are discussed on p. 79.

The replacement of terminal hair by vellus first occurs in adolescence in some 80% of Caucasoid women and about 100% of Caucasoid men, and produces that reshaping of the frontral hair margin which characteristically alters the facial outline.

Some individuals show from infancy onwards a frontal hair line with a well defined median peak, sometimes called a 'widow's peak'. This may occur as a genetic variation in pattern in subjects with a normal interpupillary distance. However, it may be much more marked in the presence of ocular hypertelorism. It has been suggested that this phenomenon results from displacement of the fields of periorbital hair growth suppression (Smith & Cohen 1973).

In the genetically predisposed the next decade may bring, by further replacement of terminal hair by vellus, the bitemporal recession which heralds the onset of common baldness. The clinical problems resulting from this pattern change are discussed on p. 104.

Hair patterns of the trunk and limbs in subjects past middle age have not been studied in great detail. Body, pubic and axillary hair becomes sparse in both sexes, but earlier in women than in men. The axillae are denuded earlier and more completely than the pubic region. The areas which last acquired terminal hair are the first to lose it.

Regional variations in hair patterns

The variations in hair pattern related to age, genetic constitution and endocrine status have been studied thoroughly in only a few regions of the body, and in a very limited number of races. The available information is summarized below, largely as an inducement to further, more detailed investigations. Few investigators, however, attempt to correlate the hair patterns in different regions in different races. Danforth & Trotter (1922), who examined soldiers on demobilization, noted that dark-haired individuals tended to have more body hair than fair-haired individuals, but that there were racial differences unrelated to pigmentation, in that fair-haired men of Italian descent had more body hair than did fair-haired Scandinavians.

The pinna

Hairiness of the pinna—the external ear—is a conspicuous racial character which has aroused much interest among geneticists and anthropologists, but has received little attention from clinicians.

The development of coarse hairs on the pinna occurs most frequently, and with the longest and densest hairs, in Indians. Normally only males are affected. The incidence and severity of the hairiness increase from the age of about 20 to over 50. By the seventh decade about 70% of men in Madras and about 30% in West Bengal are affected (Stern *et al.* 1964). In Indians the sulcus at the side of the ear bears most hairs, but the top of the ear and other sites may also be involved. The degree of hairiness ranges from a few hairs to large bushy tufts. In the Maltese (Gates & Vella 1962) and in Israeli populations (Slatis & Apelbaum 1963) the total incidence is lower than in Indians, and the top of the ear is the site most extensively affected. Hypertrichosis of the pinna has been regarded as a classical example of a sex-linked recessive trait (Dronamraju & Haldane 1962). However, many pedigrees are not compatible with inheritance by a γ-linked fully penetrant gene (Sarkar *et al.* 1961). Dronamraju (1963) favoured multifactorial inheritance. However, vellus hairs are present on the female pinna and until studies have been made on the pinnae of virilized females, sex-influenced autosomal inheritance remains a possibility (Sarkar & Ghosh 1963; Stern *et al.* 1964). There is evidence that the growth of coarse hairs on the pinna is androgen dependent. In Caucasoid males they begin to appear after the 24th year and increase in number until about the 58th year (Hamilton 1947).

A detailed investigation of the ear hair patterns in American Caucasoid and Negro males was carried out (Setty 1969). There were wide variations in the pattern and in the extent of hypertrichosis, both tending to increase with age. Over 45% of the Negroes but only 15% of the Caucasoids had no terminal hairs on their pinnae. The patterns on the two ears were not necessarily identical. The patterns in other races also have been studied. There are marked differences in the relative frequency of different patterns, but in all the hypertrichosis becomes significant, if it does so at all, by middle life.

The presence of marked hypertrichosis of the margin of the pinna in the majority of infants born to diabetic mothers (Eklund *et al.* 1960) has not been explained. Wallis (1897) found such hair in some normal infants.

Chest

The growth of terminal hair on the chest begins in the normal male soon after puberty, but the hair does not attain its greatest extent and density until the sixth decade. The pattern most frequently encountered in mature Caucasoid American males covered the sternum, with lateral extensions below the clavicles and below the nipples (Setty 1961a). This same author described and defined other patterns.

Quantitative studies of coarse sternal hairs (Hamilton *et al.* 1969) provided data which are applicable also to other androgen dependent sites. The number of sternal hairs, their mean length and shaft diameter, rose slowly from puberty to reach a peak in the 5th or 6th decade. Thereafter the number of hairs slowly declined, but there was little reduction in their size.

In some individuals with an extensive chest hair pattern, circular bare areas form above the medial to the nipples (Setty 1961b). The prevalence of this so-called 'pectoral alopecia' is not well documented. In a hospital population in the United States such bare areas were found in 46% of Negroes and 16% of Caucasoids (Gompertz 1960).

Back
The patterns of terminal hair growth on the backs of American Caucasoid males have been defined and classified (Setty 1962). Extensive covering of the back tends to accompany extensive chest hairs, but the genetic significance of striking variation in pattern is not clear.

Axillae
Terminal hair in the axillae usually appears about 2 years after the first pubic hair, but there is much individual variation and axillary hair may occasionally appear first (Tanner 1964). Coarse hairs appear at an earlier age than in the beard. In old age the follicles tend to atrophy (Hamilton & Terada 1963).

Axillary hair growth in Caucasoids and Japanese has been compared (Hamilton & Terada 1963). In both sexes axillary hair was very much more sparse in the Japanese than in the Caucasoids. Not only were there fewer hairs, but in a larger proportion of older subjects there were no hairs at all.

Abdominal wall and pubes
This region has been particularly well studied on account of the obvious relationship of its hair patterns to other pubertal developments (Pryor 1956; Thomas & Ferriman 1957).

Using the distribution of hair at and above the upper border of the pubic triangle as a criterion, Dupertuis *et al.* (1945) proposed the terms horizontal, acuminate and disperse to describe the grosser variations in pattern. They studied 1060 American Caucasoid men and 309 women. The horizontal pattern was found in 90% of women and in 38% of 18-year-old males; this pattern persisted in 17% of fully adult males. The remaining 10% of women showed an acuminate pattern, which was found also in 50% of males. Extensive—

'disperse'—abdominal hair in men aged 30–40 tended to be associated with much terminal hair on chest and thighs.

Of 3858 fit British men examined by McGregor (1961) 4.05% showed a horizontal pattern, 85.2% an acuminate or disperse pattern and 10.2% an intermediate pattern. The differences between this series and that reported by Dupertuis *et al.* (1945) can largely be explained by differences in the age composition of the two groups of subjects.

The development of pubic hair was studied in 557 Caucasoid American girls (Reynolds & Wines 1948). Sparse pigmented hair first appeared on average at the age of 11 and the full pubic triangle was complete by 13.9.

Pubic hair becomes thinned after the menopause and in those women in whom the pattern has been acuminate it becomes horizontal (Beek 1950). Large doses of oestrogen such as are prescribed in some patients with carcinoma of the prostate, may lead to the development of a horizontal abdominal hair pattern in men (Fig. 4.1).

Penis and scrotum
Penile hair patterns of four types all occur over a wide age range (Setty 1969) as do the three scrotal hair patterns (Setty 1970) which are essentially similar in American Negroes and Caucasoids.

Arms
On the arms four well-defined patterns of hair growth have been differentiated. Fairly full cover of the upper limbs, sparing only the flexor aspect of the upper arms, was found in some 70% of Caucasoid American men (Setty 1964). In another 25% there was no terminal hair on the upper arms. In 3% only the forearms bore terminal hair. Other patterns were exceptional.

In familial hypertrichosis cubiti—the hairy elbows syndrome (Beighton

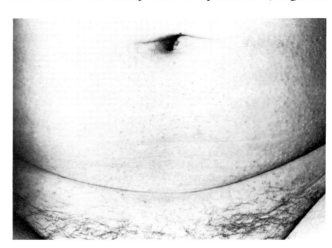

Fig. 4.1. Female pattern of abdominal hair in a male receiving oestrogen treatment (Slade Hospital, Oxford).

1970; Andreev & Stransky 1979)—hypertrichosis of the lower third of the upper arms and the upper third of the forearms is present from early infancy, becomes worse in the next year or two and then partially regresses. The mode of inheritance is uncertain (Fig. 4.2).

The fingers

There have been many anthropological studies of the incidence and patterns of hair on the backs of the fingers. Hair is present on the proximal phalanx of the index, middle, ring and little fingers of most individuals of most races, and in most the dorsum of the middle phalanx of the index finger is hairless (Ikoma 1972). Hair on the proximal phalanx of the thumb, and on the middle phalanx of the middle and ring fingers shows individual and racial variation. It was less common in a North American Indian tribe than in Japanese, and was more common still in Canadians of European descent. Genetic studies in Japan (Ikoma 1973) and Germany (Sommer 1971) showed that the trait is transmitted

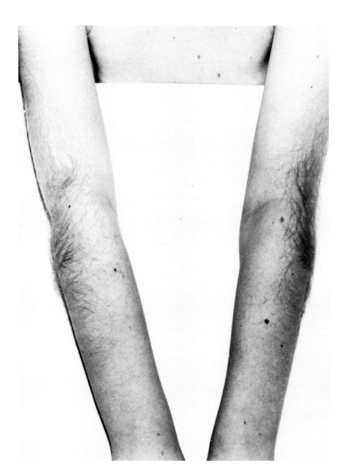

Fig. 4.2. 'Hairy elbows' in a girl aged 11 (Addenbrooke's Hospital, Cambridge).

dominantly and is controlled by multiple alleles. In identical twins there was concordance in the numbers of hairy phalanges, and in the shape, position, size and density of the hairy patches (Sommer 1971).

Thigh and leg

In adult male American Caucasoids and Negroes four patterns of terminal hair could be differentiated (Setty 1968). The thigh is completely covered with the exception of an area of variable extent on the lateral aspect of the upper thigh. The lower leg, too, may be completely covered, but far more frequently the anterolateral aspect of the lower leg, or the entire lower two-thirds of the lower leg is bare. The incidence of such bare areas, sometimes referred to as peroneal alopecia, has been found to be in the region of 35% in the US and in England (Ronchese & Chace 1939). The differences in the relative frequency of the various thigh and leg patterns were fully analysed by Setty (1968). Similar studies in other races would be helpful; the findings of Shah (1957) in women in the Bombay area of India suggest possible racial differences in the sensitivity of thigh follicles to androgen.

References

Andreev V.C. & Stransky L. (1979) Hairy elbows. *Archives of Dermatology*, **115**, 761.

Atkinson S.C., Cormia F.E. & Unrau S.A. (1959) The diameter and growth phase of hair in relation to age. *British Journal of Dermatology*, **71**, 309.

Beek C.H. (1950) A study on extension and distribution of the human body-hair. *Dermatologica*, **101**, 317.

Beighton, P. (1970) Familial hypertrichosis cubiti: hairy elbows syndrome. *Journal of Medical Studies*, **7**, 158.

Bullock W. & Sequeira J.H. (1905) On the relation of the suprarenal capsules to the sexual organs. *Transactions of the Pathological Society of London*, **56**, 189.

Danforth C.H. & Trotter M. (1922) The distribution of body hair in white subjects. *American Journal of Physical Anthropology*, **5**, 259.

Dronamraju K.R. (1963) A note on the age of onset of hypertrichosis pinnae auris in Orissa, West Bengal and Ceylon. *Journal of Geriatrics*, **58**, 324.

Dronamraju K.R. & Haldane J.B.S. (1962) Inheritance of hairy pinnae. *American Journal of Human Genetics*, **14**, 102.

Dupertuis C.W., Atkinson W.B. & Elftman H. (1945) Sex differences in pubic hair distribution. *Human Biology*, **17**, 137.

Eklund J., Hjelt L. & Lumme T. (1960) Hirsutism in the children of diabetic mothers. *Annales Paediatricae Fenniae*, **6**, 232.

Garn S.M. (1951) Types and distribution of the hair in man. *Annals of the New York Academy of Science*, **53**, 498.

Gates R.R. & Vella F. (1962) Hairy pinnae in Malta. *Lancet*, **ii**, 357.

Giacometti L. (1965) *The Anatomy of the Human Scalp in Ageing*, ed. W. Montagna. Oxford, Pergamon Press, p. 97.

Gompettz M.L. (1960) A note on the incidence of pectoral alopecia. *American Journal of Digestive Disorders*, **5**, 437.

Hamilton J.B. (1947) A secondary sexual character that develops in an organ common to both sexes but normally only in men. With a discussion of the relation of this character to endocrine stimulation. *Journal of Clinical Endocrinology*, **7**, 465.

Hamilton J.B. & Terada H. (1963) Interdependence of genetic ageing and endocrine factors in hirsutism. In *The Hirsute Female*, ed. R.B. Greenblatt. Springfield, Thomas, p. 20.

Hamilton J.B., Terada H., Mestler G.E. & Tinman W. (1969) I. Coarse sternal hairs; a male secondary sexual character that can be measured quantitatively: the influence of sex, age and genetic factors. II. Other sex-differing characters: relationship to age, to one another and to values for coarse sternal hairs. In *Hair Growth*, eds. W. Montagna & R.L. Dobson. Oxford, Pergamon Press, p. 129.

Ikoma E. (1972) An anthropological study on digital hair. *Journal of the Anthropological Society (Nippon)*, **80**, 283.

Ikoma E. (1973) A genetic study of human hair. *Japanese Journal of Human Genetics*, **18**, 259.

McGregor D. (1961) Distribution of pubic hair in a sample of fit men. *British Journal of Dermatology*, **73**, 61.

Pryor H.B. (1956) Certain physical and physiological aspects of adolescent development in girls. *Journal of Pediatrics*, **8**, 52.

Reynolds E.L. (1951) The appearance of adult patterns of body hair in man. *Annals of the New York Academy of Science*, **53**, 576.

Reynolds E.L. & Wines J.V. (1948) Individual differences in physical changes associated with adolescence in girls. *American Journal of Diseases of Children*, **75**, 329.

Ronchese F. & Chace R.R. (1939) Patterned alopecia about the calves and its apparent lack of significance. *Archives of Dermatology and Syphilology*, **40**, 416.

Sarkar S.S. & Ghosh R.R. (1963) Hairy pinnae in the Bengalee female. *Lancet*, **i**, 1432.

Sarkar S.S., Banerjee A.R., Bhattacharjee P. & Stern C. (1961) A contribution to the genetics of hypertrichosis of the ear rims. *American Journal of Human Genetics*, **13**, 214.

Setty L.R. (1961a) The distribution of chest hair in Caucasoid males. *American Journal of Physical Anthropology*, **19**, 285.

Setty L.R. (1961b) Bare areas in regions of pilosity of the chest and abdomen. *Journal of the National Medical Association*, **53**, 394.

Setty L.R. (1962) Hair patterns on the back of white males. *American Journal of Physical Anthropology*, **20**, 365.

Setty L.R. (1964) The distribution of hair of the upper limb in Caucasoid males. *American Journal of Physical Anthropology*, **22**, 143.

Setty L.R. (1968) The distribution of hair of the lower limb in white and Negro males. *American Journal of Physical Anthropology*, **29**, 51.

Setty L.R. (1969) Hair patterns of the pinnae of white and Negro males. *American Journal of Physical Anthropology*, **31**, 153.

Setty L.R. (1969) Penile hair patterns of whites and Negroes. *Journal of the National Medical Association*, **61**, 67.

Setty L.R. (1970) Scrotal hair patterns of whites and Negroes. *Journal of the National Medical Association*, **62**, 156.

Shah, P.N. (1957) Human body hair—a quantitative study. *American Journal of Obstetrics and Gynecology*, **73**, 1255.

Slatis H.M. & Apelbaum A. (1963) Hairy pinna of the ear in Israeli populations. *American Journal of Human Genetics*, **15**, 74.

Smith D.W. & Cohen M.M. (1973) Widow's peak scalp-hair anomaly and its relation to ocular hypertelorism. *Lancet*, **ii**, 1127.

Sommer K. (1971) Untersuchungen zur Genetik des Merkmals 'Fingerbehaarung'. *Humangenetik*, **11**, 155.

Stern C., Centerwell W.R. & Sarkar S.S. (1964) New data on the problem of γ-linkage of hairy pinnae. *American Journal of Human Genetics*, **16**, 455.

Szabo G. (1958) The regional frequency and distribution of hair follicles in human skin. In *The Biology of Hair Growth*, eds. W. Montagna & R.A. Ellis. New York, Academic Press, p. 33.

Tanner J.M. (1964) The adolescent growth spurt and development age. In *Human Biology*, eds. G.A. Harrison, J.S. Wiseman, J.M. Tanner & N.A. Barnicot. Oxford, Clarendon Press, p. 325.

Thomas P.K. & Ferriman D.G. (1957) Variation in familial pubic hair growth in white women. *American Journal of Physical Anthropology*, **15**, 171.

Wallis H.M. (1897) On the growth of hair upon the human ear and its testimony to the shape, size and position of the ancestral organ. *Proceedings of the Zoological Society of London*, **11**, 298.

Hirsutism

Nomenclature and introduction (references p. 74)

Hirsutism is the growth of terminal hair in part or all of the male sexual pattern. In the adult male there are marked racial and other genetic variations in the degree of hirsutism present in the individual, but such differences are rarely a matter for concern. Nevertheless men occasionally seek medical advice because they consider that they are too generously endowed with hair. They can be reassured of their normality as can also the great majority of the larger number of young men who complain of their relative lack of body hair; only rarely is hypogonadism rather than genetic constitution the explanation of their sparse hair.

Hirsutism in the male child as a manifestation of premature puberty or pseudopuberty is not discussed in this book.

Hirsutism in the female is difficult to define clinically, as distinct from anthropologically. In no race is there any sharp dividing line between the terminal hair pattern of the normal adult female and the normal adult male. There are normal females with terminal hairs along the linea alba, on the upper lip and on the breasts and there are normal males whose pubic hair has a horizontal upper margin. The proportion of normal females in whom terminal hair extends to parts of the traditional male pattern is extremely high in some Mediterranean races and extremely low in the Japanese. Girls with the Mediterranean pattern are well aware that it is normal in their community, yet when they emigrate and live in a community in which such hair growth is uncommon they come to regard themselves as abnormal and to consult their doctors. Thus hirsutism clinically covers the entire spectrum from the normal girl who in a particular environment considers herself abnormal to the girl in whom gross hirsutism is only one feature of extreme virilization.

Incidence

The normal variations in patterns of terminal hair are described above. The incidence in any given population of a degree of hirsutism which its bearer considers to be abnormal is difficult to assess. It depends on the genetic composition of the population concerned, yet when the incidence is high it is less likely to cause concern to the individual. McKnight (1964) examined 400 women students of the University of Wales, 60% of them Welsh and 40% English. No fewer than 26% had some kind of hair on the face, and in only 4% the hair was disfiguring. Terminal hair was present on the chest or breast in 17%, and on the linea alba in 35%. Taking all sites into consideration 36 (9%) were regarded as particularly hirsute. Of these 36, 16 were seriously affected. It was noted that in this latter group terminal hair on the breasts, lumbosacral region and upper back, in addition to the other sites, was frequent.

The high proportion of Welsh girls in this investigation no doubt explains the relatively high incidence of hirsutism, which is a racial characteristic of the Celts. Strictly comparable studies of other populations appear not to be available, but Pedersen's (1943) investigation of Swedish women suggests that hirsutism is considerably less frequent in that country than in Wales. McKnight (1964) points out that terminal hair on the arms and legs in particular appears to be more common in Wales than in America (Danforth & Trotter 1922) or India (Shah 1957). Our experience with Italian immigrants to Britain and with students from other Mediterranean countries suggests that in these countries hirsutism is at least as common as in Wales. Our numbers are too small, however, to allow any firm conclusions as to whether variations in the patterns of terminal hair on the limbs and back show consistent racial correlations. Shah (1957) of Bombay, India, examined 100 women (mean age 27.2 years) not complaining of hirsutism and 34 (mean age 22.2 years) who had been referred with hirsutism. This classification prejudges some of the issues under investigation. However, it is of interest that terminal hair on the thighs was found in some 80% of women regarded as hirsute but in only 30% of the non-hirsute group. Among the 'hirsute', just over 30% had terminal hair on the face, whilst none of the 'non-hirsute' group had any facial hair. These findings are so very different from others, that carefully controlled comparable studies on different racial groups can be seen to be necessary.

Aetiology

A few years ago the classification of the causes of hirsutism appeared to be relatively simple. Those many cases in which there was no evident virilization, or disturbance of the menstrual cycle or marked elevation of the urinary 17-oxosteroid excretion were labelled 'idiopathic' or if others in the family were affected the more convincing terms 'familial' or 'racial' could be applied. The smaller number of cases in which changes in ovaries or adrenals, or other endocrine disorders, could be demonstrated were classified accordingly. It was assumed that in these 'idiopathic' cases the essential abnormality was increased susceptibility of some hair follicles to normal androgenic stimulation. Such a

Table 4.1. Causes of hirsutism

1	*Racial and 'idiopathic'* (see p. 78)
2	*Ovarian*
	Polycystic ovary syndrome (p. 80)
	Tumours (p. 83)
3	*Adrenal*
	Congenital adrenal hyperplasia (p. 86)
	Cushing's syndrome (p. 86)
	Carcinoma (p. 86)
4	*Iatrogenic*
	Androgenic hormones

classification (see Table 4.1) is of course still of value provided it is never forgotten that 'idiopathic' hirsutism is not a positive diagnosis.

Doubts concerning the validity of the concept of a 'primary' form of hirsutism associated only with hair follicle sensitivity to androgens were founded first on clinical observations that hirsutism, even of the so-called idiopathic variety, shows a significant association with a tendency to male body proportions (Ferriman *et al.* 1962). Moreover, the incidence of hirsutism was found to be high in women belonging to certain athletic clubs (Michalowski & Hendzel 1966a). These same authors (1966b) noted that some degree of male baldness was present in 27.9% of 415 women with hirsutism with normal 17-oxosteroid excretion.

That the changes in so-called idiopathic hirsutism are not confined to the pilosebacous follicle was shown by Shuster *et al.* (1970) who found the skin collagen to be increased in all of 26 cases; in some the thickness of the skin also was increased. There is also an increase in the response of sweat glands to cholinergic stimuli (Shuster 1972).

References

Danforth C.H. & Trotter M. (1922) The distribution of body hair in white subjects. *American Journal of Physical Anthropology*, **5**, 259.

Ferriman D., Page B.M. & Newnham R. (1962) Studies bearing on the nature of androgyny. *Journal of Endocrinology*, **25**, 351.

McKnight E. (1964) The prevalence of 'hirsutism' in young women. *Lancet*, **i**, 410.

Michalowski R. & Hendzel G. (1966a) Hypertrichose chez les femmes sportives. *Gazette médicale francaise*, **73**, 1531.

Michalowski R. & Hendzel G. (1966b) Le syndrome hypertrichose-séborrhée-1 calvitie frontale chez les jeunes femmes. *Minerva Dermatologica*, **41**, 190.

Pedersen J. (1943) Hypertrichosis in women. *Acta Dermato-Venereologica*, **23**, 1.

Shah P.N. (1957) Human body hair—a quantitative study. *American Journal of Obstetrics and Gynecology*, **73**, 1255.

Shuster, S. (1972) Primary cutaneous virilism or idiopathic hirsuties? *British Medical Journal*, **i**, 285.

Shuster S., Black M.M. & Bottoms E. (1970) Skin collagen and thickness in women with hirsuties. *British Medical Journal*, **iv**, 772.

Genetic factors (references p. 77)

A family history of hirsutism has sometimes been said to support a presumptive diagnosis of idiopathic hirsutism. However, the syndromes of congenital adrenal hyperplasia are determined by autosomal recessive genes (p. 86) and post-pubertal onset has been noted in several members of such families (e.g. Heni & Göbel 1959). There have been few planned genetic studies of hirsutism. Lorenzo (1970) selected 90 patients with hirsutism and placed them, after investigation, in one of three groups: ovarian dysfunction, 20, adrenal dysfunction, 27, idiopathic, 43. A control group consisted of 300 women in the same age range (15–45) without hirsutism. Familial aggregation of hirsutism appeared to occur in all three groups. In all groups also the frequency of 'androgenic equivalents', e.g. menstrual disturbance, baldness and acne, correlated with the severity of the hirsutism in propositae, relatives and controls. Multifactorial inheritance seemed probable and the existence of 'idiopathic' hirsutism seemed doubtful.

Psychiatric factors (references p. 77)

Segré (1967) made the somewhat dramatic assertion that 'lack of peace of mind is . . . both a cause and a result of hirsutism'.

Andrea Cristari (1892) maintained that 'hypertrichosis' was more frequent in 'insane females' than in normal controls. A more recent investigation (Lohse & Bjarnhifdensson 1945) of schizophrenic patients in a mental hospital in Denmark showed 'hypertrichosis' to be very significantly more common in the patients than in normal controls; in the age group 15–25 100% of schizo-phrenics but only 36% of controls had hypertrichosis, by the author's criteria. These observations on psychotic patients need to be repeated, with strict quantification.

Many clinicians with experience of the investigation of patients with hirsutism are impressed by the relatively common association of a stressful episode, and in particular a depressive episode, with the onset of hirsutism (Meyer 1963). The endocrinological diagnosis may be 'idiopathic' hirsutism or, much more often, the polycystic ovary syndrome. The association of stress with the onset of hirsutism of adrenocortical origin has been reported (Bush & Mahesh 1959). Hyperprolactinaemia induced by stress may also be associated with hirsutism (p. 87).

Biochemical aspects (references p. 77)

Any attempt to provide a brief and clear survey of the biochemical basis of hirsutism is frustrated by the frequent reassessments made necessary by new advances, by the wide variations between the criteria for clinical classification employed by different investigators, and by the differences, usually ignored, in the genetic constitution of the populations studied.

Many of the earlier investigators had shown that urinary oxosteroid excretion was slightly or moderately elevated in many women with 'idiopathic' hirsutism. For example, Mahesh *et al.* (1964) found elevated exosteroid excretion in 37 of 48 hirsute women; in only 5 was this excess suppressed by dexamethasone. As assay methods for testosterone were developed, it was found (Burger *et al.* 1964) that in some women with 'idiopathic' hirsutism, the level of unconjugated testosterone in adrenal venous plasma was significantly higher than that in peripheral venous plasma.

Plasma testosterone levels were in the normal range in 40 women with 'idiopathic' hirsutism (Casey & Nabarro 1967). Adrenal and ovarian stimulation and suppression tests led these authors to conclude that the ovaries have the potential capacity to produce androgen, but do not normally do so in women with 'idiopathic' hirsutism. Selecting another of many contemporary papers it may be noted that the complications of ovary–adrenal interrelations were more fully appreciated (Lopez *et al.* 1967). The failure of dexamethasone suppression after 7 days suggested an androgenic ovary, but the failure of HCG stimulation did not exclude a polycystic ovary if adrenal overactivity was present.

Subsequently raised plasma testosterone levels were reported in the majority of women with idiopathic hirsutism. A careful investigation (Ismail *et al.* 1969) consisted of serial assays of testosterone, epitestosterone, oestrogen and pregnanediol in urine in 11 hirsute patients and 14 normal controls. In the hirsute patients overall mean levels for testosterone and epitestosterone were significantly higher than in controls, but there was considerable variation between individual women at different times. Those women in whom the hirsutism was associated with menstrual disturbances did not have higher levels than the remainder. Oestrogen and pregnanediol excretion were normal.

All of 13 consecutive hirsute women (Kirschner & Jacobs 1971) were found to have elevated testosterone production. Catheterization of ovarian and adrenal veins showed that in 9 the ovary was the major site of testosterone production, and that in 4 testosterone was produced by both adrenals and ovaries. Dexamethasone suppression was observed in all of the women in the second group, but also in 3 in the first group, which throws some doubt on the value of this test.

Urinary testosterone levels were measured (Fleetwood *et al.* 1974) in 28 hirsute women. Basal levels were elevated in 24 of the 28, and 19 of these 24 showed an abnormal response to corticotrophin stimulation. Ten of the 19 were given metyrapone and corticotrophin. In 8 of the 10 there was an abnormal increase in pregnanetriol excretion. The authors suggest that these women may have a 21-hydroxylase defect of the adrenal, whilst the two who showed no abnormal metyrapone response may have a different adrenal defect.

Useful additions to our knowledge were made by Ismail *et al.* (1974). In their 35 hirsute subjects no specific cause for the hirsutism had been discovered: in 29 of the patients the menstrual cycle was regular. Although in some patients individual plasma testosterone estimations were within normal limits, the mean of 4 plasma testosterone estimations in each patient was significantly above normal. Short-term stimulation and suppression tests gave inconsistent findings, but long-term tests showed in 5 patients that both adrenal and ovary contributed to the excess androgen, although either adrenal or ovary contributed predominantly in each patient.

Another factor in the development of hirsutism may be the dissociation of sex-hormone binding proteins, leading to an increase in unbound and therefore biologically active androgen (Burke & Anderson 1972).

The role of abnormalities in androgen metabolism in the skin itself in the production of hirsutism is considered on p. 103. That the apparent increase in the susceptibility to androgen of some follicles in some individuals may be due to such defects is probable, but it is now evident that at least a large proportion of patients, formerly labelled 'idiopathic' hirsutism have in fact increased testosterone production by the ovaries, by the adrenals, or by both. The exceptional occurrence of hirsutism confined to one side of the face (Thomason 1979) emphasizes the fact that whatever other factors are concerned the capacity of the end organ to respond is still of central importance.

References

Burger H.-G., Kent J.R. & Kellie A.E. (1964) Determination of testosterone in human peripheral and adrenal venous plasma. *Journal of Clinical Endocrinology and Metabolism,* **24,** 432.

Bush I.E. & Mahesh V.B. (1959) Adrenocortical hyperfunction with sudden onset of hirsutism. *Journal of Endocrinology,* **18,** 1.

Burke C.W. & Anderson D.C. (1972) Interrelationship of testosterone and oestradiol at 37°C, and a biological role for sex-hormone binding globules. *Journal of Endocrinology,* **53,** xxvi.

Casey, J.H. & Nabarro J.D.N. (1967) Plasma testosterone in idiopathic hirsutism and the changes produced by adrenal and ovarian stimulation and suppression. *Journal of Clinical Endocrine Metabolism,* **27,** 1431.

Cristari A. (1892) Cited in Annotation. *Lancet,* **i,** 988.

Fleetwood J.A., Leigh R.J., Hall R. and Smith P.A. (1974) Evidence for an underlying adrenocortical abnormality in hirsute women. *Clinical Endocrinology,* **3,** 457.

Heni F. & Göbel P. (1959) Familiäre postpubertaler Hirsutismus. *Endokrinologie,* **37,** 230.

Ismail A.A.A., Davidson D.W., Kirkham K.E. & Loraine J.A. (1969) Studies on sex hormone excretion in normal and hirsute women. *Acta Endocrinologica,* **61,** 283.

Ismail A.A.A., Davidson D.W., Souka A.R., Barnes E.W., Irvine W.J., Kilimsick H. & Vanderberken

Y. (1974) The evaluation of the role of androgens in hirsutism and the use of a new antiandrogen, 'Cyproterone Acetate' for therapy. *Journal of Clinical Endocrinology and Metabolism*, **39**, 81.

Kirschner M.A. & Jacobs J.B. (1971) Combined ovarian and adrenal vein catheterization to determine the site(s) of androgen overproduction in hirsute women. *Journal of Clinical Endocrinology and Metabolism*, **33**, 199.

Lohse E. & Bjarnhjfdinsson G. (1945) Frequency of hypertrichosis in schizophrenic women as compared to normal. *Acta Psychiatrica Scandinavica*, **20**, 185.

Lopez J.M., Migeon C.J. & Jones G.E.S. (1967) Hirsutism and evaluation of the dexamethasone suppression and chorionic gonadotropin stimulation tests. *American Journal of Obstetrics and Gynecology*, **98**, 749.

Lorenzo E.M. (1970) Familial study of Hirsutism. *Journal of Clinical Endocrinology and Metabolism*, **31**, 556.

Mahesh V.B., Greenblatt R.B., Aydar C.K., Roy R.A., Puebla R.A. & Ellegood J.O. (1964) Urinary steroid excretion patterns in hirsutism. 1. Use of adrenal and ovarian suppression tests in the study of hirsutism. *Journal of Clinical Endocrinology and Metabolism*, **24**, 1283.

Meyer A.E. (1963) Körperstörungen und Sexualität, dargestellt am Beispiel des genuinen Hirsutismus. *Praxis der Psychotherapie*, **8**, 262.

Segré E.J. (1967) *Androgen, Virilization and the Hirsute Female*, Springfield, Thomas.

Thomason A.J. (1975) Idiopathic unilateral familial hirsutism. *Archives of Dermatology*, **115**, 99.

Racial and idiopathic hirsutism (references p. 80)

Nomenclature and aetiology

A mild degree of hirsutism develops at puberty as an apparently physiological change in the great majority of women of some races. It is not associated with virilization, mentrual disorders or impaired fertility. The androgen metabolism of women with racial hirsutism appears not to have been investigated by modern biochemical techniques.

The term 'idiopathic' hirsutism is widely employed, but with no universally accepted definition. To some authors it means hirsutism without an obvious clinical cause, whilst to others it means hirsutism without any discernible biochemical cause. Recent work (e.g. Ismail *et al.* 1974) suggests that abnormalities of androgen metabolism are probably demonstrable in all cases. The term 'idiopathic hirsutism' is used by some authors (e.g. London 1975) for those cases for which no identifiable cause can be established. For the present this unsatisfactory term is retained for this heterogeneous group of cases, but it is already clear that many such cases will change their diagnostic labels as they evolve. A genetically determined defect in adrenal function may be latent or present as mild 'idiopathic' hirsutism; after a severely stressful episode or a pregnancy, the hirsutism may become more severe and be accompanied by menstrual disturbances.

Clinical features

Racial hirsutism is a source of anxiety to a girl only if she is living in a community

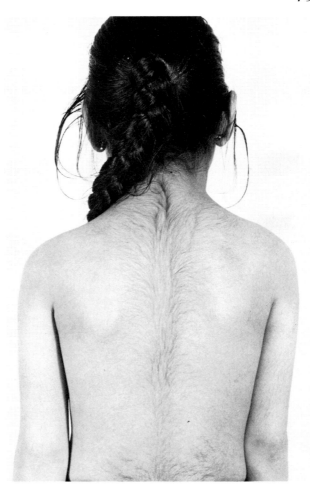

Fig. 4.3. Racial hirsutism. A normal Iranian girl aged 8 (Slade Hospital, Oxford).

in which it is uncommon or unknown (Fig. 4.3). The diagnosis is made in the presence of mild pubertal hirsutism not associated with virilization or menstrual disorders.

'Idiopathic' hirsutism is diagnosed by the exclusion of known causes of hirsutism. The number of cases to which it is now possible to apply the label is therefore steadily falling. However, the important decision has often to be made as to whether comprehensive investigations will be in the best interests of the patient.

If the hirsutism is mild and remains mild, and particularly if it involves only one site, most commonly only the upper lip (Fig. 4.4), but sometimes only the breasts, investigations are seldom helpful. The same may be said of mild hirsutism affecting proportionately all the target sites, if there is no associated seborrhoea or common baldness, and if the menstrual cycle is normal.

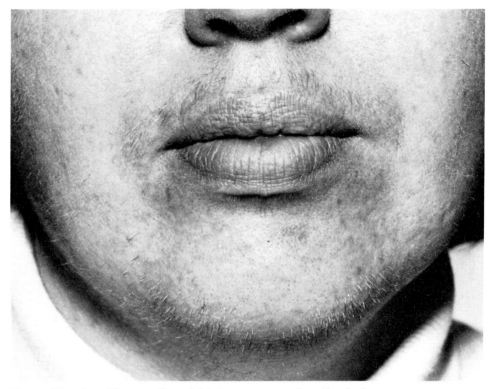

Fig. 4.4. Hirsutism of the upper lip and chin in a woman aged 35. She also has acne (Addenbrooke's Hospital, Cambridge).

References

Ismail A.A.A., Davidson D.W., Souka A.R., Barnes E.W., Irvine W.J., Killimsick H. & Vanderberken Y. (1974) The evaluation of the role of androgens in hirsutism and the use of a new antiandrogen, 'Cyproterone Acetate', for therapy. *Journal of Clinical Endocrinology and Metabolism*, **39**, 81.

London D.R. (1975) Hirsutism. *Postgraduate Medical Journal*, **51**, 236.

Ovarian syndromes

The polycystic ovary syndrome (references p. 83)

History and nomenclature. The association between hirsutism and polycystic disease of the ovaries has long been recognized (e.g. Hegar 1901). Stein & Leventhal (1935) defined a syndrome, often eponymously linked with their names, in which obesity, amenorrhoea, infertility and hirsutism occur in association with polycystic ovaries. However, the clinical and biochemical features are variable, and most authorities now prefer the broader designation, polycystic ovary syndrome.

Aetiology (Hall *et al.* 1974). The aetiology of the syndrome is uncertain; it may well be that it represents a target-organ response to a number of different stimuli. Two sisters were affected (Borghi *et al.* 1972), but many pedigrees show autosomal dominant inheritance. This syndrome is the commonest cause of familial hirsutism (Givens 1980).

In some cases the primary defect appears to be ovarian (Mahesh 1963). Abnormally the ovaries contain much androstenedione, the enzymic conversion of which to oestradiol has failed to occur. In other cases a block appears to have affected only the earlier stage of conversion of dehydroepiandrosterone to androstenedione. These two substances may then be metabolized to testosterone. But in some patients showing such changes in ovarian function, increased production of androgen by the adrenal also is demonstrable.

The possiblity that in many cases the primary defect is hypothalamic has been discussed for some years. Indirect evidence for some central disturbance is provided by cases in which the onset followed a head injury (Bartuska *et al.* 1967). We have frequently observed the syndrome to follow psychological stress, in particular an illness of depressive type.

The serum gonadotropins have been studied in many cases. In 36 women found to have polycystic ovaries (Gambull *et al.* 1973) the serum FSH was low in almost all cases, but the LH levels were either low, normal or elevated, and there was no evident correlation between the LH level and the source of androgen— ovarian, adrenal or both. It is possible that when LH secretion is abnormal, this is the result and not the cause of increased ovarian or suprarenal testosterone production (Stahl *et al.* 1974). However, it is also possible that a hypothalamic mechanism disturbs the patterns of gonadotrophin release which gives rise to the ovarian changes and that the secretion of androstenedione by the ovary further disturbs hypothalamic function and establishes a new pattern, which may become self-perpetuating.

Pathology. The ovaries are usually, but not invariably enlarged. Beneath the pearly-white thickened capsule are small follicles or cysts lined by granulosa cells. The ovarian stroma is increased in amount and the theca interna is often thickened.

Plasma testosterone is elevated, but a single estimation may be misleading because of irregular diurnal variation (Ismail *et al.* 1974). Androstenedione and/or dehydroepiandrosterone and testosterone levels are raised in ovarian vein blood and/or adrenal venous blood or both (Rivarola *et al.* 1967; Kirschner & Jacobs 1971). Urinary 17-oxosteroid excretion may be increased in about a third of cases, but not above 30 mg in 24 hours. Oestrogen levels in blood or urine are normal or slightly reduced (Barlow & Logan 1967). Serum LH is raised in about a third of cases.

Clinical features. The clinical picture as seen by the dermatologist differs obviously in the relatively greater frequency and severity of cutaneous changes, as compared with those present in patients referred in the first instance to an endocrinologist or a gynaecologist, in that virtually all the patients have hirsutism; it was present in 95% of cases reported by Prunty (1967), an endocrinologist. The hirsutism commonly begins at puberty, or within the next 10 years, it is slowly progressive and is proportionate, in that, subject only to some individual variation, it involves in equal degree all the androgen-sensitive sites. In all cases the skin becomes more greasy and in the genetically susceptible acne develops for the first time, or, when the onset of the syndrome is later, acne, which had been present in mild degree at 14 or 15, relapses and becomes severe and persistent. In about 20% of the authors' patients acne has been the presenting symptom. Hirsutism has invariably been also present, but it has sometimes been so inconspicuous that the patient did not mention it. In the genetically predisposed, too, common baldness may be a feature, and occasionally is the patient's principal anxiety. The diffuse shedding that precedes the pattern change (see p. 104) may cause much apprehension, and a misdiagnosis.

In a very few cases one or more of these cutaneous manifestations of androgenic stimulation has at first been the only evidence of polycystic disease. In the majority, however, some menstrual disturbance is found. In over 50% (Prunty 1967) there is amenorrhoea, primary or secondary; in 20% there is dysfunctional uterine bleeding. Other patients complain of irregular menstruation with increasingly severe premenstrual tension. Prunty (1967) found 40% of his patients to be obese.

Again, to quote Prunty (1967) infertility is common and is a feature of some 75% of cases.

On bimanual examination by an experienced gynaecologist enlargement of the ovaries can frequently be detected. On laparotomy or laparoscopy it is present in 95% of cases.

Diagnosis. The differential diagnosis of hirsutism is discussed on p. 88.

Treatment. To many patients infertility is the principal concern. In such cases treatment with clomiphene may be effective. Until recently management of the hirsutism has depended largely on the time-consuming and unsatisfactory mechanical procedures described on p. 89.

Antiandrogens such as cyproterone acetate (p. 112) and cimetidine (p. 114) must be regarded as still under trial, but they have given promising results in some cases, bringing about a marked reduction in hair growth and sebaceous activity (Ismail *et al.* 1974).

Wedge-resection of one or both ovaries results in a temporary reduction of plasma testosterone levels (Lloyd *et al.* 1966), but is now relatively rarely advised as a therapeutic procedure.

References

Barlow J.J. & Logan C.M. (1967) Estrogen metabolism in the polycystic ovary syndrome. *American Journal of Obstetrics and Gynecology*, 96, 687.

Bartuska D.G., Eskin B.A., Smith E.M., Dacon C. & Dratman, M.B. (1967) Brain damage, hypertrichosis and polycystic ovaries. *American Journal of Obstetrics and Gynecology*, 99, 387.

Borghi A., Maiello M. & Giusti G. (1972) Stein–Leventhal syndrome in sisters. *Acta Geneticae Medicae et Gemellologiae*, 21, 79.

Gambrell R.D., Greenblatt R.B. & Mahesh V.B. (1973) Inappropriate secretion of LH in the Stein–Leventhal syndrome. *Obstetrics and Gynaecology*, 42, 429.

Givens J.R. (1980) Polycystic ovarian disease: a common cause of hirsutism. In *Hair Trace Elements and Human Illness*, eds. A.C. Brown & R.G. Crounse, New York, Praeger, p. 283.

Hall R., Anderson J., Smart G.A. & Besser M. (1974) *Fundamentals of Clinical Endocrinology*, 2nd edn. London, Pitman Medical, p. 213.

Hegar A. (1901) Zur abnormalen Behaarung. *Beiträge zur Geburtshilfe und Gynäkologie*, 4, 21.

Ismail A.A.A., Davidson D.W., Souka A.R., Barnes E.W., Irvine W.J., Kilimsick H. & Vanderbreken Y. (1974) The evolution of the role of androgens in hirsutism and the use of a new anti-androgen 'cyproterone acetate' for therapy. *Journal of Clinical Endocrinology and Metabolism*, 39, 81.

Kirschner M.A. & Jacobs J.B. (1971) Combined ovarian and adrenal vein catheterization to determine the site(s) of androgen overproduction in hirsute women. *Journal of Clinical Endocrinology and Metabolism*, 33, 199.

Lloyd C.W., Lobotsky J., Seger E.J., Kobayishi T., Taymor M.L. & Bett R.R. (1966) Plasma testosterone and urinary 17 ketosteroids in women with hirsutism and polycystic ovaries. *Journal of Clinical Endocrinology and Metabolism*, 26, 314.

Mahesh V.B. (1963). The ovary as a source of androgens in hirsutism. In *The Hirsute Female*, ed. R.B. Greenblatt, Springfield, Thomas, p. 179.

Prunty F.T.G. (1967) Hirsutism, virilism and apparent virilism and their gonadal relationship. *Journal of Endocrinology*, 38, 85 and 203.

Rivarola M.A., Saez J.M., Jones H.W., Jones G.S. & Migeon C.J. (1967) The secretion of androgens by the normal, polycystic and neoplastic ovaries. *Johns Hopkins Medical Journal*, 121, 82.

Stahl N.L., Teeslink C.R., Beauchamps G. & Greenblatt R.B. (1973) Serum testosterone levels in hirsute women. *Obstetrics and Gynecology*, 41, 650.

Stein I.F. & Leventhal M.C. (1935) Amenorrhoea associated with bilateral polycystic ovaries. *American Journal of Obstetrics and Gynecology*, 29, 181.

Ovarian tumours causing hirsutism (references p. 84)

Ovarian tumours are a rare but important cause of hirsutism. The diagnosis should be considered particularly when hirsutism, often associated with other features of virilization, develops rapidly: however, the hirsutism is sometimes slowly and insidiously progressive over many years (Merivale & Forman 1951). The order of frequency of symptoms was found to be (Sandberg & Jackson 1963)—amenorrhoea, hirsutism, hypertrophy of the clitoris, deepening of the voice, and reduction in breast size. Most virilizing ovarian tumours occur between the ages of 20 and 40, and some have become clinically evident during pregnancy (see below); however, onset between 40 and 70 has been reported. As in all androgen-induced syndromes in women the degree to which common baldness, seborrhoea and acne are associated with the hirsutism is very variable and depends on age and genetic constitution of the individual.

There are three main types of virilizing ovarian tumours. The most frequent is the arrhenoblastoma, which usually develops in young women. The whole ovary should be removed since some 20% are malignant and recurrences and metastasis may occur (Iverson 1947).

Testosterone-secreting microadenomata of the ovary are unilateral, small and benign. They occur mainly in women under 40. Testosterone levels are in the male range. The tumours are gonadotrophin-dependent. The prognosis after surgery is good, but full recovery from hirsutism cannot be guaranteed, although it has occurred, and even frontovertical baldness has been reversed (Douglass 1947; Novak 1963). Leydig cell tumours (hilus cell tumours), which are rare, tend to occur over the age of 40. Virilization may be severe (Sachs & Spiro 1951; German *et al.* 1961). Testosterone output is increased, but 17-oxosteroid excretion is usually normal. The prognosis after surgery is excellent.

References

Douglas M. (1947) Masculinizing tumours of the ovary of the adrenal type. *American Journal of Obstetrics and Gynecology*, **53**, 190.

German E., Horowitz H., Wiele R.V. & Tocack R.M. (1961) Leydig-cell tumour of the ovary—case report and review. *Journal of Clinical Endocrinology and Metabolism*, **21**, 91.

Iverson L. (1947) Masculinizing tumours of the ovary. *Surgery, Gynecology and Obstetrics*, **84**, 213.

Merivale W.H.H. & Forman L. (1951) A case of masculinovoblastoma. *British Medical Journal*, i, 560.

Novak E.R. (1963) Virilizing tumours of the ovary. In *The Hirsute Female*, ed. R.B. Greenblatt. Springfield: Thomas, p. 195.

Sachs B.A. & Spiro D. (1951) Leydig cell tumours of the ovary: report of a case with virilism including postmortem findings. *Journal of Clinical Endocrinology and Metabolism*, **11**, 818.

Sandberg E.C. & Jackson J.R. (1963) A clinical analysis of ovarian virilizing tumours. *American Journal of Surgery*, **105**, 784.

Hirsutism in pregnancy (references pp. 85–6)

Hirsutism may develop for the first time in pregnancy, usually after the 20th week. It usually persists after delivery, but may disappear partly or completely. There appear to be no adequate studies of the endocrine basis of this not uncommon phenomenon, nor of the possible effects on the fetus of the presumably minor disturbance of androgen metabolism.

Rarely severe hirsutism occurs in pregnancy, necessarily accompanied in most cases by some degree of virilization (Judd *et al.* 1973). One report (Stoddard 1945) of two patients with severe hirsutism noted recovery post-partum and recurrence in subsequent pregnancies. Two of three patients investigated in

Finland (Turunen *et al.* 1964) were found to have abnormally low levels of placental 17β dehydrogenase, and hence an impaired capacity to inactivate testosterone. Of six children born to the three mothers, three had severe congenital malformations. A patient reported by Friedman *et al.* (1955) developed hirsutism with virilization from the 5th month of her first pregnancy, which ended in a stillbirth. The virilization regressed but recurred from the 5th month of her second pregnancy 2 years later. She was found to have hyperplasia of ovarian lutein cells.

Recently the subject of virilization in pregnancy has twice been reviewed (Novak *et al.* 1970; Fayez *et al.* 1974). The causes have been divided into two groups, as surgical or non-surgical. The surgical group consists of a variety of androgen-secreting ovarian tumours, including among others mucinous cyst-adenomas containing Leydig cells secreting testosterone, arrhenoblastomas, granulosa cell tumours, hilus cell tumours and dermoid cysts. It is noteworthy that in one patient severely virilized in the 8th month of pregnancy by a mucinous cystadenoma, all signs of virilization had regressed by the 5th month after operation (Novak *et al.* 1970). The non-surgical group accounts for an increasingly high proportion of the more recently reported cases. The conditions concerned are all apparently functional disturbances of the ovaries, though not all are self-limiting. Luteomas are believed to be caused by high levels of gonadotrophin stimulation and occur most often in Negro women who have had multiple pregnancies in rapid succession. Theca lutein cysts are a comparable ovarian response, in which the theca interior is luteinized. The multiple cysts, which may cause considerable enlargement of the ovary, can secrete large quantities of testosterone. Polycystic ovary disease (see p. 80) appears now to be the most frequent cause of hirsutism in pregnancy (Magendantz *et al.* 1972; Fayez *et al.* 1974).

Hirsutism of more than trivial severity, developing for the first time, or increasing rapidly in severity or extent during the course of a pregnancy, is an indication for full gynaecological and endocrinological investigation. The children of such pregnancies are usually normal and are born at term, but in some cases girl babies are masculinized (Fayez *et al.* 1974).

Hypertrichosis

A different phenomenon, totally unexplained, is the temporary overgrowth of the eyebrows, from the second month of pregnancy, in successive pregnancies, in several women in a family (Cedercrantz 1939).

References

Cedercrantz A. (1939) Hypertrichosis superciliarum et in fronte in graviditate apericus. *Acta dermato-venereologica*, **20**, 704.

Fayez J.A., Bunch T.R. & Miller G.L. (1974) Virilization in pregnancy associated with polycystic ovary disease. *Obstetrics and Gynecology*, **44**, 511.

Friedman I.S., Mackles A. & Daichman I. (1955) Development of virilization during pregnancy. *Journal of Clinical Endocrinology and Metabolism*, **15**, 1281.

Judd H.L., Benirschke K., De Vane G., Reuter S.R. & Yen S.C.C. (1973) Maternal virilization developing during a twin pregnancy. *New England Journal of Medicine*, **288**, 118.

Magendantz H.G., Jones D.E. & Schonberg D.W. (1972) Virilization during pregnancy associated with polycystic ovary diseases. *Obstetrics and Gynecology*, **40**, 156.

Novak D.J., Lauchlan S.C., McCawley J.C. & Faisman C. (1970) Virilization during pregnancy. *American Journal of Medicine*, **49**, 281.

Stoddard F.J. (1945) Hirsutism in pregnancy. *American Journal of Obstetrics and Gynecology*, **49**, 417.

Turunen A., Pesonen S. & Zilliacus H. (1964) Hormone assays during recurrent excessive hairgrowth in pregnancy. *Acta Endocrinologica*, **45**, 447.

Hirsutism of adrenal origin (references p. 87)

Congenital adrenal hyperplasia
The adrenal cortex is the site of synthesis, ultimately from cholesterol, of aldosterone, cortisol and testosterone. A hereditary deficiency of the enzyme concerned with any one stage of these synthetic pathways leads to a block which may result in the conversion of precursor into androgen. The commonest enzyme defects result in reduced cortisol production and hence in an increased output of ACTH and βMSH. The numerous syndromes of congenital adrenal hyperplasia show biochemical and clinical differences according to the age at which excess androgen begins to modify sexual development in the female.

Of the many distinct syndromes now recognized, only a few are relevant in the present context, as they are not uncommon and are causes of hirsutism. The defects are determined by autosomal recessive genes.

21 Hydroxylase defect. In this, the commonest of the enzyme defects, there is a block in the formation of deoxycortisol from 17α hydroxyprogesterone. There is therefore a deficiency of cortisol and increased production of androstenedione and testosterone. In the severe form there is virilization of the female fetus (Christaens *et al.* 1963); in the commoner mild form the patient appears normal at first, but soon after puberty menstruation becomes irregular and hirsutism and virilization develop (Brooks *et al.* 1960). In the affected male there is a pseudoprecocious puberty.

11β Hydroxylase defect (Gabrilove *et al.* 1965). Hirsutism and virilization may first develop in adult life. Hypertension is usually a feature.

Cushing's syndrome. Iatrogenic Cushing's syndrome is now the most common form. Bilateral adrenocortical hyperplasia (Cushing's disease) is probably secondary to a hypothalamic defect leading to increased production of ACTH. A variety of benign and malignant tumours, of which the oat-cell carcinoma of the bronchus is the most frequent, may produce ectopic ACTH. Adenomas or carcinomas of the adrenal cortex can also give rise to Cushing's syndrome. In all forms of Cushing's syndrome, except the iatrogenic induced by the administration of corticosteroids, the clinical picture depends on the combined effects of cortisol and androgens. Classical features of the syndrome are obesity of proximal distribution combined with rounding of the facial contour, purple atrophic striae, easy bruising and amenorrhoea. Hirsutism is frequent, but very severe degrees with associated virilization are seldom seen except in some adrenal tumours.

Adrenal testosterone secreting microadenomata occur at the menopause (Givens 1980). Testosterone levels are high but urinary oxosteroid secretion is normal. The tumour is gonadotrophin-dependent.

References

Brooks R.V., Mattingly D., Mills I.M. & Prunty F.T.G. (1960) Postpubertal adrenal virilization with biochemical disturbance: the congenital type of adrenal hyperplasia. *British Medical Journal*, i, 1294.

Christaens L., Fontaine G. & Lande M. (1963) Enzymopathie congénitale surrenalienne virilisante chez trois soeurs. *Archives francaises de Pédiatrie*, **20**, 169.

Gabrilove J.L., Sharman D.C. & Dorfman R.I. (1965) Adrenocortical 11β hydroxylase deficiency and virilization first manifest in the adult woman. *New England Journal of Medicine*, **272**, 1189.

Givens J.R. (1980) Polycystic ovarian disease: a common cause of hirsutism. In *Hair Trace Elements and Human Illness*, eds. A.C. Brown & R.G. Crounse. New York, Praeger, p. 283.

Hirsutism in gonadal dysgenesis (Judd *et al.* 1970)

In this rare syndrome which occurs in phenotypic females, gonadal tissue is represented by rudimentary streaks composed of an ovarian type stroma with few or no ova. These patients appear to be normal until puberty, when they fail to menstruate and their bodily proportions become eunuchoid. In 5–10% of cases hirsutism develops because the increased gonadotrophin secreted as a response to the deficiency of oestrogen stimulates androgen production by the gonadal streak tissue.

Reference

Judd H.L., Scully R.E., Atkins L., Neer R.M. & Kliman B. (1970) Pure gonadal dysgenesis with progressive hirsutism. *New England Journal of Medicine*, **282**, 881.

Hyperprolactinaemic states

Prolactin has important effects on the production of androgen by the adrenal and the gonads. It may play a regulating role in conjunction with ACTH in adrenal androgen secretion.

The secretion of prolactin is increased in depression and in some other psychiatric disturbances. It is possible that endorphins control prolactin production by altering hypothalamic dopamine turnover.

Hyperprolactinaemia may occur after severe stress. It may also occur as the result of the development of a prolactin-secreting microadenoma of the pituitary. Such adenomata are the cause of the hyperprolactinaemia–galactorrhoea–amenorrhoea syndrome. Hirsutism is present in at least 50% of these patients. The adrenal androgen production rises, but the normal ratio of 17 oxosteroids to 17 oxogenic steroids in the urine is sustained (Forbes *et al.* 1954; Seppala & Hirvonen 1975; Tyson & Pinto 1978).

Male hyperprolactinaemic states are associated with loss of libido and potency. The patient complains of diffuse shedding of scalp hair but is particularly concerned by the shedding of pubic and other body hair, which may become visibly sparse. There may be female distribution of subcutaneous fat.

References

Forbes A.P., Henneman P.H., Grisewold G.C. & Albright F. (1954) Syndrome characterized by galactorrhoea, amenorrhoea and low urinary FSH: comparisons with acromegaly and normal elastoma. *Journal of Clinical Endocrinology and Metabolism,* 14, 265.

Seppala M. & Hirvonen E. (1975) Raised serum prolactin levels associated with hirsutism and amenorrhoea. *British Medical Journal,* iv, 144.

Tyson J.E. & Pinto H. (1978) Investigation of the possible significance of prolactin in human reproduction. In *Clinics in Obstetrics and Gynaecology,* vol. 5, ed. Tyson, J.E. p. 411.

The differential diagnosis of hirsutism

It is difficult to justify the referral of a woman with hirsutism to a beauty parlour for treatment by electrolysis or some other mechanical or chemical means, without taking a careful history on the basis of which appropriate investigation can if necessary be planned. The hirsutism may be an early indication of a significant abnormality of androgen metabolism which, untreated, may lead to important irreversible changes. It is, however, equally difficult to justify subjecting a patient to expensive and worrying investigations for which there is no valid indication.

Of fundamental importance in making the decision as to which investigations are necessary or desirable, is a detailed history, with emphasis on the following features:

(i) Age of onset. Onset at puberty is characteristic of racial and 'idiopathic' hirsutism. Onset at the menopause may also occur in hirsutism of no serious significance. Onset in adult life should be regarded with greater suspicion.

(ii) Race.

(iii) Family history. A family history of pubertal hirsutism can be reassuring, but it must be remembered that adrenocortical dysfunction and the polycystic ovary syndrome can be familial.

(iv) Menstrual cycle. A normal menstrual cycle does not exclude an identifiable abnormality of androgen metabolism, but the greater the menstrual disturbance the more likely is such an abnormality to be present.

(v) Infertility or low fertility may obviously be in itself an indication for investigation, but may also be an additional indication in patients whose primary concern is hirsutism.

(vi) Other androgenetic cutaneous changes. If acne and/or common baldness are associated, they may suggest the need for investigation, although the hirsutism is of mild degree.

(vii) Weight. The presence of obesity in a hirsute young woman is an added indication for investigation. Loss of weight associated with amenorrhoea may suggest a depressive state.

(viii) Psychological state. The probability that stress can precipitate the onset of androgenetic changes in predisposed subjects has been mentioned (p. 75). The psychological effects of the skin changes on the patient have also to be considered. Some women accept without complaint a degree of hirsutism that many would consider disfiguring. Others with barely perceptible hirsutism are greatly distressed and insist that their lives are ruined by the hirsutism. It is important always to assess the role of psychological factors, primary or secondary, as an aid to accurate diagnosis and as a guide to an effective approach to treatment.

If the diagnostic criteria of idiopathic hirsutism are met, and the hirsutism is mild, it may be reasonable to plan treatment without further investigations. If, however, the history suggests a more extensive and perhaps more specific disturbance of androgen metabolism, then careful investigation is desirable. This should be carried out in a department with satisfactory facilities for the necessary biochemical screening.

Local treatment of hirsutism

If a specific and treatable endocrine abnormality has been discovered, its management is best supervized by an endocrinologist: for example control of adrenocortical hyperplasia with corticosteroids or of hyperprolactinaemia with bromocriptine.

When no specific diagnosis has been made or if specific treatment is not available, particularly if the hirsutism is associated with other disfiguring androgenetic cutaneous changes, the possibility of prescribing antiandrogens may be considered; a separate section is devoted to these drugs (p. 112).

Topical treatment with cyproterone has not proved successful, but one of the principal objections to the use of systemic cyproterone is the need to prescribe with it oestrogen to ensure effective contraception. The percutaneous administration of natural 17-beta oestradiol has none of the side effects of orally administered synthetic oestrogens. Recently 17-beta oestradiol has been administered percutaneously, a dose of 3 mg from day 16 to 25 of the menstrual cycle in hirsute patients receiving oral cyproterone acetate 50 mg daily from the fifth to the twenty-fifth day. The clinical response was good (Kuttenn *et al.* 1980).

The use of topical progesterones to inhibit the transformation of testosterone to dihydrotestosterone is still in the experimental stage (Orentreich & Rizer 1980).

When hirsutism is the only obviously significant cutaneous abnormality and when there are satisfactory grounds for accepting it as 'idiopathic' local treatments will be required. These are not very effective, but skilfully carried out can be of considerable value.

Destruction of the hair roots by X-ray has no place in the treatment of hirsutism, since any dose large enough to destroy the roots will inevitably cause radiodermatitis.

The treatment of choice is depilation by electrolysis. This and other methods of removing hair are described on pp. 424–6.

References
Kuttenn F., Rigaud C., Wright F. & Mauvais-Jarvis P. (1980) Treatment of hirsutism by oral cyproterone acetate and percutaneous estradiol. *Journal of Clinical Endocrinology and Metabolism*, **51**, 1107.
Orentreich N. & Rizer R.L. (1980) Medical treatment of androgenic alopecia. In: *Hair, Trace Elements and Human Illness*, eds. A.C. Brown & R.G. Crounse. New York, Praeger, p. 294.

Common baldness
(References p. 94)

History and nomenclature
Common baldness is a physiological event in the lives of most men and of many women of those races which carry the sex-influenced gene or genes responsible for its development. There is perhaps no other normal phenomenon that has been so widely regarded as abnormal by physician and layman alike. At least as early as the Egyptian civilization of 4000 years ago, it was already a matter for concern (Giacometti 1967).

The long history of the attempts to explain and to restrain or reverse common baldness is intrinsically interesting and is of considerable practical scientific importance. The urge to understand has led physicians uncritically to accept speculations as proven facts, and the speculative theories of earlier generations have become part of folk-lore, and have also provided the theoretical basis for the activities of those whose interest in baldness is predominantly commercial.

In past centuries attitudes to baldness appear to have been as ambivalent as they are today. In ancient Rome some considered baldness to be shameful, and according to Suetonius, Julius Caesar combed his hair to attempt to cover his denuded scalp (Cazenave 1850). No doubt then as later there were others who exalted baldness as conferring dignity; the monk Hugbald of St Amand (d. 930) went as far as to write a poem in praise of baldness (Schönfeld 1957).

The scientific study of the skin began effectively in the eighteenth century and gained momentum rapidly during the first half of the nineteenth century. Most of the earlier writers on dermatology practised primarily as surgeons or as physicians and did not confine their interest to diseases of the skin. Texts on dermatology before 1850 gave little space to the hair and most of that was devoted to ringworm infections and to alopecia areata. In the third edition of his authoritative text-book Erasmus Wilson (1852) gave a short account of calvities syn. senile baldness; he noted that it was not confined to the elderly and might 'result from mental anxiety, severe affliction or come on without apparent exciting cause'. He thought that baldness occurred on the vertex, because there 'the integument is bound down somewhat tightly on the bones of the cranium'. He was inclined to suppose that there was more subcutaneous fat beneath the scalp in women and that this accounted for their lower incidence of baldness. He mentioned heredity as one of many 'remote causes'. Since an inadequate circulation was the cause of the hair loss, treatment should aim at stimulating blood flow.

Erasmus Wilson referred to pityriasis capitis and to seborrhoea but did not relate either to baldness. However, both conditions under a bewildering variety of designations had found a place in the early classifications, including those of Plenck and of Willan, and, largely as a result of the writings of German authorities the concept became established of alopecia furfuracea (Hebra & Kaposi 1874), also known as alopecia pityrodes of Pincus. Most texts thereafter recognized senile baldness and premature baldness, which differed only in their age of onset, and, under various designations, the same pattern of alopecia associated with pityriasis or seborrhoea, by most authors alleged to be caused by these changes. However, Michelson (1885) of Königsberg wrote: 'The view of Hebra–Kaposi that a chronic seborrhoea is always the primary condition and that alopecia occurs only secondarily, has in our opinion been disproved by Pincus. Both processes are parallel effects of the same causes.' Despite Michelson's wise caution, measures alleged to control seborrhoea and pityriasis were widely believed to modify the course of the alopecia that sometimes accompanied them, and much research and even more speculation were devoted to establishing their cause.

This was the heroic age of microbiology; enthusiasm was not matched by adequate technical procedures and Koch's postulates had not yet been enunciated. In 1874 Malassez had discovered the organism later known as *Pityrosporum ovale*. Eight years later Lassar of Berlin (Lassar & Bishop 1882) claimed to have transmitted to rabbits and guinea-pigs the combination of pityriasis, seborrhoea and alopecia by rubbing into their backs the hair and scales from the scalp of a student afflicted with these disorders. Of the many workers who followed this lead the most influential was Unna of Hamburg, who summarized in his textbook (Unna 1896) his previously published work. Unna regarded the *Pityrosporum*, which he referred to as the 'bottle bacillus', as the cause of pityriasis capitis which led to alopecia pityrodes. He believed that the alopecia developed because of 'increasing difficulty in forming new hairs'. In alopecia seborrhoeica, the next stage, the bottle bacillus was relatively less abundant. 'The future must teach us which organism, and especially whether one only, is the cause of the accompanying sebotaxis.'

The most frequently quoted contemporary investigation was that of Elliott & Merrill (1895) of New York—it was still being quoted as authoritative by O'Donovan (1930). Of 320 patients with premature alopecia, in all but four this was secondary to hereditary seborrhoeic dermatitis, of which the *Pityrosporum* was accepted as the cause; the remaining four patients had hereditary premature alopecia, without seborrhoea.

Sabouraud of Paris applied his considerable intellect to these problems. His detailed and thorough investigations led him to put forward a hypothesis which provided an apparently logical explanation of observed clinical phenomena, and which was very widely accepted. It was an elaboration of the theories already mentioned. He accepted the *Pityrosporum* as the cause of pityriasis and held the invasion of the follicles by a microbacillus to be the cause of seborrhoea and the alopecia that accompanied it. In 1903 Radcliffe Crocker summed up the position. He recognized senile alopecia and idiopathic premature alopecia, but regarded seborrhoea as 'a factor' in a large proportion of cases of the former, and as the cause of nearly all cases of the latter. He recognized, thirdly, seborrhoeic alopecia and wrote, 'Personally I incline to Sabouraud's explanation, but it has not as yet quite acquired the status of a dogma.' The attraction of Sabouraud's correlation of the types and stages of baldness with microbial infections was that it offered an apparently scientific basis for treatment.

A Treatise on Diseases of the Hair by Jackson and McMurtry (1913) of New York was well received by the reviewers. In the main these authors followed Unna and Sabouraud but they also retained or revived some older theories. Senile baldness began by definition at or after 45; senile changes were the main factors, and the pressure of the aponeuroses of the occipitofrontalis muscle, and seborrhoea. Idiopathic premature alopecia was accepted as hereditary, but Pohl-Pincus (1883) was quoted, with approval for his claim that it was in fact the markedly stretched condition of the occipitofrontalis aponeuroses that was inherited. Jackson and McMurtry agreed that premature alopecia was very prevalent in those leading sedentary lives, and especially in brain workers; they quoted Jamieson, who blamed this on reflex interference with hair growth by cerebral congestion. They agreed with King (1868) that the 'continuous wearing of caps or of close fitting unventilated hats' was important, and they did not care to refute Ellinger's (1879) finding that the daily application of water was a factor in 85% of cases; as they put it, 'lack of care of the hair is an active cause'. They mention, without disapproval, Parker's (1907) opinion that a toxin developing in expired air is responsible for premature alopecia which can therefore be avoided by taking deep breaths. They are confident in their explanation of the much lower incidence of premature alopecia in women; they do not wear hats so much and these are not so close fitting; they give more attention to their hair and they avoid wetting it; their hair is not so often cut; they have less abundant hair elsewhere and there is therefore not such a drain upon the hair forming elements; and finally, they have more subcutaneous fat. In both sexes seborrhoea is a factor in at least 90% of cases of *idiopathic* premature alopecia. In the light of this statement the reader finds some difficulty in differentiating this condition from alopecia furfuracea, pityrodes of seborrhoeica which is said to be the commonest form of *symptomatic* premature alopecia. Moreover 'as seborrhoeic dermatitis and pityriasis steatoides are contagious diseases, and very prevalent' it is surprising that so few people lose their hair; most people are resistant to the parasites. As to the cause of seborrhoea, Jackson and McMurtry thought that Darier was possibly correct in considering the microbacillus secondary to seborrhoea; but in general they accepted Sabouraud's work with various reservations. Pityriasis simplex (syn. seborrhoea sicca of Unna) was caused by the *Pityrosporum*, but did not result in baldness. Pityriasis steatoides, caused by the *Pityrosporum* together with the 'coccus polymorphe à culture grise' of Sabouraud (Morococcus of Unna) did lead to hair loss. Jackson and McMurtry have been quoted at some length not with the intention of denigrating these highly reputable dermatologists, but because their opinions were shared by so many others and can be found in the standard textbooks of most countries in the first two decades of the present century, and with minor differences in emphasis, in many later texts. In 1930, in his book, *The Hair*, O'Donovan of the London Hospital exemplified perhaps the clinician attempting to come to terms with the inconsistencies of the 'scientific' knowledge of the day. On the same page he stated, 'presenile baldness associated with active seborrhoea, in my experience is rare'; and in the next paragraph, 'premature baldness is generally the result of seborrhoea'. He suggested that premature baldness was more common in men because they visited the hairdresser more often than women, but he questioned the validity of the microbial theory of seborrhoea.

Agnes Savill wrote a highly successful textbook entitled *The Hair and Scalp*. The first edition was published in 1935, and the fifth and last in 1962. In the earlier editions Dr Savill accepted without reservation the microbial hypothesis of Sabouraud. In the last edition (Savill & Warren 1962) she repeats once more the intellectually satisfying and sophisticated Sabouraud classification, but she was aware of Hamilton's (1942) classic study of the role of androgens in common baldness, to which she refers in an exercise in verbal acrobatics which allowed her with dignity to reconcile the irreconcilable.

Hamilton's (1942) paper was indeed a watershed. The evidence, to be presented in this chapter, established beyond doubt that common baldness is a normal process induced by the action of androgen on genetically predisposed follicles. If the baldness accompanies seborrhoea it is because the latter depends on similar hormonal and genetic influences. Admittedly the role of microorganisms in the aetiology of pityriasis remains uncertain, but they are not a cause of common baldness. The outstanding work of Montagna and his colleagues, in man and in other primates, confirmed and elaborated Hamilton's findings: of the nature and significance of common baldness there is no longer any doubt. Yet the theories discussed above, stripped though they are of all scientific credibility, form, together with others still more absurd, the pseudo-scientific foundations of a multi-million pound assault on public gullibility.

The contemporary nomenclature for common baldness is confusing. In some countries 'seborrhoeic alopecia' is favoured. This term is unfortunate in that it has misleading aetiological connotations. 'Male pattern alopecia' is perhaps the most widely used term, but it is descriptively misleading when applied to common baldness in women, and has encouraged the emergence of 'chronic diffuse alopecia', since the pattern of common baldness in women is not the same as in men, at least at low and moderate androgen levels. 'Pattern baldness' is unobjectionable, but has not been generally adopted. 'Androgenetic baldness' is also unobjectionable but has not found favour. 'Common baldness' has the advantage of emphasizing that, except in a minority of affected women, the loss of hair is a normal phenomenon.

References

Cazenave P.-L.A. (1850) *Traité des Maladies du Cuir Chevelu.* Paris, Baillière.

Ellinger L. (1879) Zur Aetiologie und Prophylaxe der Alopecia praematura. *Virchows Archiv für pathologische Anatomie und Physiologie,* 77, 549.

Elliott G.T. & Merrill W.H. (1895) A further study of alopecia praematura or praesenilic, and its most frequent cause—eczema seborrhoicum, and a preliminary bacteriological report on eczema seborrhoicum. *New York Medical Journal,* 62, 525.

Giacometti L. (1967) Facts, legends and myths about the scalp throughout history. *Archives of Dermatology,* 95, 629.

Hamilton J. (1942) Male hormone stimulation is a prerequisite and an incitant in common baldness. *American Journal of Anatomy,* 71, 451.

Hebra F. & Kaposi M. (1874) *On Diseases of the Skin.* Trans. W. Tay. Volume III. London, New Sydenham Society, p. 203.

King, A.F.A. (1868) On the causes of alopecia and its greater frequency in males than females. *American Journal of Medical Science,* 55, 416.

Malassez L. (1874) Note sur l'anatomie pathologique de l'alopécie pityriasique. *Archives de Physiologie,* 1, 464.

Parker D.L. (1907) Common baldness: its cause and treatment. *American Journal of Dermatology and Genito-urinary Diseases*, **11**, 261.

Pohl-Pincus J. (1883) Ueber die Alopecie und den indurativen Krankheits-Process überhaupt. *Berliner klinische Wochenschrift*, **20**, 645.

Phylogeny of common baldness

Man is not the only primate species in which baldness is a natural phenomenon associated with sexual maturity (Montagna & Uno 1968). The orang-utan (*Pongo pygmaeus*) and the chimpanzee (*Pan troglodytes*) both show some degree of baldness when they reach maturity. In the juveniles long hair extends from the level of the eyebrows to merge imperceptibly with the scalp, whereas in the adult the forehead and the frontal region of the scalp bear only fine vellus hair. Other species showing this phenomenon include the uakari (*Cacajao* sp.) and the stump-tailed macaque (*Macaca speciosa*), and the latter in particular has been extensively studied by Montagna and his colleagues at the Oregon Primate Center.

These investigations establish the essential similarity of the balding process in *Macaca* and in man. Terminal follicles are progressively transformed into 'vellus' follicles, differing from true vellus follicles in that they may still have attached to them the remnants of fibres of the arrector pili muscles. The importance of these careful comparative studies should need little emphasis. Common baldness is indeed a physiological process in those genetically predisposed to it, whether simian or human; and the role of the many factors imaginatively incriminated by some medical authorities of the past can be confidently denied.

Reference
Montagna W. & Uno H. (1968) The phylogeny of baldness. In *Biopathology of Pattern Alopecia*, ed. A. Baccareda-Boy, G. Moretti & J.R. Frey. Basel, Karger, p. 9.

Prevalence and Genetics (references p. 98)

The prevalence of common baldness in any population has not been accurately recorded, but it may be true that, at least in the Caucasoid races, it approximates to 100%, for the replacement of some terminal follicles by vellus type follicles from puberty onwards is a universal phenomenon. Recording assessments at the clinical level of evident sparsity of terminal hair, a number of investigations have been carried out, but few of them have made any real attempt at quantification. An exception is that of Hamilton (1951) of New York who examined 312 white males and 214 white females aged 20–89 and proposed a system of grading baldness, which remains valuable (see Fig. 4.5).

	Type I	Full hair.
Scalps not bald	Type II	Bitemporal recession.
	Type III	Borderline.

Type IV   Deep frontotemporal recession. Usually also some midfrontal recession. In older subjects this degree of frontotemporal loss may be associated with some vertical thinning.

Type V   Increased frontotemporal recession and marked denudation of vertex.

Type VI   Increased loss from both areas, which are becoming confluent.

Type VII   Enlarged frontotemporal and vertical areas surpassed only by band of sparse hair.

Type VIII Complete confluence of both areas.

Type I was the normal scalp in both sexes before puberty, when it was replaced by Type II in 96% of men and 79% women. Of men aged 50 or more 58% had scalps of Type V–VIII, and the extent of baldness tended to increase to the age of 70. About 25% of women developed Type IV scalps by the age of 50, after which there was no further increase. Indeed after 50 some women who have developed Type II at puberty may revert to Type I. Types V–VIII were not found in any woman.

Type I scalp was retained after puberty by most Chinese. Baldness is uncommon, mild and of late onset.

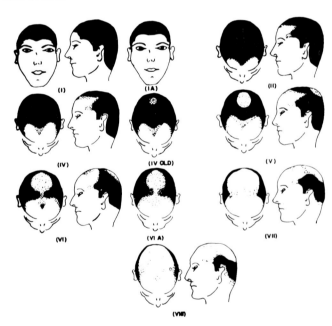

Fig. 4.5. Hamilton's classification of the pattern of common baldness in the male (Hamilton 1951).

Although, as these figures show, the male pattern of baldness occurs in females with some frequency, androgenetic alopecia in women more often assumes a diffuse form (Ludwig 1977) (Fig. 4.6).

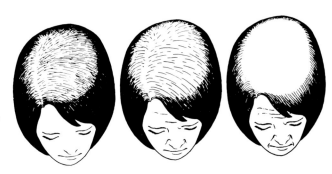

Fig. 4.6. The patterns of androgenetic alopecia commonly occurring in the female (Courtesy of Professor Ludwig and the Editor of the *British Journal of Dermatology*).

Other statistics, much less accurately recorded, tend to group together what Hamilton has classified as Types II, III and IV, and are therefore of interest only in confirming the great frequency of common baldness in other populations of Caucasoids. For example, Buschke & Grenepert (1926) in Germany found bitemporal recession in 62.5% of men aged 20–40. Beek (1946) in Holland found baldness in 27% of women aged 35–40 and 64% of those aged 40–70. Figures from Italy (Binazzi & Wierolis 1962) also serve to emphasize the frequency of baldness in women of Caucasoid descent.

The incidence and patterns of baldness in American Caucasoids and Negroes have been compared (Setty 1970). The more severe degrees of alopecia were more common in Caucasoids, and, taking all age groups together, a full head of hair—Hamilton Type I—was four times more frequent in Negroes than in Caucasoids.

This very frequency of common baldness has complicated the many attempts to establish its mode of inheritance. Moreover it is by no means clear that common baldness is genetically homogeneous, and some authorities differentiate between baldness of early onset (before 30 in men) and the same pattern of baldness becoming evident 20 years later.

Osborne (1916) thought that baldness was determined by a single pair of sex-influenced factors and Snyder & Yingling (1935) considered that both gene frequency studies and family histories supported this hypothesis. According to this theory both men and women of genotype BB are bald—and so are men, but not women, of genotype Bb. The genotype bb does not predispose to baldness in either sex.

Harris (1946) insisted that early baldness must be distinguished from late baldness, and that the former is transmitted by a single autosomal dominant gene. He assumed that the heterozygous female was normally not affected, but was uncertain about the homozygous female.

A clinical study (Smith & Wells 1964) of the first degree relatives of 56 women with ordinary baldness, showed that of those who were 30 or over, 54% of the males and 23% of the females were similarly affected. These authors considered on the basis of their material that baldness could apparently develop in the heterozygous female and they postulated either dominant inheritance with increased penetrance in the male, or multifactorial inheritance. The probability of multifactorial inheritance was supported also by Salamon (1968). However, the question remains open. It is still uncertain whether early and late onset baldness are separately inherited. It is nevertheless certain that both are inherited and that both depend upon androgenic stimulation of susceptible follicles.

There is no association between baldness and dense hair patterns on the trunk and limbs (Burton *et al.* 1979).

The association of baldness with susceptibility or resistance to certain diseases has been claimed, but the evidence is unsatisfactory; for example an increased incidence of coronary artery disease, but a fourfold decrease in the incidence of carcinoma of the bronchus, has been claimed for bald men as compared with non-bald controls (Bruchner *et al.* 1964). The association of baldness with coronary disease has not been substantiated by recent work (Cooke 1979).

The claim that baldness in men was associated with increased fertility could not be confirmed (Damon *et al.* 1965).

References

Beek C.H. (1946) Calvities frontalis bei Frauen. *Dermatologica,* **93,** 213.

Binazzi M. & Wierolis T. (1962) Les Alopécies féminines Hypooestrogéniques. *Annales de Dermatologie et de Syphiligraphie,* **89,** 382.

Bruchner H.A., Brown M. & Tretsea R.J. (1964) Baldness and Emphysema. *Journal of the Louisiana State Medical Society,* **116,** 34.

Burton J.L., Ben Halim M.M. & Meyrick, G. (1979) Male pattern alopecia and masculinity. *British Journal of Dermatology,* **100,** 507.

Buschke A. & Grenepert M. (1926) Zur Kenntnis des Sexualcharakters der Kophhaarkleiden. *Klinische Wochenschrift,* **5,** 18.

Cooke M.T. (1979) Male pattern alopecia and coronary artery disease in men. *British Journal of Dermatology,* **101,** 455.

Damon A., Burr W.A. & Gerson D.E. (1965) Baldness, fertility and number and sex ratio of children. *Human Biology,* **37,** 366.

Hamilton J.B. (1951) Patterned long hair in man: types and incidence. *Annals of the New York Academy of Science,* **53,** 708.

Harris H. (1946) The inheritance of premature baldness in man. *Annals of Eugenics,* **13,** 172.

Ludowig E. (1977) Classification of the types of androgenic alopecia (common baldness) arising in the female sex. *British Journal of Dermatology,* **97,** 249.

Osborne D. (1916) Inheritance of baldness. *Journal of Heredity,* **7,** 347.

Salamon T. (1968) Genetic factors in male pattern alopecia. In *Biopathology of Pattern Alopecia,* eds. A. Baccaradda-Boy, G. Moratti & J.R. Fray. Basel, Karger, p. 39.

Setty L.R. (1970) Hair patterns of the scalp of white and Negro males. *American Journal of Physical Anthropology*, **33**, 49.

Smith M.A. & Wells R.S. (1964) Male type alopecia, alopecia areata and normal hair in women. *Archives of Dermatology*, **89**, 95.

Snyder L.H. & Yingling H.C. (1935) The application of the gene frequency method of analysis to sex-influenced factors with especial reference to baldness. *Human Biology*, **7**, 608.

Pathology (references p. 100)

The combination of changes seen in common baldness is distinctive. The earliest change detected is focal perivascular basophilic degeneration in the lower third of the connective tissue sheath of otherwise apparently normal anagen follicles. The affected follicles become progressively smaller over a succession of hair cycles. Beneath the shrinking follicle can at first be seen the basophilic sclerotic remains of the connective tissue sheath, but eventually this too disappears. In about a third of biopsies multinucleate giant cells can be seen surrounding fragments of hair (Domnitz & Silvers 1979). The arrector pili muscle decreases in size but its atrophy lags behind that of the follicle (Maguire & Kligman 1962; Lattenand & Johnson 1975). In any area of balding, scalp follicles at all stages can be found. In the scalp which appears totally bald almost all follicles are short and small, producing at best only tiny vellus hairs. However, even in such scalps there is usually a number of quiescent terminal follicles which may sometimes be stimulated into growth to raise false hopes of 'a cure' for baldness (Montagna & Parakkal 1974). Careful studies of the differences between bald and non-bald scalp at various ages have been published by Goerttler (1965).

As the balding scalp loses its protective covering of hair so solar degenerative changes may be added to those described above (Singh & McKenzie 1961; Allegra 1968).

Soft tissue X-ray showed no correlation between the thickness of the scalp and the development of baldness (Garn *et al.* 1954), and the reduction of blood supply has been shown to follow, not precede, the baldness (Cormia & Ernyey 1961), though the degree of degenerative change in arterioles and capillaries may eventually be considerable (Allegra 1968). When the follicles become small or disappear, their now unsupported nerve networks coil and twist and come to resemble encapsulated end-organs (Giacometti & Montagna 1968).

The statement has often been made that the sebaceous glands of the scalp are enlarged and overactive in common baldness, but planimetric studies (Rampini *et al.* 1968) have shown that during the course of baldness the total number of sebaceous glands decreases significantly.

The development of baldness is associated with shortening of the anagen phase of the hair cycle and consequently with an increase in the proportion of telogen hairs, which may be detected in trichograms of the frontovertical region before evident baldness is present (Rassner *et al.* 1963; Braun-Falco &

Christophers 1968; Vogelsberg *et al.* 1980). This is no doubt the explanation of the recorded differences in the force required to extract hairs from various regions of the adult male scalp (Light 1951).

The reduction in the size of the affected follicles, which is the essential feature of ordinary baldness, necessarily results in a reduction in the diameter of the hairs they produce. This reduction is said to be greater in women than in men (Silvestri 1967). The shaft diameter was found to be reduced in women with ordinary baldness also by Jackson *et al.* (1972). Normal subjects showed a symmetrical distribution of shaft diameters with a peak at 0·08 mm; the patients showed a wide spread of shaft diameters with peaks at 0.04 and 0.06 mm.

The studies of the shaft in common baldness show no abnormality on electronmicroscopy (Puccinelli *et al.* 1968) and preliminary studies show no abnormality in its chemical composition (Salamon 1971).

References

Allegra F. (1968) Histology and histochemical aspects of the hair follicles in pattern alopecia. In *Biopathology of Pattern Alopecia*, eds. A. Baccaradda-Boy, G. Moratti & J.R. Fray. Basel, Karger, p. 155.

Braun-Falco O. & Christophers E. (1968) Hair root patterns in male pattern alopecia. In *Biopathology of Pattern Alopecia*, eds. A. Baccaradda-Boy, G. Moratti & J.R. Fray. Basel, Karger, p. 141.

Cormia F.E. & Ernyey A. (1961) Circulatory changes in alopecia. Preliminary report with a summary of the cutaneous circulation of the normal scalp. *Archives of Dermatology*, **84**, 772.

Domnitz J.M. & Silvers D.N. (1979) Giant cells in male pattern alopecia—A histologic marker and pathogenic clue. *Journal of Cutaneous Pathology*, **6**, 108.

Garn S.M., Selby S. & Young R. (1954) Scalp thickness and the fat-loss theory of balding. *A.M.A. Archives of Dermatology and Syphilology*, **70**, 601.

Giacometti L. & Montagna W. (1968) The nerve fibres in male pattern alopecia. In *Biopathology of Pattern Alopecia*, eds. A. Baccaradda-Boy, G. Moratti & J.R. Fray. Basel, Karger, p. 208.

Goerttler K. (1965) *Der menschliche Glatze im Altersformwandel der behaarten Kopfhaut*. Stuttgart, Thieme.

Jackson D., Church R.E. & Ebling F.J. (1972) Hair diameter in female baldness. *British Journal of Dermatology*, **87**, 361.

Lattenand A. & Johnson W.C. (1975) Male pattern alopecia. A histopathologic and histochemical study. *Journal of Cutaneous Pathology*, **2**, 58.

Light A.F. (1951) Patterned loss of hair in man: pathogenesis and prognosis. *Annals of the New York Academy of Science*, **53**, 729.

Maguire H.C. & Kligman, A.M. (1962) The histopathology of common male baldness. *Proceedings of the XII International Congress of Dermatology, Washington*, p. 1438.

Montagna W. & Parakkal P.F. (1974) *The Structure and Function of Skin*, 3rd edn. New York, Academic Press, p. 247.

Puccinelli V.A., Caputo R. & Casinelli T. (1968) Electron microscopic study of the hair shaft in normal and alopecic subjects. In *Biopathology of Pattern Alopecia*, eds. A. Baccaradda-Boy, G. Moratti & J.R. Fray. Basel, Karger, p. 129.

Rampini E., Bertamino R. & Moretti G. (1968) Size and shape of sebaceous glands in male pattern alopecia. In *Biopathology of Pattern Alopecia*, eds. A. Baccaraddi-Boy, G. Moratti & J.R. Fray. Basel, Karger, p. 155.

Rassner, B., Zaun H. & Braun-Falco O. (1963) Zur Pathomechanismus der männliche Glatzenbildung. *Archiv für klinische und experimentelle Dermatologie*, **216**, 307.

Salamon T. (1971) Comparative chemical investigations on hair of various areas of the capillitium in subjects with 'normal' hair and with alopecia seborrhoeica. *Folia Medica Facultatis Medicinae Universitatis Saravenensis*, **5**, 241.

Silvestri U. (1967) Studio fisico del capello in casuistica de alopecia su base seborroica. *Archivio Italiano di Dermatologia, Venereologia e Sessuologia*, **34**, 405.

Singh M. & McKenzie J. (1961) The histology and histochemistry of the diseases of hairy and non hairy parts of the human skin with special reference to baldness. *Journal of Anatomy*, **95**, 569.

Vogelsberg H., Klarner W. & Rupec M. (1980) Einige Beobachfungen zur Frage der androgene-tischen Alopezie der Frau. *Zeitschrift für Hautkrankheiten*, **55**, 125.

Pathogenesis (references p. 103)

Hypotheses formerly accepted by some scientists, but now discarded, since they lack any support from irrefutable evidence, have been summarized in the introduction to this chapter. Our knowledge of the pathogenesis of ordinary baldness is still incomplete but reliable facts are steadily accumulating and a working hypothesis can be put forward with some confidence. It must be remembered that any hypothesis proposed to explain human baldness must also be applicable to the identical condition occurring in other primates.

Hamilton's (1942) classic investigation showed that no baldness developed in 10 eunuchoids, 10 men castrated before puberty and in 34 men who had undergone orchidectomy during adolescence. The expected incidence of bald-ness in these 54 adult men was about 40%. Common baldness developed in those individuals who were genetically so predisposed when testosterone was administered; when testosterone was discontinued the baldness did not progress but it was not reversed. Certain aspects of this work were confirmed in later publications (Hamilton 1948, 1960). No subsequent investigator has been able to challenge Hamilton's findings; indeed much work in man and other primates has established beyond doubt that ordinary baldness is androgen dependent.

The possibility that men who developed baldness might produce an excess of androgen was studied, but there has been no evidence of increased output of testicular or of adrenal androgen in bald men as compared with control subjects matched for age and race. Recent findings in 25 young men with common baldness confirmed the lack of correlation between the severity of this condition and serum androgen levels (Phillipou & Kirk 1981). However, the degree of baldness correlated with urinary levels of dihydroepiandrosterone and of tetrahydrocortisone. Many patients had mild hyperadrenal activity.

Studies in women with ordinary baldness have given conflicting results, but as technical procedures have improved and as more women have been adequately studied, it has become apparent that whilst a mild degree of baldness (Types II–IV) may occur in women with normal systemic androgen metabolism, more extensive baldness is usually (Apostolakis *et al.* 1965; Binazzi & Calandra

1968; Ludwig 1968; Kuhn 1972), probably always, associated with an increased output of ovarian or adrenal androgens, or both. Normal male levels of androgen are sufficient to make manifest the degree of baldness genetically determined for the individual. Normal female levels of androgen can induce baldness only in women who are heavily genetically predisposed. In a larger proportion in whom the genetic predisposition is less strong, baldness is manifest only when androgen production is increased, and the severity of the baldness is related to the degree to which the androgen output is raised. In this group of patients hirsutism and acne may also develop, but in the lower abnormal range the genotype influences the degree and pattern of hirsutism and at all levels the genotype determines the presence or absence of acne. In a third group of women even grossly abnormal levels of androgen cause no clinically significant baldness, although all such patients are necessarily hirsute. There is no evidence that the non-sexual hormones are in any way involved in causing ordinary baldness (Stüttgen & Goerz 1968), but the changes resulting from such states as hypothyroidism may of course occur in chance association with ordinary baldness.

Accepting that androgens are the initiating factor in ordinary baldness, it remains to consider by what mechanism they induce it.

The significance of sebum

Reference has been made to the many authors, of whom Sabouraud was the best known, who observed the association of the presence of sebum with baldness and who believed that microorganisms were concerned in the production of both these phenomena. The association of sebum and baldness is a valid observation, because like baldness sebaceous gland activity is androgen dependent (Hamilton 1942). In both sexes the bald scalp appears more greasy than the fully-haired scalp: the very common use of the term seborrhoeic alopecia as a synonym for ordinary baldness effectively illustrates the extent to which it has been assumed that the sebum in some way causes the hair loss. In fact gravimetric studies of the casual levels of sebum and the hourly production of sebum in the bald scalp and hairy scalp of balding men and of the scalp of fully haired controls showed no differences between these groups (Maibach *et al.* 1968). Their subjects were all male. No similar investigation appears to have been carried out in females, but it is probable that some balding women will show greater sebum output than non-bald controls, as an inevitable result of their raised androgen levels. However, it is clear that increased sebum output does not in itself result in hair loss, but is an associated androgen-dependent phenomenon.

As early as 1926 Eliassow suggested an abnormality in the composition of sebum might influence hair growth. Later workers (Bloom *et al.* 1955) could find no abnormality in the content of squalene or of free or esterified fatty acids in the sebum of balding subjects. More recently a number of investigators, e.g.

Kuchinska (1973), (reviewed by Thiele (1975)), have suggested that the auto-oxidation of hair lipids gives rise to substances which have depilatory activity. The evidence that such substances play any part in ordinary baldness is unconvincing. Kuchinska's (1967) observation that washing the hair appears to reduce the rate of hair loss for the subsequent 24 hours is readily explained by the fact that washing the hair removes club hairs nearing the end of normal telogen, and thus temporarily changes the trichograms and reduces physiological hair-fall for a few days (see p. 13). Moreover, if auto-oxidation products are depilatory why do they act only on certain follicles?

The metabolism of the hair follicles

The weight of evidence strongly supports the opinion that the essential inherited factor responsible for ordinary baldness concerns the manner in which certain follicles in the frontovertical region of the scalp respond to androgens. However, regional variations in the metabolism of testosterones by hair follicles do not adequately explain observed differences in androgen-mediated hair growth (Schwiekert & Wilson 1974). Reviewing the now very extensive literature on this subject Montagna & Parrakal (1974) suggest that the initial stage in the process of balding is probably the accumulation in the condemned follicles of 5α dihydrotestosterone. This is the tissue-active androgen which activates sebaceous glands but inhibits the metabolism of hair follicles (Adachi 1973). The conversion of testosterone to dihydrotestosterone (DHT) is catalysed by 5α reductase, but Adachi has shown that it is not this enzyme which controls the conversion. What factors exert this control, and what mechanisms are involved after the accumulation of DHT remains to be established. The findings in published investigations offer abundant material for speculation, but are to some extent contradictory (Allegra *et al.* 1970; Fazekas & Sandor 1973; Crovato *et al.* 1973). The clinical observation that a depressive illness may advance the onset of androgen-induced cutaneous changes in the genetically predisposed (see p. 75) cannot yet be satisfactorily explained.

References

Adachi K. (1973) The metabolism and control mechanism of human hair follicles. *Common Problems in Dermatology*, **5**, 37.

Allegra F., Giacometti L., Uno H. & Adachi K. (1970) Studies of common baldness in the stump-tailed *Macaque*. III. DNA synthesis in regressing hair. *Acta Dermato-Venereologica*, **50**, 169.

Apostolakis M., Ludwig E. & Voigt K.-D. (1965) Testosteron-Oestrogen, und Gonadotropenausscheidung bei diffuser unerblicher Alopecia. *Klinische Wochenschrift*, **43**, 9.

Binazzi M. & Calandra P. (1968) Testosterone elimination in female patients with acne, chronic alopecia and hirsutism. *Italian General Review of Dermatology*, **8**, 241.

Bloom R.E., Woods S. & Nicolaides N. (1955) Hair fat composition in early male pattern alopecia. *Journal of Investigative Dermatology*, **24**, 97.

Crovato F., Moretti G. & Butamino R. (1973) 17 Betahydroxysteroid dehydrogenases in hair

follicles of normal and bald scalp. A histochemical study. *Journal of Investigative Dermatology*,
    60, 126.

Eliassow A. (1926) Cholesterinstoffwechsel und Haarwuchs. *Dermatologische Wochenschrift*, **83**,
    1463.

Fazekas A.G. & Sandor T. (1973) The metabolism of dehydroepiandrosterone by human scalp hair
    follicles. *Journal of Clinical Endocrinology*, **36**, 582.

Hamilton J.B. (1942) Male hormone stimulation is prerequisite and an incitement in common
    baldness. *American Journal of Anatomy*, **71**, 451.

Hamilton J.B. (1948) The role of testosterone secretions as indicated by the effect of castration in
    man and by studies of pathological conditions and the short life-span associated with maleness.
    Recent Progress in Hormone Research, **3**, 257.

Hamilton J.B. (1960) Effect of castration in adolescent and young adult males upon further
    changes in the proportions of bare and hairy scalp. *Journal of Clinical Endocrinology*, **20**, 1309.

Kuchinska R. (1967) Die Beinflüssung des Haarausfalls durch Kosmetische Präparate. *Kosme-
    tischen Monatschrift*, **16**, 12.

Kuchinska R. (1973) Chemische Aspekte des Haarausfalls and ihre kosmetologischen Bedeutung.
    Kosmetologie, **5**, 177.

Kuhn B.H. (1972) Male pattern alopecias and/or androgenic hirsutism in females. Part III.
    Definition and etiology. *Journal of the American Medical Women's Association*, **27**, 357.

Ludwig E. (1968) The role of sexual hormones in pattern alopecia. In *Biopathology of Pattern
    Alopecia*, eds. A. Baccaradda-Boy, G. Moratti & J.R. Fray. Basel, Karger, p. 50.

Maibach H.I., Feldman R., Payne B. & Hutshell T. (1968) Scalp and forehead sebum production in
    male pattern alopecia. In *Biopathology of Pattern Alopecia*, eds. A. Baccaradda-Boy, G. Moratti &
    J.R. Fray. Basel, Karger, p. 171.

Montagna W. & Parakkal P.F. (1974) *The Structure and Function of Skin*, 3rd edn. New York,
    Academic Press.

Papa C.M. & Kligman A.M. (1965) Stimulation of hair growth by topical application of androgens.
    Journal of the American Medical Association, **191**, 521.

Phillipou G. & Kirk J. (1981) Significance of steroid measurements in male pattern alopecia. *Clinical
    and Experimental Dermatology*, **6**, 53.

Savin R.C. (1968) The ineffectiveness of testosterone in male pattern baldness. *Archives of
    Dermatology*, **98**, 512.

Schwiekert H.U. & Wilson J.D. (1974) Regulation of human hair growth by steroid hormones. I.
    Testosterone metabolism in isolated hairs. *Journal of Clinical Endocrinology*, **38**, 811.

Stüttgen G. & Goerz G. (1968) Non sexual hormones and male pattern alopecia. In *Biopathology of
    Pattern Alopecia*. Basel, Karger, p. 61.

Thiele F.A.J. (1975) Chemical aspects of hair loss and its cosmetological significance. *British
    Journal of Dermatology*, **92**, 355.

Clinical features (reference p. 110)

Until further genetic studies have clarified the situation ordinary baldness of
early and of late onset are regarded as variants of a single clinical syndrome. The
very high incidence of some degree of common baldness, and the great frequency
of many disorders of hair growth, in particular the temporary and reversible
disturbances of the hair cycle, inevitably results in the frequent fortuitous
association of one or more disorders with common baldness.

The essential clinical feature of common baldness in both sexes is the replacement of terminal hairs by progressively finer hairs, which are eventually very short and virtually unpigmented. This process may begin at any age after puberty and may become clinically apparent by the age of 17 in the normal male and by 25 to 30 in the endocrinologically normal female. The reduction in the size of the follicles is accompanied by shortening of anagen and therefore necessarily by increased shedding of telogen hairs. This shedding often attracts the patient's attention and induces him or her to seek advice. The replacement of terminal by smaller hairs occurs characteristically in a distinctive pattern, which spares the posterior and lateral scalp margins, even in the most advanced cases, and even in old age. The sequence of patterns in the male has been well described by Hamilton (see Fig. 4.5). Bitemporal recession is followed by balding of the vertex. Eventually more uniform frontal recession joins the bald areas and the entire frontovertical region bears only inconspicuous secondary vellus hair, which may also finally be lost. Variations in the pattern are governed at least in part by genetic factors, as can be confirmed in any collection of family portraits. The rate of progression too is probably determined largely by heredity; however, in the absence of evidence it would be wrong to exclude the possible influence of other factors.

The use of the term 'male pattern alopecia' must be held partly responsible for the frequent failure to appreciate that in its earlier stages common baldness in women need not conform to the 'male pattern'. As in the male, increased shedding of telogen hairs accompanies the reduction of shaft diameter, but the follicles first affection are more widely distributed over the frontovertical region. As a result many secondary vellus hairs are interspersed with hairs still normal, and others only slightly reduced in diameter. Partial baldness is sometimes first apparent on the vertex, but is more commonly diffusely distributed over the frontovertical region. Hair loss in this pattern has been regarded as a distinct entity (Guy & Edmundson 1960) often known as 'chronic diffuse alopecia'. We entirely agree with those authors (Maguire & Kligman 1963; Ludwig 1964; Vadasz & Debreczeni 1967) that the most frequent presentation of common baldness in women is as a diffuse alopecia. Ludwig (1977) has classified the succession of patterns occurring in women confirming the distinctive clinical features of 'female pattern alopecia' (Fig. 4.6, p. 97).

In women who are endocrinologically normal the rate of progression of common baldness is usually very slow, but nevertheless a severe degree of baldness, though still 'diffuse', may be present by the 7th decade. However, many women with ordinary baldness, particularly if it is of early onset, produce an excess of testosterone (Pierard *et al.* 1968). According to their genetic constitution this may give rise to hirsutism and/or recurrence or aggravation of existing acne or to no detectable abnormality other than the baldness. The entire clinical spectrum is seen according to the degree of androgenic stimulation and the capacity of follicles and sebaceous glands to respond to it. As a result of the

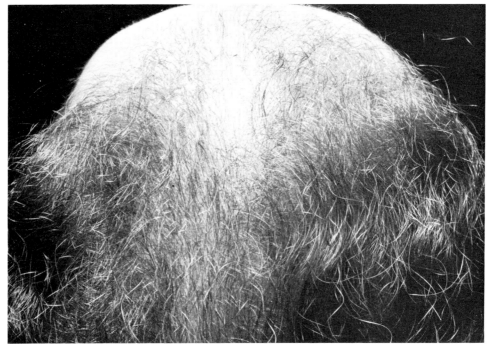

Fig. 4.7. Male pattern baldness in a woman with an ovarian tumour (John Radcliffe Hospital).

physiological response of the sebaceous glands to androgen a complaint of
increasing greasiness of the scalp is often made by women with common
baldness (Fig. 4.9). In all women with common baldness of rapid onset, even if it
be an isolated abnormality, and in women with common baldness of gradual
onset but accompanied by menstrual disturbance, hirsutism or recrudescence of
acne, a full medical history and examination are essential, and in many cases
endocrinological investigation is desirable. We have observed baldness of Type
IV in women without hirsutism. More extensive baldness (Types V–VIII) is
always accompanied by hirsutism and we have seen only once baldness of Type
VIII, in a woman grossly masculinized by an ovarian tumour (Fig. 4.7).

Diagnosis (references p. 110)

In the male over 25 the characteristic pattern of the baldness usually makes
diagnosis a simple matter, provided that the possible coexistence of hair loss of a
different type is constantly borne in mind. Such a possibility is suggested by a
history of recent rapid deterioration. It is frequently necessary to see the patient
on several occasions over a period of some weeks before a definite conclusion can
be reached, and investigations to exclude the known causes of diffuse hair loss (p.

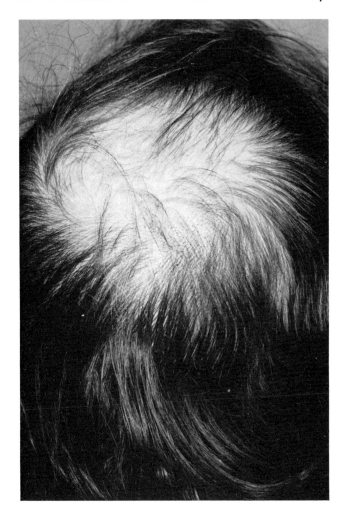

Fig. 4.8. Androgenetic alopecia of well over 20 years' duration in a woman aged 60 (Addenbrooke's Hospital, Cambridge).

120) may be required. It should also be remembered that balding men are not immune to syphilis or to alopecia areata.

In the younger male, the diagnosis may be difficult. He often complains principally not of baldness, but of increased shedding, particularly when he washes his hair. In such patients it is not always easy to determine whether shedding is really excessive or whether introspection born of depression has made him abnormally apprehensive of physiological shedding. Sometimes he may complain of baldness which is not evident to the observer. Such patients should not be dismissed with casual reassurance, but should be re-examined at intervals, after a detailed medical and social history has been taken. A strong family history may support a diagnosis of common baldness, but the absence of such a history does not exclude the diagnosis. The presence or absence of

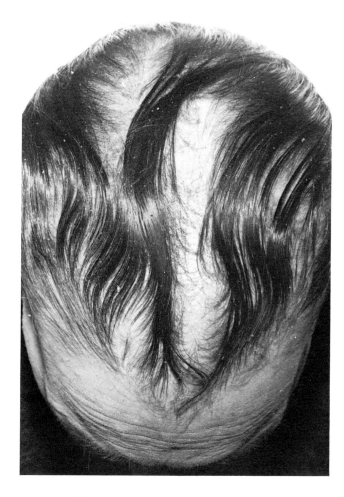

Fig. 4.9. Androgenetic alopecia in a woman accompanied
by gross seborrhoea (Addenbrooke's Hospital, Cam-
bridge).

seborrhoea is not of diagnostic significance, for this is a genetic variable, and
seborrhoea is evidence merely of normal sexual maturation in a susceptible
subject.

A small but distinctive group of young adult males present a history of
increased shedding of head hair and also some loss of body hair in particular
pubic hair. The patient is usually depressed and gives a history of recent severe
stress. He may also complain of loss of libido and of partial impotence. Sometimes
the distribution of subcutaneous fat approaches the female pattern. Serum
prolactin is elevated (p. 87).

In women, the diagnosis of common baldness may be difficult. In all cases it
should be regarded as one of three cutaneous manifestations of androgenic
stimulation and the presence of acne and/or of hirsutism should be noted. In the
presence of such changes endocrinological assessment may be desirable. In their

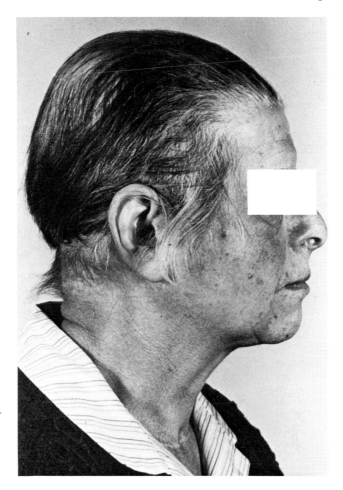

Fig. 4.10. Androgenetic alopecia in the male pattern in a woman with elevated plasma testosterone (Slade Hospital, Oxford).

absence, particularly if there is a strong family history of baldness, the diagnosis may present no problems. However, the most frequent presentation is as a diffuse fronto-vertical thinning; the patient may volunteer the information that her hair has become finer and greasier. As in men the association of common baldness with other forms of hair loss is frequently encountered, and many cases require careful evaluation over a period of weeks. An accurate diagnosis is of importance in prognosis, and at times a biopsy may be useful.

References
Braun-Falco O. & Zaun H. (1962) Zum Wesen des chronischer diffuser Alopecie bei Frauen. *Archiv für klinische und experimentelle Dermatologie,* **215,** 165.
Guy W.B. & Edmundson W.F. (1960) Diffuse cyclic hair loss in women. *Archives of Dermatology,* **81,** 205.
Ludwig E. (1964) Die androgenetische Alopecie bei der Frau. *Archiv für klinische und experimentelle Dermatologie,* **219,** 558.

Ludwig E. (1977) Classification of the types of androgenic alopecia (common baldness) occurring in the female sex. *British Journal of Dermatology*, **97**, 247.

Maguire H.C. & Kligman A.M. (1963) Common baldness in women. *Geriatrics*, **18**, 329.

Pierard J., Kint A. & de J. Backer (1968) Sur le role probable de l'hormone male dans l'alopécie féminine. *Archives Belges de Dermatologie et Syphiligraphie*, **24**, 409.

Vadasz E. & Debreczeni M. (1967) Untersuchungen zur Ätiologie der androgenetischen Alopecie der Frau. *Hautarzt*, **18**, 454.

Treatment (references p. I I 2)

Effective treatment which will at least prevent the further transformation of terminal into vellus hair can be offered to many of the women in whom the additional severity of their baldness, beyond the physiological level, is the result of abnormal androgen metabolism. The available procedures, surgical and medical, are discussed below.

In men, and in the many older women, in whom the baldness is a natural consequence of their genetic make-up, and who are endocrinologically normal, no specific treatment is available. Each patient needs careful medical assessment to ensure that the diagnosis is beyond doubt. He or she should then be given a detailed explanation of the nature and significance of common baldness. Most men, if they are mildly affected, will accept the situation philosophically. Many, however, when baldness first becomes manifest at a stressful stage of their career, may attempt to lay the blame for any lack of success, socially or at work, on their baldness, even when this is of minimal extent. Such patients should be encouraged to discuss their problems in full. In the course of doing so they often become aware that they have not seen their baldness in its proper perspective, and are soon enabled to do so. However, in some patients this lack of perspective is only one of many manifestations of a depressive illness which may require treatment.

Surgery

There are some men however, who, because of the nature of their occupations, for example as entertainers or as salesmen, reasonably regard their baldness as a considerable disability. For such patients hair transplantation deserves serious consideration. One study of 50 patients who had undergone hair transplants (Clabaugh *et al.* 1973) showed that as compared with control subjects they were vain and assertive and mildly antisocial. Six would have been excluded from operation had they been tested earlier, but they had presented no special problems post-operatively. Our experience suggests, nevertheless, that patients for operation should be very carefully selected. The operation is expensive, and its results, especially in the long term, are not invariably entirely satisfactory. The patient whose real problem is his personality, rather than his baldness, should not be accepted.

Surgical treatment involves the transplantation to the bald areas of multiple small full thickness grafts from those areas of scalp still bearing predominantly terminal hairs (Orentreich 1959; Ayers 1964; Friedrich 1970). The success of the procedure depends on proper selection of patients, and on the skill and experience of the operator. Reported complications include infection, bleeding, fistula formation and scarring (Lepaw 1973). An excellent practical account of the technique is given by Unger (1978).

Wigs

In women the baldness is usually too diffuse for transplantation surgery to be feasible. If the hair loss is extensive, only a wig will conceal it.

There are various procedures by which small wigs are interwoven with presenting terminal hair; the cosmetic result is sometimes satisfactory. The patient who seeks advice from his doctor before embarking on some such procedure should be assessed in the same way as the patient considering surgery—is his baldness really his problem? If it is, he should be advised to obtain from the firm he intends to employ a written statement of the probable cost of the initial procedure and of subsequent regular maintenance. Tension on the patient's surviving terminal hair has occasionally led to patchy scarring alopecia (Perlstein 1969).

Topical applications

There is no topical application, chemical or physical (e.g. ultraviolet or other radiation, or massage) which has been proved to alter the long-term course of ordinary baldness. However, a lotion containing 0.025% 17α oestradiol reduced the proportion of telogen hairs in 63% of patients and therefore reduced the rate of hair shedding; it did not result in the regrowth of hair (Orfanos & Vogels 1980).

The claim that topical testosterone induced the growth of terminal hairs in bald scalp (Papa & Kligman 1965) has not been confirmed (Savin 1968). Many different stimuli will induce temporary growth of certain resting follicles in some subjects, raising hopes which are false, for no cosmetically useful recovery occurs.

Conclusions

The patient who appears to have common baldness should not be dismissed with the summary statement that nothing can be done for him. The accuracy of the diagnosis should be established beyond doubt and any associated disorders of hair growth should be treated. He should receive a full explanation, and be helped to identify and face up to his problems.

If he also has seborrhoea or pityriasis capitis (p. 451) these should be controlled.

References

Ayers S. (1964) Conservative surgical management of male pattern baldness. *Archives of Dermatology*, **90**, 492.

Clabaugh W., Norwood O'T. & Pearson J. (1973) Personality studies in patients receiving hair transplants for treatment of male pattern baldness. *Cutis*, **12**, 113.

Friedrich H.C. (1970) Indikation und Technik der operativ-plastischer Behandlung des Haarverlustes. *Hautarzt*, **21**, 197.

Lepaw M.I. (1973) Hair implant complications. *Cutis*, **11**, 88.

Orentreich N. (1959) Autografts in alopecias and other selected dermatological conditions. *Annals of the New York Academy of Sciences*, **83**, 463.

Orfanos C.E. & Vogels L. (1980) Lokeltherapie der Alopecia androgenetica mit 17α Oestradiol. *Dermatologica*, **161**, 124.

Papa C.M. & Kligman A.M. (1965) Stimulation of hair growth by topical applications of androgen. *Journal of the American Medical Association*, **191**, 521.

Perlstein H.H. (1969) Traction alopecia due to hair weaving. *Cutis*, **5**, 440.

Savin R.C. (1968) The ineffectiveness of testosterone in male pattern baldness. *Archives of Dermatology*, **98**, 512.

Unger W. (1978) *Hair Transplantation*. Basle, Dekker.

Treatment of androgenetic cutaneous changes with cyproterone acetate (references p. 114)

The anti-androgen cyproterone acetate was synthesized in 1953 by Wiechert. Its antiandrogenic activity was demonstrated in experimental animals and it was used initially in the treatment of male sexual offenders. (For a summary of the history of the early trials of this drug see Hammerstein and Cupceancu 1969). Since 1969 the drug has been used extensively in the treatment of androgenetic cutaneous changes in women. It is given to women in whom such changes occur in the absence of any significant elevation of the parameters of androgen metabolism, to the much more uncommon patients in whom the non-specific elevation of these parameters leads them to be included with the first group in the category 'idiopathic hirsutism', and also to women with the polycystic ovary syndrome. Cyproterone blocks the binding of testosterone by target-cell receptors; it also has a progestational effect and it inhibits the gonadotropic effect in the anterior pituitary.

The first series of cases of hirsutism to be treated with cyproterone acetate (Hammerstein & Cupceancu 1969) consisted of 49 women, who were given cyproterone acetate 100–200 mg from the 5th to the 14th day of the menstrual cycle combined with 50 μg ethinyl oestradiol from the 5th to the 25th day. Three-quarters of the women experienced a significant reduction in hirsutism, and acne and seborrhoea were promptly and effectively controlled. There was little effect on alopecia. Lassitude and some loss of libido were occasional side effects. Similar results were obtained by Dewhurst *et al.* (1977).

Ebling *et al.* (1977) studied one patient quantitatively. Her sebaceous secretion rate fell after two cycles of treatment from over 3 mg/10 cm^2/hour to below 1.5 mg.

Both growth rate and shaft diameter of hair on her thighs were reduced.

Other investigators have also obtained improvement in hirsutism and acne in 66–75% of women treated, but no consistent endocrinological differences have been established between those women who responded and those who did not (Hammerstein 1975).

Recent trials have confirmed the highest success rates in acne and hirsutism, but the response to androgenetic alopecia is also great enough in many women to give marked clinical benefit. The rate of telogen shedding is reduced and in some cases there is some regrowth of terminal hair. The reduced greasiness of the scalp contributes to the improvement, for it improves the texture of the hair and makes it easier to control (Anderson & Browning 1978; Ekoe *et al.* 1980, Peereboom-Wynia & Bockhorst 1980). The maximum reduction of sebaceous activity is achieved within 3 months, but maximum reduction in the hirsutism is not achieved until after 6–8 months of treatment.

Administration of cyproterone acetate in the lower dose of 2 mg with ethinyl oestradiol 50 µg daily from the 5th to the 25th days of the cycle for a period of 12 months (Schmidt-Elmandorff & Steyer 1977) also brought about a marked improvement in acne, seborrhoea and hirsutism. The highest rates of improvement were recorded in the more severe cases; hirsutism improved in 37.4% of mild cases but in 60.9% of severe cases. Maximum improvement in hirsutism was observed only after 10 months' treatment. The response of the hirsutism to the 100 mg dose of cyproterone appears to be more rapid (Braendl *et al.* 1974), but further studies are required, particularly in relation to the incidence of side effects in the low- and high-dose regimes. Kaiser *et al.* (1976) used the low-dosage regime with similar good results. They found that in a few refractory cases it was an advantage to give 50 mg additional cyproterone acetate for the first 10 days of each treatment cycle.

After a year or more, when the treatment is discontinued, a rebound relapse is liable to occur. Kaiser *et al.* (1976) suggest that this can be avoided by giving a non-androgenic progestogen for at least 3–6 months; megestrol acetate 2 × 0.35 mg daily is recommended.

Side effects
Side effects are most frequent and most severe during the first 3 months of treatment. During the subsequent months of treatment many will lessen or disappear. The most frequent side effects are dysmenorrhoea, breast tenderness, headache and decreased libido.

More serious side effects, such as thrombophlebitis, are rare. Hepatitis is uncommon, but liver function tests at intervals are desirable.

The manufacturers know of no cases in which the combination of oestradiol and cyproterone acetate have failed to act as an effective contraceptive, but nevertheless it is wise to employ other methods of contraception during the first two or three treatment cycles.

Contraindications

These are essentially the same as for the contraceptive hormones. The cyproterone regimes should be avoided in the obese, or hypertensive, in the heavy smoker or with any history of thrombophlebitis.

References

Anderson J.A.R. & Browning M.C.K. (1978) An assessment of (1) cyproterone acetate and (2) ethinyl oestradiol and lynoestrenol (Minilyn) in the treatment of idiopathic hirsutism. *British Journal of Dermatology*, **99**, 545.

Braendl W., Boess H., Buckwoldt M., Leven C. & Bellendorf G. (1974) Wirkung und neben Wirkung von Cyproterone acetat. *Archiv für Gynäkologie*, **216**, 335.

Dewhurst C.J., Underhill R., Goldman S. & Mansfield M. (1977) The treatment of hirsutism with cyproterone acetate (an anti-androgen). *British Journal of Obstetrics and Gynaecology*, **84**, 119.

Ebling F.J., Thomas A.K., Cooke I.D., Randall V.A., Skinner J. & Cawood M. (1977) Effect of cyproterone acetate on hair growth, sebaceous secretion and endocrine parameters in a hirsute subject. *British Journal of Dermatology*, **97**, 371.

Ekoe T.M., Burchardt P. & Reredi B. (1980) Treatment of hirsutism, acne and alopecia with cyproterone acetate. *Dermatologica*, **160**, 338.

Hammerstein J. (1978) Endocrinological findings in hirsute women with equivalent response to treatment with cyproterone acetate and ethinyl oestradiol. *Acta Endocrinologica*, **78**, Suppl. 193, 100.

Hammerstein J. & Cupceancu B. (1969) Behandlung des Hirsutismus mit Cyproteronacetat. *Deutsche medizinische Wochenschrift*, **94**, 829.

Kaiser E., Loch E.G., Winckelmann G., Schröpl F., Dietz M. & Hartmann P. (1976) Behandlung mit antiandrogen bei der Frau. *Die Medizinische Welt*, **27**, 1863.

Peereboom-Wynia J.D.R. & Bockhurst J.C. (1980) Effect of cyproterone acetate orally on hair density and diameter and endocrine factors in women with idiopathic hirsutism. *Dermatologica*, **160**, 7.

Schmidt-Elmendorff H. & Steyer N. (1977) Klinische Erfahrungen mit einen niedrig dosienter Antiandrogen (Cyproteronacetate) und Äthinylöstradiol bei Frauen mit Viriliseinenperschinungen. *Geburtshilfe und Frauenheilklinik*, **37**, 297.

Treatment with cimetidine

Cimetidine blocks androgen receptors. It has been used in the treatment of androgenetic cutaneous changes. It does not affect serum androgen levels or the levels of urinary excretion of 17 oxosteroids. Cimetidine 300 mg was given five times each day for 3 months to five severely hirsute women: four with polycystic ovaries and one with 'idiopathic' hirsutism (Vigorsky *et al.* 1980). In four of the patients there was a reduction rate of hair growth of $64 \pm 11\%$. There were no side effects. This treatment requires further evaluation.

Reference

Vigorsky R.A., Mehlman I., Glass A.R. & Smith C.E. (1980) Treatment of hirsute women with cimetidine. *New England Journal of Medicine*, **303**, 1042.

Chapter 5
Diffuse Alopecia: Endocrine, Metabolic and Chemical Influences on the Follicular Cycle

History and Nomenclature
(References p. 122)

The diffuse shedding of hair has been often referred to as 'symptomatic alopecia', or, by older authors, as defluvium capillorum. However, some authors, e.g. Sabouraud (1932), restricted the latter term to sudden diffuse loss of hair following shortly after a severe emotional shock, and others have applied it to all forms of alopecia.

Kligman (1961), in a lucid and influential article, studied the pathodynamics of one common pattern of response of hair follicles to a variety of insults and named it telogen effluvium. Kligman cannot be held responsible for the frequent misuse of this term by some authors.

During the 1950s many authors described 'chronic diffuse alopecia' in women (e.g. Sulzberger *et al.* 1960). This syndrome was differentiated from acute diffuse reversible alopecia, attributable in most cases to a readily identifiable cause. We agree with Ludwig (1966–7) and others who find that the majority of such patients have common (androgenetic) baldness, undiagnosed because of the misleading use of the term 'male pattern alopecia'.

We are here concerned with the clinical syndrome of diffuse alopecia in either sex. Many of the conditions which can give rise to the various forms of the syndrome are discussed in greater detail in other chapters.

Pathogenesis

The daily shedding of telogen hairs diffusely distributed over the scalp is a physiological process. The follicles which have shed their hairs normally re-enter anagen, and the trichogram remains unchanged and no alopecia results. If, however, a significant number of hair follicles prematurely enter catagen and thence telogen, the excessive shedding of hair inevitably takes place some 2–3 months later: the hair is temporarily sparse but regrows normally if the insult is not repeated. This is the mechanism of 'telogen effluvium', which may be induced by childbirth, high fever, haemorrhage, sudden starvation, accidental or surgical trauma, severe emotional stress, and by certain drugs.

The sudden diffuse shedding of telogen hairs is one of the responses of the hair follicles to the unknown insult or insults of alopecia areata (p. 291).

Follicles which shed their hairs at the end of a normal telogen may temporarily fail to re-enter anagen. Diffuse thinning of the scalp hair then develops slowly in the absence of any increase in the rate of hair shedding. This form of diffuse alopecia is seen in iron deficiency (Quinones & Garcia Munoz 1963; Aquilera Maruri 1966). Malnutrition, whether primary or secondary, is accompanied by diffuse shedding of telogen hairs, usually in association with changes in shaft diameter and in pigmentation (see p. 127). The mechanism of hair loss in hypothyroidism and hypopituitarism may well be similar, but has not been adequately studied (see p. 126). The metabolic disturbances that accompany severe impairment of liver function may be associated with increased shedding of telogen hairs (Zaun *et al.* 1969).

The gross metabolic disturbance following resection of a large part of the liver for a massive hepatoma was associated with severe alopecia. In one such case (Starzl *et al.* 1975) hair loss developed within a few days post-operatively. The liver gradually regenerated, and the hair regrew in 9 months.

Hair loss in patients with malignant disease has been relatively little investigated by modern methods; it is diffuse, with increased shedding of telogen hair. It was formerly attributed to a hypothetical 'cancer toxin', but it may well be the result of iron deficiency or hypoproteinaemia. Alopecia has occurred as an early sign of Hodgkin's disease (Klein *et al.* 1973).

The problem of so-called idiopathic chronic diffuse alopecia in women has already been mentioned. Most such women have ordinary baldness, periods of progression of which are always preceded and accompanied by increased shedding of telogen hairs (p. 102). It is perhaps necessary to remember, however, that as common baldness is common in many races, it frequently occurs in association with hair loss of other origins. Multifactorial alopecia is often encountered (Steigleder & Mahrle 1973) and a double or even a treble diagnosis is appropriate.

Diffuse alopecia caused by drugs or other chemicals has been considered in some detail on pp. 133–141 and will here be discussed only as a problem in differential diagnosis.

The role of psychological factors in diffuse alopecia is very difficult to assess. There is circumstantial evidence that acute stress may precipitate acute reversible hair loss (Sabouraud 1932; Kligman 1961) but the relationship of the patient's psychological state to chronic diffuse alopecia is controversial. Androgenetic common baldness in women may be associated with depression (Eckert 1975); the patient may blame the alopecia for the depression, but in our experience there are patients in whom depression antedates or exactly coincides with the onset of alopecia (see p. 175). Depression may of course lead a patient to become aware of and concerned about hair shedding of physiological degree.

The association of alopecia with organic lesions of the central nervous system has been the subject of many case reports, but no consistent picture emerges. Head injuries, particularly in children, have been followed by diffuse alopecia, often associated with reversible hirsutism, which may be asymmetrical (Tarnow 1971). Total alopecia has been seen in association with postencephalitic damage to the brain stem, and with a glioma of the hypothalamus (Hoff & Riehl 1937–8). Recurrent annual hair loss in a patient with syringo-encephalia and syringobulbia remains mysterious (Mikula & Steidl 1961). Our almost complete ignorance of the effects of the central nervous system on hair growth is further emphasized by the report of frequent episodes of generalized piloerection in a patient with a deep parietal glioblastoma (Brody *et al.* 1960).

Incidence

The incidence of diffuse alopecia is high in both sexes, but most episodes of increased shedding are transitory and cause little or no concern. Shedding whether acute or chronic which leads to a significant degree of baldness is also common and although large numbers of such patients are referred to dermatologists these represent only a small proportion of those affected, many of whom do not even consult their own doctors. Hospital statistics are therefore biased, but no others are available.

Alexander (1965) studied 98 women with diffuse alopecia, excluding cases in which the hair loss was of 'male pattern'. She found that the alopecia had followed fever in 10, childbirth in 10, and was a manifestation of alopecia areata in 9. Drugs were incriminated in 5 cases. External trauma from self-inflicted cosmetic procedures was involved in no fewer than 36 cases, and in an additional 6 the physical or chemical trauma had been inflicted by hairdressers. In 5 the alopecia was associated with anaemia and in 1 case it was caused by syphilis. Sixteen patients remained unclassified. Bergfeld (1978) confirmed the importance of trauma. Patchy baldness with broken hairs and eventually some scarring may be produced by the excessively frequent application of hair dyes over a long period (Brown & Brayles 1980).

Eckert and her colleagues (1967) excluded cases of alopecia areata from their series of 150 women with diffuse alopecia. They found 7 patients with alopecia of the male pattern. Cosmetic trauma was the cause of the hair loss in 11, and 7 had seborrhoeic dermatitis and 2 had ichthyosis involving the scalp. In 14 the alopecia had followed parturition, in 4 it was post-febrile. Two patients had systemic lupus erythematosus and 8 were iron deficient. In 6 cases amphetamines were incriminated. Endocrine disorders were present in 21 cases; hypothyroidism in 16, hyperthyroidism in 2, and hypopituitarism in 3. Three patients developed alopecia after oophorectomy, but, as the authors point out, there is no evidence that the menopause is a factor in diffuse alopecia. In no fewer than 68 patients no associated factors, local or systemic, could be found.

In these papers the number of cases in which no cause for the alopecia was evident ranged from 16% to over 45%. In over 350 cases of diffuse alopecia in women at Cambridge more than 60% had the diffuse type of common baldness (see p. 105 for diagnostic criteria). In 5% no cause whatsoever could be established, but many of these cases may well also have had common baldness.

The scarcity of publications on diffuse alopecia in men is due to the fact that the large proportion who have common baldness are readily recognized as such, although sometimes only tardily in young men who present with diffuse shedding and have as yet no patterned baldness. After common baldness the most frequent causes of diffuse alopecia in young males are alopecia areata, fevers and drugs, and in older males drugs and malignant disease.

Aetiology

Post-febrile alopecia (Fig. 5.1)
It is said that the fever must exceed 39°C (Sabouraud 1932) and in our experience it is usually above this figure. In the days before antibiotics typhoid and tuberculosis were the classical causes. Recurrent bouts of fever have a more marked effect than a single bout, for each damages follicles at the same susceptible stage of their cycles. Fever of any origin has a similar effect; diffuse alopecia may follow febrile episodes in ulcerative colitis (Schwenzner & Walther 1961) and we have seen it after influenza, malaria, glandular fever, pneumonia and brucellosis. Erysipelas which involves the scalp may lead to early shedding of hair from the affected region and more delayed loss from the remainder of the scalp (Sabouraud 1932). Post-febrile alopecia begins 8–10 weeks after the first damaging bout of fever; it may be severe but is never total. Full recovery is the rule, but is not invariable particularly when the fever has been prolonged or recurrent (Alexander 1965).

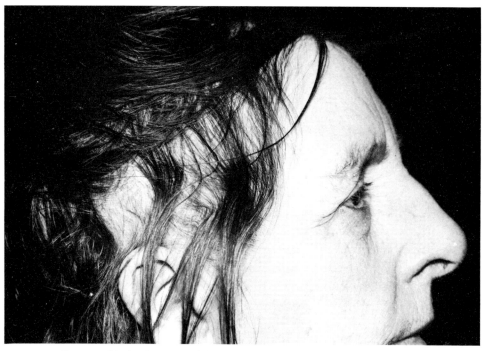

Fig. 5.1. Diffuse postfebrile alopecia (Addenbrooke's Hospital, Cambridge).

Post-partum alopecia

Some postpartum increase in hair loss is probably constant, but hair loss sufficient to cause anxiety to the patient is not uncommon, and occasionally quite severe alopecia may occur. The increased loss of hair becomes obvious 1 month after childbirth in some women but only after 2–3 months in the majority, and may occasionally be delayed until after 4 months (Schiff & Kern 1963; Skelton 1966). For unknown reasons the loss is usually most marked in the frontal and temporal regions, but may be generalized; it is never total. Full spontaneous recovery takes 3–12 months.

Drug-induced alopecia (see also p. 133)

In the presence of diffuse alopecia a careful history of all recent medication is essential, and the possibility of industrial or accidental exposure to chemicals must be considered. Microscopy of shed and growing hairs may reveal the type of injury to the follicles and thus help to incriminate a particular type of chemical.

Stress-induced alopecia

Many patients with chronic diffuse alopecia will attempt to correlate periods of increased shedding with emotional stress, but the association is difficult to prove.

Acute episodes of shedding following 2–3 months after acute stress are, however, less suspect; we have seen such hair loss in several young women who had been passengers on a disturbing flight from London to the Far East.

Severe hair loss beginning 2 weeks after severe stress, and tending to become total, as reported by Sabouraud (1932) and other authors, requires further study; some at least of such cases may be alopecia areata.

The telogen shedding of early common baldness if associated with depression, and more particularly with gain in weight and menstrual irregularities, requires careful investigation (p. 105).

Alopecia and food deprivation

Alopecia and the other hair changes associated with primary or secondary malnutrition are not easily overlooked. Acute voluntary starvation in young women is common and may be overlooked as a cause of hair loss. Obese adolescents sometimes inflict upon themselves a diet of salads and fruit, even when they do not have anorexia nervosa. In 20 obese patients on a total fast or on a 200 calorie diet, oedema, hair loss and weakness were noted, but not when small amounts of protein were taken (Rooth & Carlström 1970).

Hypoprotinaemia

Hypoprotinaemia of metabolic as well as of dietary origin may lead to the premature onset of telogen in some follicles. This possibly accounts for the temporary diffuse loss of hair which may follow blood loss, including voluntary blood donation.

Iron deficiency

Iron deficiency, even in the absence of anaemia, may be a factor in diffuse alopecia, but it is a common condition and its fortuitous association with common baldness is therefore to be expected. However, if iron deficiency is discovered it should be treated and its cause should be established.

Alopecia in hypothyroidism

The hair may gradually become dry, and diffusely sparse. The diagnosis is suspected on account of other signs or symptoms of thyroid deficiency and confirmed by estimation of serum thyroxin. Full recovery of the hair may take place with adequate replacement therapy, but is not invariable. If the hypothyroid state has been of long duration some follicles are likely to have been destroyed. Moreover, the presence of hypothyroidism does not of course exclude common baldness.

Alopecia in malignant disease in renal failure and in hepatic insufficiency

The diffuse hair loss has no distinctive features.

Diffuse alopecia areata

Rapid onset of diffuse alopecia of some severity may be the first sign of alopecia areata, particularly in young patients (Fig. 5.2). Diagnostic changes may be lacking, for alopecia areata may cause merely widespread precipitation into telogen. The diagnosis can then only be suspected, and perhaps confirmed by the subsequent course.

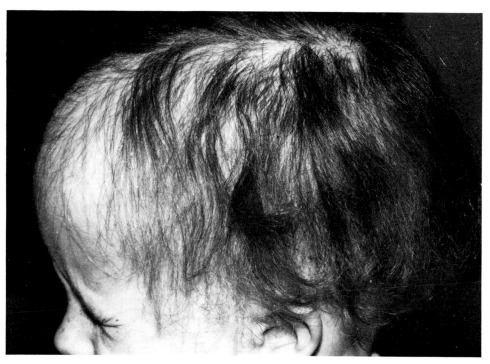

Fig. 5.2. Diffuse alopecia in a child. The cause was not established. The diffuse form of alopecia areata is probable, but a toxic origin could not be excluded. Spontaneous recovery took place (Addenbrooke's Hospital, Cambridge).

Syphilis

Diffuse hair loss may occur in secondary syphilis, in which the classical 'moth-eaten' appearance is not always present (see p. 429).

Traumatic alopecia

We do not apply the term diffuse alopecia to the patchy or widespread damage to hair shafts by physical or chemical agents but many authors (Alexander 1965; Eckert *et al.* 1967) include it among the diagnostic possibilities. Certainly it must be excluded on a careful history, supported by microscopy of the damaged hairs and it must be remembered that misguided 'treatment' of diffuse alopecia of any origin may add variations to the clinical picture.

In psychologically disturbed women the compulsive plucking of hair may denude the scalp almost completely, leaving only a carpet of 1 cm stumps.

Diagnosis

The diagnosis of diffuse alopecia is time consuming and often canot be accomplished in a single consultation. A detailed general medical history is essential. First, common baldness must be excluded (see p. 105). Then, on history and with the appropriate investigation, the other known causes of diffuse hair loss must be systematically excluded. Microscopy of growing and of shed hair should always be carried out. It may reveal evidence of physical and chemical damage to hair shafts; it may show dystrophic anagen hairs, the fractured hairs of cytotoxic injury, or the unsuspected presence of a congenital defect of shaft formation which has rendered the hair unduly susceptible to trauma.

Treatment

Treatment is the treatment of the cause, when this can be established.

References

Alexander S. (1965) Diffuse alopecia in women. *Transactions of the St John's Hospital Dermatological Society*, **51**, 99.

Aquilera Maruri C. (1966) Alopecia diffusa feminina e hiposideremia. *Actas Dermo-Sifiliograficas*, **57**, 169.

Bergfeld W. (1978) Diffuse hair loss in women. *Cutis*, **22**, 190.

Brody I.A., Odom G.L. & Kunkle E.C. (1960) Pilomotor seizures. *Neurology*, **10**, 993.

Brown A.C. & Brayles J.A. (1980) Accumulative scarring of the scalp due to hair dyes. In *Hair, Trace Elements and Human Illness*, eds. A.C. Brown & R.G. Crounse. New York, Praeger, p. 348.

Eckert J. (1975) Diffuse hair loss and psychiatric disturbance. *Acta Dermato-Venereologica*, **55**, 147.

Eckert J., Church R.E., Ebling F.J. & Munro D.S. (1967) Hair loss in women. *British Journal of Dermatology*, **79**, 543.

Hoff H. & Riehl G. (1937–8) Zur Frage der durch Erkrankung des Zentralnervensystems bedingter Alopecie. *Archiv für Dermatologie und Syphilologie*, **176**, 191.

Klein A.W., Rudolph R.I. & Leyden J.J. (1973) Telogen effluvium as a sign of Hodgkin's disease. *Archives of Dermatology*, **108**, 702.

Kligman A.M. (1961) Pathologic dynamics of reversible hair loss in humans. I. Telogen effluvium. *Archives of Dermatology*, **83**, 175.

Ludwig E. (1966–7) Uber das endokrine Substrat der diffusen weiblichen (androgenetischen) Alopecie. *Archiv für klinische und experimentelle Dermatologie*, **227**, 468.

Mikula F. & Steidl L. (1961) Ein Beitrag zur Ätiopathogenase der periodischer Alopezie. *Dermatologische Wochenschrift*, **143**, 543.

Quinones P.A. & Garcia Munoz C.M. (1963) El Metabolismo del Hierro en las Alopecias—Alopecias Difusas femininas y 'Ferropenia latente'. *Actas Dermo-Sifiliograficas*, **54**, 425.

Rooth G. & Carlström S. (1970) Therapeutic fasting. *Acta medica Scandinavica*, **187**, 455.

Sabouraud R. (1932) *Diagnostic et Traitement des Affections du Cuir Chevelu*. Paris, Masson, p. 342.

Schiff B.L. & Kern A.B. (1963) Study of postpartum alopecia. *A.M.A. Archives of Dermatology*, **87**, 609.

Schwenzner G. and Walther H. (1961) Alopecia diffusa bei Colitis ulcerosa und nach allgemeiner zytostatischer Therapie mittles Endoxan. *Zeitschrift für Haut und Geschlectskrankheiten*, **31**, 211.

Skelton J.B. (1966) Postpartum alopecia. *American Journal of Obstetrics and Gynecology*, **94**, 125.

Starzl T.E., Putnam C.W., Groth C.G., Corman J.L. & Taubman J. (1975) Alopecia, ascites and incomplete regeneration after 85–95% liver resection. *American Journal of Surgery*, **129**, 587.

Steigleder G.K. & Mahrle G. (1973) Haarausfall als polyätiologisches Symptom. *Fortschritte der praktischen Dermatologie und Venereologie*, **7**, 237.

Sulzberger M.B., Witten V.H. & Kopf A.W. (1960) Diffuse alopecia in women. *A.M.A. Archives of Dermatology*, **81**, 556.

Tarnow G. (1971) Haarkleidstörungen nach schweren Hirntraumen. *Journal of Neuro-Visceral Relations*, Suppl. x, 549.

Zaun H., Müting D. & Steinmann I. (1969) Wachstumsstörungen der Kopfhaare als Folge von Hepatopathien. *Archiv für klinische und experimentelle Dermatologie*, **235**, 386.

The hair in pregnancy
(References p. 124)

When the extent and complexity of the endocrine changes of pregnancy are considered (Hytten & Leitch 1971) their relatively small effects on hair growth seem surprising. However, there is certainly considerable individual variation in these effects and further quantitative investigations are needed.

Many women maintain that their hair is particularly attractive and healthy during pregnancy. Trichograms show no increase in density, but during the second half of pregnancy, the percentage of anagen hairs increases from the normal 85% to about 95% (Lynfield 1960; Pecoraro *et al.* 1969); in other words, the normal shedding of telogen hairs is reduced. At this same stage of pregnancy the percentage of hairs of large shaft diameter is higher than in non-pregnant women of the same age (Pecoraro *et al.* 1969).

The rate of hair growth is slightly reduced during pregnancy (Pecoraro *et al.* 1969; Bosse 1971). A few women complain that the hair is sparse, especially in the parietal regions. It appears that some of those follicles which enter a normal telogen phase may fail to re-enter anagen (Bosse 1971), and this rather than increased shedding accounts for the clinically evident thinning.

After parturition the follicles in which anagen has been prolonged, rapidly enter catagen and thus telogen. Increased shedding is evident after a few weeks (1–4 months) and may continue for several months, since shedding that will restore the pre-pregnancy equilibrium is supplemented by further shedding precipitated by the psychophysical trauma of labour, with blood loss, low plasma protein, and sometimes also anticoagulants, as contributory factors (Bosse 1971). Full recovery is usual and no treatment is available or necessary.

All the changes so far described tend to be less severe in subsequent pregnancies (Pecoraro *et al.* 1969).

Other changes in hair growth in pregnancy are uncommon. The rate of growth of body hair is not normally affected (Trotter 1935). However, hirsutism may develop, usually during the last trimester (see pp. 84–5). In such cases irreversible frontovertical baldness accompanies it in genetically predisposed subjects.

References

Bosse K. (1971) Haarwachstum und Schwangerschaft. *Schriften der Alfred-Marchionini-Stiftung*, **2**, 59.

Hytten F.E. & Leitch I. (1971) *The Physiology of Human Pregnancy*, 2nd edn. Oxford, Blackwell Scientific Publications.

Lynfield Y.L. (1960) Effect of pregnancy on the human hair cycle. *Journal of Investigative Dermatology*, **35**, 323.

Pecoraro V., Barman J.M. & Astore I. (1969) The normal trichogram of pregnant women. In *Advances in Biology of Skin*, vol. IX, *Hair Growth*, eds. W. Montagna & R.L. Dobson. Oxford, Pergamon Press, p. 203.

Trotter M. (1935) The activity of hair follicles with reference to pregnancy. *Surgery, Gynecology and Obstetrics*, **60**, 1092.

Oral contraceptives and the hair
(References p. 125)

Oral contraceptives of the most widely favoured combined type contain a small dose of oestrogen, usually 0.05 mg of mestranol or ethinyloestradiol, combined with any one of several progestogens, of different potency, and in a dose which varies four- or fivefold. Pills of the sequential type contain much larger doses of oestrogen during both phases of the sequence. Published observations on the effects of 'the pill' on hair growth have unfortunately often been uncontrolled, and have often also failed to take into account the nature of the hormones or their dose. Reports such as those of Cormia (1967) and Greenwald (1970) are difficult to evaluate. Both authors noted diffuse alopecia in five women whilst they were taking, or after they stopped taking, a contraceptive pill. Other causes of hair loss were not excluded.

Zaun & Gerber (1969) studied 50 women who were taking a contraceptive pill of the combined type. Many patients showed no significant change in the proportion of anagen to telogen scalp follicles. Twenty-five showed a temporary increase in the proportion of telogen follicles, but the ratio returned to normal by the 6th month. Eleven patients whose telogen percentage was certainly high showed a steady return to normal. Dystrophic changes in hair roots were occasionally seen. In a similar investigation of 51 women taking a sequential contraceptive pill, essentially the same changes were observed but there were no dystrophic hairs (Zaun & Ruffing 1970). In neither group of patients were there clinically evident changes while the pill was being taken. This lack of clinically evident effects has been confirmed by other (Griffiths 1973). The observation (Cormia 1967; Greenwald 1970) that many women show increased shedding of hair from 2 weeks to 3–4 months after they stopped taking an oral contraceptive has also been confirmed (Dawber & Connor 1971; Griffiths 1973). This hair loss simulates that which is commonly seen after parturition; it seldom results in more than a mild degree of diffuse alopecia, but it varies greatly in degree: recovery occurs spontaneously.

In genetically predisposed women those pills with a high content of potent progestogen may induce acne, hirsutism (Zaun 1972) and baldness of the common type. The difficulty in diagnosing early common baldness has been stressed (p. 105). If the patient insists that her hair is getting sparser, especially in the frontovertical region, hirsutism and seborrhoea should be sought. If these other androgen-induced changes have developed or progressed since the pill has been taken, a pill of low progestogen potency should be substituted.

References

Cormia F.E. (1967) Alopecia from oral contraceptives. *Journal of the American Medical Association*, **201**, 635.

Dawber R.P.R. & Connor B.L. (1971) Pregnancy, hair loss and the pill. *British Medical Journal*, **iv**, 234.

Greenwald A.E. (1970) Anovulatorias y alopecie. *Dermatologia ibero latino-americana*, **12**, 29.

Griffiths W.A.D. (1973) Diffuse hair loss and oral contraceptives. *British Journal of Dermatology*, **88**, 31.

Zaun H. & Gerber T. (1969) Die Wirkung monophasisder Ovulationshemmer auf das Wachstem der Kopfhaare. *Archiv für klinische und experimentelle Dermatologie*, **234**, 353.

Zaun H. & Ruffing H. (1970) Untersuchungen uber der Einfluss antikonzeptioner Zuriphasen— Hormonpräparate auf das Wachsstem der Kopfhaare. *Archiv für klinische und experimentelle Dermatologie*, **238**, 197.

Zaun H. (1972) *Ovulationshemmer in der Dermatologia*. Stuttgart, Thieme.

Thyroid influences on hair growth
(References p. 127)

Epidermal thickness is reduced in patients with hypothyroidism, and the rates of epidermal cell division and anabolic activity in the epidermis are increased in thyrotoxicosis (Holt *et al.* 1976). The changes observed in both hypothyroid and hyperthyroid states are reversible when the euthyroid state is restored. Epidermal receptors for thyroid hormone appear to be specific for tri-iodothyronine (Holt & Marks 1977).

Hypothyroidism

In severe hypothyroidism of long duration the skin appendages are almost completely absent (Berkheiser 1955). When the changes are rather less severe (Saito *et al.* 1976) the number of appendages in the atrophic epidermis is reduced and horny plugs are seen in orifices of sweat ducts and follicles.

There is no consistent correlation between the degree and duration of hypothyroidism and the severity of alopecia, probably because the thyroid, apart from its direct effect on the hair cycle, has other metabolic activities which can directly or indirectly affect hair growth (Saito *et al.* 1976). Whilst a dry skin and diffuse sparsity of scalp and body hair are commonly seen in cretins (Butterworth 1954) and in myxoedema, diffuse alopecia may be the only cutaneous sign of hypothyroidism (Church 1965). The cases of hypothyroid alopecia must likely to come to the notice of the dermatologist are cases of this type, including those in whom the hypothyroidism has been induced by antithyroid drugs or by iodides (Chapman & Main 1967).

The alopecia in hypothyroidism is of very gradual onset and is diffuse. The microscopy of plucked hairs shows a marked increase in the proportion in telogen. The telogen ratio drops rapidly when thyroxin is administered and resting follicles re-enter anagen (Freinkel & Freinkel 1972). The routine history taken from the patient with diffuse hair loss without obvious cause, should include questions concerning gain in weight, cold tolerance and energy and initiative. Even in the absence of such symptoms of hypothyroidism the serum protein-bound iodine, and the thyroid radio-iodine uptake and the blood thyroxin level should be estimated.

An unusual clinical manifestation of hypothyroidism is myxoedema of the scalp, presenting as diffuse thickening with the consistency 'of a rubber pillow' (Frankel & Frankel 1964). The scalp hair was normal. The diagnosis was confirmed histologically and biochemically.

Hypothyroid alopecia responds promptly to replacement therapy with thyroxin, unless it is of very long duration and some follicles have atrophied. However, alopecia in a patient who is biochemically hypothyroid is not necessarily wholly or even partly the result of impaired thyroid function. We have frequently seen patients with common baldness who have been treated for long periods with thyroxin on the basis of borderline biochemical findings, or even of a so-called 'clinical diagnosis' of hypothyroidism based on gain in weight and perhaps on elevated serum cholesterol level, neither of which is an acceptable diagnostic criterion.

An unusual and unexplained temporary diffuse alopecia occurred in a child aged 10 months with myxoedema, 17 days after starting treatment with thyroid (Achten *et al.* 1960).

Thyrotoxicosis
Severe thyrotoxicosis is said to cause diffuse alopecia of the scalp. We have not seen cases in which this cause for the hair loss could be established beyond doubt.

Nor can we confirm the claim that decreased axillary hair is a feature of about 50% of cases of thyrotoxicosis (Williams 1947).

References

Achten G., Ledoux-Corbusier M., Van der Meiren L. & Wolter R. (1960) Défluvium chez un enfant myxoedémateux traité. *Archives Belges de Dermatologie et de Syphiligraphie*, **16**, 209.

Berkheim G.W. (1955) Adult hypothyroidism. Report of an Advanced Case. *Journal of Clinical Endocrinology and Metabolism*, **15**, 44.

Butterworth T. (1954) Dermatological aspects of cretinism. *Archives of Dermatology and Syphilology*, **70**, 565.

Chapman R.S. & Main R.A. (1967) Diffuse thinning of the hair in iodine-induced hypothyroidism. *British Journal of Dermatology*, **79**, 103.

Church R.E. (1965) Hypothyroid hair loss. *British Journal of Dermatology*, **77**, 661.

Frankel E.B. & Frankel A.R. (1964) Localized myxoedema of the scalp and hypothyroidism. *Archives of Dermatology*, **90**, 460.

Freinkel R.K. & Freinkel N. (1972) Hair growth and alopecia in hypothyroidism. *Archives of Dermatology*, **106**, 349.

Holt P.J.A., Lazarus J. & Marks R. (1976) The epidermis in thyroid disease. *British Journal of Dermatology*, **95**, 513.

Holt P.J.A. & Marks R. (1977) The epidermal responses to changes in thyroid status. *Journal of Investigative Dermatology*, **68**, 299.

Saito R., Hori Y. & Kuribayashi T. (1976) Alopecia in hypothyroidism. In *Biology and Diseases of the Hair*, eds. T. Kobori & W. Montagna. Baltimore, University Park Press, p. 279.

Williams R.H. (1947) Thyroid and adrenal interrelations with special reference to hypotrichosis axillaris in thyrotoxicosis. *Journal of Clinical Endocrinology and Metabolism*, **7**, 52.

Nutritional influences on hair growth
(References p. 129)

Many states of malnutrition have important effects on hair growth. The most widespread is protein–calorie malnutrition, which is common in many developing countries, but is not unknown in countries with a high standard of living. The more specific dietary deficiencies, affecting hair growth, are to some extent the product of sophisticated techniques of artificial feeding.

Protein–calorie malnutrition (PCM)

PCM is classified in four degrees of severity:
  (i) Nutritional growth retardation ⎤
  (ii) Kwashiorkor   ⎦ deficiency of good quality protein.
  (iii) Marasmic kwashiorkor ⎤
  (iv) Nutritional marasmus ⎦ protein and calorie deficiency.

In PCM the hair becomes dry and lifeless in appearance. Partial loss of pigment from black hair gives patches which are reddish or pale in colour (Hennington *et al.* 1958). The hair roots show a prompt response to protein deficiency. The proportion of roots in telogen increases. Those roots in anagen show dystrophic changes with reduction in the diameter of the hair-bulb and contour of the shaft (Bradfield 1968; Bradfield *et al.* 1969). Both internal and external root sheaths are markedly reduced (Crounse *et al.* 1970). There is a gross reduction in the rate of hair growth (Sims 1968). Other clinical aspects of kwashiorkor are discussed by Gillman & Gillman (1951) and by Lowy & Meilman (1975).

Secondary protein deficiency has occurred after severe diarrhoea some years after a gastrectomy (Silverblatt & Brown 1960) and in ulcerative colitis (Melnikoff 1957). In both patients black hair became reddish and sparse.

In marasmus the hair is also fine and dry but almost no anagen follicles remain, and if the marasmic state continues, the hair becomes very sparse as the telogen hairs are shed.

Marasmus is severe chronic malnutrition, in which the child adapts to the stress by failing to grow (Bradfield 1974). Follicles in telogen conserve nitrogen. In kwashiorkor a relatively acute shortage of protein interrupts a period of more normal growth. Linear growth of hair may continue, but the calibre of the hair shaft is reduced, and some anagen follicles become dystrophic. Intermediate stages are also seen (Bradfield & Bailey 1968; Bradfield *et al.* 1969). Bradfield (1974) advocated the microscopy of hair specimens for field surveys of the frequency, severity and chronicity of PCM in a population. The value of the study of changes in hair root morphology in nutrition surveys was later assessed statistically (Johnson *et al.* 1976). Significant differences in shaft diameter and in anagen/telogen ratio were found only between well-nourished and severely malnourished children. The different stages of PCM could not be reliably differentiated in a field survey by the examination of hair morphology. Nevertheless such changes constitute an important physical sign in the individual child.

Essential fatty acid deficiency
Deficiency of essential fatty acids is liable to arise in patients who receive prolonged parenteral alimentation. Cutaneous changes caused by this deficiency have been reported in infants (Caldwell *et al.* 1972) and adults (Riella *et al.* 1975; Skolnik *et al.* 1977). After 2–4 months of deficient alimentation the patient develops redness and scaling in the scalp and eyebrows. Most hair is shed, and what remains is dry, unruly and lighter in colour.

The suspected diagnosis can be confirmed by demonstrating a high serum level of the fatty acid eicosatrianoic acid, and a low concentration of arachidonic acid.

The cutaneous changes are reversed by the topical application of safflower oil, which contains 60–70% linoleic acid (Skolnik *et al.* 1977).

Zinc deficiency
Zinc deficiency occurs as a result of an inborn defect of zinc absorption, or from

dietary deficiency of this element, or as the result of long-continued parenteral alimentation.

Acrodermatitis enteropathica

This uncommon hereditary disorder of zinc metabolism is determined by an autosomal recessive gene (Moynahan 1974). The onset of symptoms often coincides with weaning. There are erythema and scaling plaques, partially covered with bullae and vesicles. These skin changes characteristically occur around the mouth and anus and on the extremities. The hair may be sparse, dry and brittle or may be completely shed. The child is listless and apathetic and growth is retarded. The symptoms respond rapidly to zinc sulphate 50 mg three times daily.

Environmental zinc deficiency

In the absence of an adequate intake of zinc, such as occurs in some areas of Egypt and Iran as a result of a diet of unleavened wholemeal wheat bread, high in phosphate, growth and sexual maturation are retarded in some prepubertal males (Ronaghy *et al.* 1974). Hair growth in such individuals has not been investigated, but there are no gross clinical changes.

Zinc deficiency after parenteral alimentation

Acute zinc deficiency is characterized by a dermatitis resembling that of acrodermatitis enteropathica, and associated with diarrhoea, apathy and alopecia (Kay & Tasman-Jones 1975). Chronic zinc deficiency in patients receiving only parenteral feeding (Wexler & Pace 1977) gave rise to skin changes after about 2 months. Redness and scaling developed in the nasolabial folds and at the corner of the mouth. Red scaly patches appeared on the knees, bullae on the hands and feet, then perianal erosions and sparseness of the scalp hair and eyebrows. In another patient similar but less severe changes occurred after 16 months of hyperalimentation. Many other cases have been reported (Weisman *et al.* 1976). The symptoms which should suggest the possibility of zinc deficiency are perioccipital redness and scaling, bullae and hair loss. The subject has been fully reviewed by Weismann (1980).

References

Bradfield R.B. (1968) Changes in hair root morphology and hair diameter associated with protein-calorie malnutrition. In *Protein Deficiencies and Calorie Deficiencies*, eds. R.A. McCance & E.M. Widdowson. London, Churchill, p. 213.

Bradfield R.B. (1974) Hair tissue as a medium for the differential diagnosis of protein calorie malnutrition: a commentary. *Journal of Pediatrics*, **84**, 294.

Bradfield R.B. & Bailey M.A. (1968) Hair root response to protein undernutrition. In *Advances in Biology of Skin*, vol. IX, *Hair Growth*, eds. W. Montagna & R.C. Dobson. Oxford, Pergamon Press, p. 109.

Bradfield R.B., Cordano A. & Graham G.G. (1969) Hair-root adaptation to marasmus in Andean Indian children. *Lancet*, **ii**, 1395.

Caldwell M.D., Jonsson H.T. & Otherson H.B. (1972) Essential fatty acid deficiency in an infant receiving prolonged parenteral alimentation. *Journal of Pediatrics*, **8**, 894.

Crounse R.G., Bollet A.J. & Owens S. (1970) Tissue assay of human protein malnutrition using scalp hair roots. *Transactions of the Association of American Physicians*, **83**, 185.

Gillman J. & Gillman T. (1951) *Perspectives in Human Malnutrition*. New York, Grune & Stratton.

Hennington V.M., Caroe E., Derbes V. & Kennedy B. (1958) Kwashiorkor. *Archives of Dermatology*, **78**, 157.

Johnson A.A., Latham M.C. & Ron D.A. (1976) An evaluation of the use of changes in hair root morphology in the assessment of protein–calorie malnutrition. *American Journal of Clinical Metabolism*, **29**, 502.

Kay R.G. & Tasman-Jones C. (1975) Acute zinc deficiency in man during intravenous alimentation. *Australia and New Zealand Journal of Surgery*, **292**, 879.

Lowy G. & Meilman I. (1975) Kwashiorkor, aspectes clinicos e dermatologicos. *Medicina cutanea, I.L.E.*, **3**, 181.

Melnikoff G.M. (1957) Temporary reddening of the hair in ulcerative colitis. *American Journal of Digestive Diseases (and Nutrition)*, **2**, 738.

Moynahan E.J. (1974) Acrodermatitis enteropathica. A lethal inherited human zinc deficiency disorder. *Lancet*, **ii**, 399.

Riella M.C., Broviac J.W., Wells M. & Scribner B.H. (1975) Essential fatty acid deficiency in human adults during total parenteral nutrition. *Annals of Internal Medicine*, **83**, 786.

Ronaghy H.A., Reinhold J.G., Mahloudji M., Ghavasni P., Spivey Fox N.R. & Halsted J.A. (1974) Zinc supplementation of malnourished schoolboys in Iran: increased growth and other effects. *The American Journal of Clinical Nutrition*, **27**, 112.

Silverblatt C.W. & Brown H.E. (1960) 'Kwashiorkor-like' syndrome associated with burning feet syndrome in an adult male. *American Journal of Medicine*, **28**, 847.

Sims R.T. (1968) The measurement of hair growth as an index of protein synthesis in malnutrition. *British Journal of Nutrition*, **22**, 229.

Skolnik P., Eaglstein W.H. & Ziboh V.A. (1977) Human essential fatty-acid deficiency. *Archives of Dermatology*, **113**, 939.

Weismann K. (1980) Zinc metabolism and the skin. In *Recent Advances in Dermatology*, eds. A. Rook & J.A. Savin. Edinburgh, Churchill Livingstone, p. 109.

Weismann K., Hjorth N. & Fischer A. (1976) Zinc depletion syndrome with acrodermatitis during long-term intravenous feeding. *Clinical and Experimental Dermatology*, **1**, 237.

Wexler D. & Pace W. (1977) Acquired zinc deficiency disease of the skin. *British Journal of Dermatology*, **96**, 669.

Malabsorption
(References p. 131)

There are numerous causes of malabsorption states (Dyer & Dawson 1968) and there are wide quantitative and qualitative variations in the nature and degree of absorption failure. It follows that the clinical manifestations of malabsorption may be equally diverse.

Classical symptoms, not all present in every patient, are frequent loose, pale and bulky stools. Weight loss is usual. If the malabsorption begins in childhood there will be short stature and hypogonadism. Cutaneous changes are common

(Wells 1962) but are rarely progressive. Most frequent are dryness, ichthyosis and follicular keratosis. The scalp is dry and the hair somewhat sparse. The tongue may be sore, red and smooth.

Less frequently there may be eczema, extensive but without distinctive features (Friedman & Hare 1965). Still less frequently the eczema occurs in large, scaly plaques, which are followed by conspicuous pigmentation. If these plaques are in the scalp there may be extensive temporary shedding of the hair in the affected areas (Lachapelle & Rook 1967), and this circumscribed severe loss is superimposed on the already existing diffuse sparsity of dry, fine scalp hair.

Detailed studies by modern methods of the hair changes in malabsorption states have not been reported. At present from the practical point of view malabsorption should be suspected when sparse hair and growth retardation are associated with symptoms mentioned above and each case should be thoroughly investigated. The response to appropriate treatment, e.g. a gluten-free diet, is impressive.

References

Dyer N.H. & Dawson A.M. (1968) Malabsorption. *British Medical Journal*, ii, 161.
Friedman M. & Hare P.J. (1965) Gluten-sensitive enteropathy and eczema. *Lancet*, i, 521.
Lachapelle J-M. & Rook A.J. (1967) Les manifestations cutanées des états de malabsorption. *Archives Belges de Dermatologie et de Syphiligraphie*, 23, 267.
Wells G.C. (1962) Skin disorders in relation to malabsorption. *British Medical Journal*, ii, 937.

Pancreatic disease of the tropics

A form of pancreatic disease affecting predominantly young adult males occurs widely in East Africa (Klaus 1980). Its cause is unknown.

The principal manifestations of pancreatic disease of the tropics are steatorrhoea, upper abdominal pain, the symptoms of diabetes mellitus and malnutrition. Malabsorption may result in weakness, oedema and ascites.

In Uganda about one-third of patients with this disease develop a distinctive cutaneous syndrome. Small irregular areas of fine scaling gradually become generalized and are associated with pigment dilution, the black skin becoming light brown.

The hair becomes soft, fine and silky and reddish-brown in colour. Diffuse alopecia develops on the vertex and pubic and axillary hair become sparse.

Reference

Klaus S.N. (1980) Acquired pigment dilution of the hair and skin. *International Journal of Dermatology*, 19, 508.

Chronic renal failure and maintenance haemodialysis (Lubach 1980)

Chronic renal failure is frequently associated with cutaneous changes. Pigmentation is increased and the skin generally is dry and pruritic. Maintenance haemodialysis does not reverse these changes and often gives rise to additional abnormalities, particularly of the hair and nails. The scalp hair becomes dry and brittle and rather sparse and there is thinning of body hair, including pubic and axillary hair. The nails are brittle and may be deformed.

Reference
Lubach D. (1980) Dermatologische Veranderungen bei Patienten mit Langzeithämodialyse. *Hautarzt*, 31, 82.

Cronkhite–Canada syndrome

History and nomenclature
This rare but well-defined syndrome is conveniently linked eponymously to Cronkhite & Canada (1955) as its pathogenesis is still uncertain.

Pathology
Diffuse gastrointestinal polyposis has been regularly reported, but it has been suggested (Johnson *et al.* 1972) that the essential abnormality is a diffuse, potentially reversible gastroenterocolitis with the formation of inflammatory pseudopolyps. Malabsorption and exudative enteropathy are constant features and hypoproteinaemia may be extreme (Shibuya 1972; Mielke 1973).

The twenty or so reported cases have been of several different races, and aged between 40 and 75 at the onset of symptoms.

Clinical features
The principal symptoms are severe diarrhoea, weakness, oedema, and loss of weight. The first cutaneous symptoms may precede but commonly follow the onset of the diarrhoea.

Loss of head hair is usually diffuse and may be severe. In one case (Johnston *et al.* 1962) it was described as 'extensive alopecia areata'. In some cases it becomes total (Nishiyama *et al.* 1965). Body hair becomes sparse. The pathodynamics of the hair loss have not been adequately studied.

All or almost all finger and toe nails show a distinctive though not pathognomonic dystrophy. The humped appearance suggests the formation of ventral nail in the absence of normal nail formation by the matrix (Cunliffe & Anderson 1967).

Pigmentation of variable degree and extent is not a constant feature. It may affect the palmar aspect of the fingers and may be widespread, but does not involve the mucous membranes.

References

Cronkhite L.W. & Canada W.J. (1955) Generalized gastrointestinal polyposis: an unusual syndrome of polyposis, pigmentation, alopecia and onychatrophia. *New England Journal of Medicine*, **252**, 1011.

Cunliffe W.J. & Anderson J. (1967) Case of Cronkhite–Canada syndrome and associated jejunal diverticulosis. *British Medical Journal*, iv, 601.

Johnson G.K., Soergel K.H., Hensby G.T., Dodds W.J. & Hogan W.J. (1972) Cronkhite–Canada syndrome: gastrointestinal pathophysiology and morphology. *Gastroenterology*, **63**, 140.

Johnston M.N., Vosburgh J.W., Wiens A.T. & Walsh G.C. (1962) Gastrointestinal polyposis associated with alopecia, pigmentation and atrophy of the fingernails and toenails. *Annals of Internal Medicine*, **56**, 935.

Mielke F.W. (1973) Diffuse polyposis ventriculi, polyposis intestinali—Cronkhite–Canada syndrome. *Zeitschrift für Gastroenterologie*, **11**, 529.

Nishiyama S., Mori S. & Harada S. (1965) Gastrointestinale polyposis mit universelle Alopecie, Onychodystrophie und Pigmentation der Haut. *Archiv für klinische und experimentelle Dermatologie*, **221**, 144.

Shibuya C. (1972) An autopsy case of Cronkhite–Canada's syndrome—generalized gastrointestinal polyposis, pigmentation, alopecia and onychatrophia. *Acta pathologica japonica*, **22**, 171.

Alopecia and pigmentary changes induced by chemicals
(References p. 134)

Many chemicals which are capable of inducing alopecia are in frequent use in therapeutics. To some other chemicals man is only rarely and accidentally exposed; others are occupational hazards. Together they account for a small but increasing proportion of cases of diffuse alopecia. The role of environmental chemical contamination in causing alopecia and other disturbances of hair growth is probably underestimated. Exposure to boric acid, for example (see below), is seldom considered amongst diagnostic possibilities. There are in the literature a number of reports of single cases or groups of cases in which alopecia has accompanied polyneuritis and optic atrophy (Euzière *et al.* 1951; Symonds 1953) and in which a toxic cause was suspected but never proved. In unexplained hair loss exposure to a chemical should always be considered as a possible cause.

The mode of action of many of these chemicals on the hair cycle is known and the clinical features and course of the alopecia can be correlated with the nature of the changes produced in the growing follicles. Flesch (1963) reviewed the subject at length and differentiated drugs which inhibit mitosis, those that disturb keratinization and those which precipitate premature catagen in growing follicles, and these distinctions are clinically important, but a single drug may interfere with hair growth in different ways according to the degree of damage it inflicts. The clinical effect of a given dose is influenced by the ratio of anagen to telogen follicles in the scalp when it is administered; the greater the proportion of anagen follicles, the greater the hair loss. The A/T ratio is generally higher in the young but the proportion of telogen hairs is increased in many diseases, including many neoplastic diseases.

However, in the case of many drugs the mode of action is not known and the non-specific nature of increased shedding of telogen hairs can be related to the administration of the drug only circumstantially. All dermatologists see patients in whom diffuse alopecia clearly related to an acute febrile illness has been wrongly attributed to the drugs prescribed to treat it. On the other hand it is probable that drugs as a cause of increased shedding of hair are often overlooked.

Although a provisional classification of the mechanisms of drug action on hair follicles is possible, there are so many drugs the mode of action of which is unknown, that it is more practical to classify the drugs into groups according to their pharmacological activity.

References

Euzière J., Pages P. & Coulier C. (1951) Polynévrites récidivantes avec alopécie et atrophie optique. *Revue neurologique*, **84**, 343.

Flesch P. (1963) Inhibition of keratinizing structures by systemic drugs. *Pharmacological Reviews*, **15**, 653.

Symonds W.J.C. (1953) Alopecia, optic atrophy and peripheral neuritis of probably toxic origin. *Lancet*, **ii**, 1338.

Cytostatic agents (references p. 136)

Inhibition of mitosis in the hair papilla leads to narrowing of the hair shaft, which fractures readily at this point, or to complete failure of hair formation. In either case so-called 'anagen alopecia' results and dystrophic hairs are shed within days of the first administration of an adequate dose of the drug. But the same drug may produce broken shafts and anagen shedding in some follicles and premature catagen, followed by telogen shedding in others (Zaun 1964). A study of the trichograms of 40 patients receiving cytostatic drugs (Orfanos & Gerstin 1976) showed that qualitative changes such as broken shafts, disordered keratin structure and melanin distribution were regularly found, the proportion of such hairs and of telogen hairs varying with the drug and with the dose. In a further study (Gerstin & Orfanos 1976) 49 of the patients receiving cytostatic drugs developed hair loss. In most the hair loss developed 10 days to 6 weeks after starting treatment. Of these patients 31 were carefully followed; 6 developed total baldness of the scalp; 29 developed some generalized hair loss and this became universal in 4. The rate of hair growth was reduced and the male patients needed to shave less frequently.

Cyclophosphamide (also known as Endoxan) has been very thoroughly investigated (Braun-Falco 1961). With this drug and with methotrexate and actinozine D (Crounse & Van Scott 1960) 4–6 days after an adequate dose there was diminution of the diameter of the bulb or of the keratogenic zone leading to constriction and fracture of the hair. Continued therapy with two or more cytostatic drugs has a greater effect than a larger dose of only one. The occasional delay of the onset of alopecia to 3 months after the start of cytostatic therapy has been reported (Falkson & Schulz 1960, 1964). There are examples of the so-called 'universal' alopecia, in which telogen shedding predominates.

Colchicine produces similar changes (Malkinson & Lynfield 1959; Harms 1980). With high dosage there is anagen alopecia and matrix atrophy. With low dosage there is increased telogen shedding. High dosage of desacetyl methyl colchicine led to loss of 90% of scalp hair in 2 weeks (Mikkelson *et al.* 1956). The sensitivity of cells to injury by colchicine depends on the mitosis rate: the statement that this drug does not cause depilation in Negroids (Brown & Seed 1945) requires further investigation.

Cytostatic drugs taken to induce abortion have produced anagen alopecia, with diagnostic broken, tapered hair shafts (Maibach & Maguire 1964), which could be of medicolegal importance.

Cantharidine administered with criminal intent, or taken accidentally, causes an anagen alopecia, with fracture of dystrophic anagen hairs (Pinetti & Biggio 1967).

The administration of cytostatic drugs is often a life-saving procedure which has to be carried out despite the inevitability of side effects, but measures to diminish the severity of alopecia should not be neglected. With cyclophosphamide loss of hair is less with continuous low dosage than with intermittent high dosage (Stoll 1974). With doxorubicine alone, or in combination with cyclophosphamide, the application of ice packs to the scalp for 30 minutes before the drug was injected produced considerable benefit, and some patients did not require wigs (Luce *et al.* 1973; Edelstyn *et al.* 1977; Dean *et al.* 1979). A slightly different technique using a cooling gel pack for 15 minutes before, and at least 30 minutes after doxorubicine treatment, was effective in preventing hair loss or reducing it to a cosmetically acceptable level (Anderson *et al.* 1981).

The combination of azathioprine and prednisone, commonly prescribed for renal transplant patients, leads to general thinning and breaking of scalp hair, beginning after 1–3 weeks. When the hair is allowed to regrow it may be darker, greyer or more curly than before immunosuppression (Koranda 1974).

The interesting observation has been recorded (Cassady & Jaffe 1974) that in three patients in whom the hair had regrown after shedding caused by irradiation, it was protected from the epilatory effect of subsequent radiotherapy.

The accidental ingestion of the bulbs of *Gloriosa superba*, a member of the lily family (Gooneratne 1966), which contains colchicine, was followed by a severe acute alopecia.

Cytostatic agents capable of provoking acute anagen alopecia occur in a number of leguminous plants which may be accidentally eaten by man. Various spines of *Lecythis* contain selenocystothionine (Kerdel Vegas 1964). *Leucaena glauca* contains mimosine, which has caused alopecia in women (Crounse *et al.*

1962). Abain, present in the seeds of *Abrus precatorius*, has a similar effect (Vignolo-Lutasi 1962). As the coloured seeds of this plant are worn in necklaces the possibility of accidental exposure, especially in children, may arise in countries in which the plant itself does not occur.

References

Anderson J.E., Hunt J.M. & Smith I.E. (1981) Prevention of doxorubicin-induced alopecia by scalp cooling in patients with advanced breast cancer. *British Medical Journal*, **282**, 423.

Braun-Falco O. (1961) Kliniik und Pathomechanismus der Endoxan-Alopecie als Beitrag zur Wesen cytostatischer Alopecie. *Archiv für klinische und experimentelle Dermatologie*, **212**, 194.

Brown W.O. & Seed L. (1945) Effect of colchicine on human tissues. *American Journal of Clinical Pathology*, **65**, 189.

Cassady J.R. & Jaffe N. (1974) Protection from chemotherapeutic epilation by pure irradiation. *Radiology*, **112**, 197.

Crounse R.G. & Van Scott E.J. (1960) Changes in scalp hair roots as a measure of toxicity from cancer therapeutic drugs. *Journal of Investigative Dermatology*, **35**, 83.

Crounse R.G., Maxwell J.D. & Blank H. (1962) Inhibition of growth of hair by mimosine. *Nature*, **194**, 694.

Dean J.C., Salmon S.E. & Griffith, K.S. (1979) Prevention of doxorubicine-induced hair-loss with scalp hypothermia. *New England Journal of Medicine*, **301**, 1427.

Edelstyn G.A., MacDonald M. & MacRae K.D. (1977) Doxorubicine-induced hair loss and its possible modification by scalp cooling. *Lancet*, **ii**, 253.

Falkson G. & Schulz E.J. (1960) Endoxan alopecia. *British Journal of Dermatology*, **72**, 296.

Falkson G. & Schulz E.J. (1964) Skin changes caused by cancer chemotherapy. *British Journal of Dermatology*, **76**, 309

Gerstein E. & Orfanos C.G. (1976) Haarausfall nach Zytostatica. *Artzliche Kosmetologie*, **6**, 54.

Gooneratne B.W.N. (1966) Massive generalized alopecia after poisoning by *Gloriosa superba*. *British Medical Journal*, **i**, 1023.

Harms M. (1980) Haarausfall und Haarverändermazen. *Haararzt*, **31**, 161.

Kerdel Vegas F. (1964) Generalized hair loss due to the ingestion of 'Coco de Mono' (*Lecythis ollaria*). *Journal of Investigative Dermatology*, **42**, 91.

Koranda F.C. (1974) Hair changes in immunosuppressed patients. *First Human Hair Symposium*, ed. A.C. Brown. New York, Medcom Press. p. 91.

Luce J.K., Raffetto T.J., Crisp I.M. & Grief G.C. (1973) Prevention of alopecia by scalp-cooling in patients receiving adriamycin. *Cancer Chemotherapy Reports*, **57**, 108.

Maibach H.I. & Maguire H.C. (1964) Acute hair-loss from drug-induced abortion. *New England Journal of Medicine*, **270**, 1112.

Malkinson F.D. & Lynfield Y.L. (1959) Colchicine alopecia. *Journal of Investigative Dermatology*, **33**, 371.

Mikkelson W.M., Salin R.W. & Duff I.F. (1956) Alopecia totalis after desacetylmethylcolchicine therapy of acute gout. *New England Journal of Medicine*, **255**, 766.

Orfanos C.G. & Gerstein E. (1976) Haarausfall nach Zytostatica. *Artzliche Kosmetologie*, **6**, 96.

Pinetti P. & Biggio P. (1967) Contributo alla conoscenza delle alopecie tossiche con particolare riguardo alle alopecie conseguenti ad avvelenamento da cantaridina. *Rassegna Medica Sarda*, **70**, 433.

Stoll B.A. (1974) Evaluation of cyclophosphamide dosage schedules in breast cancer. *British Journal of Cancer*, **24**, 475.

Vignolo-Lutasi, K. (1962) Uber die experimentelle Alopecie durch Abain. *Archiv für Dermatologie und Syphilologie*, **111**, 549.

Zaun H. (1964) Tierexperimentelle Untersuchungen zur Pathophysiologie der 'gemischten' Alopecie. *Archiv für klinische und experimentelle Dermatologie*, **221**, 75.

Anticoagulants (references p. 137)

Heparin, the heparinoids and the coumarins all cause diffuse alopecia in some 50% of patients. It usually begins after about 8 weeks (3–20 weeks) and lasts for about 6 months (Fischer *et al.* 1953). The incidence of alopecia shows some variation in different series (Hirschback *et al.* 1954). It tends to be highest when large doses have been given over a short period (Tudhope *et al.* 1958). A synthetic heparinoid, a polyhexuronic ester, produced alopecia in 70%, beginning after 3–4 weeks; up to 75% of hair was lost from the vertex, but less from the sides and back of the scalp (Field *et al.* 1961). The precise mode of action of anticoagulants on the hair follicle is uncertain. From studies in man and in the rat (Miki 1960a, b) an antimitotic effect on anagen follicles has been suggested.

Coumarin, in the form of Warfarin, is used as a rat-poison. Children have developed alopecia after eating poisoned food, put down as bait (Cornbleet & Hoit 1957).

References

Cornbleet T. & Hoit L. (1957) Alopecia from coumarin. *Archives of Dermatology*, **75**, 440.

Field J.B., Attyah A.M., Ramsay G.D. & Levitt H. (1961) The chemical intoxication caused by a heparinoid. *American Journal of Medical Science*, **241**, 637.

Fischer R., Bircher J. & Reith T. (1953) Der Haarausfall nach antikoagulierender Therapie. *Schweizeriche Medizinische Wochenschrift*, **82**, 509.

Hirschback J.S., Madison F.W. & Pischiotta A.V. (1954) Alopecia and other toxic effects of heparin and synthetic heparoids. *American Journal of Medical Science*, **227**, 278.

Miki Y. (1960a) Alopecia from heparin. *Medical Journal of Osaka University*, **11**, 315.

Miki Y. (1960b) The effect of heparin on hair growth of rats. *Medical Journal of Osaka University*, **11**, 325.

Tudhope G.R., Cohn H. & Meikle R.W. (1958) Alopecia following treatment with dextran sulphate and other anticoagulant drugs. *British Medical Journal*, i, 1034.

Thallium (references p. 139)

Thallium salts have been widely used to kill rodents and cockroaches, and contaminated food stores have caused outbreaks of poisoning in dogs and cats and in man. They have been used in homicide (Truhaut 1958), and have been prescribed in medicine, first to control sweats in tuberculosis, and later to produce epilation in the treatment of ringworm. An early report of hair loss (Combemale 1898, cit. Heyroth 1947) was the consequence of the prescription of thallium to a tuberculous patient. There is an extensive early literature on such disasters (Buschke & Peiser 1931).

Investigations in the rat (Thyresson 1951) showed that thallium was taken up by anagen follicles and disturbed keratinization. Tactile hairs in rats (Thyresson 1952) showed vacuolization of matrix cells after about 3 days; later the hair shafts showed nodular enlargements through which some shafts broke. The addition of 1–2% cystine to the diet of rats (Gross *et al.* 1948) delayed the development of alopecia in chronic thallium poisoning and reduced the mortality in acute poisoning.

In accidental poisoning in dogs and cats (Skelley & Gabriel 1964) hair loss began after 12–14 days; in some cases erythema and necrosis of the skin occurred, especially around the muzzle and in the large flexures.

Thallium salts are no longer prescribed in medicine, and are not contained in pesticides available in Britain, but in many parts of the world outbreaks of poisoning have occurred from contamination of food, for example in Brussels (Achten 1962), Texas (Grulee & Clark 1951; Chamberlain *et al.* 1958; Reed *et al.* 1963), New York (Frank & Hirsch 1952) and California (Munch *et al.* 1933). With growing awareness of the dangers of these tasteless poisons, large-scale outbreaks are likely to be less frequent, but pesticides containing the salts are still available in many countries; an attempted suicide by thallium poisoning was reported from Brazil (Ribeiro Estrella *et al.* 1970).

A report on the histopathology of the skin in chronic thallium poisoning in man (Schwartzman & Kirschbaum 1962) emphasized the degree of epidermal injury and the early induction of telogen. In more acute poisoning the hair shafts break within the follicle. The tapered lower end of the broken hair shows a distinctive dark zone (Ludwig 1961; Eberhartinger 1962). A study of the dynamics of thallium alopecia (Arnold *et al.* 1964) confirmed that the initial alopecia is due to intrafollicular breaking of growing hairs, but a week after the onset of the alopecia 80% of follicles were in catagen.

The symptoms of thallium poisoning are very variable. Nausea and vomiting may occur early, and weakness, ataxia and tremor somewhat later, but alopecia, fatigue and pains in the legs are the most frequent manifestations (Munch *et al.* 1933; Chamberlain *et al.* 1958). In the more acute forms the initial gastrointestinal symptoms are rapidly followed by delirium, convulsions and coma (Report 1957). In patients exposed to smaller doses there may be fatigue, weight loss and aching limbs, but alopecia may be the only symptom (Hubler 1959, 1966). The hair loss which is diffuse and may become total develops in the 2nd and 3rd week (Grulee & Clark 1951); it is a most important diagnostic feature, whether it occurs alone or with vaguer and non-specific symptoms (Gettler & Weiss 1943).

In one Texas outbreak (Reed *et al.* 1963) 13% of 72 cases were fatal. Death results from damage to the central nervous system and to the kidneys, and some survivors have permanent neurological defects (Steinberg 1961; Reed *et al.* 1963). Most victims of less severe poisoning make a complete recovery (e.g. Nordman 1957). Generalized hyperaminoacidosis of renal type has been reported in some cases (Fischl 1966).

Unexplained diffuse alopecia, if the commoner causes can be excluded, should lead to a suspicion of thallium poisoning even if no source of thallium can be traced. The suspicion is verified if the alopecia is accompanied by neurological symptoms or signs (Webster *et al.* 1958). Thallium is excreted in the urine and faeces over a period of many weeks; any thallium present is abnormal.

References

Achten G. (1962) L'Intoxication thallique. *Archives Belges de Dermatologie et Syphiligraphie*, **18**, 300.

Arnold W., Herzberg J.J., Ludwig E. & Sturde H. (1964) Die Dynamik des Haanausfalls bei Thallium-Vergiftung. *Archiv für klinische und experimentelle Dermatologie*, **218**, 396.

Buschke A. & Peiser B. (1931) Die biologische Wirkung und die praktische Bedeutung des Thalliums. *Ergebnisse der allgemeiner Pathologie*, **25**, 1.

Chamberlain P.H., Stavinoha W.B., Davis H., Kniker W.T. & Panos T.C. (1958) Thallium poisoning. *Pediatrics*, **22**, 1170.

Eberhartinger C. (1962) Die diagnostische Bedeutung von Haarveränderungen bei Thalliumvergiftung. *Wiener medizinische Wochenschrift*, **112**, 329.

Fischl J. (1966) Aminoacidosis in thallium poisoning. *American Journal of the Medical Sciences*, **251**, 40.

Frank S.B. & Hirsch D.R. (1952) Thallium intoxication. Report of two cases. *Journal of the American Medical Association*, **150**, 586.

Gettler A.O. & Weiss L. (1943) Thallium poisoning. III. Clinical toxicology of thallium. *American Journal of Clinical Pathology*, **13**, 422.

Gross P., Runne E. & Wilson J.W. (1948) Studies on the effect of thallium poisoning on the rat. The influence of cystine and methionine on alopecia and survival periods. *Journal of Investigative Dermatology*, **10**, 119.

Grulee C.G. & Clark E.H. (1951) Thallotoxicosis in a preschool nursery. *American Journal of Diseases of Children*, **81**, 47.

Heyroth F.F. (1947) Thallium. *Reports of the U.S. Public Health Service*, Supplement 197.

Hubler W.R. (1959) Partial alopecia due to thallium. *A.M.A. Archives of Dermatology*, **80**, 137.

Hubler W.R. (1966) Hair loss as a symptom of chronic thallotoxicosis. *Southern Medical Journal*, **59**, 436.

Ludwig E. (1961) Pathognomonische Haarbefunde bei Thallium-Vergiftung und dem Deutung. *Hautarzt*, **12**, 456.

Munch J.G., Ginsberg H.M. & Nixon C.E. (1933) The 1932 thallotoxicosis outbreak in California. *Journal of the American Medical Association*, **100**, 1315.

Nordman R. (1957) Thallium-Vergiftung bjei einem Kind. *Neue Österreiches Zeitschrift für Kinderheilkunde*, **2**, 297.

Reed D., Crawley J., Faro S.N., Pieper S.J. & Kurland L.T. (1963) Thallotoxicosis. *Journal of the American Medical Association*, **183**, 516.

Report to the Council on Drugs of the American Medical Association (1957) Thallotoxicosis—a recurring problem. *Journal of the American Medical Association*, **165**, 1566.

Ribeiro Estrella R., Azulay R.D., Peixoto P.R. & de Azevedo Marinho D.E. (1970) Alopecia por Sulfato de Tálio. *Annais brasilieros de Dermatologia e Sifilografia*, **45**, 333.

Schwartzman R.M. & Kirschbaum J.O. (1962) The cutaneous histopathology of thallium poisoning. *Journal of Investigative Dermatology*, **39**, 169.

Skelley J.F. & Gabriel K.L. (1964) Thallium intoxication in the dog. *Annals of the New York Academy of Science*, **111**, 612.

Steinberg H.J. (1961) Accidental thallium poisoning in adults. *Southern Medical Journal*, **54**, 6.

Thyresson N. (1951) Experimental induction of thallium poisoning in the rat. *Acta Dermato-Venereologica*, **31**, 3 and 133.

Thyresson N. (1952) Effect of thallium on the growth of tactile hairs in the white rat. *Acta Dermato-Venereologica*, Suppl. 29, 370.

Truhaut R. (1958) L'intoxication par le thallium. *Annales de Médecine légale*, **38**, 189.

Webster J.R., Huff S. & Gecht M.C. (1958) Thallotoxicosis. *A.M.A. Archives of Dermatology*, **78**, 278.

Thyreostatic drugs

These drugs may cause hair loss by inducing hypothyroidism, but there are reports also of diffuse hair loss in patients who were still hyperthyroid, such as the patient (Wilburne 1951) in whom first methylthiouracil and then propyl-thiouracil produced diffuse hair loss and yellowish pigmentation of previously white hair. Levy (1950) reported pronounced hair loss in a woman whose basal metabolic rate was reduced from +55 to 0 by propylthiouracil.

Seven patients with thyrotoxicosis treated with thiouracil developed a myxoedematoid syndrome of which diffuse alopecia was one component (Lundbaek 1946).

Carbimazole produced hair loss in five patients, 4–40 weeks after starting treatment (Papadopoulos & Harden 1966). The mechanism was not studied.

References

Levy L.K. (1950) Loss of hair following use of propylthiouracil. *Journal of the American Medical Association*, **147**, 860.

Lundbaek K. (1946) Toxic, allergic and myxedematoid symptoms in the treatment of thyrotoxicosis with antithyroid substances. *Acta medica Scandinavica*, **124**, 266.

Papadopoulos S. & Harden R.N. (1966) Hair loss in patients treated with carbimazole. *British Medical Journal*, **ii**, 1502.

Wilburne M. (1951) Hair loss and pigmentation due to thiouracil derivatives. *Journal of the American Medical Association*, **147**, 379.

Borax

Borates may be ingested accidentally as a result of the excessive use of proprietary mouth-washes containing boric acid (Stein *et al.* 1973), or from occupational exposure to sodium borate (Tan 1970). The alopecia is diffuse and of gradual onset. Serum boric acid levels are elevated.

References

Stein K.M., Odom R.B., Justice G.R. & Martin G.C. (1973) Toxic alopecia from ingestion of boric acid. *Archives of Dermatology*, **108**, 95.

Tan T.G. (1970) Occupational toxic alopecia due to borax. *Acta Dermato-Venereologica*, **50**, 55.

Hypocholesteraemic agents

Triparanol and other drugs given to reduce hypercholesterolaemia also reduce cholesterol biosynthesis in epidermis (Flesch 1963). The skin gradually becomes dry and ichthyotic. The hair becomes sparse, dry, and paler in colour (Achor *et al.* 1961; Winkelmann *et al.* 1963). Cataracts may develop (Kirby *et al.* 1962).

References

Achor R.W.P., Winkelmann R.K. & Perry H.O. (1961) Cutaneous side effects from use of triparanol (Mer-29): preliminary data on ichthyosis and loss of hair. *Proceedings of Staff Meetings of the Mayo Clinic*, **36**, 217.

Flesch P. (1963) Inhibition of keratinizing structures by systemic drugs. *Pharmacological Reviews*, **15**, 653.

Kirby T.J., Achor R.W.P., Perry H.O. & Winkelmann R.K. (1962) Cataract formation after triparanol therapy. *Archives of Ophthalmology*, **68**, 486.

Winkelmann R.K., Perry H.O., Achor R.W.P. & Kirby T.J. (1963) Cutaneous syndromes produced as side effects of triparanol therapy. *Archives of Dermatology*, **87**, 372.

Hypervitaminosis A

The ingestion of excessive doses of vitamin A is usually the consequence of misguided medical prescribing or of cranky self-medication, but acute vitamin A poisoning has occurred in polar explorers eating the livers of seals and huskies (Cleland & Southcott 1969). In acute poisoning a febrile illness with headache, drowsiness, vertigo, vomiting and diarrhoea, is followed by generalized exfoliation and loss of hair.

Chronic hypervitaminosis A in adults was first described by Sulzberger & Lazar (1951) in a woman who for 18 months had taken 600,000 i.u. of vitamin A daily. She had a dry, rough, scaly skin, with sparse, coarse, brittle scalp hair, and absent eyebrows, lashes, pubic and axillary hair and vellus. These changes were reversed when she stopped taking the vitamin A. Other cases (Gerber *et al.* 1954; Raaschou-Nielsen 1961; Stimson 1961; Soler-Bechara & Soscia 1963) have shown similar changes. Fatigue, weight loss, bone and joint pains, and headache, have been the other principal manifestations.

References

Cleland J. & Southcott R.V. (1969) Hypervitaminosis A in the Australasian Antarctic Expedition of 1911–1914. *Medical Journal of Australia*, **i**, 1337.

Gerber A., Raab A.P. & Sobel A.E. (1954) Vitamin A poisoning in adults. *American Journal of Medicine*, **16**, 729.

Raaschou-Nielsen W. (1961) Chronic intoxication with vitamin A in adults. *Dermatologica*, **123**, 293.

Solen-Bechara J. & Soscia J.L. (1963) Chronic hypervitaminosis A. *Archives of Internal Medicine*, **112**, 462.

Stimson W.H. (1961) Vitamin A intoxication in adults. *New England Journal of Medicine*, **265**, 369.

Sulzberger M.B. & Lazar M.P. (1951) Hypervitaminosis A. Report of a case in an adult. *Journal of the American Medical Association*, **140**, 788.

Chloroprene

Condensation products of monomeric chloroprene have caused diffuse reversible alopecia in workers manufacturing synthetic rubber (Polemann 1954; Lijhancova 1967). Hair loss occurred also in workers engaged in the polymerization of chlorobutadin to elastomers of the neoprene class (Ritter & Carter 1948). It is of interest that vitamin A is an isoprene derivative.

References

Lijhancova G. (1967) Berufsbedingte Haarausfall durch Chloroprene. *Berufsdermatosen,* **15**, 280.

Polemann G. (1954) Depilationswirkung ungesättigter Verbindemger als Beitrag zur Alopezie-problem. *Dermatologica,* **108**, 98.

Ritter W.L. & Carter A.S. (1948) Hair loss in neoprene manufacturers. *Journal of Industrial Hygiene (and Toxicology),* **30**, 192.

Levodopa

Levodopa has been held responsible for severe diffuse alopecia developing 6 weeks to 3 months after starting a daily dose of 2.5–3 g (Marshall & Williams 1971).

Reference

Marshall A. & Williams M.J. (1971) Alopecia and levodopa. *British Medical Journal,* **ii**, 47.

Propranolol

Propranolol may cause diffuse alopecia after an interval of about 3 months (Martin *et al.* 1973; Hilder 1979).

References

Hilder R.J. (1979) Propranolol and alopecia. *Cutis,* **24**, 63.

Martin C.M., Southwick E.G. & Maibach H.I. (1973) Propranolol-induced alopecia. *American Heart Journal,* **86**, 236.

Butyrophenone

Butyrophenone has been used in the management of schizophrenia. Cutaneous changes were produced in those patients receiving high doses (Simpson *et al.* 1964). The skin became dry and ichthyotic, and the hair, which was shed diffusely, also became lighter in colour.

Reference

Simpson G.M., Blair J.H. & Cranswick C.H. (1964) Cutaneous effects of a new butyrophenone drug. *Clinical Pharmacological Therapy,* **5**, 310.

Potassium thiocyanate

This drug, formerly prescribed in the treatment of hypertension, can cause diffuse alopecia, beginning after about 3 months' treatment (Hollander *et al.* 1949).

Reference

Hollander L., Evans G.F. & Krugh F.J. (1949) Multiple cutaneous effects of potassium sulfocyanate. *A.M.A Archives of Dermatology and Syphilology,* **59**, 112.

Antimalarial drugs

Mepacrin (quinacrin) widely prescribed during World War II, caused a severe lichenoid eruption in some individuals. When the scalp was involved an irreversible cicatricial alopecia resulted (Bauer 1981).

Chloroquine has caused bleaching of normally blonde or reddish hair (Marten 1957; Saunders *et al.* 1959). The bleaching was first apparent in the eyebrows or at the temples.

References

Bauer F. (1981) Quinacrin hydrochlorides drug eruption. *Journal of the American Academy of Dermatology*, **4**, 239.

Marten R.H. (1957) Hair bleaching during chloroquine treatment. *Transactions of the St John's Hospital Dermatological Society*, **39**, 45.

Saunders T.S., Fitzpatrick T.B., Seiji M., Brunet P. & Rosenbaum E.E. (1959) Decrease in human hair color and feather pigment of fowl following chloroquine diphosphate. *Journal of Investigative Dermatology*, **33**, 87.

Mercury (including acrodynia)

Occupational exposure to mercury is now strictly regulated in most countries, and mercury poisoning occurs either accidentally or from cosmetics. Some bleaching creams contain mercury and there may be sufficient percutaneous absorption to cause diffuse loss of hair and systemic symptoms such as weight loss and restlessness. In one such case the nails were hyperpigmented (Wüstner & Orfanos 1975).

Medicaments containing mercury were until recently frequently prescribed for infants as teething powders, as antibacterial applications and for a variety of infections.

The symptoms of mercury poisoning in infancy were known as 'pink disease' but the syndrome was named acrodynia by Chardon in 1830. It was gradually accepted during the late 1940s and early 1950s that mercury was the cause of the disease (Fanconi & Botzteja 1948; Warkany & Holland 1953; Warkany 1966).

Affected children, usually between 6 months and 2 years of age, first suffer from unexplained febrile symptoms, restlessness and hypotonia. The hands and feet and the nose become swollen and pink and soon peel. Sweating is profuse. Some shedding of hair occurs diffusely and alopecia may be severe. The nails may also be shed.

The diagnosis is confirmed by estimating the level of mercury in the urine.

References

Chardon, Fils (1830) De l'acrodynie. *Revue Médicale Française*, **3**, 51.

Fanconi G. & Botzteja A. (1945) Die Feersche Krankheit. *Helvetica Paediatrica Acta*, **3**, 264.

Warkany J. & Holland (1953) Acrodynia and mercury. *Journal of Paediatrics*, **42**, 365.

Warkany J. (1966) Acrodynia—postmortem of a disease. *American Journal of Diseases of Children,* 112, 146.

Wüstner H. & Orfanos C.E. (1975) Nagelsverfarbung und haarausfall: leitsymptome einer quecksilbervergiftung durch kosmetische bleichmittel. *Deutsche medizinische Wochenschrift,* 100, 1694.

Bromocriptine

Bromocriptine, used in hyperprolactinaemia and in acromegaly, caused increased hair loss from the beginning of treatment in all of fourteen women but in none of ten men. The hair loss did not become severe even after 3 years of treatment (Blum & Leiba 1980).

Reference

Blum I. & Leiba S. (1980) Increased hair loss as the side effect of bromocriptine treatment. *New England Journal of Medicine,* 303, 1418.

Thiamphenicol

Thiamphenicol caused diffuse alopecia in 10 of 155 patients; in two the baldness became complete. Eight weeks after the end of treatment the hair had regrown in six but the alopecia persisted in two; one patient had died, and one had been lost to observation (Manchlin *et al.* 1974).

Reference

Manchlin S., Novotny Z., Koller F. & Ruefli P. (1974) Cytostatic side effects of thiamphenicol: alopecia and reversible cytopenia. *Schweizerische medizinische Wochenschrift,* 104, 384.

Mephenesin

Mephenesin has caused depigmentation of dark hair (Spillane 1963).

Reference

Spillane J.D. (1963) Brunette to blonde. Depigmentation of human hair during oral treatment with mephenesin. *British Medical Journal,* i, 997.

Trimethadione

This chemical is said to have produced diffuse alopecia in children (Holowach & Sanders 1960).

Reference

Holowach J. & Sanders H.V. (1960) Alopecia as a side effect of the treatment of epilepsy with trimethadione. *New England Journal of Medicine,* 263, 1187.

Paraaminosalicylate

This has caused a lichenoid eruption leaving cicatricial alopecia (Piñol Aguadé *et al.* 1968).

Reference

Piñol Aguadé J., Castells Mas A., Lecha M., Mascaro J.M., Gimarz-Camerase J.M., Harch P. de, Gras J., Tuset N. & Castalls Rodallas A. (1968) Gran dermatitis liquenoide con Alopecia irreversible z beta alanuria en pacientes tratados con tuberculostaticos. *Medicina cutanea*, 3, 275.

Bismuth

When it was in frequent use in the treatment of syphilis, bismuth is said to have provoked diffuse alopecia (Göltner 1961).

Reference

Göltner E. (1961) Versenatbehandlung einer Alopezie nach Wismuththerapie. *Zeitschrift für Haut und Geschlechskrankheiten*, 31, 164.

Diagnosis of alopecia caused by chemicals

Before loss of hair is attributed to a chemical, it must be established that the type of alopecia is that which the chemical is known to induce (e.g. anagen, telogen, dystrophic) and that the time intervals between exposure to the chemical and onset of hair loss are appropriate.

If the suspected chemical has not previously been incriminated as causing alopecia, recovery of the hair loss on discontinuing the exposure and further recurrence on reexposure may be required before the evidence can be considered convincing.

Chapter 6
Hereditary and Congenital Alopecia and Hypotrichosis

History and nomenclature
(References p. 150)

Case reports of individuals who have been almost or totally hairless throughout life can be found in the early literature, but these reports and some more recent ones are of limited value, because they include no histological information and an inadequate account of associated defects; there is at the most a note to the effect that the nails and teeth were or were not normal.

There have been numerous attempts to classify the conditions characterized by congenital alopecia or hypotrichosis. Bonnet (1892) proposed a classification which was widely used for the next 40 years, and which was said to be based on embryological principles.

(a) Congenital absence of hair, with associated defects of teeth and nails.
(b) Congenital absence of hair with normal teeth and nails.
(c) Congenital absence of hair with partial or complete recovery at puberty.

Cockayne (1933) in attempting a more critical analysis of the literature, was aware that this oversimplification was no longer helpful. Each of Bonnet's groups can be shown to contain a number of genetically distinct entities as well as many cases which cannot yet be categorized. Although there are now many conditions which are so well defined that they can be diagnosed on clinical features alone, there are many more which are still of questionable status, and will remain so until adequate histological studies of the scalp and electronmicroscopic studies of shafts of any hairs that may be present have been combined with analysis of the chemical and physical properties of such hairs, and the detailed examination of the patient for structural and metabolic defects involving other organs.

As a working classification which allows the known syndromes to be identified, and provides a provisional status for those not yet characterized, the following modification of Muller's (1973) proposals has been found useful.

(A) Congenital alopecia or hypotrichosis without associated defects.
(B) Congenital alopecia or hypotrichosis as a major feature of well-defined hereditary syndromes.
(C) Congenital alopecia or hypotrichosis as a major feature of uncharacterized syndromes.
(D) Congenital alopecia or hypotrichosis as a minor or inconstant feature of hereditary syndromes.

Any classification of congenital and hereditary alopecias must be tentative. However, recent work (Baden & Kubilus 1980) suggests that it may be possible to differentiate congenital alopecias which are due to an abnormality in the formation of the follicle, from those due to an abnormality in some component of the hair.

The ectodermal dysplasias
(References p. 150)

The term 'ectodermal dysplasia' was originally applied to anhidrotic ectodermal dysplasia (p. 152) in which hair, teeth, nails and sweat glands are defective. As more and more syndromes have been described their nomenclature has become confused and complex and 'ectodermal dysplasia' has been applied loosely and inconsistently to a wide variety of states.

Freire-Maia (1977) has drawn attention to these difficulties of classification and nomenclature and has suggested a provisional classification based on the ectodermal derivatives which show a primary defect—conditions in which the ectodermal changes are secondary, as in xeroderma pigmentosum are thus excluded from the ectodermal dysplasias. According to Freire-Maia's classification (1) is a hair dysplasia, (2) a dental dysplasia, (3) a nail dysplasia, (4) a sweat gland defect, and (5) a defect of other ectodermal structures. Anhidrotic ectodermal dysplasia thus falls into sub-group 1, 2, 3, 4, hidrotic ectodermal dysplasia into sub-group 1, 2, 3, and any syndrome in which hair dysplasia is the only defect, into sub-group 1 (Solomon & Keuer 1980).

Hereditary alopecia without associated defects

Recessive forms

There are several apparently distinctive genotypes. Most commonly reported is a total and permanent absence of hair, probably determined by an autosomal recessive gene. Two brothers (Calvo Melendro 1955) whose parents were consanguineous, came of a family in which 261 individuals could be traced through over a century; 3.04% were affected. Lundbäck (1944) reported nine cases in two families. The hair was normal at birth, but was soon shed and never replaced. Hair follicles were absent, but sebaceous glands were normal in number, but small. In the family reported by Birke (1954) two of three children of consanguineous parents were bald from birth; a third child was born with some head hair, which was soon lost. A biopsy showed short follicles containing horny plugs; there were no milia or papules. Two of four German siblings showed essentially the same clinical, and histological changes (Kauftheil 1926) as did the patients reported by Kraus (1903). A similar condition, with universal absence of hair was reported in three of four Jugoslav siblings (Bunton & Fettich 1974) and in three of five Punjabi siblings (Sein 1936). Other authors who

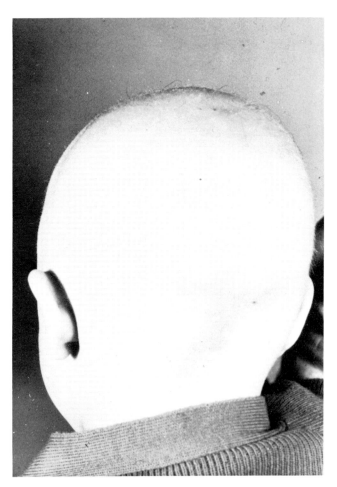

Fig. 6.1. Congenital alopecia without associated defects (Slade Hospital, Oxford).

have reported one or more cases of what appears to be the same condition include Bettmann (1902), Stein (1925), Klövekorn (1928), Henckel (1935), Janssen & Kox (1947), Friederich (1930), Tillman (1952), Linn (1964), Shy & Treister 1968) and Cantu *et al.* (1980). The siblings reported by Porter (1973) probably had the same syndrome; histological and histochemical investigations suggested that the essential defect was dyskeratosis of the hair shaft.

Dominant forms

Several pedigrees have been published showing autosomal dominant inheritance of hypotrichosis as an apparently isolated defect. There are differences in the clinical features and more than one genotype is involved.

Peterson (1915) described a family in which nine individuals were affected in three generations. From about the age of 5 the previously normal scalp hair was replaced by short, sparse hair of a lighter colour.

Jeanselme & Rimé (1924) observed a family in which fourteen individuals in four generations were affected. Towards the end of the first year normal hair was shed and was partially replaced by sparse and brittle hair in all hairy regions including the brows and lashes.

A pedigree covering eight generations of a Spanish family was well documented by Toribio & Quiñones (1974). The hair was normal until the age of 5–12 years when retardation of hair growth was first noted and diffuse thinning began. By the age of 25 only a few hairs remained on the scalp, but hair elsewhere was not affected. Histologically the number of follicles is found not to be decreasd but they fail progressively to re-enter anagen. The hair shafts appear normal with the light microscope and in the electronmicroscope show focal cuticular defects which are not distinctive and may be the result of normal weathering.

A similar condition in four generations of a family was reported by Bentley-Phillips & Grace (1979). The hair was apparently normal until the age of 7–13 when there was progressive shedding of scalp hair, and eyebrows and lashes were lost. Eventually only a few wispy hairs remained in the atrophic scalp. Teeth, nails and eyes were normal. In the scan electronmicroscope the hairs show weathering with partial or complete absence of cuticular scales.

A few other pedigrees also suggest apparent dominant transmission of congenital alopecia (Pajtas 1950; Tillman 1952).

Madarosis

The congenital absence or underdevelopment of the eyelashes occurs sporadically, but autosomal dominant inheritance has been reported (Bergsma 1979). The eyebrows and scalp hair may also be absent, but nails and sweat glands are normal.

References

Baden H.P. & Kubilus J. (1980) Analysis of hair from alopecia congenita. *Journal of the American Academy of Dermatology*, **3**, 623.

Bentley-Phillips B. & Grace H.J. (1979) Hereditary hypotrichosis. *British Journal of Dermatology*, **101**, 331.

Bergsma D. (1979) Madarosis. In *Birth Defects Compendium*, 2nd edn., ed. D. Bergsma. London, Macmillan, p. 676.

Bettman S. (1902) Uber angeborenen Haarmangel. *Archiv für Dermatologie und Syphilologie*, **60**, 348.

Birke G. (1954) Uber Atrichia congenita und ihren Erbgang. *Archiv für Dermatologie und Syphilologie*, **197**, 322.

Bonnet R. (1892) Ueber Hypotrichosis congenita universalis. *Anatomische Hefte*, **1**, 233.

Bunton S. & Fettich J. (1974) Atrichia congenita universalis. *Acta Dermato-venereologica Jugoslav*, **1**, 97.

Calvo Melendro J. (1955) Atriquia congenita total y permanente. *Medicina clinica*, **24**, 253.

Cantu J.M., Sanchez-Corona J., Gonzalez-Mendoza A., Martinez R.M. & Garcia-Crez D. (1980) Autosomal recessive inheritance of atrichia congenita. *Clinical Genetics*, **17**, 209.

Cockayne A.E. (1933) *Inherited Abnormalities of the Skin and its Appendages*. Oxford, Oxford University Press, p. 229.

Freire-Maia, N. (1977) Ectodermal dysplasia revisited. *Acta Genetico Medico e Gemellologia*, **26**, 121.

Friederich H.C. (1930) Zur Kenntniss der Kongenitale Hypotrichosis. *Dermatologische Wochenschrift*, **121**, 408.

Henckel K.O. (1935) Hypotrichosis congenita bei eineigen Drillingen. *Klinische Wochenschrift*, **14**, 428.

Janssen T.A.E. & Kox W. (1947) Alopecia universalis congenita and hypoplasia renum in a newborn. *Acta paediatrica (Stockholm)*, **34**, 289.

Jeanselme & Rimé (1924) Un cas d'alopécie congénitale familiale. *Bulletin de la Société française de Dermatologie et de Syphiligraphie*, **31**, 79.

Kauftheil L. (1926) Uber einen Fall von Atrichia congenita. *Dermatologische Zeitschrift*, **48**, 267.

Klövekorn (1928) Totale kongenitale alopecie. *Archiv für Dermatologie und Syphilologie*, **155**, 328.

Kraus A. (1903) Beiträge zur Kenntnis der Alopecia congenita familiaris. *Archiv für Dermatologie und Syphilologie*, **66**, 369.

Linn H.W. (1964) Congenital atrichia. *Australian Journal of Dermatology*, **7**, 223.

Lundbäck H. (1944) Total congenital hereditary alopecia. *Acta Dermato-venereologica*, **25**, 189.

Muller S.A. (1973) Alopecia: syndromes of genetic significance. *Journal of Investigative Dermatology*, **60**, 475.

Pajtas J. (1950) Totale familiäre hereditäre Hypotrichosis in 4 Generationen. *Dermatologica*, **101**, 90.

Peterson H. (1915) Kongenitale familiäre hereditäre Alopezie auf der Basis irres Hypothyroidismus. *Dermatologische Zeitschrift*, **22**, 202.

Porter P.S. (1973) Genetic disorders of hair growth. *Journal of Investigative Dermatology*, **60**, 493.

Sein M. (1936) Congenital and familial absence of hair from the whole surface of the body. *Lancet*, **ii**, 564.

Shy W.S. & Treister M. (1968) Isolated Congenital Hypotrichosis. i. Recessive Hairlessness in Man. ii. Mendelian Inheritance in Man, 2nd edn., ed. V.A. McKusick. Baltimore, Johns Hopkins Press.

Solomon L.M. & Keuer E.J. (1980) The ectodermal dysplasias. *Archives of Dermatology*, **116**, 1295.

Stein R.O. (1925) Alopecia totalis congenita. *Zeitschrift für Haut und Geschlechtskrankheiten*, **18**, 520.

Tillman W.G. (1952) Alopecia congenita: report of two families. *British Medical Journal*, **ii,** 428.
Toribio J. & Quiñones P.A. (1974) Hereditary hypotrichosis simplex of the scalp. *British Journal of Dermatology*, **91,** 687.

The hair in ectodermal dysplasias
(Reference p. 152)

The term ectodermal dysplasia is used here as defined by Solomon & Keuer (1980).

The following criteria must be met: the disease is congenital; it is diffuse and involves the epidermis and at least one of the appendages; it is not progressive. The hair defect is in almost all ectodermal dysplasias a reduction in the number and size of the follicles, producing hypotrichosis or alopecia, but in some, e.g. the Chand syndrome, the hair is curly but otherwise normal.

The ectodermal dysplasias, thus defined, are here classified provisionally in accordance with Freire-Maia's suggestion (see p. 147):

Subgroup 1,2,3,4   *Hair, teeth, nails and sweating defects*
  Anhidrotic ectodermal dysplasia
  Rapp–Hodgkin hypohidrotic ectodermal dysplasia
  Ectrodactyly, ectodermal dysplasia and cleft lip or palate
  Popliteal web syndrome
  XTE syndrome

Subgroup 1,2,3   *Hair, teeth, nail defects*
  Clouston's hidrotic ectodermal dysplasia
  Trichodento-osseous syndrome
  Ellis–van Creveld syndrome
  AEC syndrome
  Basan syndrome
  Tooth–nail syndrome

Subgroup 1,3,4   *Hair, nails and sweating defects*
  Freire-Maia syndrome

Subgroup 1,2   *Hair and teeth defects*
  Orofaciodigital syndrome I
  Sensenbrenner syndrome
  Trichodental syndrome

Subgroup 1,3   *Hair and nail defects*
  CHAND syndrome
  Onychotrichodysplasia with neutropenia

Subgroup 1   *Hair defects*
    Trichorhinophalangeal syndromes I and II
    Dubowitz syndrome
    Moynahan syndrome

Reference
Solomon L.M. & Keuer E.J. (1980) The ectodermal dysplasias. *Archives of Dermatology*, **116**, 1295.

Anhidrotic ectodermal dysplasia (Christ–Siemens–Touraine syndrome)
The inheritance of this uncommon syndrome is usually determined by a sex-linked recessive gene (Kerr *et al.* 1966). Sweat gland and other skin appendages are absent or few in number. The full syndrome occurs only in males. Scalp hair is short, fine and very sparse and often light in colour, but may increase in quantity after puberty (Reed *et al.* 1970). In the electronmicroscope (Porter & Aoyagi 1974) the hairs show unusual overlapping and furrowing of cuticular scales, occasional irregular bulging of the shaft, and some longitudinal ridging. Eyebrows and eyelashes may also be sparse or absent but may be relatively little affected. Body hair may be sparse or absent. The prominent square forehead, saddle nose, the thick lower lip and the pointed chin produce a distinctive facies. The skin around the eyes is finely wrinkled and may be pigmented. The teeth may be absent or few in number, characteristically the canines and incisors are conical. The absent or reduced sweating leads to heat intolerance, and unexplained pyrexia may be the presenting symptom in infancy. Carrier females may be clinically normal but may show in some degree one or more of the features of the syndrome, e.g. conical teeth, hypotrichosis or heat intolerance. Otherwise apparently normal carriers may show dermatoglyphic abnormalities, the presence of which may be of value in diagnosis (Verbov 1970).

Anhidrotic ectodermal dysplasia may sometimes depend on an autosomal recessive gene, in which case the full syndrome may be found in the female. It is not yet certain whether, as is probable, cases so inherited differ in some respects from those determined by a sex-linked recessive gene (Passarge *et al.* 1966; Crump & Danks 1971).

References
Crump I.A. & Danks D.M. (1971) Hypohidrotic ectodermal dysplasia. *Journal of Pediatrics*, **78**, 466.
Kerr C.B., Wells R.S. & Cooper K.E. (1966) Gene effect in carriers of anhidrotic ectodermal dysplasia. *Journal of Medical Genetics*, **3**, 169.
Passarge E., Nuzum C.T. & Schubert W.K. (1966) Anhidrotic ectodermal dysplasia as autosomal recessive trait in an inbred kindred. *Humangenetik*, **3**, 181.
Porter P.S. & Aoyagi T. (1974) Classification of genetic abnormalities of hair growth. *First Human Hair Symposium*, ed. A. Brown. New York, Medcom, p. 205.

Reed W.B., Lopez D.A. & Landing B. (1970) Clinical spectrum of anhidrotic ectodermal dysplasia. *Archives of Dermatology*, **102**, 134.
Verbov J. (1970) Hypohidrotic (or anhidrotic) ectodermal dysplasia. An appraisal of diagnostic methods. *British Journal of Dermatology*, **83**, 341.

Rapp–Hodgkin hypohidrotic ectodermal dysplasia

In this syndrome, the inheritance of which is determined by an autosomal dominant gene, hypohidrosis may be severe enough to lead to heat intolerance. The hair is sparse and the nails are narrow and dystrophic. Short stature, a cleft lip and palate and hypospadia are other features. The hair is light in colour and of the texture of steel wool.

References

Rapp R.S. & Hodgkin W.E. (1968) Anhidrotic ectodermal dysplasia: autosomal dominant inheritance with palate and lip anomalies. *Journal of Medical Genetics*, **5**, 219.
Summitt R.L. & Hiatt R.L. (1971) Hypohidrotic ectodermal dysplasia with multiple associated anomalies. *Birth Defects*, **7**, 121.
Wamarachue N., Hall B.D. & Smith D.W. (1972) Ectodermal dysplasia with multiple defects (Rapp–Hodgkin type). *Journal of Pediatrics*, **81**, 1217.

EEC syndrome

The association of Ectrodactyly (lobster-claw deformity), Ectodermal dysplasia, and Cleft lip and palate in a syndrome of autosomal dominant inheritance is now well documented (Brill *et al.* 1972). However, the expressivity of the gene is very variable and there are numerous reported of cases or pedigrees of complex syndromes which are probably genetically distinct but which show some of the main features of the EEC syndrome. All cases in which ectrodactyly or syndactyly and/or cleft lip or palate are associated with ectodermal defects are worthy of full investigation so that the genetic pattern of these syndromes may be elucidated.

Cases reported as the EEC syndrome show sparse hair, malformed teeth with early caries, ectrodactyly, cleft lip and/or palate, lacrimal duct stenosis and renal anomalies, but not all defects are present in all affected individuals within a single family (Brill *et al.* 1972; Preuss & Fraser 1973).

Other cases are reported in which hypotrichosis as one manifestation of ectodermal dysplasia is associated with cleft lip or palate and a variety of other defects, and the presence of such an association should suggest the need for a search of the rapidly growing genetic literature in which such syndromes are gradually being characterized.

References

Brill C.R., Hsu L.Y.F. & Hirschhorn K. (1972) The syndrome of ectrodactyly, ectodermal dysplasia and cleft lip and palate: report of a family demonstrating a dominant inheritance pattern. *Clinical Genetics*, **3**, 295.
Preuss M. & Fraser F.C. (1973) The lobster claw defect with ectodermal defects, cleft lip and palate, tear duct anomaly and renal anomalies. *Clinical Genetics*, **4**, 369.

Popliteal web syndrome

History and nomenclature. This rare syndrome was first reported by Trilet in 1869, but has been widely recognized only in the last two decades (Roselli & Gulienetti 1961). It has been referred to as the popliteal pterygium syndrome or alternatively as the popliteal web syndrome.

Aetiology. Most pedigrees show autosomal dominant inheritance determined by a gene of variable expressivity (Hecht & Jarvinen 1967), but Bartsocas & Papas (1972) suggest that a form with more severe manifestations including mental retardation may be determined by an autosomal recessive gene.

Clinical features. The principal features of the syndrome are a cleft palate, with or without a cleft lip, lip-pits, popliteal and other webs, hypodontia, enamel defects and toe-nail dysplasia. Genital and perineal defects vary greatly in degree. There may be a large clitoris, a bifid scrotum or aplasia of the labia majora. Syndactyly has been present in some cases. An inconsistent feature is absence of eyebrows and eyelashes, with brittle, short, sparse, light-coloured head hair.

References

Bartsocas C.S. & Papas C.V. (1972) Popliteal pterygium syndrome. *Journal of Medical Genetics*, **9**, 222.

Hecht F. & Jarvinen J.M. (1967) Hereditable dysmorphic syndrome with normal intelligence. *Journal of Pediatrics*, **70**, 927.

Roselli D. & Gulienetti R. (1961) Ectodermal dysplasia. *British Journal of Plastic Surgery*, **14**, 190.

Xeroderma, talipes and enamel defect: XTE syndrome

This autosomal dominant syndrome is characterized by dry skin, readily forming blisters in the spring season, talipes and defective enamel. The sweat glands are small and few in number. The scalp hair is coarse and sparse, the eyelashes are absent and the nails are dystrophic.

Reference

Moynahan E.J. (1970) XTE syndrome (Xeroderma, Talipes and Enamel defect): a new heredofamilial syndrome. Two cases. Homozygous inheritance of a dominant gene. *Proceedings of the Royal Society of Medicine*, **63**, 447.

Clouston's hidrotic ectodermal dysplasia (references p. 155)

This hereditary syndrome, which is not excessively rare, is determined by an autosomal dominant gene (Clouston 1929, 1939; Williams & Fraser 1967). A structural gene for a matrix polypeptide is probably implicated (Gold & Scriver 1971). Keratinization is disturbed, resulting in abnormal hair and nails and reduced surface desquamation, most evident on palms and soles. The alopecia is such a striking feature of this syndrome that many pedigrees have been published under the diagnosis of congenital alopecia (e.g. Bazant-Gavalowski 1921; Stevanovic 1959).

Detailed studies of the hair (Gold & Scriver 1972) showed reduced elasticity and tensile strength. Birefringence also was reduced; the shaft had a loose structure and the normal parallel longitudinal striation was distorted. However, on X-ray diffraction the α helical structure of the keratin fibres was intact. Biochemically, serine, proline and cystine residues were decreased and tyrosine and phenylalamine residues were increased. A reduced disulphide content was not compensated by a thiol increase. It was postulated that there was depletion of matrix proline and disruption of, or failure of some disulphide bonds in the remaining keratin. In the electronmicroscope (Wilsch *et al.* 1977) numerous structural abnormalities are seen in variation in diameter, splitting of the cuticle, fracture without node formation, and an abnormal cuticular pattern.

Head hair is very sparse, fine, pale and brittle; it may be totally absent. Eyebrows are sparse or absent and eyelashes are few and small. Pubic and axillary hair, and vellus, are sparse or absent. Although the hair changes are inconstant and variable they are present at least in some degree in the majority of cases (Clouston 1929; Lopez *et al.* 1970; Dethlep & Tronnier 1972). In only 20% of individuals with nail changes is the hair apparently normal (Wilkinson 1974). Sweating is normal. There is often some keratoderma of palms and soles, which may be red, scaly and fissured.

General physical development and sexual maturation are normal, but some degree of mental retardation is frequent. The teeth are usually normal. The nails are consistently dystrophic from birth, being thickened, ridged and discoloured or, less frequently, thin and brittle.

The diagnosis is made on the association of alopecia with nail dystrophy, with or without palmoplantar keratoderma, but with normal sweating and no distinctive dental defect. The biochemical and biophysical defects of the hair appear to be diagnostic.

References

Bazant-Gavalowski K. (1921) Hypotrichosis universalis congenita. *Archiv für Dermatologie und Syphilologie*, **137**, 174.

Clouston H.R. (1929) A hereditary ectodermal dystrophy. *Canadian Medical Association Journal*, **21**, 18.

Clouston H.R. (1939) The major forms of hereditary ectodermal dysplasia. *Canadian Medical Association Journal*, **40**, 1.

Dethlep B. & Tronnier H. (1972) Beitrag zum Krankheitsbild der hydrotischen (Minor-) Form des Ectodermalen Dysplasia. *Hautarzt*, **23**, 541.

Gold R.J.M. & Scriver C.R. (1971) The characterization of hereditary abnormalities of keratin. *Birth Defects, Original Article Series*, **7**, 91.

Gold R.J.M. & Scriver C.R. (1972) Properties of hair keratin in an autosomal dominant form of ectodermal dysplasia. *American Journal of Human Genetics*, **24**, 549.

Lopez D.A., Reed W.B., Berke M. & Morales R.A. (1970) Displasio ectodermico congenita de tepo hidrotico. *Medicina cutanea*, **4**, 335.

Stevanovic D.V. (1959) Alopecia congenita. *Acta Genetica*, **9**, 127.

Wilkinson R.D. (1974) Hidrotic ectodermal dysplasia of clouston: clinical and histopathological features. *First Human Hair Symposium*, ed. A. Brown. New York, Medcon, p. 61.

Williams M. & Fraser F.C. (1967) Hidrotic ectodermal dysplasia—Clouston's family revisited. *Canadian Medical Association Journal*, **96**, 36.

Wilsch L., Haneke E. & Schaidt G. (1977) Structural hair abnormalities in hidrotic ectodermal dysplasia. *Archives of Dermatological Research*, **259**, 101.

Trichodento-osseous syndrome (TDO syndrome)

All children who subsequently show the distinctive features of this syndrome are born with a full head of tightly curled air, which tends to become straighter during childhood. Microscopically the structure of the shaft is seen to be normal. The eyelashes also are curly.

The teeth are small and widely spaced, pitted on account of defective enamel, and soon eroded and discoloured. Early caries is inevitable. Dolichocephaly combined with frontal bossing and a square jaw give a distinctive facies. Bone density is slightly to moderately increased. Physical development is normal.

The syndrome is determined by an autosomal dominant gene.

References

Lichtenstein J., Warson R., Jorgenson R., Dorst R.P. & McKusick V.A. (1972) The Tricho-Dento-Osseous (TDO) syndrome. *American Journal of Human Genetics*, **24**, 569.

Melnick N., Shields E.D. & El-Kafrawy A.H. (1977) Trichodentoosseous syndrome: a scanning electron microscopic analysis. *Clinical Genetics*, **12**, 17.

Robinson G.C., Miller J. & Worth H.M. (1966) Hereditary manual hypoplasia: its association with characteristic hair structure. *Pediatrics*, **37**, 498.

Ellis–van Creveld syndrome, syn. chondroectodermal dysplasia

The principal features of this autosomal recessive syndrome are chondrodysplasia of the long bones giving rise to acromelic dwarfism, congenital heart disease in about 50%, and ectodermal dysplasia. The latter includes oligodontia and attachment of the upper lip to the anterior gingival margin, small hypoplastic nails and sparse hair, but the hair defect may be mild in degree.

Reference

Gorlin R.J., Pindborg J.J. & Colen M.M. (1976) Chondroectodermal dysplasia. In *Syndromes of the Head and Neck*, 2nd edn., eds. R.J. Gorlin, J.J. Pindborg and M.M. Cohen. New York, McGraw-Hill, p. 80.

AEC syndrome

This newly described autosomal dominant syndrome has been identified in seven patients in four families (Hay & Wells 1976). Ankyloblepharon is associated with Ectodermal defects, and Cleft lip and palate.

The hair is wiry and sparse, or absent. On electronmicroscopy the hair shafts show changes similar to those found in the Marie Unna syndrome i.e. longitudinal fluting and focal defects of the cuticle. The nails are absent or dystrophic. The teeth are pointed and widely spaced and are soon eroded or lost, and sweating is diminished. The broad nasal bridge and sunken maxilla produce a facies which is striking rather than pathognomonic.

Inconstantly associated defects include lacrimal duct stenosis, supernumerary nipples, syndactyly and deformities of the auricle.

Reference

Hay R.J. & Wells R.S. (1976) The syndrome of ankyloblepharon, ectodermal defects and cleft lip and palate: an autosomal dominant condition. *British Journal of Dermatology*, **94**, 277.

Basan syndrome

Aetiology. This rarely reported hereditary ectodermal defect is determined by an autosomal dominant gene.

Clinical features. Body hair, eyebrows and eyelashes are sparse throughout life. Scalp hair may at first be normal in quantity, but coarse, and is shed during the second decade. The skin generally is very dry, with sweating reduced to a degree sufficient to give rise to moderate intolerance of heat.

The mucous membranes are dry, and severe dental caries develops early.

Reference

Basan M. (1965) Ektodermal dysplasia. Fehlendes Papillanmuster. Nagelveränderungen und Vierfingerfurche. *Archiv für klinische und experimentelle Dermatologie*, **222**, 546.

Tooth and nail syndrome

In this autosomal dominant syndrome hypodontia, with peg-shaped milk teeth and agenesis of permanent teeth, is accompanied by hypoplastic nails. The hair is sparse with some twisting but not pili torti.

In one family (Ellis & Dawber 1980) there was 50% reduction of palmar sweat pore patency, but the number of sweat pores was normal. Sweating was normal on the trunk and limbs.

References

Ellis J. & Dawber R.P.R. (1980) Ectodermal dysplasia syndrome: a family study. *Clinical and Experimental Dermatology*, **5**, 295.

Giansanti J.S., Long S.M. & Rankin J.L. (1974) The 'tooth and nail' type of autosomal dominant ectodermal dysplasia. *Oral Surgery*, **37**, 576.

Oro-Facio-Digital syndrome I

Aetiology. The inheritance of this syndrome is determined by an X-linked dominant gene, linked in the male.

Clinical features. Oral and skeletal defects dominate the syndrome. The tongue is lobed, the lower lateral incisor teeth fail to develop and the palate is cleft.

In 90% of cases there is brachydactyly, syndactyly or clinodactyly. There are numerous milia on the skin at birth and the hair is frequently fine, sparse and dry.

Abnormalities of the skin and hair are not features of Oro-Facio-Digital syndrome II.

Reference
Gorlin R.J. & Psaume J. (1962) Orodigitofacial dysostosis: a new syndrome: a study of 22 cases. *Journal of Pediatrics*, **61**, 520.

Sensenbrenner syndrome Sensenbrenner *et al.* (1975)
This rarely reported syndrome is probably determined by an autosomal recessive gene. The affected children are small and dolichocephalic. The facies is unusual with frontal bosses, hypertelorism, epicanthic folds, antimongoloid palpebral fissues, full rounded cheeks and eversion of the lower lip. The hair is short and very fine. The teeth are small, grey and widely spaced.

Reference
Sensenbrenner J.A., Dorst J.P. & Owens R.P. (1975) New syndrome of skeletal, dental and hair anomalies. *Birth Defects*, **11**, 372.

Trichodental syndrome
In a large pedigree the inheritance of this syndrome was determined by an autosomal dominant gene. The scalp hair is fine, dry and lustreless and grows slowly. In the electronmicroscope the cuticular scale pattern is abnormal. The outer halves of the eyebrows are missing. There is hypodontia.

Reference
Salinas C.F. & Spector M. (1980) Trichodental syndrome. In *Hair, Trace Elements and Human Illness*, eds. A.C. Brown & R.G. Crounse. New York, Praeger, p. 290.

Curly hair, ankyloblepharon nail dysplasia syndrome (CHANDS)
This autosomal dominant syndrome is characterized by curly hair, dysplastic nails and ankyloblepharon.

Reference
Baughman F.A. (1971) CHANDS: the Curly Hair–Ankyloblepharon–Nail Dysplasia syndrome. *Birth Defects Original Article Series*, **7**, 100.

Onychotrichodysplasia with neutropenia
In this syndrome, apparently determined by an autosomal recessive gene, sparse hair and dystrophic nails are associated with mild mental retardation and with chronic neutropenia.

Reference

Hernandez A., Olivares F. & Carter J.N. (1979) Autosomal recessive onychotrichodysplasia chronic neutropenia and mental retardation: delineation of the syndrome. *Clinical Genetics*, **15**, 147.

Trichorhinophalangeal syndrome, Type I
The inheritance of this syndrome is usually determined by an autosomal dominant gene of variable expressivity, but there may also be a recessive form. The principal features are (a) a distinctive facies provided by a pear-shaped nose and a high philtrum, with a receding chin (Fig. 6.2); (b) brachyphalangeal

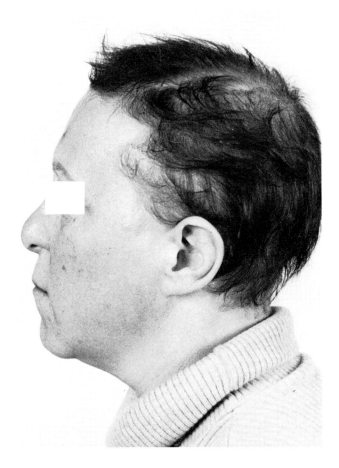

Fig. 6.2. Trichorhinophalan-geal syndrome Type I showing distinctive facies (Professor Hunter, Edinburgh).

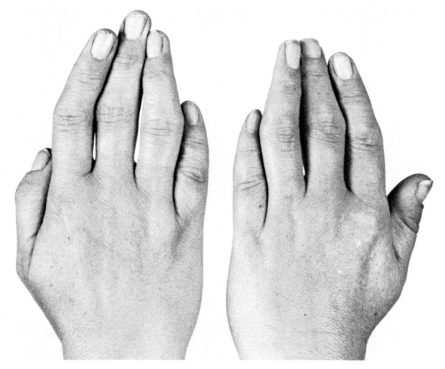

Fig. 6.3. Trichorhinophalangeal syndrome Type I—brachyphalangeal dysostosis (Professor Hunter, Edinburgh).

dysostosis, which results in fusiform swelling of the proximal interphalangeal joints (Fig. 6.3); and (c) fine, brittle, sparse hair (Fig. 6.4). The sparse hair is often the symptom for which the parents seek medical advice. The medial halves of the eyebrows are denser than the lateral halves.

Reference
Giedion A., Burdea M., Fruchter Z., Meloni T. & Trox V. (1973) Autosomal-dominant transmission of the tricho-rhino-phalangeal syndrome. *Helvetica paediatrica Acta,* **28,** 249.

Trichorhinophalangeal syndrome, Type II
All reported cases of this syndrome have been sporadic. The nose is bulbous, the philtrum is elongated and prominent, the upper lip is thin and the ears are large and protruding. The scalp hair is sparse. There is some degree of microcephaly and mild to moderate mental retardation.

Multiple cartilaginous exostoses develop from childhood.

Reference
Hall J.G. (1979) Tricho-rhino-phalangeal syndrome type II. In *Birth Defects Compendium,* 2nd edn., ed. D. Bergsma. London, Macmillan, p. 1043.

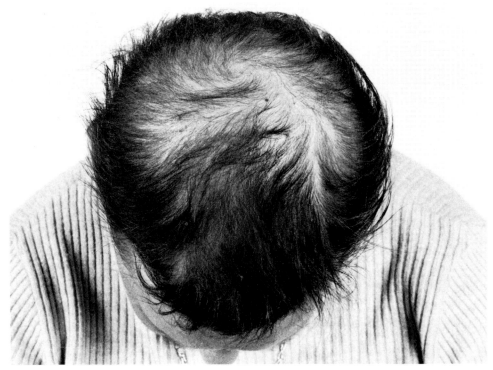

Fig. 6.4. Trichorhinophalangeal syndrome Type I—fine brittle sparse hair (Professor Hunter, Edinburgh).

Moynahan syndrome

This very rare syndrome is characterized by absence of hair at birth, and the development of very sparse fine hair later.

Epilepsy and severe mental retardation are present.

Reference

Moynahan E.J. (1979) Moynahan Syndrome. In *Birth Defects Compendium*, 2nd edn., ed. D. Bergsma. London, Macmillan, p. 723.

Hereditary hypotrichosis: Marie Unna type
(References pp. 164–5)

History and nomenclature

Marie Unna of Hamburg published in 1925 an account of a family in which 27 individuals in seven generations were affected by a previously unreported type of hypotrichosis. Ludwig (1953) found three more cases among the descendants of a member of this same family and Borelli (1954) found two more in another branch of the family. The syndrome is distinctive and most subsequent authors have associated it eponymously with Marie Unna.

Cases have now been reported from Hungary (Kemeny & Csontos 1967), Jugoslavia (Stevanovic 1970), Britain (Peachey & Wells 1971) and the United States (Solomon *et al.* 1971).

Ullmo's (1944) patients were a brother and sister with similar hair changes, but as they also had keratosis pilaris and mental retardation, may not have had the same syndrome.

Aetiology
The inheritance of this form of hypotrichosis is determined by an autosomal dominant gene. This mode of inheritance has been noted in all pedigrees in which the diagnosis is beyond question. There may be minor differences between families (Peachey & Wells 1971) but the main features of the syndrome are remarkably consistent.

Pathology
The histological changes in the balding scalp are not pathognomonic. The number of follicles is markedly reduced; granulomatous reactions may be seen around partially destroyed follicles. Solomon *et al.* (1971) found proliferation of the internal root sheath and horn cyst formation in the lower third of some follicles, but Stevanovic (1970) noted proliferation of the external root sheath in the region of the keratogenous zone, with a tendency for it to bulge into the internal root sheath.

With the light microscope the hairs are coarse and flattened, and are twisted at irregular intervals. The shaft diameter may be up to 100 μm as compared with 65–75 μm in normal relations (Ludwig 1953).

In the scan electronmicroscope the hair shafts are ridged and the scale pattern is lost, particularly in the valleys between the ridges (Peachey & Wells 1971) (Fig. 6.5). On routine electronmicroscopy (Solomon *et al.* 1971) there are intracellular fractures of cuticular cells and an increase in interfibrillar matrix. On chemical analysis a small decrease in cysteine–cystine and an increase in methionine are found.

Clinical features
The hair may be normal at birth and be shed during infancy, but more frequently is sparse or absent at birth, and remains fine and sparse for the first years of life. During the 3rd year coarse twisted hair grows on the scalp, but with the approach of puberty is progressively lost from the vertex and scalp margins (Fig. 6.6). The ultimate extent of the scarring alopecia shows some variation, and it tends to be more severe in males. It is often patchy (Fig. 6.7).

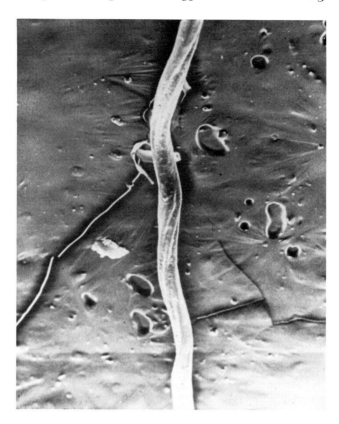

Fig. 6.5. Hair from Marie Unna syndrome: scanning electronmicrograph (Slade Hospital, Oxford).

Eyebrows and eyelashes and body hair are absent or scanty from birth, and after puberty, axillary and pubic and beard hair is also sparse.

Affected individuals are usually otherwise normal; facial milia were present at birth in all of eight cases in one family (Solomon *et al.* 1971).

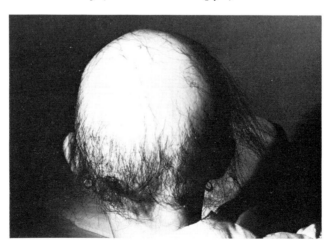

Fig. 6.6. Extensive alopecia in the Marie Unna syndrome (Slade Hospital, Oxford).

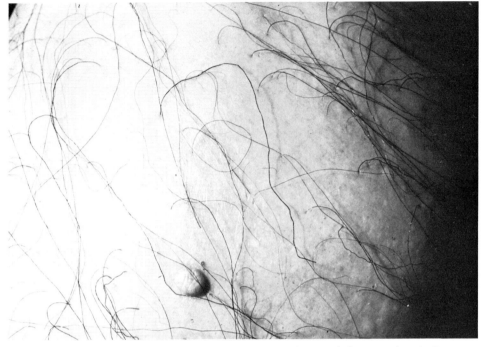

Fig. 6.7. Sparse hair of horse-hair texture in Marie Unna syndrome (Slade Hospital, Oxford).

Differential diagnosis

Despite the reported variations in the age of onset and degree of severity of the alopecia, the growth of coarse twisted hair in early childhood and its subsequent destruction with scarring on the vertex and the scalp margins, cannot be confused with any other syndrome. The histopathological changes are not diagnostic. The defects in the structure of the hair shaft support the clinical diagnosis.

Treatment

There is no effective treatment, but avoidance of trauma may bring some cosmetic benefit as the abnormal hairs are brittle and are also easily extracted. When folliculitis is troublesome, long-term antibiotic treatment may be useful (Peachey & Wells 1971).

References

Borelli S. (1954) Hypotrichosis congenita hereditaria Marie-Unna. *Hautarzt*, **5**, 18.
Kemeny P. & Csontos E. (1967) Hypotrichosis congenita hereditaria (Unna syndrome). *Kindercörtzliche Praxis*, **35**, 29.

Ludwig E. (1953) Hypotrichosis congenita hereditaria. Typ. M. Unna. *A.M.A. Archives of Dermatology and Syphilology*, **196**, 261.

Peachey R.D.G. & Wells R.S. (1971) Hereditary hypotrichosis (Marie-Unna type). *Transactions of the St John's Hospital Dermatological Society*, **57**, 157.

Solomon L.M., Esterly M.B. & Medenica M. (1971) Hereditary trichodysplasia: Marie Unna's hypotrichosis. *Journal of Investigative Dermatology*, **57**, 387.

Stevanovic D.V. (1970) Hereditary hypotrichosis congenita: Marie Unna type. *British Journal of Dermatology*, **83**, 331.

Ullmo A. (1944) Un nouveau type d'agénésie et de dystrophie pilaire familiale et héréditaire. *Dermatologica*, **90**, 75.

Unna M. (1925) Uber Hypotrichosis congenita hereditaria. *Dermatologische Wochenschrift*, **81**, 1167.

Hallermann–Streiff syndrome
(References p. 166)

History and nomenclature

It was the curious pattern of sutural alopecia which first attracted attention to this syndrome (Aubry 1893). It was subsequently described by others under various designations which emphasized the ocular defects (see Lamy *et al.* 1965). Two of at least four such reports were published by Hallermann (1948) and Streiff (1950) who differentiated the syndrome from mandibulofacial dysostosis. François (1958) reviewed the literature thoroughly and gave a good description of the syndrome, which is now known as mandibulo-oculo-facial dyscephaly or, eponymously, as the Hallermann–Streiff syndrome, the Hallermann–Streiff–François syndrome, or the François syndrome.

Aetiology

This complex of ectodermal and mesodermal defects is not proved to be hereditary, and most cases have been sporadic. However, it has been reported in a father and son (Guyard *et al.* 1962), and may be determined by a dominant gene, most cases being new mutations.

Pathology

The atrophic skin shows loosely woven collagen and frequent abnormal elastic fibres (François & Pierard 1971). The hair shafts show, in the scan electron-microscope, circumferential grooving of the cuticle, which in places is deficient (Golomb & Porter 1975).

Clinical features

Dyscephaly, a beaked nose and a hypoplastic mandible give the patient a bird-like profile. Physical and mental development is retarded. Microphthalmia and congenital cataracts are the concomitant of many ocular defects (François

1958). Dental defects also are frequent and numerous (Hutchinson 1971); teeth may be absent, hypoplastic or irregularly implanted.

The scalp hair may be normal at birth but soon becomes diffusely sparse and brittle, with frontal baldness, baldness of lateral and posterior scalp margins or, most characteristically, following the lines of the cranial sutures. Eyebrows and eyelashes are scanty or absent and pubic and axillary hair also may be sparse (Golomb & Porter 1975).

The skin of the face is atrophic, particularly in the central area, where telangiectasia may be marked. The subcutaneous veins may be conspicuously visible.

Diagnosis
The association of the hair loss with the distinctive facies should establish the diagnosis. In progeria the alopecia is diffuse and the cutaneous atrophy is generalized.

Treatment
Little can be offered but regular ophthalmic and dental supervision and the provision of a wig.

References
Aubry M. (1893) Variété singulaire d'alopécie congénitale: Alopécie suturale. *Annales de Dermatologie et de Syphiligraphie,* **4,** 399.
François J. (1958) A new syndrome: dyscephalia with bird face and dental anomalies, nanism, hypotrichosis, cutaneous atrophy, micro-ophthalmia and congenital cataract. *Archives of Ophthalmology,* **60,** 842.
François J. & Pierard J. (1971) François dyscephalic syndrome and skin manifestations. *American Journal of Ophthalmology,* **71,** 1241.
Golomb R.S. & Porter P.S. (1975) A distinct hair shaft abnormality in the Hallermann–Streiff syndrome. *Cutis,* **16,** 122.
Guyard M., Perdriel G. & Cerutti F. (1962) Sur deux cas de syndrome dyscéphalique à tête d'oiseau. *Bulletin de la Société ophtalmique de France,* **62,** 433.
Hallermann W. (1948) Vogelgesicht und Cataracta congenita. *Klinische Monatschrifte fur Augenheilkunde,* **113,** 315.
Hutchinson D. (1971) Oral manifestations of oculomandibulodyscephaly with hypotrichosis. *Oral Surgery,* **31,** 234.
Lamy M., Jammet M.-L., Marateaux P. & Ajjan N. (1965) Le Dyscephalu. *Archives françaises de Pédiatrie,* **22,** 929.
Streiff E.B. (1950) Dysmorphie mandibulo-faciale (tête d'oiseau) et altérations oculaires. *Ophthalmologie,* **120,** 79.

Atrichia with papular lesions
(References p. 167)

History and nomenclature
Under this descriptive term Damsté & Prakken (1954) of Amsterdam described in

their patients a distinctive association of atrichia with numerous follicular keratinous cysts. A few years later Loewenthal & Prakken (1961) reported another very similar case. The few cases since published have been observed in Germany, in Spain or in Latin American countries. The mode of inheritance is uncertain but two Mexican patients were sisters (Castillo *et al.* 1974). Two affected brothers were the children of an incestuous relationship (Fonseca Moreton *et al.* 1972). Three German patients were brothers (Czarnecki & Stiegl 1980). Autosomal recessive inheritance is therefore probable.

Although all cases show lack of hair in association with keratinous cysts, there is considerable variation between them and it cannot yet be established whether one or more genotypes are concerned.

Pathology
The papules are keratin-filled follicular cysts. The scalp shows normal sebaceous glands and horn plugs in the follicular orifices (Castillo *et al.* 1974).

Clinical features
The first of the three cases of Damsté & Prakken (1954) was a woman aged 26. She had been born with normal hair which was soon shed and never replaced. She had sparse eyebrows, normal lashes and no body hair. She began to develop horny papules on her face at 18 and they gradually spread to other parts of the body. In the two other patients described by these authors the hair loss was similar but the papules began to appear at the age of 5 or 6. In some cases the papules have developed as early as the second year (Castillo *et al.* 1974). The papules are pin-head sized, smooth and white (Loewenthal & Prakken 1961).

The patient reported by Ledo *et al.* (1973) was a boy who showed essentially the same features as did the two Spanish brothers (Fonseca Moreton *et al.* 1972), who had also severe acne.

The three patients reported by Czarnecki & Stiegl (1980) were hairless from birth, and developed follicular cysts from the age of 7; they also showed retarded ossification and abnormal dental implantation.

Physical and mental development have been normal except in two sisters (Castillo *et al.* 1974) who were mentally retarded.

A case reported under this diagnosis from the Argentine (Krinaa 1955) gives insufficient detail for classification. The patient was bald from birth and had also atrophoderma vermiculata of the cheeks. His grandmother and maternal aunt were similarly affected.

A Japanese patient also had extensive polyposis throughout the gastrointestinal tract (Ishii *et al.* 1979).

References
del Castillo V., Ruiz-Maldonado R. & Carnvale A. (1974) Atrichia with papular lesions and mental retardation in two sisters. *International Journal of Dermatology*, **13**, 261.

Czarnecki N. & Stiegl S. (1980) Atrichia congenita mit Hornzysten—Variante einer partiellen ektodermalen Dysplasia. *Zeitschrift für Hautkrankheiten,* **55,** 210.

Damsté J. & Prakken J.R. (1954) Atrichia with papular lesions: a variant of congenital ectodermal dysplasia. *Dermatologica,* **108,** 14.

Fonseca Moreton A., Aguilar R., Franil P., Balsa T., Oubiña N. & Prado C. (1972) Atriquia familiae con pápulas. *Medicins cutanea,* **6,** 407.

Ishii Y., Kremhara T. & Nagata T. (1979) Atrichia with papular lesions associated with gastrointestinal polyposis. *Journal of Dermatology (Tokyo),* **6,** 111.

Krinaa J. (1955) Atriquia congenita familiae con lesiones papulosas y atrofodermia vermiculata de las surjillas. *Archivos Argentinos de Dermatologia,* **5,** 196.

Ledo A., Jaqueti G. & Gallago J.R. (1973) Atriquia con lesiones papulosas. *Medicina cutanea,* **7,** 339.

Loewenthal J.A. & Prakken J.R. (1961) Atrichia with papular lesions. *Dermatologica,* **122,** 85.

Hair in the premature ageing syndromes

Sparse scalp and body hair is a feature of progeria. Scalp hair is sparse and fine in metageria, and premature greying followed by loss of hair are usual in Werner's syndrome—pangeria.

A prematurely aged appearance is usual in poikiloderma congenitale and in some forms of birdheaded dwarfism and in Cockayne's syndrome.

Progeria (De Busk 1972)

The inheritance of progeria is possibly determined by an autosomal recessive gene, but affected subjects do not reproduce, and proof is lacking. During the first year the child appears to be more or less normal, though there may be scleroderma-like changes on the abdomen, flanks or thighs and mid-facial cyanosis. During the second year somatic growth becomes retarded and subcutaneous fat is progressively lost. Alopecia becomes total, apart from a few downy blonde or white hairs, and eyebrows and lashes are sometimes shed. The child comes to resemble a little old man and early death from premature arteriosclerosis is inevitable.

Metageria

This recently described autosomal recessive syndrome (Gilkes *et al.* 1974) is characterized by normal physical and mental development, lack of subcutaneous fat, and a thin face with a prominent broad nose. During the second decade mottled pigmentation and telangiectases develop. The scalp hair is fine and sparse.

References

De Busk F.L. (1972) The Hutchinson-Gilford progeria syndrome. *Pediatrics,* **80,** 697.

Gilkes J.J.H., Sharvill D.E. & Wells R.S. (1974) The premature ageing syndromes. *British Journal of Dermatology,* **91,** 243.

Werner's syndrome syn. pangeria
The inheritance of this uncommon but widely distributed syndrome is determined by an autosomal recessive gene. It has been described also as pangeria of
the adult and as pangeria (Gilkes *et al.* 1974), terms which underline its status as
one of the spectrum of syndromes characterized by features of premature ageing.

Growth ceases at about the age of 12 years, and the stature remains small.

Greying of the hair at the temples usually begins between the ages of 12 and
14, but onset as early as 8 has been recorded (Maeder 1949). The greying
gradually becomes more extensive and may be complete by 20, and is soon
associated with progressive alopecia, bitemporal at first, but gradually more
diffuse, and the increasing sparsity of the hair is accentuated by a reduction in
the diameter of the hair shaft. The ultimate extent of the alopecia is very variable.
The body hair also is sparse, and hypogonadism is usual, but not constant.

Other skin changes are usually first noticed between 18 and 30. The lower
legs and feet, the forearms and hands are most severely affected, the face and
neck less so. The shiny, tense, adherent skin shows mottled pigmentation and
telangiectasia. Subcutaneous fat is lost on the face and limbs, and the bird-like
facies and spindly limbs contrast with an often obese trunk. Ulcers of the legs are
frequent. Cataract develops in some cases between 20 and 35. Diabetes occurs in
over 20%, and abnormal glucose tolerance in many more. Early generalized
arteriosclerosis shortens life, as does the high incidence of malignant disease
(Schumacher *et al.* 1969).

References
Gilkes J.J.H., Sharvill D.E. & Wells R.S. (1974) The premature ageing syndrome. *British Journal of Dermatology*, **91**, 243.
Maeder G. (1949) Le Syndrome de Rothmund et le Syndrome de Werner. *Annales d'Oculistique*, **182**, 809.
Schumacher K., Rodermund O.E. & Doerfman R. (1969) Das Werner-Syndrom. *Archiv für klinische Medizin*, **216**, 116.

Poikiloderma congenitale (Rothmund–Thomson syndrome)
This hereditary syndrome is determined by an autosomal recessive gene. In early
infancy erythema of the face and ears and of the extensor aspects of the limbs is
followed by mottled pigmentation, depigmentation, atrophy and telangiectasia.

Associated defects may include hypogonadism and cataracts. Scalp, axillary
and pubic hair may be sparse or almost absent (Fig. 6.8) and eyebrows and
eyelashes are often scanty (Rook *et al.* 1959; Gorlin *et al.* 1976).

References
Gorlin R.J., Pindborg J.J. & Cohen M.M. (1976) *Syndromes of the Head and Neck*, 2nd edn. New York, McGraw-Hill, p. 652.
Rook A., Davis R.A. & Stevanović D. (1959) Poikiloderma congenitale. Rothmund–Thomson Syndrome. *Acta Dermato-venereologica*, **39**, 392.

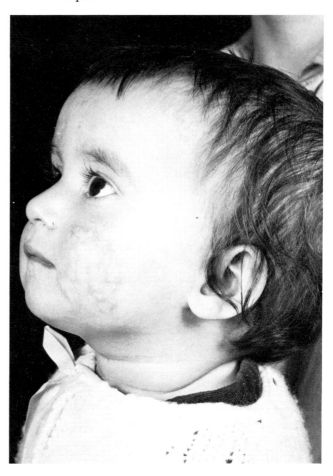

Fig. 6.8. Poikiloderma congenitale—sparse fine hair (Dr
Harvey Baker, London Hospital).

Bird-headed dwarfism (Fitch *et al.* 1970)
A beaked nose, micrognathia and low-set ears give these children a distinctive
bird-like facies. Dwarfism and microcephaly are characteristic. The hair becomes
grey prematurely and hair loss in the male pattern is well advanced by 18.

Reference
Fitch N., Pinsky L. & Lachance R.C. (1970) A form of bird headed dwarfism with premature
    senility. *American Journal of Diseases of Children*, **120**, 210.

Cockayne's syndrome (Lasser 1972)
Growth retardation becomes evident during the second year. The limbs are long,
with large hands and feet. Photosensitivity results in the early development of
solar degenerative changes which increase the aged appearance. Mental as well
as physical retardation is usual. The scalp hair is sparse and fine.

Reference
Lasser A.E. (1972) Cockayne's syndrome. *Cutis,* 10, 143.

Hair defects and skeletal abnormalities

Hypotrichosis is a feature of several syndromes in which skeletal abnormalities occur:

Cartilage–hair hypoplasia
Chondrodysplasia punctata
Focal dermal hypoplasia
Hypomelia–hypotrichosis–facial haemangioma syndrome

Cartilage–hair hypoplasia
This syndrome is determined by an autosomal recessive gene. It is unexpectedly frequent in Finland (Virolainen *et al.* 1978). A metaphyseal dysostosis from cartilage hypoplasia results in a high degree of dwarfism (McKusick *et al.* 1965). Many affected children showed increased susceptibility to certain infections, and an impaired cell-mediated response (Lux *et al.* 1970, Virolainen *et al.* 1978).

The hair is short, sparse, fine and silky, and lighter in colour than in unaffected siblings. There is considerable variation in hair shaft calibre, but if many hairs are measured the hairs of patients are significantly finer and show less variation than those of control subjects (Dapuzzo & Jon 1972). In some affected individuals there may be almost complete baldness.

The appearance of the hair in the electronmicroscope is normal, apart from decreased diameter and increased spaces between overlapping cuticular cells (Brown 1971; Blackston & Brown 1980). The tensile strength of the hair is disproportionately reduced (Coupe & Lowry 1970). Stress–strain curves are markedly abnormal. The filamentous and matrix proteins of the hair have no gross structural defects, and it has been suggested that decreased reactivity of some disulphide bonds may be responsible for the hair's abnormal properties (Kelling *et al.* 1973).

References
Blackston R.D. & Brown A.C. (1980) Cartilage–hair hypoplasia. In *Hair, Trace Elements and Human Illness,* eds. A.C. Brown & R.G. Crounse. New York, Praeger, p. 257.
Brown A.C. (1971) Congenital hair defect. *Birth Defects, Original Article Series* VII, 52.
Coupe R.L. & Lowry R.B. (1970) Abnormality of the hair in cartilage–hair hypoplasia. *Dermatologica,* 141, 329.
Dapuzzo V. & Jon E. (1972) Metaphysale Dysostose und Hypoplasie der Haar: Knorpel-Haar Hypoplasie. *Helvetica Pediatrica Acta,* 27, 241.
Kelling C., Goldsmith L.A. & Baden H.P. (1973) Biophysical and biochemical studies of the hair in cartilage–hair hypoplasia. *Clinical Genetics,* 4, 500.

Lux S.E., Johnston R.B., August C.S., Say B., Penchaszadeh V.B., Rosen F.S. & McKusick V.A.
    (1970) Chronic neutropenia and abnormal cellular immunity in cartilage–hair hypoplasia.
    New England Journal of Medicine, **282**, 231.
McKusick V.A., Eldridge R., Hostatler J.A., Ruangwrt U. & Egeland J.A. (1965) Dwarfism in the
    Amish. *Bulletin of the Johns Hopkins Hospital*, **116**, 285.
Virolainen M., Savilahti E., Kaitela I. & Perhecutana J. (1978) Cellular and humoral immunity in
    cartilage–hair hypoplasia. *Pediatric Research*, **12**, 961.

Chondrodysplasia punctata

Punctate calcification of the long bones, carpal and tarsal bones, the processes of
the vertebrae and the ischiopubic bones is present as a radiological change in
infancy. During childhood there is asymmetrical shortening of the long bones,
with epiphyseal defects in regions which formerly showed punctate calcification.

These skeletal abnormalities form part of two, possibly three syndromes in
which changes of skin and scalp occur in a significant proportion of cases
(Sprenger *et al.* 1971).

Chondrodysplasia punctata—Conradi–Hänemann type. Many cases are sporadic,
but autosomal dominant inheritance is usual (Bergstrom *et al.* 1972). X-linked
dominant inheritance also is reported (Happle 1980).

At birth and in early infancy in about 25% of cases extensive erythema and
scaling are frequently present, and are succeeded by ichthyosis. A saddle nose, a
high arched palate are also found and congenital cataracts are present in 20%.
Characteristic stippling of the epiphyses is seen on radiological examination, but
tends to disappear after the age of 6 months (Bodian 1966; Tasker *et al.* 1970).

Relatively few reports have been published of children over the age of 5 with
this disease, but a high proportion of such patients have shown follicular
atrophoderma of the distal extremities, and coarse head hair with patchy
cicatricial alopecia (Comings *et al.* 1968; Edidin *et al.* 1977). The hair is lustreless
and irregularly twisted. Eyebrows and lashes are sparse and irregular.

Chondrodysplasia punctata—rhizomelic type (Sprenger *et al.* 1971). The inheritance of this disorder is determined by an autosomal recessive gene. The skin
changes occur with approximately the same frequency as in the above
syndrome, but there are also lymphoedema of the face and microcephaly.
Cataracts are present in 80%.

Most affected children die in infancy; those that survive to childhood are
severely retarded.

References
Bergstrom K., Gustavson K.-H. & Jorulf H. (1972) Chondrodystrophia calcificans congenita
    (Conradi's disease) in a mother and her child. *Clinical Genetics*, **3**, 158.
Bodian E.L. (1966) Skin manifestations of Conradi's disease. *Archives of Dermatology*, **94**, 743.

Comings D.E., Papazian C. & Schoeme H.R. (1968) Conradi's disease. *Journal of Pediatrics*, **72**, 63.

Edidin D.V., Esterly N.P., Banzais A.K. & Fretzin D.F. (1977) Chondrodystrophia punctata. *Archives of Dermatology*, **113**, 1931.

Happle R. (1980) X-gekoppelt dominante Chondrodystrophia punctata. *Monatschrift für Kinderheilkunde*, **128**, 203.

Sprenger J.W., Opitz J.M. & Bidder U. (1971) Heterogeneity of Chondrodysplasia punctata. *Humangenetik*, **11**, 190.

Tasker W.C., Mastri A.R. & Gold A.P. (1970) Chondrodystrophia calcificans congenita (Dysplasia epiphysalis punctata). *American Journal of Diseases of Children*, **119**, 122.

Focal dermal hypoplasia

This is a rare syndrome probably transmitted by an autosomal dominant gene, with lethality in the male (Ruiz-Maldonado *et al.* 1974) for almost all cases have been female.

The destructive skin lesions are of three types; there are irregular linear streaks of telangiectasia, atrophy and pigmentation; groups, often linear, of soft fatty nodules, and papillomas of the lips and sometimes of the vulva and anus. Skeletal malformations and ocular defects complete the main characteristics of the syndrome.

The scalp hair is usually sparse and brittle and may be lacking completely from small areas of aplasia cutis, which may be present also in the pubic region (Goltz *et al.* 1970). In some cases there may be more extensive cicatricial alopecia (Gomez Orbaneja & de Castro Torres 1967). Two girls (Howell 1965) had generally sparse hair, with linear or oval areas of cicatricial alopecia.

The incidence of hypotrichosis in the syndrome is difficult to estimate reliably. The analysis of 41 case reports (Ishibashi & Kurihara 1972) gave an incidence of 24%, but if only those reports in which the state of the hair is specifically mentioned are included, the incidence is over 80%.

References

Goltz R.W., Henderson R.R., Hitch J.M. & Ott J.E. (1970) Focal dermal hypoplasia syndrome. *Archives of Dermatology*, **101**, 1.

Gomez Orbaneja J. & de Castro Torres A. (1967) Un nuevo caso de hipoplasia dérmica focal. *Actas Dermo-Sifiliograficas*, **58**, 93.

Howell J.B. (1965) Nevus angiolipomatas vs. focal dermal hypoplasia. *Archives of Dermatology*, **92**, 328.

Ishibashi A. & Kurihara Y. (1972) Goltz's syndrome: focal dermal dysplasia syndrome. *Dermatologica*, **144**, 156.

Ruiz-Maldonado R., Carnevale A., Tamayo L. & Milonas de Montiel E. (1974) Focal dermal hypoplasia. *Clinical Genetics*, **6**, 36.

Hypomelia–hypotrichosis–facial haemangioma syndrome

Four cases of this distinctive syndrome, probably inherited as an autosomal recessive trait, were described by Herrmann *et al.* (1969) in two pairs of siblings. The limb defects suggested the designation 'pseudothalidomide syndrome'. The report of a further, sporadic, case (Hall & Greenberg 1972) emphasized the constancy of its principal features. These are limb reduction defects, a mid-facial capillary naevus, and sparse silver-blonde hair.

The nasal bridge is high, the alae and septum are hypoplastic and the nares are retroverted. These defects in combination with micrognathia give a distinctive facies.

No reports on the electronmicroscopic appearance or chemical composition of the hair have been published.

References

Hall B.D. & Greenberg M.H. (1972) Hypomelia, hypotrichosis–facial hemangioma syndrome. *American Journal of Diseases of Children*, **123**, 602.

Herrmann J., Feingold M. & Tuffli G.A. (1969) A familial dysmorphogenetic syndrome of limb deformation, characteristic facial appearance, and associated anomalies: the pseudothalido-mide or SC syndrome. *Birth Defects, Original Article Series*, **5**, 81.

Hypotrichosis in other hereditary syndromes

Hypotrichosis is reported in some patients with dyskeratosis congenita and has also been associated with hypomelanosis of Ito, and, exceptionally, with xeroderma pigmentosum.

Dyskeratosis congenita
Pachyonychia congenita
Xeroderma pigmentosum
Bazex's syndrome
Hypomelanosis of Ito
Dubowitz syndrome

Dyskeratosis congenita

The inheritance of this syndrome is determined by an autosomal recessive gene. Most reported cases have been males, but the full syndrome and partial forms have occurred also in females.

The affected child is usually apparently normal for its first 5 years. During the next 10 years the essential features make their appearance—nail dystrophy and destruction following episodes of infection: leukoplakia leading eventually to carcinoma: reticulate pigmentation most marked on neck and thighs (Bazex & Dupré 1957). Haematological abnormalities are frequent.

The hair is often normal, but may be fine and dry and sparse (Bazex & Dupré 1957). Premature canities has been reported (Connan & Trague 1981; Sorrow & Hitch 1963). Two patients had cicatricial alopecia (Milgrom *et al.* 1964; Nazarro *et al.* 1971).

References

Bazex A. & Dupré A. (1957) Dyskeratose congénital. *Annales de Dermatologie et de Syphiligraphie*, **84**, 497.

Connan J.M. & Trague R.H. (1981) Dyskeratosis congenita. Report of a large kindred. *British Journal of Dermatology*, **105**, 321.

Milgrom H., Stoll H.L. & Crissey J.T. (1964) Dyskeratosis congenita. *Archives of Dermatology*, **89**, 345.

Nazzaro P., Argenturi R., Bassetti F., Leonetti F. & Fuzio M. (1971) La discheratosi congenita di Zinsser–Cole–Engman. *Bolletino dell'Instituto Dermatologico S. Gallicano*, **7**, 3.

Sorrow J.M. & Hitch J.M. (1963) Dyskeratosis congenita. *Archives of Dermatology*, **88**, 340.

Pachonychia congenita

The inheritance of this rare syndrome is determined by an autosomal dominant gene of variable expressivity. Present in all cases, and in some degree even at birth, is the pachyonychia, which is strictly a thickening of the nail bed which imparts a pronounced transverse curve to the overlying nail.

Other features are palmoplantar keratoderma, at pressure points, and hyperhidrosis. Leukoplakia, sometimes leading to malignancy, develops on the oral, nasopharyngeal or anal mucous membranes from the second decade onwards.

Hypotrichosis, which may be severe, is present in over 10% of cases (Moldenhauer & Ernst 1968), and may be associated with 'kinky' hair (Soderquist & Reed 1968) or other defects of the hair shafts. Hypotrichosis may be generalized (Vogt *et al.* 1971) or confined to the scalp.

References

Moldenhauer E. & Ernst K. (1968) Das Jadassohn-Lewandowsky Syndrom. *Hautarzt*, **19**, 441.

Soderquist N.A. & Reed W.B. (1968) Pachyonychia congenita with epidermal cysts and other congenital dyskeratoses. *Archives of Dermatology*, **97**, 31.

Vogt H.-J., Calap J. & Müller-Jensen K. (1971) Jadassohn–Lewandowsky–Syndrom mit Miterophthalmos. *Hautarzt*, **22**, 294.

Xeroderma pigmentosum

This term is applied to a group of hereditary disorders all characterized in varying degree by increased susceptibility to light damage, with the early onset of pigmentary changes, atrophy, keratoses and malignant tumours on light-exposed skin (Reed *et al.* 1969). The hair is usually clinically normal, but no biochemical or biophysical studies have been reported. One patient with xeroderma pigmentosum had no hair (Diem & Fritsch 1973), but the association of these defects may have been fortuitous.

References

Diem E. & Fritsch P. (1973) Xeroderma pigmentosum, universelle. Haarlösigkeit und assoziente neuro-oculäre Symptomatik. *Hautarzt*, **24**, 204.

Reed W.B., Landing B., Sugarman G., Cleaver J.E. & Melnyk J. (1969) Xeroderma pigmentosum. *Journal of the American Medical Association*, **207**, 2073.

Bazex's syndrome (Bazex *et al.* 1964)
The mode of inheritance of this complex syndrome is uncertain. The characteristic features are follicular atrophoderma, localized anhidrosis or generalized hypohidrosis, multiple basal-cell carcinomas, and hypotrichosis. In one family in which eight individuals in three generations were known to be affected (Viksnins & Berlin 1977) the hair was normal, but in other reported cases the sparsity of hair has been a striking feature (Cabrera *et al.* 1980; Plosila *et al.* 1981). The hair shafts are defective and may show pili torti (Meynadier *et al.* 1979).

The follicular atrophoderma is present on the dorsa of hands and feet and on the elbows. There may be multiple facial milia at birth. Basal-cell carcinomas of the face develop from adolescence or early adult life.

References
Bazex A., Dupré A. & Christol B. (1964) Génodermatose complexe de type indeterminé associant une hypotrichose, un état atrophodermique généralisé et des dégénérescences cutanées multiples (épithéliomas basocellulaires). *Bulletin de la Société française de Dermatologie et de Syphiligraphie*, **71**, 206.

Cabrera H.N., Ferreyra M. & Costa J.A. (1980) Sindrome de Bazex–Dupré–Christol. *Revista Argentina de Dermatología*, **61**, 97.

Meynadier J., Guilhou J.-J., Barnéon G., Malbos S. & Guillot B. (1979) Atrophodermie folliculaire, hypotrichose, grains de milium multiples associés à des dystrophies ostéocartilagineuses minimes. *Annales de Dermatologie et de Syphiligraphie*, **106**, 497.

Plosila M., Kiistala R. & Niemi K.-M. (1981) The Bazex Syndrome; follicular atrophoderma, with multiple basal cell carcinomas, hypotrichosis and hypohidrosis. *Clinical and Experimental Dermatology*, **6**, 31.

Viksnins P. & Berlin A. (1977) Follicular atrophoderma and basal cell carcinomas. *Archives of Dermatology*, **113**, 948.

Hypomelanosis of Ito
This rare syndrome was first reported from Japan, where it is perhaps less uncommon than elsewhere, under the name of 'incontinentia pigmenti achromians'. It is characterized by the development in infancy or later in childhood of depigmentation which is like a negative image of the pigmentation of 'incontinentia pigmenti' (p. 339). Most cases occur in females and some have ocular and dental defects.

In one reported case (Hamada *et al.* 1967) the scalp hair was said to be sparse.

References
Hamada T., Saito T., Sugai T. & Morita Y. (1967) Incontinentia pigmenti achromians (Ito). *Archives of Dermatology*, **96**, 673.

Jelinek J.E., Bart R.S. & Schiff G.M. (1973) Hypomelanosis of Ito. *Archives of Dermatology*, **107**, 596.

Dubowitz syndrome (Dubowitz 1965)

Aetiology. The inheritance of this rarely reported syndrome is determined by an autosomal recessive gene.

Clinical features. Low birthweight and retardation of post-natal growth and some degree of mental retardation are associated with a distinctive facies. The hair is sparse and fine. There is a high sloping forehead and flat supra orbital ridges and a broad nasal bridge. The palpebral fissues are short and the mouth is small. Eczema may develop.

Reference
Dubowitz V. (1965) Familial low birthweight, dwarfism with an unusual facies and a skin eruption. *Journal of Medical Genetics,* **2**, 12.

Johanson–Blizzard syndrome
Sparse, fine, hypopigmented hair is associated with aplasia cutis of the scalp and with multiple defects.

Dystrophia myotonica, syn. Steinert's disease (Slatt 1961)
This rare disorder is inherited as an autosomal dominant trait. It becomes clinically apparent during the third decade with myotonia and muscle wasting. Premature greying of the hair accompanies frontoparietal baldness and reduction in body hair. The subcutaneous fat is diminished. The skin becomes dry as sebum secretion is reduced. There is testicular atrophy.

    The average age of onset is 27 years, but the disease can be recognized in infancy (Bell & Smith 1972).

References
Bell D.B. & Smith D.W. (1972) Myotonic dystrophy in the neonate. *Journal of Pediatrics,* **81**, 83.
Slatt B. (1961) Myotonia dystrophia: a review of 17 cases. *Canadian Medical Association Journal,* **85**, 250.

Hypotrichosis in chromosomal abnormalities

Down's syndrome
In Down's syndrome (mongolism) which occurs once in about 700 births, and the incidence of which increases with the age of the mother, some 95% of cases are due to trisomy 21, and the remainder to other chromosomal abnormalities.

    The most frequent cutaneous changes are vascular (Desmons *et al.* 1974): fixed erythema of the cheeks and livedo reticularis of the limbs. Keratosis pilaris and other keratotic lesions are common. The skin is soft and velvety in infancy, but during childhood becomes progressively drier and more scaly.

    Skin infections occur frequently and infection and trauma partly account for the chronic cheilitis seen in well over 50%, and increasing in incidence with age (Butterworth *et al.* 1960).

The hair may be normal, but is often fine and may become sparse and dry. The most comprehensive study of the hair on Down's syndrome was reported by Vivot (1968) in his thesis. His figures show that sparsity of pubic and axillary hair is less often found than some authors have suggested, but the horizontal pattern of pubic hair is usual in both sexes. He confirms the high incidence of alopecia areata in Down's syndrome. This is unexplained; the incidence of eczema, asthma and hay fever is lower in these children than in their unaffected siblings (Coghlan & Evans 1964).

References
Butterworth T., Leoni E.P., Burmon H., Wood M.G. & Shear L.P. (1980) Cheilitis of mongolism. *Journal of Investigative Dermatology*, **35**, 247.
Coghlan M.K. & Evans P.R. (1964) Infantile eczema, asthma and hay fever in Mongolism. *Guy's Hospital Reports*, **113**, 223.
Desmons F., Bar J. & Brandt A. (1973) Les signes cutanés du mongolisme (Trisomie 21). *Bulletin de la Société française de Dermatologie et de Syphiligraphie*, **80**, 232.
Vivot N.A. (1968) *Alteraciones cutaneas en el Sindrome de Down (Mogolismo)*. Buenos Aires, Direccion Nacional de Sanidad Escolar.

Klinefelter's syndrome
The karyotype of this syndrome is 47XXY: it occurs once in about 400 male births.

There are no clinical manifestations before puberty, which tends to be delayed. The testes remain small, but the external genitalia usually develop normally, although they may be small in some patients. Fertility is low. In one series of 50 cases (Becker *et al.* 1966) diminished facial and body hair was common, as was a horizontal pubic escutcheon. Gynaecomastia frequently occurs. The urinary gonadotrophin excretion is above normal.

The sparsity of facial hair sometimes brings these patients to a dermatologist, since the wearing of full beards has again become fashionable amongst the young in some countries.

The diagnosis can be confirmed by establishing the karyotype.

Reference
Becker K.L., Hoffman D.L., Albert A., Underdahl L.O. & Mason H.L. (1966) Klinefelter's syndrome. *Archives of Internal Medicine*, **118**, 314.

Chapter 7
Defects of the Hair Shaft

Introduction

Structural defects of the hair shaft may be sufficient in degree to cause significant cosmetic disability, or they may render the hair abnormally susceptible to injury by minor degrees of trauma. They may also be the result of hereditary or acquired metabolic disorders, to the diagnosis of which they afford valuable clues.

Price (1979) classifies anomalies of the shaft into those which are associated with increased fragility, and those which are not. This distinction is useful because only the former present clinically as patchy or diffuse alopecia. Price's classification will be followed throughout the present chapter.

Reference
Price V.H. (1979) Strukturanomalien des Haarschaftes. In *Haar und Haarkrankheiten*, ed. C.E. Orfanos. Stuttgart, Fischer, p. 387.

Structural defects of the shaft with increased fragility

Monilethrix (references p. 185)

History and nomenclature
Walter Smith of Dublin first published in 1879 a description of 'A Rare Nodose
Condition of the Hair', for which Radcliffe Crocker subsequently suggested the
term monilethrix, which has been generally accepted. Luce in France independently described the same defect in his Paris thesis entitled 'Un cas curieux
d'alopécie innominée'. Alternative names to monilethrix such as Spindelhaare
and Alopecia pilorum intermittens have failed to find favour. Many other cases
were reported during the next 2 years and the condition was firmly established as
an entity at the International Medical Congress in London in 1881. Nevertheless
some early reports, and even some more recent ones, confuse monilethrix with
other shaft defects.

Aetiology
The hereditary nature of monilethrix was recognized soon after the condition
was first identified. Autosomal dominant transmission has been demonstrated in
numerous large pedigrees (Alexander & Grant 1958; Bartosova & Jorda 1973;
Beare 1956; Norgaard 1957; Rodemund 1969; Salamon & Schneyder 1962;
Solomon & Green 1963; Tomkinson 1932).

The alleged occurrence of normal carriers of the dominant gene has not been
proven, for a parent with only 5% of abnormal follicles is easily passed as normal
(Deraemaeker 1957). The gene appears to have high penetrance but variable
expressivity.

Cockayne (1933) reviewed the evidence that monilethrix may be determined
also by an autosomal recessive gene. Several pedigrees suggested this possibility
and some more recently published pedigrees do likewise (Hanhart 1955). If the
existence of a second genotype is established, it is likely that phenotypic
differences can be shown to be present.

Pathology
The hair shaft is beaded and brittle as the result of a developmental defect.
Elliptical nodes 0.7–1.0 mm apart are separated by internodes at which the
medulla is lacking. The width of the nodes and the distance between them show
some variation within a single family but interfamily variation is probably not
significant (Korn-Heydt *et al.* 1967). In the scanning electronmicroscope (Fig.
7.1) the nodes and some of the internodes show a normal imbricated scale
pattern, but most internodes show longitudinal ridging (Dawber & Comaish
1970). This ridging is acquired and progressive as internodes move away from

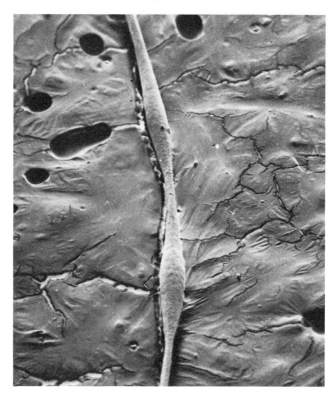

Fig. 7.1. Monilethrix. Scanning electromicrograph (Slade Hospital, Oxford).

the scalp (Dawber 1980). X-ray diffraction studies (Malt 1965) show α keratin less well accentuated than in normal hair.

Histologically the follicle shows wide and narrow zones corresponding to the nodes and internodes, but the general structure of the follicle is otherwise essentially normal (Borda & Abulafia 1952; Salamon & Schneyder 1962). However, the follicles are abnormally distributed and there is no whorl formation.

Attempts have been made to investigate the mechanism of node formation and to relate it to the diurnal rate of hair growth. Behrend (1885) suggested that the nodes were formed at night and the internodes by day. Martin-Scott (1950) was unable to confirm this. Klingmüller (1954) claimed to have found a 48-hour cycle in two patients. Baker (1962) studied four cases in one family in which inheritance was of autosomal dominant type; he found that a complete nodal complex was formed in 24 hours. Comaish (1969) studied two patients autoradiographically and found no daily rhythm and no simple time-cycle; the rate of growth of beaded hair was greater than that of normal hair in the same subject. A recent study (Lubach & Triantos 1979) also showed no regular rhythm of node formation.

Intermittent administration of an antimitotic agent can give rise to zones of constriction alternating with zones of normal diameter (Van Scott *et al.* 1957). Mimosine causes similar changes in sheep (Reis *et al.* 1975).

Studies in the electronmicroscope (Dawber 1977) have shown that increased susceptibility of the hair shaft to the effects of trauma—premature weathering—is an important factor in the failure of the hair to attain a normal length.

Clinical features
Monilethrix shows considerable variation in age of onset, severity and course. There is not yet sufficient information to establish whether these variations are in part consistently correlated with different genotypes. There is, however, much variation even within the more commonly reported autosomal dominant form, but some of it is merely apparent: vigorous hair brushing may reveal a defect, the presence of which would otherwise have been overlooked.

The hair may be obviously abnormal at birth but is most commonly normal, and is progressively replaced by abnormal hair during the first months of life (Beare 1956): in other cases the normal hair is succeeded by horny follicular papules from the summit of which emerge brittle beaded hairs (Fig. 7.2). The follicular keratosis and the abnormal hairs are most frequent on the nape and occiput but may involve the entire scalp. However, the keratosis is not directly related to the beading and either change may precede the other and the keratosis is sometimes absent. In a typical case the short stubble of broken hairs and rough horny plugs give a distinctive appearance. However, the apparent onset of monilethrix may occur in early childhood or even as late as 17 (Gilchrist 1898). Severe alopecia may develop (Fig. 7.3) or only a few affected hairs may be present, which may be overlooked unless they are carefully sought.

In some cases the eyebrows and eyelashes, pubic and axillary hair and

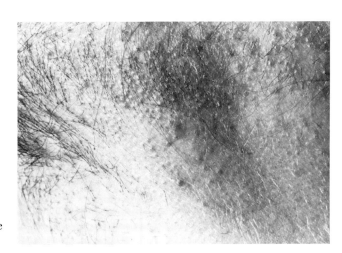

Fig. 7.2. Manilethrix. Follicular keratosis of the nape (Slade Hospital, Oxford).

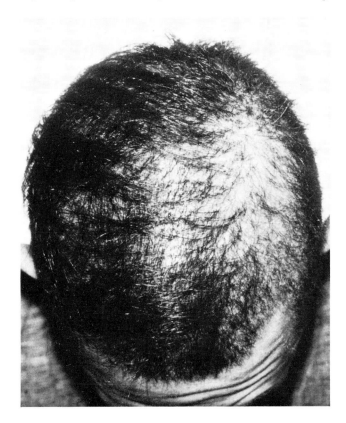

Fig. 7.3. Monilethrix. Moderately severe alopecia (Dr G. Holti, Newcastle).

general body hair may be affected, or one or more of these sites may show few or many abnormal hairs, when the scalp is normal.

In cases of early onset the degree of baldness tends to increase during childhood, but only to a limited extent if trauma is avoided. In many patients the condition persists with little change throughout life (Alexander & Grant 1958), though there may be some temporary improvement in pregnancy (Solomon & Green 1963) (Fig. 7.4). Spontaneous improvement or complete recovery have occurred (Heydt 1964; Solomon & Green 1963). Temporary improvement has followed an epilating dose of X-rays (Ingram 1934) and has been reported during pregnancy (Summerly & Donaldson 1962). Griseofulvin also has temporarily restored normal hair growth (Keipert 1973).

Associated defects
Only one of 134 patients with monilethrix had oligophrenia and schizophrenia: genetic linkage is improbable (Korn-Heydt 1967). However, other investigators (Salamon & Schneyder 1962) thought the association with oligophrenia and with nail and tooth defects was significant. Two affected girls also had a delayed

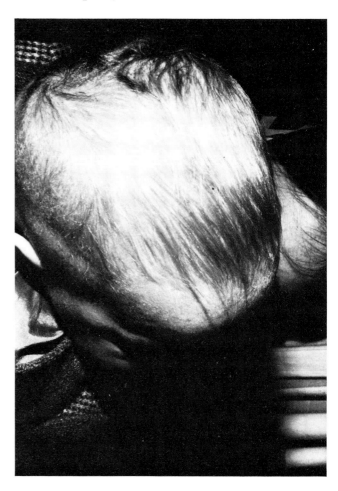

Fig. 7.4. Monilethrix. Growth of normal new hair during pregnancy (Dr E.M. Donaldson).

and incomplete second dentition (Strandberg 1922). It is possible that such associations may be a feature of the recessive phenotype, since oligophrenia and poor physical development were noted also in two siblings with monilethrix (Sfaello & Hariga 1967). In another family in which the authors (Bartosova & Jorda 1973) suggested that inheritance was of the autosomal recessive type, two of five affected individuals were oligophrenic, and one epileptic. An association with juvenile cataract has been reported on a number of occasions (Thiel 1959).

   Reports on abnormalities in amino acid metabolism are conflicting. Argininosuccinicaciduria was reported in a number of cases (Grosfeld *et al.* 1964; Barthowick *et al.* 1967; Sobolewska & Wilmanska 1968; Rondon Lugo *et al.* 1977), but a technical error was subsequently detected (Efron & Hoefnagel 1966). No abnormality in the urinary amino-acid pattern was found in a family presenting the autosomal dominant type investigated by Summerly & Donaldson

(1962) or in an isolated case in a sickly child (Mäder & Rose 1969). An apparent excess of aspartic acid and of arginine in the urine of an affected mother and daughter (Marques Llagaria *et al.* 1973) remains unexplained.

Diagnosis
The differential diagnosis from other developmental shaft defects must be based on careful microscopical study of affected hairs.

Treatment
None is available. Reduction of hairdressing trauma may be followed by some improvement in the less severely affected cases.

References
Alexander J. O'D. & Grant P.W. (1958) Monilethrix. *Scottish Medical Journal*, **3**, 351.
Baker H. (1962) An investigation of monilethrix. *British Journal of Dermatology*, **74**, 24.
Barthowick K., Pawkaczyk B., Sochacka K. & Spalona M. (1967) Monilethrix. *Przeglad Dermatologiczny*, **54**, 689.
Bartosova L. & Jorda V. (1973) Monilethrix. *Ceskoslovenská Dermatologie*, **48**, 232.
Beare J.M. (1956) Monilethrix. *Ulster Medical Journal*, **25**, 98.
Behrend G. (1885) Ueber Knotenbildung am Haarshaft. *Berliner Klinische Wochenschrift*, **22**, 270.
Borda J.M. & Abulafia J. (1952) Monilethrix. *Archivos Argentinos de Dermatologia*, **2**, 337.
Cockayne E.A. (1933) *Inherited Abnormalities of the Skin and its Appendages.* Oxford, Oxford University Press, p. 144.
Comaish S. (1969) Autoradiographic studies of hair growth and rhythm in monilethrix. *British Journal of Dermatology*, **81**, 443.
Dawber R.P.R. (1977) Weathering of hair in monilethrix and pili torti. *Clinical and Experimental Dermatology*, **2**, 271.
Dawber R.P.R. (1980) Weathering of hair in some genetic hair shaft abnormalities. In: *Hair: Trace Elements and Human Illness*, eds. A. Brown & R.G. Crosin. New York: Praeger.
Dawber R.P.R. & Comaish S. (1970) Scanning electronmicroscopy of normal and abnormal hair shafts. *Archives of Dermatology*, **101**, 316.
Deraemaeker R. (1957) Monilethrix: Report of a family with special reference to some problems concerning inheritance. *American Journal of Human Genetics*, **9**, 195.
Efron M.L. & Hoefnagel D. (1966) Argininosuccinic acid in monilethrix. *Lancet*, **i**, 321.
Gilchrist T.C. (1898) A case of monilethrix with an unusual distribution. *Journal of Cutaneous Diseases*, **16**, 157.
Grosfeld J.C.M., Mighorst J.A. & Moolhuysen T.M.G.F. (1964) Argininosuccinic aciduria in monilethrix. *Lancet*, **ii**, 789.
Hanhart E. (1955) Erstmaliger Hinweis auf das Vorkommen iners Monohybrid-rezessivere Erbgangs bei Monilethrix (Moniletrichosis). *Archiv Julius-Klaus Stiftung für Vererbungsforschung*, **30**, 1.
Heydt G.E. (1964) Intrafamiliäre Expressivitätshaarkanger des Monilethrix-Gens. *Archiv für klinische und experimentelle Dermatologie*, **219**, 415.
Ingram J.T. (1934) Monilethrix. *British Journal of Dermatology*, **46**, 272.
Keipert J.A. (1973) The effect of griseofulvin on hair growth in monilethrix. *Medical Journal of Australia*, **ii**, 1236.
Klingmüller G. (1954) Monilethrix mit 48 Stunden-Rhythmus. *Hautarzt*, **5**, 23.

Korn-Heydt G.E. (1967) Uber einem Fall von Monilethrix mit Schwadsinen und Schizophrenia. *Archiv für klinische und experimentelle Dermatologie*, **228**, 445.

Korn-Heydt G.E., Dinger R. & Ihen P. (1967) Statistische Untersuchungen zur intra und inter familiären Variabilität des Monilethrix-Gens. *Archiv für klinische und experimentelle Dermatologie*, **229**, 256.

Lubach D. & Triantos N. (1979) Untersuchungen über die Monilethrix. *Hautarzt*, **30**, 253.

Mäder A.K. & Rose H.-J. (1969) Monilethrix und Argininbernsteinsaüre-Ausscheidung. *Dermatologische Monatschrift*, **155**, 409.

Malt R.A. (1965) Keratin in monilethrix. *Journal of Investigative Dermatology*, **44**, 364.

Marques Llagaria E., Calap Calatynd J. & Torres Peris V. (1973) Monilethrix: Estudio aproposito de dos casos familiares. *Actas Dermo-Sifiligraficas*, **64**, 203.

Martin-Scott I. (1950) Monilethrix. *British Journal of Dermatology*, **62**, 35.

Norgaard O. (1957) Monilethrix i Fem Generationer. *Nordisk Medicin*, **58**, 1082.

Reis P.J., Downes A.M. & Chapman R.E. (1976) The influence of chemical defleecing agents in the properties of wool. In *Proceedings, 5th International Wool Research Conference, Aachen, 1975*, ed. K. Ziegler. Aachen, Deutsches Wollforschungsinstitut Technische Hochschule, Vol. 4, pp. 24–34.

Rodemund O.E. (1969) Zur Monilethrix. *Zeitschrift für Haut und Geschlectskrankheiten*, **44**, 291.

Rondon Lugo A.J., Piquero J., Moullo J. & Hernandez P. (1977) Caso de Monilethrix con aminoaciduria anormal. *Dermatologia Venezolana*, **15**, 43.

Salamon T. & Schneyder U.W. (1962) Uber die Monilethrix. *Archiv für klinische und experimentelle Dermatologie*, **215**, 105.

Sfaello Z. & Hariga J. (1967) Monilethrix associé à la debilité mentale: étude d'une famille. *Archives Belges de Dermatologie et Syphiligraphie*, **23**, 363.

Smith W.G. (1879) A rare nodose condition of the hair. *British Medical Journal*, **11**, 291.

Sobolawska G. & Wilmanska J. (1968) Monilethrix and argininosuccinuria. *Przeglad Dermatologiczny*, **55**, 157.

Solomon I.L. & Green O.C. (1963) Monilethrix. *New England Journal of Medicine*, **269**, 1279.

Strandberg J. (1922) A contribution to our knowledge of Aplasia moniliformis. *Acta Dermatovenereologica*, **3**, 650.

Summerly R. & Donaldson E.M. (1962) Monilethrix. *British Journal of Dermatology*, **74**, 387.

Tomkinson J.G. (1932) Monilethrix: group of 22 cases. *British Medical Journal*, **ii**, 1009.

Thiel E. (1959) Monilethrix und Frühstar. *Hautarzt*, **10**, 271.

Van Scott E.J., Reinertson R.P. & Steinmuller R. (1957) The growing hair roots of the human scalp and morphologic changes therein following amethopterin therapy. *Journal of Investigative Dermatology*, **29**, 197.

Pseudomonilethrix

It is not uncommon to see patients who complain that their hair is of poor quality or brittle, and if the patient in question is a young child microscopy of the hair to exclude the classical shaft defects is a routine procedure. It should be a routine procedure also in the older child or adult. Bentley-Phillips & Bayles (1973, 1975) have found a syndrome which they named 'pseudo-monilethrix' to be relatively frequent in South Africans of European or Indian descent. The status of the syndrome is uncertain; some of the shaft deformities may be artefactual.

The patients present with alopecia from the age of 8 onwards, and their lack of hair can be shown to be the result of a defect, the inheritance of which is determined by an autosomal dominant gene, which renders the hair so fragile that it readily breaks with the trauma of brushing, combing or other hairdressing procedures.

On microscopy one, or occasionally two, of three abnormalities can be seen. These are (a) pseudomonilethrix—irregular nodes, which on electronmicroscopy prove to be the protruding edges of depressions in the shaft; (b) irregular twists of 25–200° without flattening of the shaft; (c) breaks with brush-like ends, in apparently normal shafts. There is no keratosis pilaris.

The reduction of hairdressing trauma may be followed by a marked improvement in the condition.

References

Bentley-Philips B. & Bayles M.A.H. (1973) A previously undescribed hereditary hair anomaly (pseudo-monilethrix). *British Journal of Dermatology*, **89**, 159.
Bentley-Phillips B. & Bayles M.A.H. (1975) Pseudomonilethrix. *British Journal of Dermatology*, **92**, 113.

Pili torti (references p. 193)

History and nomenclature

The first definite description of pili torti was given by Schütz in 1900, although earlier authors, notably Unna and Lassar, had referred to the condition. Schütz's paper was entitled 'Pili moniliformis', and reflects the confusion between twisting and beading of the hair shaft, which has still not been completely eliminated from the literature. In 1922 Rieche proposed the term trichokinesis which is still favoured by some German authors. Ormsby & Mitchell (1924, 1925) twice presented the same patient to the Chicago Dermatological Society. On the first occasion the diagnosis was 'atrophia pilorum'; monilethrix. Forster, in discussing the case, drew attention to the fact that the hairs were twisted and not beaded. On the second occasion the diagnosis was simply 'atrophia pilorum'. A very typical case of pili torti was described by Freund in 1925. In 1932 Galewsky suggested the term 'pili torti' which in the same year was adopted by Ronchese in America and has since been widely accepted.

In 'pili torti', the hairs are 'flattened and at irregular intervals, completely rotated through 180° around their long axis (Hellier *et al.* 1940). This may be regarded as a definition of classical pili torti (Fig. 7.5). The increasing use of the scanning electronmicroscope (Fig. 7.6) is, however, making it clear that twisted hairs occur in many distinct forms, and that the twisting may be associated with a number of other shaft defects. Many more studies will be needed before the significance and specificity of minor variations can be established. As new syndromes are characterized a residue of cases remains in which twisted hair is apparently the sole defect; many reported cases cannot be classified retrospectively since even the known syndromes cannot be excluded on the inadequate data.

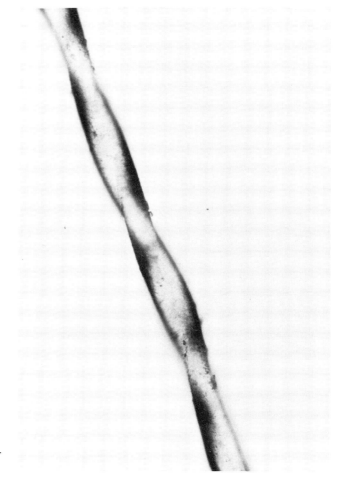

Fig. 7.5. Pili torti. Light microscopic appearance.

Syndromes of which twisted hair is a feature

   Menkes' syndrome (p. 195): light-coloured twisted hair as a manifestation of a hereditary defect of intestinal copper transport: the inheritance is of sex-linked recessive type.

   Björnstad's syndrome (p. 194): twisted hair with sensorineural deafness: probable autosomal dominant inheritance.

   Bazex syndrome (p. 176): twisted hair, with basal carcinomas of the face and follicular atrophoderma.

   Crandall's syndrome (p. 194): twisted hair and deafness are associated with hypogonadism: probable sex-linked recessive inheritance.

   Hypohidrotic ectodermal dysplasia (p. 152): twisted hairs associated with characteristic facies and dental defects.

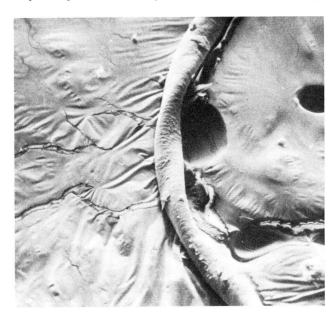

Fig. 7.6. Pili torti. Scanning Electronmicrograph (Slade Hospital, Oxford).

Pseudomonilethrix (p. 186): twisted hair is associated in the individual or the family with apparently beaded hairs of autosomal dominant inheritance.

When patients with these syndromes are excluded, only pili torti remains, but there is evidence that they do not constitute a homogeneous entity; the hairs show considerable variation from patient to patient in their ability to withstand breaking and pulling forces: otherwise expressed the hairs in some patients weather badly, but in others they do not (Dawber 1977).

A syndrome has been reported (Pollitt *et al.* 1968) in which siblings with mental retardation had pili torti and trichorrhexis nodosa. Their hair-keratin was deficient in cystine (p. 204). However, dystrophic pili torti may occur with a normal cystine content (Lyon & Dawber 1977).

Aetiology

In those cases in which classical pili torti of early onset appears to have occurred as an isolated defect, inheritance has usually been determined by an autosomal dominant gene (Appel & Messina 1942; Gedda & Cavalieri 1962). No explanation is available for the apparently high incidence in females. There are many reports of apparently sporadic cases. Some of these could be explained if one parent was affected so mildly that the diagnosis was overlooked. However, there are also cases in which the siblings of normal but consanguineous parents have been affected and in which recessive inheritance must be suspected (Pierini & Borda 1947). There is at present insufficient evidence to allow any dogmatic statements as to possible differences between the two phenotypes.

Pili torti of post-pubertal onset is genetically distinct (Beare 1952; Ullmo 1944). The inheritance of this form is apparently also of autosomal dominant type.

Local inflammatory processes which distort the follicles can result in distorted and twisted hairs, such as may be found around the edges of patches of cicatricial alopecia (Fig. 7.9) (Kurwa & Abdel-Aziz 1973); in these cases, the asymmetrical scarring of the inner root sheath leads to failure of the latter to control cell movement and hair shape; since these are local, twisting develops (Fig. 7.9). Localized pili torti has appeared to follow a scalp infection (Scott 1950). In another case (Schlammadinger 1938) permanent waving probably did no more than reveal the presence of a previously undetected defect.

Pathology
The earlier reports emphasized that the affected hairs were flattened and twisted through 180° around their long axis; at irregular intervals along the shaft (Hellier *et al.* 1940). Electronmicroscopic studies have shown that structural defects other than flattening may accompany and indeed probably determine the development of twists. For example, ridging and fluting of the shafts has been described (Björnstad 1941). The X-ray diffraction pattern of hairs from one case (Hellier *et al.* 1940) was of normal α keratin type, but there must be deviations from parallelism of the polypeptide chains. The load-extension curve resembled that of the wool of merino sheep; the hairs broke more easily than normal, but there was much variation between different hairs.

Histologically the only abnormality is some curvature of the hair follicles. With the scanning electronmicroscope the cuticle of the hair shaft appears normal (Dawber & Comaish 1970).

Clinical features
The hair is usually normal at birth, but is gradually replaced by abnormal hair which becomes clinically evident as early as the 3rd month, or not until the 2nd or 3rd year. In one case a child was bald until 5 and then grew sparse twisted hairs (Clarke & Glicksberg 1941).

There is wide variation from case to case in the fragility of the hair, and hence in the clinical picture.

Affected hairs are brittle and may break off at a length of 5 cm or less, or grow longer in areas of the scalp least subject to trauma (Fig. 7.7). There may therefore be only a short coarse stubble over the whole scalp or there may be circumscribed baldness, irregularly patchy (Siskind 1947) or occipital (Nichamin 1958). Affected hairs have a spangled appearance in reflected light. In mild cases the abnormal hairs have to be carefully sought, for there may be few and the hair may appear grossly normal. Such is sometimes the case after puberty, as normal

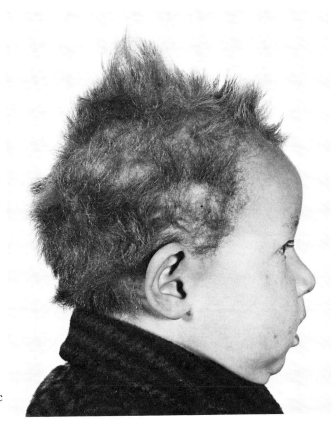

Fig. 7.7. Pili torti of dystrophic type (Dr John Lyon, Ipswich).

hairs may replace most of the pili torti during the later years of childhood. However, some patients remain severely affected throughout life.

The involvement of sites other than the scalp has often been reported, but is an inconstant feature, most often seen in the more sever cases. The eyebrows may be sparse and twisted (Freund 1925; Mitchell-Heggs & May 1947).

Other ectodermal defects may be associated with pili torti. Keratosis pilaris is the most frequent of them, but nail dystrophies, dental abnormalities, corneal opacities and mental retardation have all been reported, though not simultaneously. One girl aged 16 (Friederich & Seitz 1955) had sparse, twisted hair on the scalp, eyebrows, eyelids, axillae and pubis. She had dystrophic nails of thumbs and big toes, generalized hypohidrosis and a corneal dystrophy.

A boy aged 15 (Zaun & Burg 1969) had soft blonde hair until the age of 3, when his hair became darker, coarse and brittle. The scalp hair was twisted and so were some of the sparse brittle vellus hairs on his limbs, and the eyebrows which appeared only at 13 and remained sparse. This may be the same syndrome described by Whiting *et al.* (1980) as corkscrew hair.

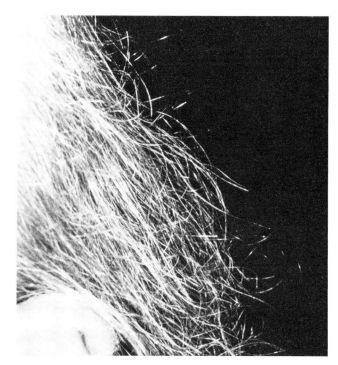

Fig. 7.8. Pili torti—showing 'spangling' effect (Dr R.E. Bowers, Gloucester).

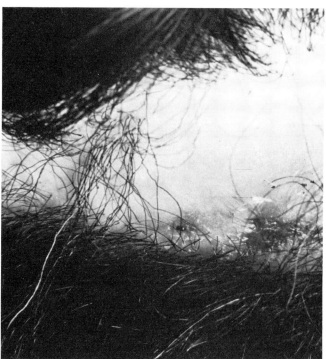

Fig. 7.9. Pili torti—acquired pili torti in cicatricial alopecia (Slade Hospital, Oxford).

The post-pubertal type of pili torti presents as a patchy alopecia (Beare 1952; Kurwa & Abdel-Aziz 1973). Eyebrows and lashes, beard and body hair are sparse. The affected hairs are black.

Diagram

The diagnosis should be suspected if the hair is brittle and dry. The typical spangled appearance in reflected light (Fig. 7.8) is present only if the hair is at least moderately severely affected, yet is not so brittle that it breaks to leave only a sparse stubble.

Microscopical examination of several hairs must be made to confirm the diagnosis. The associated defects of other syndromes with twisted hair should be sought.

Treatment

There is no effective treatment, but reduction of the physical and chemical trauma of hairdressing procedures may allow a considerable increase in length of the hair to take place.

References

Appel B. & Messina S.J. (1942) Pili torti hereditaria. *New England Journal of Medicine*, **226**, 912.

Beare J.M. (1952) Congenital pilar defect showing features of pili torti. *British Journal of Dermatology*, **64**, 366.

Björnstad R.T. (1941) Ein Fall von 'Pili Torti'. *Acta Dermatovenereologica*, **22**, 242.

Clarke G.E. & Glicksberg E.L. (1941) Pili torti. *Archives of Dermatology and Syphilology*, **43**, 836.

Dawber R.P.R. (1977) Weathering of hair in monilethrix and pili torti. *Clinical and Experimental Dermatology*, **2**, 271.

Dawber R.P.R. & Comaish S. (1970) Scanning electron microscopy of normal and abnormal hair shafts. *Archives of Dermatology*, **101**, 316.

Freund E. (1925) Su un'anomalia congenita dei capelli finora non descritta. *Giornale Italiano de Dermatologia e Sifilografia*, **66**, 514.

Friederich H.C. & Seitz R. (1955) Uber eine Forme der ektodermalen Dysplasie unter dem Bilde der Pili torti mit Augurbeteiligung und Störung der Schweisssekretion. *Dermatologische Wochenschrift*, **131**, 277.

Galewsky E. (1932) Pili torti. *Archiv für Dermatologie und Syphilologie*, **167**, 659.

Gedda L. & Cavalieri R. (1962) Relievi genetici delle Distrofie congenita dei capelli. *Cronache dell'Istituto Dermopatico dell'Immacolata*, **17**, 3.

Hellier F.F., Astbury W.J. & Bell F.O. (1940) A case of pili torti. *British Journal of Dermatology*, **52**, 173.

Kurwa A.R. & Abdel-Aziz A.-H.M. (1973) Pili torti—congenital and acquired. *Acta Dermatovenereologica*, **53**, 585.

Lyon J.B. & Dawber R.P.R. (1977) A sporadic case of dystrophic pili torti. *British Journal of Dermatology*, **96**, 197.

Mitchell-Heggs G.B. & May W.R. (1947) Pili torti. *Proceedings of the Royal Society of Medicine*, **40**, 481.

Nichamin S.J. (1958) Twisted hairs (pili torti). *American Journal of Diseases of Children*, **95**, 612.

Ormsby O. & Mitchell J.H. (1924) Atrophia pilorum. Monilethrix. *Archives of Dermatology and Syphilology*, **10**, 398.
Ormsby O.S. & Mitchell J.H. (1925) Atrophia pilorum. *Archives of Dermatology and Syphilology*, **12**, 146.
Pierini L.E. & Borda J.M.C. (1947) Pili torti. *Revista Argentina dje Dermatosifilogia*, **31**, 75.
Pollitt R.J., Jenner F.A. & Davies M. (1968) Sibs with mental and physical retardation, with abnormal amino-acid composition of the hair. *Archives of Disease in Childhood*, **43**, 211.
Ronchese F. (1932) Twisted hairs (pili torti). *Archives of Dermatology and Syphilology*, **26**, 98.
Schlammadinger J. (1938) Pili torti. *Dermatologische Zeitschrift*, **78**, 206.
Schütz J. (1900) Pili moniliformis. *Archiv für Dermatologie und Syphilologie*, **53**, 69.
Scott O.L.S. (1950) Localised pili torti. *Proceedings of the Royal Society of Medicine*, **43**, 68.
Siskind W.M. (1947) Pili torti. *Archives of Dermatology and Syphilology*, **56**, 540.
Ullmo A. (1944) Un nouveau type d'Agnosie et du dystrophie pilaire familiale et héréditaire. *Dermatologica*, **90**, 74.
Whiting D.A., Jenkins T. & Witcomb M.J. (1980) Corkscrew hair—a unique type of congenital alopecia in pili torti. In *Hair, Trace Elements and Human Illness*, ed. A.C. Brown & R.G. Crounse. New York, Praeger, p. 238.

Björnstad's syndrome; Crandall's syndrome

In 1935 Björnstad of Oslo reported five patients in whom pili torti was associated with sensorineural hearing loss. Four of the five were females; members of their families appear not to have been examined but the aunt of one patient is said to have had pili torti and hearing loss, and the brother of another probably had pili torti. A brother of the male patient had both pili torti and deafness. The loss of hair usually began in infancy but in one case it was not noticed until the age of 8. There was a correlation between the severity of the hair defect and the degree of hearing loss. On microscopy the hair shafts showed longitudinal ridging and irregular twisting. A further affected brother and sister suggests that the mode of inheritance is probably autosomal recessive (Voigtlander 1979).

Three brothers were reported with this same association of deafness and pili torti (Reed *et al.* 1967). Two of the brothers were re-investigated after they had reached puberty and were found to have secondary hypogonadism (Crandall *et al.* 1973) with deficiency of luteinizing and of growth hormones. The pedigree suggests that inheritance of this syndrome is determined by an autosomal recessive gene.

Other than that they share two features in common these syndromes must be regarded as distinct.

References

Björnstad R.T. (1965) Pili torti and sensory neural loss of hearing. *Proceedings of the Fennoscandinavian Association of Dermatologists, Copenhagen*, p. 3.
Crandall B.F., Samec L., Sparkes R.S. & Wright S.W. (1973) A familial syndrome of deafness, alopecia and hypogonadism. *Journal of Pediatrics*, **82**, 461.
Reed W.B., Stone V.M., Boder E. & Ziprkowski L. (1967) Hereditary syndrome with auditory and dermatological manifestations. *Archives of Dermatology*, **95**, 456.
Voigtlander V. (1979) Pili torti with deafness (Björnstad syndrome). *Dermatologica*, **159**, 50.

Menkes' kinky-hair syndrome (syn. Trichopoliodystrophy) (references p. 196)

Aetiology
The inheritance of this syndrome is determined by a sex-linked recessive gene. Although the condition was not recognized until 1962 (Menkes *et al.* 1962) it is estimated to occur once in about 35,00 live births.

A partial block in the intestinal absorption of copper (Lott *et al.* 1975) leads to gross copper deficiency to which the pathological changes are believed to be attributable (Danks *et al.* 1972b).

Analysis of the abnormal hair showed a ninefold increase in the free sulphydryl content as compared with normal control subjects (Danks *et al.* 1972b). Similar but less marked changes have been found in the wool of copper-deficient sheep (Gillespie 1964).

Pathology (Menkes *et al.* 1962; Aguilar *et al.* 1966; Danks *et al.* 1971; Mollekaer 1974).
The internal elastic lamina of arteries is fragmented, resulting in tortuosity and wide variation in their calibre. The brain shows gliosis and cystic degeneration. The metaphyses of the long bones show changes resembling those of scurvy.

The serum levels of copper and of caeruloplasmin are low; as is the copper content of the hair (Singh & Bresnan 1973).

Study of the hairs shows several different patterns of hair-twisting (Dupré & Enjobras 1980). There may be multiple loose twists in a single direction, or close twists in a single direction, or two or three twists in one direction, followed by two or three in the opposite direction or a single twist of 180° in one direction followed by a single twist in the other.

Clinical features

Hair. Hair present at birth is normal (Wesenberg *et al.* 1969; Danks *et al.* 1972a; Collie *et al.* 1980). As this is shed it is replaced by short, brittle, light coloured, kinky hair, which on microscopy has the features of pili torti. During the early weeks only a few hairs are abnormal. Trichorrhexis nodosa has also been observed (Menkes *et al.* 1962) but this is a non-specific abnormality which occurs readily in structurally defective hair shafts. Monilethrix was mentioned in three case reports (Bray 1965; Billings & Degnan 1971; French *et al.* 1972), but the examination of a large number of specimens from several families showed only 'pili torti' (Danks *et al.* 1972a).

Skin. The skin generally is pale; the pallor was strikingly evident in an affected child of Negro parentage (Volpintesta 1974). The facies is recognizable: the cheeks are plump, the expression lacks emotive mobility, and the eyebrows are horizontal and twisted (Danks *et al.* 1972a).

Systemic. During the first 2 months the child may be apparently normal. There is progressive psychomotor retardation from the 3rd month and the child is drowsy and lethargic. Temperature regulation is impaired and there is a high susceptibility to infection. Convulsions, usually myoclonic jerking movements, are frequent. Survival for more than a year or two is unusual.

Diagnosis
Before the characteristic hair changes appear at about 3 months the diagnosis may be suspected on the basis of the systemic symptoms and the facies. The suspicion may be strengthened by the radiological findings (Wesenberg *et al.* 1969) and confirmed by the estimation of the serum copper.

The heterozygote (Danks *et al.* 1972a)
The obligate heterozygote may have pili torti but her hair may be normal. The serum copper is normal. Skin fibroblasts from heterozygotes show metachromasia in primary culture, and this test may prove to be valuable in detecting carriers amongst the female relatives of a patient.

Treatment (Danks *et al.* 1972b; Bucknall *et al.* 1973; Lott *et al.* 1975)
Treatment with parenteral copper may become feasible as detailed knowledge of the metabolic defect accumulates.

References
Aguilar M.J., Chadwick D.L., Okuyama K. & Kamoshita S. (1966) Kinky-hair disease: I. Clinical and pathological features. *Journal of Neuropathology and Experimental Neurology*, **25**, 507.
Billings, D.M. & Degnan M. (1971) Kinky hair syndrome. *American Journal of Diseases of Children*, **121**, 447.
Bray P.F. (1965) Sex-linked neurodegenerative disease associated with monilethrix. *Pediatrics*, **36**, 417.
Bucknall W.E., Haslam R.H.A. & Holtzman N.A. (1973) Kinky hair syndrome: response to copper therapy. *Pediatrics*, **52**, 653.
Collie W.R., Goka T.J., Moore C.N. & Howell R.R. (1980) Hair in Menkes disease. A Comprehensive Review. In *Hair, Trace Elements and Human Illness*, ed. A.C. Brown & R.G. Crounse. New York, Praeger, p. 197.
Danks D.M., Cartwright E., Campbell P.E. & Mayne V. (1971) Menkes kinky hair syndrome: a heritable disorder of connective tissue. *Lancet*, **ii**, 1089.
Danks D.M., Campbell P.E., Stevens B.J., Mayne V. & Cartwright E. (1972a) Menkes's kinky hair syndrome: an inherited defect in copper absorption with widespread effects. *Pediatrics*, **50**, 188.
Danks D.M., Stevens B.J., Campbell P.E., Gillespie J.M., Walker-Smith J., Blomfield J. & Turner B. (1972b) Menkes' kinky-hair syndrome. *Lancet*, **i**, 1100.
Dupré A. & Enjobras O. (1980) Syndrom de Menkes an Pilotorten alternant. *Annales de Dermatologie et Vénéréologie (Paris)*, **102**, 269.

French J.H., Sherard E.S., Lubell H., Brotz M. & Moore C.L. (1972) Trichopoliodystrophy. I. Report of a case and biochemical studies. *Archives of Neurology*, **26**, 229.

Gillespie J.M. (1964) The isolation and properties of some soluble proteins from wool. VIII. The proteins of copper deficient wool. *Australian Journal of the Biological Sciences*, **17**, 282.

Lott I.T., Di Paolo R., Schwartz D., Janonska S. & Kaufer J.N. (1975) Copper metabolism in the steely-hair syndrome. *New England Journal of Medicince*, **292**, 197.

Menkes J.H., Alter M., Steigleder G.K., Weakley D.R. & Sung J.H. (1962) A sex-linked recessive disorder with retardation of growth, peculiar hair and focal cerebral and cerebellar degeneration. *Pediatrics*, **29**, 764.

Mollekaer A.M. (1974) Kinky hair syndrome. *Acta Paediatrica Scandinavica*, **63**, 289.

Singh S. & Bresnan M.J. (1973) Menkes kinky hair syndrome. *American Journal of Diseases of Children*, **125**, 572.

Volpintesta E.J. (1974) Menkes kinky hair syndrome in a black infant. *American Journal of Diseases of Children*, **128**, 244.

Wesenberg R.L., Gwinn J.L. & Barnes G.R. (1969) Radiological findings in the kinky-hair syndrome. *Radiology*, **92**, 500.

Netherton's syndrome (bamboo hair) (references p. 199)

History and nomenclature

The hereditary association of an ichthyosiform erythroderma with hair shaft defects of 'trichorrhexis nodosa' type was noted by Touraine & Solente in 1937. In 1949 Comel described and named ichthyosis linearis circumflexa, without referring to hair defects. The distinctive features of this ichthyosiform syndrome had in fact been recorded in 1922 by Rille (Frühwald 1964). Netherton (1958) observed the bamboo-like nodes in the fragile hairs of a girl 'with erythematous scaly dermatitis'. It has gradually become apparent that ichthyosis linearis circumflexa and 'bamboo hairs' (trichorrhexis invaginata) are two features of a single syndrome (Mevorah *et al.* 1974). Most cases of Netherton's syndrome have had ichthyosis linearis circumflexa (ILC) but some have ichthyosis vulgaris (Brodin & Porter 1980; Curban 1973), or both conditions (Schneider *et al.* 1962) or ichthyosiform erythroderma. All cases of ILC in which hair changes have been carefully sought have been found to show them. The syndrome is associated with the atopic state in about 75% of cases, which may explain the occasional association with ichthyosis vulgaris. In one pedigree ILC and ichthyosis vulgaris were found to segregate (Schneider *et al.* 1962).

ILC is thus an almost constant feature of the syndrome, with hair shaft defects of various types and degrees of severity. Until the nature of the underlying abnormality is fully understood the eponym Netherton's syndrome is acceptable. Some authorities (Hurwitz *et al.* 1971) question the variability of the syndrome.

Aetiology

The inheritance of Netherton's syndrome appears to be determined by an autosomal recessive gene of variable expressivity, but the apparent differences in the severity of the hair defect may be related to the trauma to which it is exposed. Girls are affected more often than boys.

Pathology

The histological changes have until recently been considered not to be diagnostic, but it has now been shown by Mevorah & Frank (1974) that in the figurate lesions there is eosinophilic degeneration of cells in the upper malpighian layers. The eosinophilic material, probably a glycolipoprotein, is seen also in the overlying parakeratotic horny layer. In the electronmicroscope the severity of the localized disturbance of keratinization is confirmed (Frenk & Mevorah 1972); the desmosome–tonafilament complex is reduced, membrane coating granules and keratolysation are lacking and dense round bodies are present. The horny layer has lost its lamellar structure.

Scan electronmicroscopy of the hair shafts shows focal defects which produce the development of torsion nodules, invaginated nodules (trichorrhexis invaginata) (Fig. 7.10) and trichorrhexis nodosa (Orfanos *et al.* 1971).

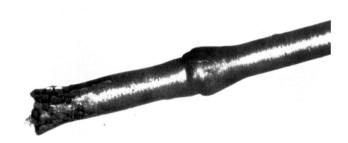

Fig. 7.10. Trichorrhexis invaginata in Netherton's syndrome.

Clinical features (Netherton 1958; Altman & Stroud 1969). The patient may present primarily either with cutaneous changes or complaining of sparse and fragile hairs. Generalized scaling and erythema are present from birth or early infancy, but the degree, extent and persistence of the erythema are very variable. In some cases the erythema may be slight and transient. On the trunk and limbs the fine dry scales are associated with a polycyclic and serpiginous eruption the horny margin of which slowly changes its pattern (Fig. 7.11). Rarely there may be small subcorneal bullae in this margin (Dimitrowa & Georgirwa 1961).

Atopic manifestations are superimposed in some patients (Porter & Starke 1968) when generalized dryness and flexural lichenification may be the predominant skin changes.

The hair defects may be detected only if deliberately sought, but in most cases are readily apparent clinically (Stevanovic 1969; Randell & Wall 1972; Salamon *et al.* 1972). The hair is short, dry, lustreless and brittle, and the eyebrows and

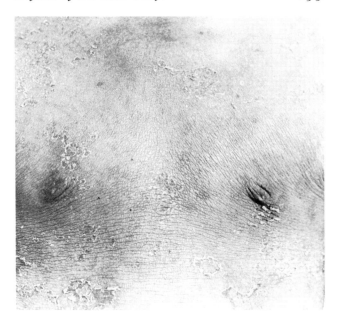

Fig. 7.11. Ichthyosis linearis circumflexa in Netherton's syndrome (Slade Hospital, Oxford).

lashes are sparse or absent. Weathering and misguided 'treatment' and vigorous hairdressing may influence the severity of the cosmetic disability.

Treatment
The protection of the hair from avoidable physical and chemical trauma may result in considerable cosmetic benefit.

References
Altman J. & Stroud J. (1969) Netherton's syndrome and ichthyosis linearis circumflexa. *Archives of Dermatology*, **200**, 550.
Brodin M.M.B. & Porter P.S. (1980) Netherton's syndrome. *Cutis*, **26**, 185.
Curban G.V. (1973) Iction linear circumflexa. *Anais Brasilieros de Dermatologia e Sifilografia*, **48**, 43.
Dimitrowa J. & Georgirwa S. (1961) Ichthyosis linearis circumflexa mit subkornealen Bläschen. *Dermatologische Wochenschrift*, **144**, 1041.
Frenk E. & Mevorah B. (1972) Ichthyosis linearis circumflexa Comèl with Trichorrhexis invaginata (Netherton's syndrome). *Archiv für Dermatologische Forschung*, **245**, 42.
Frühwald R. (1964) Zur Frage der Comelschen Krankheit. *Dermatologische Wochenschrift*, **150**, 289.
Hurwitz S., Kirsch N. & McGuire J. (1971) Reevaluation of ichthyosis and hair shaft anomalies. *Archives of Dermatology*, **103**, 266.
Mevorah B. & Frenk E. (1974) Ichthyosis linearis circumflexa Comèl with trichorrhexis invaginata (Netherton's syndrome). *Dermatologica*, **149**, 193.
Mevorah B., Frenk E. & Brooke E.M. (1974) Ichthyosis linearis circumflexa Comèl. *Dermatologica*, **149**, 201.
Netherton G.W. (1958) A unique case of trichorrhexis nodosa—'bamboo hairs'. *A.M.A. Archives of Dermatology*, **78**, 483.

Orfanos C.E., Mahrle G. & Salamon T. (1971) Netherton-Syndrom. *Hautarzt*, **22**, 397.

Porter P.S. & Starke J.C. (1968) Netherton's syndrome. *Archives of Disease in Childhood*, **43**, 319.

Randell P.L. & Wall L.M. (1972) Netherton's syndrome—case report. *Australian Journal of Dermatology*, **13**, 119.

Salamon T., Lazovic O. & Stenek S. (1972) Uber das Netherton-Syndrom. *Hautarzt*, **23**, 66.

Schneider W., Coppenrath R. & Bock H.D. (1962) Ichthyosis linearis circumflexa bei familiären Auftreten von Ichthyosis vulgaris. *Archiv für klinische und experimentelle Dermatologie*, **215**, 79.

Stevanović D.V. (1969) Multiple defects of the hair shaft in Netherton's disease. *British Journal of Dermatology*, **81**, 851.

Touraine A. & Solente (1937) Erythrokeratodermie du cuir chevelu et 'Trichorrhexis nodosa' familiales. *Bulletin de la Société française de Dermatologie et de Syphiligraphie*, **44**, 1011.

Trichorrhexis nodosa

History and nomenclature

According to Jackson & McMurtry (1913) this defect of the hair shaft was first recognized by Samuel Wilks of Guy's Hospital in 1852, but his first published account of the condition appeared in his *Lectures on Pathological Anatomy* in 1857. Meanwhile Beigel of Vienna had published a description in 1855. A variety of terms have been proposed but trichorrhexis nodosa, suggested by Kaposi, has been generally favoured. Terms which have been frequently used more or less as synonyms are trichoclasis and fragilitas crinium, but both terms merely describe a consequence of the essential abnormality, the formation of nodes, through which rupture of the hair shaft readily occurs. Moreover, trichorrhexis nodosa is not the sole cause of fragile hair.

Aetiology

The literature of the past century has repeatedly revived the controversy as to whether trichorrhexis nodosa is a developmental defect, sometimes hereditary, the consequence of acquired nutritional or metabolic disturbance, or solely a response to trauma, physical or chemical (Chernosky 1974). Nor has there been any agreement concerning the incidence of trichorrhexis; some authors have considered it to be common, others rare. It is in fact the commonest defect of the hair shaft.

Trichorrhexis is best regarded as a distinctive response of the hair shaft to injury. If the degree or frequency of the injury be sufficient it can be induced in normal hair. The cuticular cells become disrupted allowing the cortical cells to splay out to form nodes (Dawber & Comaish 1970). If, however, the hair is abnormally fragile trichorrhexis may follow relatively trivial injury. The trauma of hairdressing procedures has often been incriminated (Cajkovac 1938; Chernosky & Owens 1966). Scratching may produce identical changes in the hairs in the genitocrural region (Chernosky & Owens 1966).

The severity of experimentally induced trichorrhexis nodosa was related to the degree of trauma, in patients with or without pre-existing trichorrhexis

(Owens & Chernosky 1966). In one patient the cumulative effect of shampooing, brushing, sea bathing and sunlight led to seasonal recurrences each summer (Papa *et al.* 1972). In another the provocative trauma was a chemical hair straightener (Jolly & Carpenter, 1967).

Some authors have differentiated a generalized form from a much rarer localized form, often beginning early in life and sometimes genetically determined (Touraine & Clerfeuille 1938). In fact the distribution depends on the localization and nature of the trauma (Friederich 1950).

That congenital and hereditary defects of the hair shaft can predispose to trichorrhexis nodosa is well established. Some children have other characterized defects of hair shaft structure (Dorn 1956). Trichorrhexis nodosa may occur in pseudomonilethrix (p. 186), in Netherton's syndrome (p. 197) or with pili annulati (Leider 1950) (p. 208).

Trichorrhexis nodosa is a feature of the rare metabolic defect argininosuccinic aciduria, in which it is associated with mental retardation (Allan *et al.* 1958). There is a deficiency of the enzyme argininosuccidase (Levin *et al.* 1961). Some twenty patients have been reported (Brenton *et al.* 1974). The patients can be classified in three groups, according to the age of the onset of the symptoms (Shih 1972). Where symptoms begin at birth early death is usual: gradual onset during the first months of life is characterized by physical and mental retardation and enlargement of the liver. Onset from the second year onwards is also characterized by psychomotor retardation and also by episodes of ataxia. The hair tends to be dry, brittle and lustreless and may show trichorrhexis nodosa (Rauschkolb *et al.* 1967) but not all patients with this metabolic disorder develop it (Cederbaum *et al.* 1973). As soon as the diagnosis is established a special diet should be provided (Shih 1972).

Trichorrhexis nodosa may occur in certain families as an apparently isolated defect of the hair; node formation and fracture are induced by minimal trauma and develop during the early months of life. Such a defect associated with abnormalities of teeth and nails was determined by an autosomal dominant gene in one family (Rousset 1952). Wolff *et al.* (1975) have described as trichorrhexis congenita the presence from birth of trichorrhexis nodosa confined to the scalp, in a boy with normal teeth and nails.

In a case of generalized trichorrhexis nodosa in male adult (Leonard *et al.* 1980) electron histochemical study showed evidence of a disorder in the formation of α-keratin chains within the globular matrix of the hair cortex with respect to cystine. This cortical change together with vacuoles found in the endocuticle appear to be the defects which allow the formation of trichorrhexis nodosa in response to relatively trivial trauma.

Pathology

In simple trichorrhexis nodosa the shaft may appear normal with the light or

electronmicroscope except at the nodes; or the shaft, apart from the proximal
1 cm, may show signs of abnormal wear and tear (Dawber & Comaish 1970). At
the nodes the cortex bulges and is split by longitudinal fissures. If fracture occurs
transversely through a node, i.e. trichoclasis, the end of the hair resembles a
small paint brush (Figs. 7.12, 7.13).

Clinical features
In trichorrhexis nodosa complicating a congenital defect of the hair shafts the

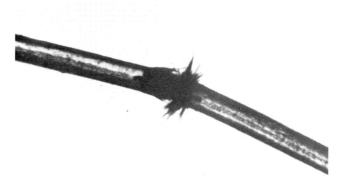

Fig. 7.12. Trichorrhexis nodosa—light microscope (Slade
Hospital, Oxford).

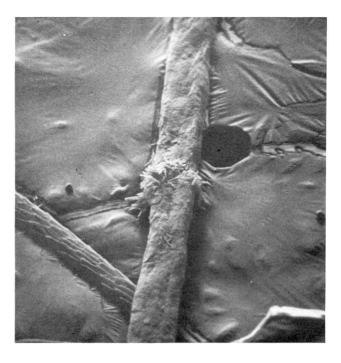

Fig. 7.13. Trichorrhexis
nodosa in the scanning
electronmicroscope (Slade
Hospital, Oxford).

hair breaks so easily that large or small portions of the scalp show only broken stumps and alopecia may be quite gross.

In the much commoner conditions in which trauma plays a proportionately larger role and the predisposing inadequacy of the shaft a proportionately smaller one, there are three principal clinical presentations (Price 1975).

Proximal trichorrhexis nodosa occurs in Negroes. The hair is short in areas subjected to the greatest trauma, and trichorrhexis, trichoptilosis and trichoclasis are seen on microscopy.

Distal trichorrhexis nodosa occurs in other races. Often it is discovered incidentally and only a few whitish nodules are seen near the ends of scattered hairs. If many hairs are affected the patient may complain that the hair is dry, dull or brittle. On examination hairs with white nodules are seen among others which have fractured through the nodes.

The third clinical form was well described by Sabouraud (1921) but it appears now to be rare. In a localized area of scalp, moustache or beard, some hairs are broken, and others show from one to five or six nodules. It is said that trauma of any sort can be excluded, and that spontaneous recovery eventually occurs.

Diagnosis

The congenital forms must be differentiated from other shaft defects. The distal acquired form may simulate dandruff or even pediculosis. In all cases diagnosis depends on careful microscopy and if possible scanning electronmicroscopy.

Treatment

The avoidance of all unnecessary trauma may be followed by marked improvement.

References

Allan J.D., Cudsworth D.C., Dent C.E. & Wilson V.K. (1958) A disease, probably hereditary, characterized by severe mental deficiency and a constant gross abnormality of aminoacid metabolism. *Lancet*, i, 182.

Brenton D.P., Cudsworth D.C., Harthy S., Lundy S. & Kuzemko J.A. (1974) Argininosuccinicaciduria: clinical, metabolic and dietary study. *Journal of Mental Deficiency Research*, 18, 1.

Cajkovac S. (1938) Ein Beitrag zur Frage der Schädigung des Haarschaftens. *Dermatologische Zeitschrift*, 77, 305.

Casals D.A. & Castellanos P.G. (1950) Trichorrexie noueuse circonscrite en plaque unique. *Annales de Dermatologie et de Syphiligraphie*, 10, 668.

Cederbaum S.D., Shaw K.N.F., Valente M. & Cotton M.E. (1973) Argininosuccinic acidurea. *American Journal of Mental Deficiency*, 77, 395.

Chernosky M.E. (1974) Acquired trichorrhexis nodosa. *The First Human Hair Symposium*, ed. A.C. Brown. New York, Medcom Press, p. 36.

Chernosky M.E. & Owens D.W. (1966) Trichorrhexis nodosa. *Archives of Dermatology*, 94, 577.

Dawber R.P.R. & Comaish S. (1970) Scanning electron microscopy of normal and abnormal hair shafts. *Archives of Dermatology*, 101, 316.

Dochao L. de A. & Vidal A.Z. (1950) Tricoclasia idiopatica. *Actas Dermo-Sifiliográficas*, **41**, 347.

Dorn H. (1956) Dominant-geschlachts-chromosomen-gebundener Erbgang bei Trichoclasie. *Zeitschrift für Haut und Geschletskrankheiten*, **20**, 129.

Friederich H.C. (1950) Eine Beitrag zur Pathogenese der Trichorrhexis nodosa circumscripta. *Zeitschrift für Haut und Geschletskrankheiten*, **8**, 163.

Jackson G.T. & McMurtry C.W. (1913) *A Treatise on the Diseases of the Hair*. London, Kimpton, p. 131.

Jolly H.W. & Carpenter C.L. (1967) Trichorrhexis nodosa following hair straightener. *Cutis*, **3**, 359.

Leider M. (1950) Multiple simultaneous anomalies of the hair. *Archives of Dermatology and Syphilology*, **62**, 510.

Leonard J.N., Gunner C.L. & Dawber R.P.R. (1980) Generalized trichorrhexis nodosa. *British Journal of Dermatology*, **103**, 85.

Levin B., Mackay H.R.M. & Oberholzer V.G. (1961) Argininosuccinic aciduria, an inborn error of aminoacid metabolism. *Archives of Disease in Childhood*, **36**, 622.

Owens D.W. & Chernosky M.E. (1966) Trichorrhexis nodosa. *Archives of Dermatology*, **94**, 568.

Papa C.M., Mills O.H. & Hanshaw W. (1972) Seasonal trichorrhexis nodosa. *Archives of Dermatology*, **106**, 888.

Polemann G. (1950) Zur Kenntnis der traumatischen Trichoklasie und der idioputischen Trichoklasie Jackson–Sabouraud. *Archiv für Dermatologie und Syphilologie*, **190**, 535.

Price V. (1975) Office diagnosis of structural hair anomalies. *Cutis*, **15**, 231.

Rauschkolb E.W., Chernovsky M.E., Knox J.M. & Owens D.W. (1967) Trichorrhexis nodosa—an error of aminoacid metabolism. *Journal of Investigative Dermatology*, **48**, 260.

Rauschkolb E.W., Freeman R.G. & Farrell G. (1968) Hair fragility. *Cutis*, **4**, 1315.

Rousset M.J. (1952) Génodermatose difficilement classable (trichorrhexis nodosa) prédominant chez les mâles dans quatre générations. *Bulletin de la Société française de Dermatologie et de Syphiligraphie*, **59**, 298.

Sabouraud R. (1921) Trichoclasie, trichorrhexie et trichophilose. *Annales de Dermatologie et de Syphiligraphie*, **2**, 445.

Shih V.E. (1972) Early dietary management in an infant with argininosuccinase deficiency: preliminary report. *Journal of Pediatrics*, **80**, 645.

Touraine A. & Clerfeuille G. (1938) Les diverses variétés de trichorrhexie noueuse. *Bulletin de la Société française de Dermatologie et de Syphiligraphie*, **45**, 636.

Wolff H.H., Vigl E. & Braun-Falco O. (1975) Trichorrhexis congenita. *Hautarzt*, **26**, 576.

Trichothiodystrophy (references p. 207)

History and nomenclature

This term was coined (Price *et al.* 1980a, b) to describe brittle hair with an abnormally low sulphur content. It is not yet certain whether the different syndromes of which it is a feature represent a single rather variable entity, or distinct entities sharing this feature.

Pollitt's patients (Pollitt *et al.* 1968) were mentally and physically retarded. The Mexican family, whose origin in the town of Sabinos has led to this name being attached to the syndrome from which they suffer, have mental retardation, nail dysplasia, and reduced fertility (Arbisser *et al.* 1976; Howell *et al.* 1980). Members of the Amish community with trichothiodystrophy are mildly retarded mentally, and are of small stature (Watson *et al.* 1973; Jackson *et al.* 1974;

Baden *et al.* 1976). One patient with this hair defect (Brown *et al.* 1970) was otherwise physically and mentally normal. The patients reported by Jorizzo *et al.* (1980) had lamellar ichthyosis, which has been a feature of some other reported cases (e.g. Price *et al.* 1980).

Where it has been possible to establish the mode of inheritance this has been of autosomal recessive type.

Pathology
The hair is brittle. With trauma it may break cleanly (trichoschisis) (Fig. 7.14) or may form nodes somewhat resembling trichorrhexis nodosa but without conspicuous release of individual spindle cells (Price *et al.* 1980).

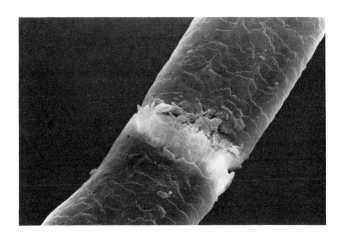

Fig. 7.14. Trichoschisis in trichothiodystrophy (Dr Van Neste, Lille).

In the scanning electron microscope the hairs are seen to be flattened, and sometimes folded over themselves. The shaft is irregular with ridging and fluting and the cuticular scales are patchily absent (Fig. 7.15).

With the polarizing microscope the hairs show alternating bright and dark zones (Fig. 7.16).

The sulphur content of the hair is much reduced.

Clinical features
The hair is sparse, short and brittle, but the degree of alopecia varies considerably (Fig. 7.17). In the Sabinos cases it is often almost total. There may be lamellar ichthyosis. The nails may be dystrophic.

Mental and physical development may be normal but one or both may be slightly, moderately or severely retarded.

Until further cases have been studied the relationship between the syndromes showing trichothiodystrophy is a matter for speculation.

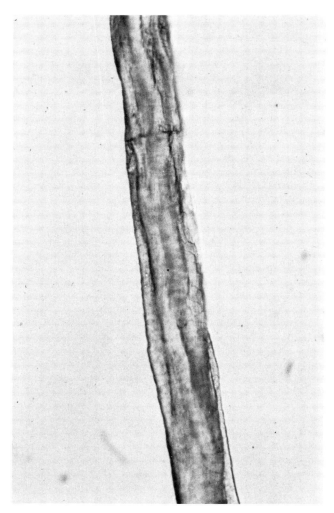

Fig. 7.15. Trichothiodystrophy. In the scanning electron-microscope the hairs are seen to be flattened and irregularly ridged and fluted (Dr Van Neste, Lille).

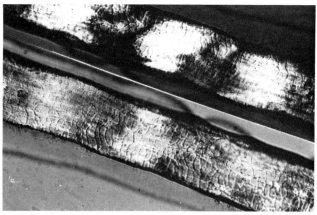

Fig. 7.16. Trichothiodystrophy: alternating bright and dark zones in the polarizing microscope (Dr Van Neste, Lille).

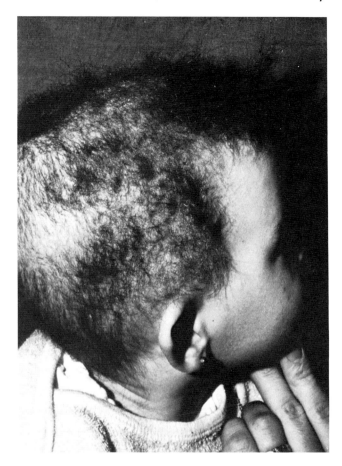

Fig. 7.17. Moderately severe alopecia in trichothiodystrophy (Dr Van Neste, Lille).

References

Arbisser A.I., Scott C.I. Jr, Howell R.R., Ong P.S. & Cox H.L. Jr (1976) A syndrome manifested by brittle hair with morphologic and biochemical abnormalities, developmental delay and normal stature. *Birth Defects, Original Article Series,* **12,** 219.

Baden H.P., Jackson C.E. & Weiss L. (1976) The physico-chemical properties of hair in the BID syndrome. *American Journal of Human Genetics,* **28,** 514.

Brown A.C., Belser R.B., Crounse R.G. & Wehr B.F. (1970) A congenital hair defect: trichoschisis with alternating birefringence and low sulphur content. *Journal of Investigative Dermatology,* **54,** 496.

Howell R.R., Collie W.R., Cavasos O.I., Arbisser A.I., Fraustadt U., Marcks S.N. & Parsons D. (1980) The Sabinos brittle hair syndrome. In *Hair, Trace Elements and Human Illness,* eds. A.C. Brown & R.G. Crounse. New York, Praeger, p. 210.

Jackson C.T., Weiss J.L. & Watson J.H.L. (1974) 'Brittle' hair with short stature, intellectual impairment and decreased fertility: an autosomal recessive syndrome in an Amish kindred. *Pediatrics,* **54,** 201.

Jorizzo J.L., Crounse R.G. & Winter C.E. (1980) Lamellar ichthyosis, dwarfism, mental retardation and hair shaft abnormalities. *Journal of the American Schools of Dermatology,* **2,** 309.

Pollitt R.J., Jenner F.A. & Davies M. (1968) Sibs with mental and physical retardation and trichorrhexis nodosa with abnormal associated composition of the hair. *Archives of Diseases in Childhood*, **43**, 211.

Price V.H., Odom R.B., Jones F.T. & Ward W.H. (1980a) Trichthiodystrophy: sulfur-deficient brittle hair. In *Hair, Trace Elements and Human Illness*, eds. A.C. Brown and R.G. Crounse. New York, Praeger, p. 220.

Price V.H., Odom R.B., Ward W.H. & Jones F.T. (1980b) Trichothiodystrophy: sulfur-deficient brittle hair as a marker for a neuroectodermal symptom complex. *Archives of Dermatology*, **116**, 1375.

Watson J.H.L., Weiss L. & Jackson C.E. (1973) Scanning electron microscopy of human hair in a syndrome of trichoschisis with mental retardation. In *The First Human Hair Symposium*, ed. A.C. Brown. New York, Medcom Press, p. 120.

Marinesco–Sjögren syndrome

This rare syndrome, of autosomal recessive inheritance, has as its principal features (Norwood 1964) cerebellar ataxia, dysarthria, retarded physical and mental development and congenital cataracts. The teeth are abnormally formed and the lateral incisors may be absent. The nails are flat, thin and fragile.

The hair is sparse, fine, light in colour, short and brittle. On microscopy transverse fractures—trichoschisis—can be seen at the sites of impending fractures. In polarized light the hair is irregularly birefringent. Scalp biopsy shows normal anagen follicles, but with incomplete keratinization of the internal root sheath (Porter 1971).

References

Norwood W.F. (1964) The Marinesco–Sjögren syndrome. *Journal of Pediatrics*, **65**, 431.

Porter P.S. (1971) The genetics of human hair growth. *Birth Defects, Original Article Series*, **7**, 69.

Structural defects of the shaft without increased fragility

Ringed hair (references p. 211)

History and nomenclature
The first description of ringed hair is often ascribed to Karsch of Münster (1846), but the pigmentary defect in his patient was more complex, with rings of irregular width as only one of several abnormal features. Erasmus Wilson in 1867 presented to the Royal Society an account of the condition now known as ringed hair, or as pili annulati or leucotrichia annularis.

Aetiology
The inheritance of ringed hair has been shown in many extensive pedigrees to be determined by an autosomal dominant gene (Ehrhardt 1932; Reyn 1934, Juon 1942; Harris & Kalmus 1948; Ashley & Jacques 1950). One pedigree (Ebbing

1957) is compatible with autosomal recessive inheritance, and there are reports (e.g. McCleary & Montgomery 1955) of apparently sporadic cases. However, the expressivity of the dominant gene is variable, and mild cases without any great increase in hair fragility are easily overlooked. Blue naevus and ringed hair were associated in some members of a family, but the two conditions segregated (Dawber 1972).

Pathology and pathogenesis
With the light microscope abnormal dark bands alternate with normal, light bands (Fig. 7.18); in reflected light the colours of normal and abnormal bands are

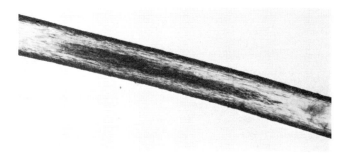

Fig. 7.18. Ringed hair: alternating bright and normal bands (Slade Hospital, Oxford).

reversed. The light appearance of the abnormal bands in reflected light is due to air spaces in the cortex (Cady & Trotter 1922). The rate of growth has been measured in one case (Dawber 1972) and found to be 0.16 mm/day, which is less than half the average normal rate. Breaking stress analysis showed no significant abnormality in ringed hair, but fractures were always in the abnormal bands.

Electronmicroscopic studies (Price *et al.* 1968) showed that the clusters of air-filled cavities (Fig. 7.19), randomly distributed throughout the cortex in the abnormal bands, lie partly within cortical cells and between macrofibrils, or in the case of larger cavities appear to replace cortical cells. There is perhaps a defect in the formation of the microfibril matrix complex (Musso 1970). Recent work has indicated that both these suggestions are correct. Hairs from the family described by Dawber (1972) showed an abnormal surface cuticle which appeared 'cobble-stoned' on scanning electronmicroscopy. The work of Gummer & Dawber (1981) using electron histochemical methods confirmed this; cuticular cells are thrown into folds.

On biochemical analysis (Dawber 1972) the cystine content of affected hair was low, but its sulphur content was normal. The pathogenesis of ringed hair remains uncertain. The abnormal bands appear to be produced at random and not cyclically in relation to specific periods of growth (Dawber 1972).

In Ebbing's (1957) patients in whom recessive inheritance of the trait seemed

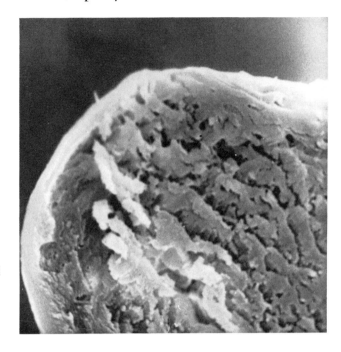

Fig. 7.19. Ringed hair: cortical spaces seen in the abnormal bands in the scanning electronmicroscope (Slade Hospital, Oxford).

probable, the bands were regularly spaced. It remains to be seen whether this will prove to be a constant feature of a recessive form.

Clinical features
Ringed hair is associated with a very variable degree of fragility. When the fragility is slight and relatively few hairs are affected the condition may be discovered only when deliberately sought. If many hairs are affected and fragility is great then short hair may attract attention in early life and the spangled appearance of the shafts in reflected light can be readily detected (Fig. 7.20). The axillary hair is occasionally affected (Montgomery & Binder 1948). The fractures in some brittle hairs take the form of trichorrhexis nodosa (Leider 1950).

Diagnosis
The diagnosis is readily established on microscopy of affected hair. A defect in which partially twisted shafts have an elliptical cross section has been named pseudopiliannulati because such hair may give an impression of alternating light and dark bands (Price *et al.* 1970).

Prognosis and treatment
The prognosis is good in the sense that the severity of the defect does not increase with age, but the cosmetic appearance depends largely on restraint in the use of

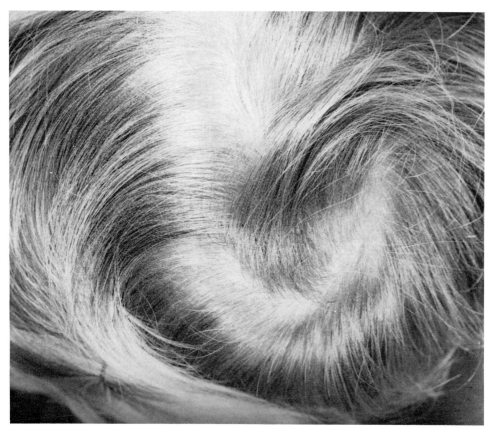

Fig. 7.20. Ringed hair (Addenbrooke's Hospital, Cambridge).

hairdressing procedures. If the hair can be spared chemical and physical trauma, including unnecessary brushing, it may grow to an acceptable length.

References

Ashley L.M. & Jacques R.S. (1950) Four generations of ringed hair. *Journal of Heredity*, **41**, 82.

Cady L.O. & Trotter M. (1922) Study of ringed hair. *Archives of Dermatology and Syphilology*, **6**, 301.

Dawber R. (1972) Investigation of a family with pili annulati associated with blue naevus. *Transactions of the St John's Hospital Dermatological Society*, **58**, 51.

Ebbing H.C. (1957) Gibt es auch bei Ringelhaaren (Pili annulati) einen einfach-rezessiven Erbgang. *Homo*, **8**, 35.

Ehrhardt S. (1932) Ringelhaare in der Familie E. *Münchene medizinische Wochenschrift*, **79**, 949.

Gummer C.L. & Dawber R.P.R. (1981) Pili annulati: electron histochemical studies on affected hairs. *British Journal of Dermatology*, **105**, 303.

Harris H. & Kalmus H. (1948) On the manifestation of ringed hair in a mother and daughter. *Annals of Eugenics*, **14**, 209.

Juon M. (1942) Eine Brobachtung familiären Auftratung von Pili annulati. *Dermatologica*, **86**, 117.

Karsch A. (1846) De Capillitiri humani coloiebus quardan. Cit. by Landois (1866).

Landois L. (1866) Das plötzliche Ergrauer der Haupthaare. *Archiv für pathologische Anatomie und Physiologie*, **35**, 575.

Leider M. (1950) Multiple simultaneous anomalies of the hair. *Archives of Dermatology and Syphilology*, **62**, 510.

McCleary J. & Montgomery H. (1955) Ringed hair. Report of a case. *A.M.A. Archives of Dermatology*, **71**, 526.

Montgomery R.M. & Binder A.I. (1948) Ringed hair. *Archives of Dermatology and Syphilology*, **58**, 177.

Musso L.A. (1970) Pili annulati. *Australian Journal of Dermatology*, **11**, 67.

Price V.H., Thomas R.S. & Jones F.T. (1968) Pili annulati. *Archives of Dermatology*, **98**, 640.

Price V.H., Thomas R.S. & Jones F.T. (1970) Pseudophili annulati. *Archives of Dermatology*, **102**, 54.

Reyn A. (1934) Pili annulati occurring as a family disorder. *British Journal of Dermatology*, **46**, 168.

Wilson E. (1867) A remarkable alteration of appearance and structure of human hair. *Proceedings of the Royal Society*, **15**, 406.

Woolly hair (references p. 215)

History and nomenclature

Woolly hair is more or less tightly coiled hair occurring over the entire scalp or part of it, in an individual not of Negroid origin. The clinical syndromes of which woolly hair is a feature have been much confused by many authors. The recent investigation by Hutchinson *et al.* (1974) has done much to clarify the position; the classification proposed by these authors is followed here. It remains possible, however, that woolly hair is a feature also of other syndromes not yet characterized.

Classification and aetiology

(1) Hereditary woolly hair. The inheritance of this disorder is determined by an autosomal dominant gene. It has been reported in six generations of a Rhineland family (Hoffmann 1953).

(2) Familial woolly hair. The genetic evidence is inconclusive but the condition has occurred in siblings whose parents were normal. Autosomal recessive inhritance is probable (Furando *et al.* 1979).

(3) Acquired progressive kinking of the hair is of unknown origin.

(4) Symmetrical circumscribed allotrichia appears to be a distinct syndrome (Knierer 1955).

(5) Woolly hair naevus. This is a circumscribed developmental defect, present at birth, and apparently not genetically determined.

Hereditary woolly hair (Fig. 7.21)

Pathology. In some pedigrees the shaft diameter in affected individuals is reduced (Hutchinson *et al.* 1974); the hair is fragile and may show trichorrhexis nodosa.

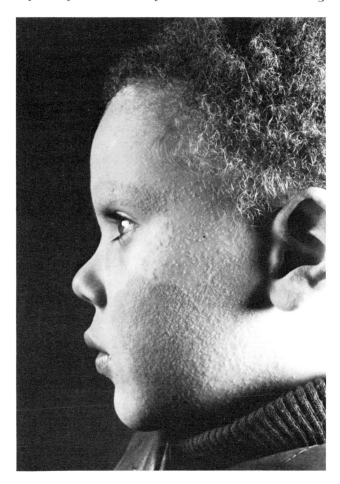

Fig. 7.21. Hereditary woolly hair associated with keratosis pilaris atrophicans (Dr J.S. Pegum). A full report of this patient will be published by Dr Pegum.

Pili torti and pili annulati have been reported as associated defects, but in different families.

Clinical features. Excessively curly hair is evident at birth or in early infancy; it has sometimes been described as Negroid in appearance (Mohr 1932; Hoffmann 1953), but tending to become less so in adult life (Schlaginhaufen 1945). Anderson (1936) considered that the hair, though tightly coiled was not Negroid. The degree of variation in severity within a family is inconstant (Hutchinson *et al.* 1974). There is no consistent association with any hair colour (Schokking 1934). The hair shaft may be twisted (Verbov 1978).

In some cases the hair is brittle and breaks readily, probably as a result of trichorrhexis nodosa. The hair in sites other than the scalp is usually normal but Hoffmann (1953) found it to be sparse and thin.

Familial woolly hair

Pathology. There is a marked reduction in the diameter of hair shafts which may be poorly pigmented. The hair is brittle and on scanning electronmicroscopy shows signs of cuticular wear and tear (Hutchinson *et al.* 1974).

Clinical features. So few cases have been reported that generalizations are unwarranted. In three cases (Hutchinson *et al.* 1974) fine, tightly curled, poorly pigmented hair was present from birth; in two of them the hair never achieved a length of more than 2 or 3 cm. Eyebrows and body hair were sparse.

In the case reports of Gottheil (1919) and of Sweitzer (1948) few details are given but the principal findings appear to have been essentially similar.

Salamon's (1963) patients had sparse dark brown, curly hair, and may have had the same condition, but the report again fails to give a sufficiently detailed description.

Acquired progressive kinking of the hair (Fig. 7.22)

History and nomenclature. Acquired progressive kinking (APK) of the scalp hair, described by Wise & Sulzberger in 1932, appears to be extremely rare, but many cases may not be recorded. Some have been confused with the woolly hair naevus, but APK is differentiated clinically by its onset in adolescence or adult life and its progressive extension over a period of years.

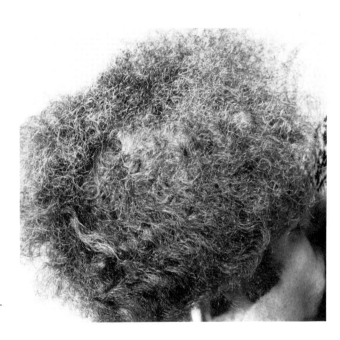

Fig. 7.22. Acquired progressive kinking of the hair in a man aged 28. The condition had been noticed at about the age of 15 (Addenbrooke's Hospital, Cambridge).

Aetiology and pathology. The aetiology of APK is unknown; there is as yet no evidence that it is genetically determined. The hairs in the affected region of the scalp show both structural and functional abnormalities (Coupe & Johnston 1969). They may be finer (Wise & Sulzberger 1932) or coarser than in the normal scalp, and they show irregularly distributed kinks and half-twists. The duration of anagen is reduced.

Clinical features. The patient gradually becomes aware that the hair in one region of the scalp is becoming kinky and that a progressive change in texture is accompanied by a decreased rate of growth, as a result of which he rarely requires a hair cut.

On examination the hair on one or more regions of the scalp is wiry, kinky and unruly, dry and lustreless. There are no sharply defined boundaries between normal and abnormal hair. In some of the cases described, the acquired kinking preceded the development of common male baldness.

Symmetrical circumscribed allotrichia

History and nomenclature. Among cases reported as woolly hair naevus are some for which Norwood (1981) has proposed the term 'whisker hair' but which are identical with the cases reported by Knierer (1955) as symmetrical circumscribed allotrichia.

Clinical features. From adolescence onwards the hair in an irregular band extending around the edge of the scalp from above the ears towards the occipital region becomes coarse and whisker-like. A similar case was recorded by Bovenmyer (1979).

Woolly hair naevus

Pathology. The hair in the affected region of the scalp is finer than elsewhere. Electronmicroscopy of the abnormal hair showed the absence of cuticle; trichorrhexis nodosa was present (Crosti & Menni 1979).

Clinical features. The hair in a circumscribed area of the scalp is tightly curled from birth or from early infancy (Born 1957). The size of the affected areas usually increases only proportionately with general growth, but it may extend for 3 or 4 years (Post 1958). The abnormal hair may be slightly paler in colour than that of the rest of the scalp.

In over half of the reported cases a pigmented or epidermal naevus has been present but not in the same site. In Streitman's (1959) case, for example, a woolly hair naevus of the right occipital region was associated with a linear epidermal naevus of the left cheek, the left side of the neck and the left hand. A woolly hair naevus has been associated also with ocular defects (Jacobson & Lewis 1975).

Other cases have been reported by Wise (1927), Anderson (1943), Grant (1960) and Domonkos (1962).

References

Anderson E. (1936) An American pedigree for woolly hair. *Journal of Heredity*, **27**, 444.

Anderson N.P. (1943) Woolly-haired naevus of the scalp. *Archives of Dermatology and Syphilology*, **47**, 286.

Born W. (1957) Über Umschriebene Kräuselnaevi Innerhalb Sonst Glatten Kopfhaars. *Dermatologica*, **115**, 119.

Bovenmyer D.A. (1979) Woolly hair naevus. *Cutis*, **24**, 322.

Coupe R.L. & Johnston M.N. (1969) Acquired progressive kinking of the hair. *Archives of Dermatology*, **100**, 191.

Crosti C. & Menni S. (1979) Woolly hair naevus. Observasioni su su tre casi clinici. *Giornale Italiano de Dermatologio/Minerva Dermatologica*, **114**, 45.

Domonkos A.N. (1962) Woolly hair naevus. *Archives of Dermatology*, **85**, 568.

Furando J., Gertalos M.R. & Fontarnau R. (1979) Woolly hair. Estudo Histologica e ultrastrucuturale en quatro casos. *Actas Dermosithiligraphicas*, **70**, 203.

Gottheil W.S. (1919) Peculiar woolly hair. *Journal of Cutaneous Diseases*, **37**, 489.

Grant P.W. (1960) A case of woolly hair naevus. *Archives of Disease in Childhood*, **35**, 512.

Hoffmann E. (1953) Über einen Kräuselnaevus innerhalb sonst glatten Kopfhaares im Vergleich zum erblichen Kraushaar und zur Lockenbildung nach Röntgenepilation. *Dermatologica*, **197**, 281.

Hutchinson P.E., Cairns R.J. & Wells R.S. (1974) Woolly hair. *Transactions of St John's Hospital Dermatological Society*, **60**, 160.

Jacobson K.V. & Lewis M. (1975) Woolly hair naevus with ocular involvement. *Dermatologica*, **151**, 249.

Knierer W. (1955) Allotrichia circumscripta symmetrica capillitii. *Dermatologische Wochenschrift*, **132**, 794.

Mohr O.L. (1932) Woolly hair, a dominant mutant character in man. *Journal of Heredity*, **23**, 345.

Norwood C.T. (1981) Whisker-hair—an update. *Cutis*, **27**, 651.

Post C.F. (1958) Woolly hair nevus. *A.M.A. Archives of Dermatology*, **78**, 488.

Salamon T. (1963) Über eine Familie mit recessiver Kraushaarigkeit, Hypotrichose und anderen Anomalien. *Hautarzt*, **13**, 540.

Schaginhaufen O. (1945) Helicotrichie in einem schweizerischen Stammbaum. *Archiv der Julius Klaus-Stiftung*, **20**, 201.

Schokking C.P. (1934) Another woolly-hair mutation in man. *Journal of Heredity*, **25**, 337.

Streitman B. (1959) Beitrag zur Kenntnis des Kräuselhaarnaevus. *Dermatologische Wochenschrift*, **139**, 185.

Sweitzer S.E. (1948) Woolly hair naevus. *Archives of Dermatology and Syphilology*, **58**, 643.

Verbov J. (1978) Woolly hair study of a family. *Dermatologica*, **157**, 42.

Wise F. (1927) Woolly hair naevus: a peculiar form of birthmark of the hair of the scalp, hitherto undescribed, with a report of two cases. *Medical Journal and Record*, **125**, 545.

Wise F. & Sulzberger M.B. (1932) Acquired progressive kinking of the scalp hair accompanied by changes in its pigmentation. *Archives of Dermatology and Syphilology*, **25**, 99.

Uncombable hair syndrome

Aetiology

This very distinctive hair-shaft defect appears to have been first described by Dupré *et al.* (1973). Since then at least a dozen cases have been reported, some of them under the name of 'spun glass hair' (Stroud & Mehregan 1974). The mode of inheritance is uncertain as although siblings were affected in two families (Grupper *et al.* 1974; Ferrandiz *et al.* 1980), in another it occurred in a father and his son (Yulzari *et al.* 1978).

Pathology

With the light microscope the hairs may appear more or less normal: very minor non-pathognomonic defects are mentioned by some authors (Grupper *et al.* 1974). Histological examination of the scalp, if the section cuts one or more follicles transversely, may show the shafts to be triangular. In the scanning electronmicroscope the triangular configuration of the shaft is clearly seen, and also a well-defined longitudinal depression (Ferrando *et al.* 1977; Dupré & Bonafé 1978) (Fig. 7.23). The terms 'pili trianguli et canaliculi' have been proposed for these defects. The pili canaliculi are present in all cases, pili trianguli in the majority and pili torti in a few (Ferrando *et al.* 1980). The defect resembles the 'straight hair naevus' of which it may be a diffuse form.

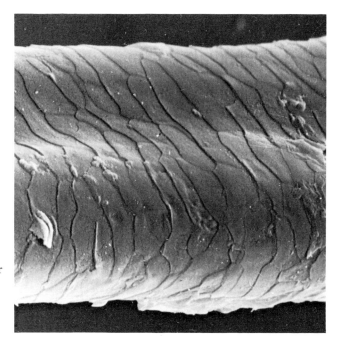

Fig. 7.23. Uncombable hair: longitudinal depression in hair shaft seen in the scanning electronmicroscope (Dr Van Neste, Dr Tennstedt and Dr J-M. Lachapelle).

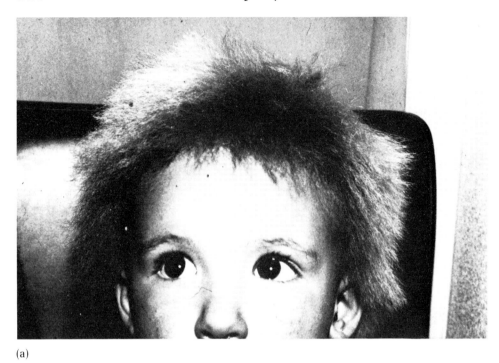

(a)

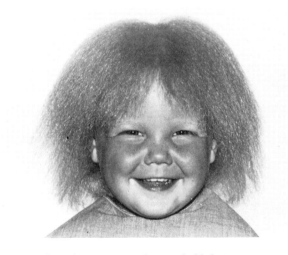

(b)

Fig. 7.24. Variations in the clinical appearance of uncombable hair:
(a) Hair brittle and short (Dr J. Ferrando);
(b) Longer unmanageable hair (Dr. G. Holti).

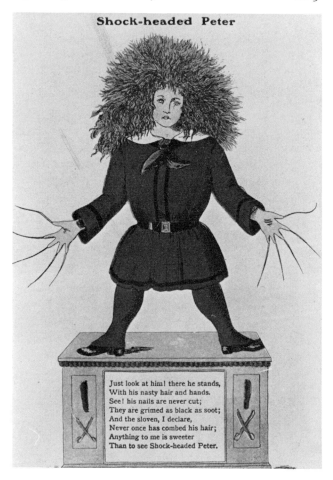

Shock-headed Peter

Just look at him! there he stands,
With his nasty hair and hands.
See! his nails are never cut;
They are grimed as black as soot;
And the sloven, I declare,
Never once has combed his hair;
Anything to me is sweeter
Than to see Shock-headed Peter.

Fig. 7.25. 'Shock-headed Peter', a character in a traditional German nursery rhyme. It seems possible that this character was originally based on a case of uncombable hair.

Clinical features (Stroud & Mehregan 1974; Dupré *et al.* 1978)

The child's parents may become aware during the early months of infancy that its hair is abnormal, but more commonly the abnormality is first noticed at the age of about 3 years. On the other hand the onset, or at least awarenes of the presence of the abnormality, may be as late as 12 years (Ferrando *et al.* 1980).

The hair is normal in quantity and sometimes also in length, but its wildly disorderly appearance totally resists all efforts to control it with brush or comb (Figs. 7.24, 7.25). In some cases these efforts lead to the hair breaking, but increased fragility is not a constant feature. The hair is often a rather distinctive silvery blond colour. The eyebrows and eyelashes are normal.

During childhood a considerable degree of spontaneous improvement may occur.

Differential diagnosis

The clinical appearance is usually distinctive. With light microscopy the diagnosis cannot be reliably established unless triangular hairs are seen. The appearances in the electronmicroscope are distinctive.

References

Dupré A., Rochiccidi P. & Bonafé J.-L. (1973) 'Cheveux incoiffables': anomalie congénitale des cheveux. *Bulletin de la Société française de Dermatologie et de Syphiligraphie,* **80,** 111.

Dupré A. & Bonafé J.-L. (1978) A new type of pilar dysplasia. The uncombable hair syndrome with pili trianguli et canaliculi. *Archives of Dermatological Research,* **261,** 217.

Dupré A., Bonafé J.-L., Litoux F. & Victor M. (1978) Le syndrome des cheveux incoiffables. Pili trianguli et canaliculi. *Annales de Dermatologie et de Vénéréologie (Paris),* **105,** 627.

Dupré A. & Bonafé J.-L. (1979) A propos du syndrome des cheveux incoiffables. *Annales de Dermatologie et de Vénéréologie (Paris),* **106,** 617.

Ferrándiz C., Peyrí J., Henkes J., Ferrando J. & Fontarnáu R. (1980) 'Pili canaliculi' familiar. *Actas Dermo-sifiliograficas,* **71,** 227.

Ferrando J., Gratacos M.R., Fontarnau R. & Castells Rodellas A. (1977) Síndrome de los cabellos 'impeinables'. *Medicina cutanea Ibero-Latino-Americana,* **5,** 39.

Ferrando J., Fontarnau R., Gratacos M.R. & Mascaro J.M. (1980) Pili canaliculi ('Cheveux incoiffables' ou 'Cheveux en fibre de verre'). Dix nouveaux cas avec étude au microscope électronique à balayage. *Annales de Dermatologie et de Vénéréologie (Paris),* **107,** 243.

Grupper C., Attal C. & Gougne B. (1974) Syndrome des cheveux incoiffables. *Bulletin de la Société française de Dermatologie et de Syphiligraphie,* **81,** 299.

Stroud J.D. & Mehregan A.H. (1974) 'Spun-glass' hair, a clinico-pathological study of an unusual hair defect. *First Human Hair Symposium,* ed. A.C. Brown. New York, Medcom Press, p. 43.

Yulzari M., Laurent R., Makki S. & Agache P. (1978) Syndromes des cheveux incoiffables. Deux nouveaux cas familiaux avec étude au microscope électronique à balayage. *Annales de Dermatologie et de Vénéréologie (Paris),* **105,** 633.

Straight hair naevus

In the straight hair naevus the hairs in a circumscribed area of a Negro scalp are straight, and are round in cross section. The abnormal hair may be associated with an epidermal naevus (Day 1967; Gibbs & Berger 1970), but in one case (Downham *et al.* 1976) hair was shed at the age of 5–6 months from a circumscribed patch of apparently normal scalp and regrew straight and was still doing so when the patient was 15. In the scanning electromicroscope the cuticular scales were small and their pattern was disorganized.

References

Day T.L. (1967) Straight-hair nevus, ichthyosis hystrix, leucokeratosis of the tongue. *Archives of Dermatology,* **96,** 606.

Downham T.F., Chapel T.A. & Lupulescu A.P. (1976) Straight-hair nevus syndrome: a case report with scanning electron microscope findings of hair morphology. *International Journal of Dermatology,* **15,** 498.

Gibbs R.L. & Berger R.A. (1970) The straight-hair nevus. *International Journal of Dermatology,* **9,** 47.

Other abnormalities of the shaft

Trichoptilosis

History and nomenclature
The term trichoptilosis was suggested by Devergie in 1872 to describe longitudinal splitting of the hair shaft. The patient will often refer to the condition as 'split ends'.

Aetiology
Trichoptilosis is the commonest macroscopic response of the hair shaft to the cumulative effects of chemical and physical trauma (Friederich & Fröb 1949). It can readily be produced experimentally by vigorous brushing of normal hair, and it occurs in the nodes of pili torti.

Pathology
The distal end of the hair shaft is split longitudinally into two or several divisions. The split commonly extends 2 or 3 cm along the shaft, but may be more prolonged. Other microscopic evidence of hair damage may be present.

Clinical features
Trichoptilosis is often an incidental finding in a woman who complains that her hair is dry and brittle. Sometimes self-examination, prompted by cosmetic advertisements, has led her to make her own diagnosis. Trichorrhexis nodosa and trichoclasis are often present in the same patient.

Treatment
Careful explanation is necessary to encourage the patient to avoid further chemical trauma, for unless she does so the condition will inevitably recur. If the split ends are unsightly they may be cut.

Reference
Friederich H.C. & Fröb G. (1949) Zur Pathogenese der Trichoptilosis. *Dermatologische Wochenschrift*, 120, 674.

Trichomalacia (references p. 222)

History and nomenclature
In 1942 Miescher of Zurich described as trichomalacia a patchy alopecia in which some follicles are plugged and contain soft, deformed, swollen hairs. Miescher & Schmuziger (1957) and Haensch & Blaich (1960) attributed the changes to the repeated trauma resulting from a hair-pulling tic, and subsequent

histological studies in trichotillomania (see p. 262) confirm this opinion. However, in one case in a mentally retarded child, Nuller & Girardet (1957) thought trauma could be excluded as a cause.

The condition described by Pinkus (1965) in a strain of mice appears not to be identical, although there are many points of histological similarity.

Pathology
Above the bulb the cells of the hair shaft appear to be disconnected and the hair is shapeless or partially disintegrated. High in the follicle the shaft is thin and may be coiled. Birefringence of affected hairs is reduced or absent (Pinkus 1965). In any affected area of scalp a proportion of hairs remain normal.

Clinical features
These are those of trichotillomania. If a non-traumatic form of trichotillomania occurs in man, it has not yet been reliably reported.

References
Haensch R. & Blaich W. (1960) Trichomalacia und Trichotillomania. *Archiv für klinische und experimentelle Dermatologie*, **210**, 447.

Miescher G. (1942) Trichomalacie. *Archiv für Dermatologie und Syphilologie*, **183**, 117.

Miescher G. & Schmuziger P. (1957) Trichomalacie und Trichotillomanie. *Dermatologica*, **114**, 199.

Nuller R. & Girardet P. (1957) Contribution à l'etiologie de la trichomalacie. *Dermatologica*, **115**, 717.

Pinkus H. (1965) Transient alopecia in weanling BD mice (trichomalacia). In *Biology of the Skin and Hair Growth*. Eds. A.G. Lyne & B.F. Shaw. Sydney, Angus & Robertson, p. 747.

Pohl–Pinkus constriction (references p. 223)

In some individuals a zone of decreased shaft diameter coincides in time with a surgical operation or an illness, or the administration of folic acid antagonists, or other drugs which inhibit mitosis; it was first described by Pohl in 1894; he later changed his name to Pinkus. The proportion of hairs so affected is variable and it seems probable that hairs in early anagen are most susceptible to a period of hypoproteinaemia or disturbed protein synthesis. This phenomenon was present in 21 of 100 patients (Sims 1967); whether the illness or operation had been associated with pyrexia was not a relevant factor. The most marked changes were seen after haemorrhage from peptic ulcers. The lower incidence of the phenomenon than in an earlier study in Berlin (Pinkus 1917) may be attributable to the generally improved nutritional status of the patients.

These constrictions in the hair shaft have been considered to be analogous to the transverse furrows in the nails (Beau's lines) which also coincide with episodes of ill-health. However, in a patient in whom regularly recurring changes were present in nails and hair shafts (Fabry 1965) the latter showed an increase in diameter, and not a constriction corresponding to each furrow in the nails.

References

Fabry H. (1965) Gleichzeitiges rhythmisches Auftreten von Querfurchen der Nägel und gruppierten Knotenbildungen der Haare. *Zeitschrift für Haut und Geschlectskrankheiten*, **39**, 336.

Pinkus F. (1971) *Die Einwirkung von Krankheiten auf das Kopfhaar des Menschen*. Berlin, Karger.

Sims R.T. (1967) Reduction of hair shaft diameter associated with illness. *British Journal of Dermatology*, **79**, 43.

Trichonodosis (references p. 224)

History and nomenclature
The first description of knotting of the hair is said (McCarthy 1940) to have been given by Duncan Bulkley of New York in 1881. Michelson (1884) proposed the term noduli laqueati, and noted that naturally curly hair was most frequently affected. Galewsky (1906) coined the term trichonodosis, which is now generally employed; his patients were a father and son, and he therefore suggested that a genetic factor might be implicated. However, Kren (1907) found the condition in 35 of 64 consecutively examined patients with skin disease.

Aetiology
The knotting of the hair shafts is induced by trauma. Short curly hair of relatively flat diameter is most readily affected (Dawber 1974). Knots were found most frequently in Negroid hair and in short, curly Caucasoid hair; none was seen in long, straight hair. In another investigation (English & Jones 1973) trichonodosis was found in 36 of 134 normal subjects; all those, male and female, with long kinky hair, over 50% of men with short kinky hair and 30% of males or females with long curly hair.

Pathology
The only abnormalities are secondary to the knotting and are localized to that part of the shaft which forms the knot (Dawber 1974). In the scanning electronmicroscope the cuticle shows longitudinal fissuring and fractures, and cuticular scales are lost (Fig. 7.26).

Clinical features (McCarthy 1940; Pratt 1947)
Trichonodosis is usually an incidental finding, for it is inconspicuous and must be deliberately sought. One or a few hairs only are affected. The trauma of brushing or combing may cause the shaft to break at the site of the knot.

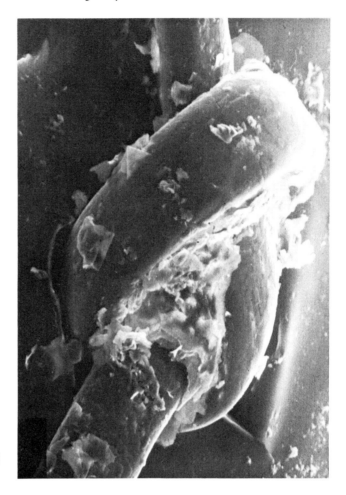

Fig. 7.26. Trichonodosis.
Knotting of scalp hair
(reduced from × 500 in the
scanning electronmicroscope)
(Slade Hospital, Oxford).

Pubic and other body hair may show knotting, as a result of rubbing and scratching in the presence of pediculosis (Scott 1951).

References
Dawber R.P.R. (1974) Knotting of scalp hair. *British Journal of Dermatology,* **91,** 169.
English D.T. & Jones H.E. (1973) Trichonodosis. *Archives of Dermatology,* **107,** 77.
Galewsky E. (1906) Uber eine noch nicht beschreibene Haarerkrankung (Trichonodosis). *Archives für Dermatologie und Syphilologie,* **81,** 195.
Kren O. (1907) Trichonodosis. *Wiener klinische Wochenschrift,* **20,** 916.
McCarthy L. (1940) *Diagnosis and Treatment of Diseases of the Hair.* London, Kimpton, p. 103.
Michelson P. (1884) Anomalien des Haarwechstums und der Haarfärbung in Handbuch der speziellen. *Pathologie und Therapie,* **14,** 89.
Pratt A.G. (1947) Trichonodosis. *Archives of Dermatology and Syphilology,* **56,** 262.
Scott M.J. (1951) Trichonodosis. Report of a case. *Archives of Dermatology and Syphilology,* **63,** 769.

Trichostasis spinulosa

History and nomenclature
Galewski in 1911 appears to have been the first to describe this condition. In 1912 Franke proposed the term pinselhaar (thysanothrix) and further cases were described the following year. Hochstetter (1913) and Nobl (1913) reported cases and the latter suggested the term trichostasis spinulosa, which most authors now favour. The condition was thought to be uncommon until Mitchell (1925) and Burgess (1932) showed that it is of frequent occurrence, but easily overlooked. When it was specifically sought 51 cases were seen in one month in Madras (Kailasam *et al.* 1979).

Aetiology
The aetiology of trichostasis spinulosa has aroused much speculation, seldom supported by investigation. A suggested failure to expel normally formed vellus hairs (Hochstetter 1913), perhaps the result of follicular hyperkeratosis, induced by exogenous chemicals (Poschacher 1925) has not been confirmed, and many authors have supported Burgess' (1932) belief that the defect is of developmental origin. Ladany (1954) thought trichostasis was no more than a variant of the comedo, and pointed out that 85% of comedones contain from one to ten or more vellus hairs. Trichostasis is now regarded as a normal age-related process with retention of telogen hairs in large sebaceous follicles (Goldschmidt *et al.* 1974).

Trichostasis is found most commonly in the middle aged or elderly, and is said by most authors to occur particularly on the nose and face (Ladany 1954). Other sites were perhaps not always examined, for others have found it to be not uncommon on the trunk and limbs, and in young as well as older adults (Starkany & Gaylarde 1971). Cases have been reported from most European countries, from North America, from India and from Japan (Ishikawa 1969).

Pathology
The affected follicles contain up to 50 vellus hairs embedded in a keratinous plug. A mild perifolliculitis is often present. The condition must be differentiated from the 'multiple hairs' of Flemming-Giovannini in which up to 7 hairs grow from a composite papilla with a common outer root sheath (Pinkus 1951).

Clinical features (Frain-Bell 1956; Ishikawa 1969).
Those reported to be affected have ranged in age from 17 to over 60. The lesions, which closely resemble comedones, may occur predominantly on the nose, forehead and cheeks, or the face may be spared and the nape, the back, shoulders, upper arms and chest may be affected. The lesions vary greatly in number. On inspection with a hand lens the 'comedones' seem to be unusually prominent and in some cases a tuft of hairs may be seen projecting through the

horny plug. They have been observed in solar elastosis of the nape of the neck (Braun-Falco and Vakilzadeh 1967).

Treatment

Keratolytic preparations have often been recommended, but we have found them to be of little value. The most effective treatment is retinoic acid (Mills & Kligman 1973) which should be used as in the treatment of acne. Depilatory wax has also been successfully employed (Sarkany & Gaylarde 1971).

References

Braun-Falco O. & Vakilzadeh F. (1967) Trichostasis spinulosa. *Hautarzt*, **18**, 501.
Burgess J.F. (1932) Trichostasis spinulosa. *Archives of Dermatology and Syphilology*, **25**, 40.
Frain-Bell W. (1956) Trichostasis spinulosa. *Transactions of St John's Hospital Dermatological Society*, **36**, 41.
Franke F. (1912) Das Pinselhaar: Thysanothrix. *Dermatologische Wochenschrift*, **55**, 1269.
Galewski K. (1911) Uber eine eigenartige Verhorungsanomalie der Follikel und deren Haare. *Archiv für Dermatologie und Syphilologie*, **106**, 215.
Goldschmidt H., Hajyo-Tomoka M.J. & Kligman A.M. (1974) Trichostasis spinulosa: a common inapparent follicular disorder of the aged. *First Human Hair Symposium*, ed. A.C. Brown. New York, Medcom Press, p. 50.
Hochstetter B. (1913) Uber eine seltene anomalie des Haarwechsels. *Dermatologische Zeitschrift*, **20**, 316
Ishikawa K. (1969) Trichostasis spinulosa. *Hautarzt*, **20**, 367.
Kailasam V., Kailasam A. & Thambiah A.S. (1979) Trichostasis spinulosa. *International Journal of Dermatology*, **18**, 297.
Ladany E. (1954) Trichostasis spinulosa. *Journal of Investigative Dermatology*, **23**, 33.
Mills O.H. & Kligman A.M. (1973) Topically applied tretinoin in the treatment of trichostasis spinulosa. *Archives of Dermatology*, **108**, 378.
Mitchell J.H. (1925) Trichostasis spinulosa or pinselhaar. *Archives of Dermatology*, **11**, 80.
Nobl G. (1913) Trichostasis spinulosa. *Archiv für Dermatologie und Syphilologie*, **114**, 611.
Pinkus H. (1951) Multiple hairs (Flemming–Giovannini). *Journal of Investigative Dermatology*, **17**, 291.
Poschacher A. (1925) Uber trichostasis spinulosa. *Acta Dermatovenereologica*, **6**, 107.
Sarkany I. & Gaylarde P.M. (1971) Trichostasis spinulosa and its management. *British Journal of Dermatology*, **84**, 311.

Pili multigemini

History and nomenclature

The term pili multigemini describes an uncommon developmental defect of hair follicles as a result of which multiple matrices and papillae form hairs which emerge through a single pilosebaceous canal. The condition was described by Flemming in 1883 and named and studied by Giovannini in a series of papers from 1907 to 1910 (Giovannini 1910). It then attracted little notice until Pinkus drew attention to it in 1951.

The incidence of multigeminate hairs in the general population is unknown.

Numerous follicles showing this defect have been seen in a patient with cleidocranial dysostosis (Mehregan & Thompson 1979).

Pathology
From two to eight matrices and papillae, each with its internal root sheath, form hairs which are often flattened, ovoid or triangular in configuration and may be grooved. In the follicular canal contiguous hairs may adhere, bifurcate and then re-adhere. This abnormality has been separately described as pili bifurcati (Weary *et al.* 1973) and may also occur as an isolated defect in otherwise normal follicles.

Clinical features
Multigeminate follicles occur mainly on the face, especially along the lines of the jaw. Tufts of hair may be seen emerging from a few or many follicles. Their discovery is often a matter of chance but the patient may complain of recurrent inflammatory nodules, leaving scars.

Treatment
Treatment is unsatisfactory. If the hairs are plucked, they regrow (Mehregan & Thompson 1979).

References
Flemming W. (1883) Ein Drillingshaar mit gemeinsamer innerer Wurzelscheide. *Monatschefte für Praktische Dermatologie*, **2**, 163.
Giovannini S. (1910) I peli con papilla composita. *Anatomischer Anzeiger*, **37**, 39.
Mehregan A.H. & Thompson W.S. (1979) Pili multigemini. Report of a case in association with cleidocranial dysostosis. *British Journal of Dermatology*, **100**, 315.
Pinkus H. (1951) Multiple hairs (Flemming–Giovannini). *Journal of Investigative Dermatology*, **17**, 291.
Weary P.E., Hendricks A.A., Wawner F. & Ajgaonkar G. (1973) Pili bifurcati. A new anomaly of hair growth. *Archives of Dermatology*, **108**, 403.

Weathering of the hair shaft (references pp. 231–2)

All hair fibres undergo some degree of cuticular and secondary cortical breakdown from root to tip before being shed during the telogen or early anagen phase of the hair cycle. The term weathering of hair has been limited by some authorities to structural changes in the hair shaft due to cosmetic procedures; indeed, both *in vivo* and *in vitro* studies carried out by cosmetic scientists have shown the type of damage that factors such as combing, brushing, bleaching and permanent waving can cause (Swift & Brown 1972; Brown & Swift 1975; Robinson 1976). However, in considering the degeneration of hair fibres, cosmetic and other influences such as natural friction, wetting and ultraviolet

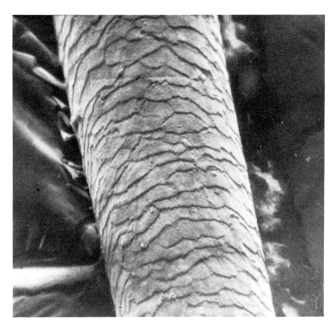

Fig. 7.27. Normal cuticle, near the scalp surface.

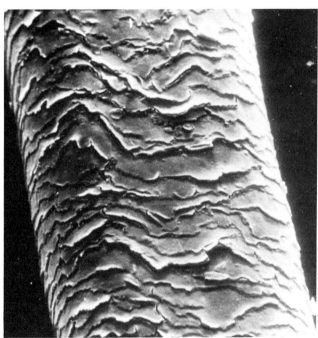

Fig. 7.28. Weathering, lifting and breaking of the free edges of cuticular cells a few centimetres from the scalp surface.

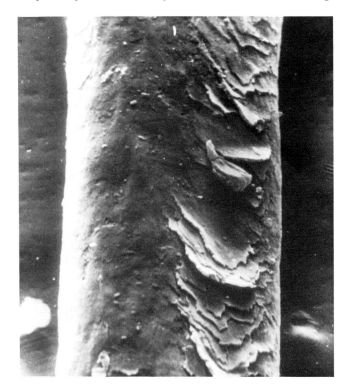

Fig. 7.29. Weathering: areas denuded of cuticle.

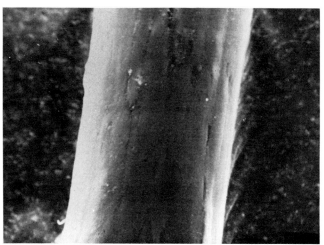

Fig. 7.30. Weathering: complete loss of cuticular scales.

radiation are so interwoven that it is more useful in practice to define weathering as the progressive degeneration of hair from root to tip due to a variety of environmental and cosmetic factors. Scalp hair, having a long anagen phase and being subject to more frictional damage and cosmetic treatment, shows more deep cuticular and cortical degeneration than fibres from other sites.

Weathering of scalp hair has been studied in greater detail than hair from other sites. The progressive changes from root to tip are shown in Figs. 7.27–7.33. At the root end surface cuticle cells are closely apposed to deeper layers (Fig. 7.27). Within a few centimetres of the scalp, the free margin of these cells lifts up and breaks irregularly (Fig. 7.28) (Garcia *et al.* 1978). Increasing scale loss leads to surface areas denuded of cuticle (Fig. 7.29). Many fibres show complete loss of overlapping scales well proximal to the tip (Fig. 7.30). This is particularly common on long hair shafts which frequently also have a frayed tip. Proximal to terminal fraying, longitudinal fissures may be present between exposed cortical cells (Figs. 7.31, 7.32). Hairs subjected to considerable friction damage may show transverse fissures and some nodes of the type seen in

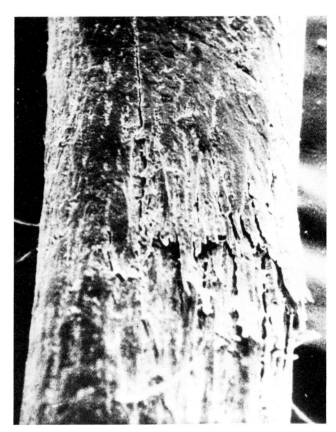

Fig. 7.31. Weathering: fissues between exposed cortical cells.

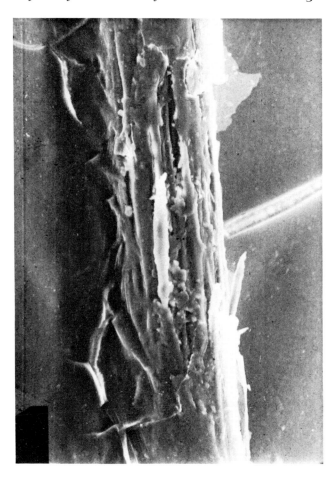

Fig. 7.32. Weathering: more advanced longitudinal fissuring.

trichorrhexis nodosa (Dawber & Comaish 1970; Chernosky 1974). Hair that has been bleached or permanently waved may show shaft distortion (Fig. 7.33); apart from the biochemical weakening of such fibres, the altered shape increases the propensity for friction damage to occur.

Trichorrhexis nodosa (p. 200) is the severest form of weathering. Many of the changes seen in normal hair towards the tip are visible more proximally in congenitally weakened hair (Rauschkolb *et al.* 1966; Pollitt *et al.* 1968; Pollitt & Stonier 1971; Lyon & Dawber 1977) and in trichorrhexis nodosa caused by over-use of cosmetic treatments.

In some hair structural abnormalities such as monilethrix and pili torti, specific weathering patterns may be seen (Dawber 1980).

References

Brown A.G. & Swift J.A. (1975) Hair breakage; the scanning electron microscope as a diagnostic tool. *Journal of the Society of Cosmetic Chemists*, **26**, 289.

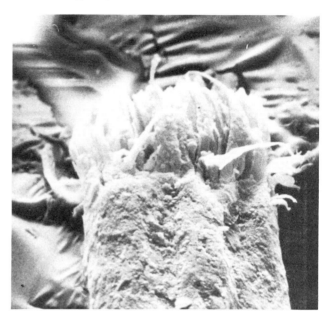

Fig. 7.33. Weathering: breakage of a severely distorted shaft.

Chernosky M.E. (1974) Acquired trichorrhexis nodosa. In *The First Human Hair Symposium*, ed. A.C. Brown. New York, Medcom Press.

Dawber R.P.R. & Comaish S. (1970) Scanning electron microscopy of normal and abnormal hair shafts. *Archives of Dermatology*, **101**, 316.

Dawber R.P.R. (1980) Weathering of hair in some genetic hair dystrophies. In *Hair, Trace Elements and Human Illness*, eds. A.C. Brown & R.G. Crounse. Praeger Scientific Publishers, New York.

Garcia M.L., Epps J.H. & Yare R.S. (1978) Normal cuticle wear patterns in human hair. *Journal of the Society of Cosmetic Chemists*, **29**, 155.

Lyon J.B. & Dawber R.P.R. (1977) A sporadic case of dystrophic pili torti. *British Journal of Dermatology*, **96**, 197.

Pollitt R.J., Jenner F.A. & Davies M. (1968) Sibs with mental and physical retardation and trichorrhexis nodosa with abnormal amino-acid composition of the hair. *Archives of Diseases of Childhood*, **42**, 211.

Rauschkolb E.W., Chernosky M.E. & Knox J.M. (1967) Trichorrhexis nodosa, an error of amino-acid metabolism. *Journal of Investigative Dermatology*, **48**, 260.

Robinson V.N.E. (1976) A study of damaged hair. *Journal of the Society of Cosmetic Chemists*, **27**, 155.

Swift J.A. & Brown A.G. (1972) The critical determination of fine changes in the surface architecture of human hair due to cosmetic treatment. *Journal of the Society of Cosmetic Chemists*, **23**, 695.

Chapter 8
Hypertrichosis

Introduction

Hypertrichosis is the growth of hair excessive for the site and for the age of the patient. Androgen-induced hirsutism is excluded by definition.

Congenital hypertrichosis lanuginosa
(References p. 234)

History and nomenclature
This extremely rare syndrome has been known for at least 400 years yet fewer than 50 cases have been reported. As Cockayne (1933) pointed out in reviewing the earlier literature, affected individuals cannot escape notice and were formerly collected by kings for the entertainment of their courtiers or exhibited by showmen for the amusement of the public, as 'dog-faced' or 'monkey-faced' freaks. The number of cases reported with adequate scientific detail is too small to allow any dogmatic assertions, and it is possible that the term congenital hypertrichosis lanuginosa covers more than one disorder; hypertrichosis universalis congenita is accept as a synonym.

Aetiology
Congenital hypertrichosis lanuginosa appears to be determined by an autosomal dominant gene, but some reported cases have been allegedly sporadic. However, the degree of variability of expression of the gene has not been investigated (Beighton 1970). Only one pedigree (Janssen & Lange 1946) suggests possible autosomal recessive inheritance. The dominant form has been reported in several different races.

The atavistic hypothesis no longer receives much support. The follicles certainly appear to retain throughout life the fetal capacity to form only lanugo,

233

but the dynamics of hair growth in these patients has not been investigated and the nature of any underlying biochemical defect is unknown.

Clinical features (Felgenhauer 1968, 1969; Beighton 1970)
The child is usually noticed to be excessively hairy at birth, particularly on the face, on which long, fine hairs join the eyebrows to the scalp hair. During infancy and early childhood the entire skin, except the palms and soles, is covered by silky hair which may be as long as 10 cm. Some affected individuals have apparently been normal at birth, and the general hypertrichosis has not developed until the 2nd–7th years. In addition to these variations in time of onset, there are marked differences between individuals in the relative hairiness of different regions of the body. It is not clear whether all these cases are the varying expressions of a single genotype. In Ray's (1966) patient, for example, the chest was not affected. In some cases (e.g. Gardner 1964; Beighton 1970) the hairiness of the trunk and limbs has diminished slightly in later childhood, but only to a very limited extent, whilst the hair on the face has remained unchanged. At puberty the pubic, axillary and beard hairs retain the characteristics of lanugo.

Some patients have had large, thick, coarse eyebrows and very long eyelashes, and these were a feature in the otherwise normal father of one patient (Beighton 1970).

Dental defects, notably a deficiency in the number of teeth, have been present in some families (Danforth 1925), but are not invariable.

The patients usually have otherwise good health, but are confronted with a formidable cosmetic problem. However, physical and mental retardation and photophobia were present in a boy, whose mother also had hypertrichosis (Freire Maia *et al.* 1976). The child had hyperdontia (retention of deciduous teeth).

The condition reported by Janssen & Lange (1946) affected three of the children of a normal mother. They were profusely hairy at birth, and died in the first few days of life. The number of hair follicles was said to be greater than normal.

Differential diagnosis
In cases in which the hypertrichosis develops in early childhood diagnosis may be difficult in the absence of a family history. To be differentiated are iatrogenic hypertrichosis (p. 254) and the rare syndrome of hypertrichosis with gingival hyperplasia.

References
Beighton P. (1970) Congenital hypertrichosis lanuginosa. *Archives of Dermatology,* 101, 669.
Cockayne A.E. (1933) *Inherited Abnormalities of the Skin and its Appendages.* Oxford, Oxford University Press, p. 245.

Danforth C.H. (1925) Studies on hair with special reference to hypertrichosis. *Archives of Dermatology and Syphilology*, **12**, 380.

Felgenhauer W.-R. (1968) *Hypertrichosis lanuginosa universalis*. M.D. thesis. University of Geneva.

Felgenhauer W.-R. (1969) Hypertrichosis lanuginosa universalis. *Journal de Génétique Humaine*, **17**, 1.

Freire Maia M., Felizali J. & Figueredo A.C. (1976) Hypertrichosis lanuginosa in a mother and son. *Clinical Genetics (Kobenhavn)*, **10**, 303.

Gardner A.L.K. (1964) A case of hypertrichosis universalis. *East African Medical Journal*, **41**, 345.

Janssen T.A.E. & Lange C. de (1946) Hypertrichosis (trichostasis) lanuginosa. *Nederlandsch Tijdschrift voor Geneeskunde*, **90**, 198.

Ray A.K. (1966) Hypertrichosis universalis with simian characteristics. *Journal of Medical Genetics*, **3**, 156.

Congenital circumscribed hypertrichosis

The growth of hair inappropriately long and coarse for the site may occur in circumscribed areas as a feature of a naevoid abnormality.

Congenital melanocytic naevi

Coarse hair often accompanies melanocytic naevi present at birth. Such naevi may be extensive and grossly disfiguring. The German term 'Tierfellnevus' (animal skin naevus) is graphically descriptive (Fig. 8.1). The naevus may be flat with a more-or-less dense covering of hair, but is often raised and is sometimes irregularly nodular. Nodule formation is not necessarily evidence of malignant change (Krinitz & Wozniak 1972) but should raise this suspicion, for malignant melanoma develops in a significant proportion of these lesions. Early excision, if necessary in stages, is advisable on both prophylactic and cosmetic grounds, if it is technically practicable.

Reference

Krinitz, K. & Wozniak K.-D. (1972) Malignes Melanom und Tierfellnevus. *Dermatologische Medizinschrift*, **158**, 130.

Becker's naevus (references p. 238)

The pigmented hairy epidermal naevus of Becker is not uncommon and has been reported in Caucasoids and Negroids (Copeman & Wilson Jones 1965). The majority of those affected are male.

Pathology. Histologically there is increased basal pigmentation of the somewhat acanthotic epidermis. The dermis is consistently thickened and contains bundles of smooth muscle (Haneke 1979). In the electronmicroscope giant melanosomes are evident and the dermal venules are surrounded by multiple layers of basement membrane (Bharvan & Chang 1979). There are increased numbers of melanin-laden melanophores in the dermis (Frenk & Delacrétaz 1970).

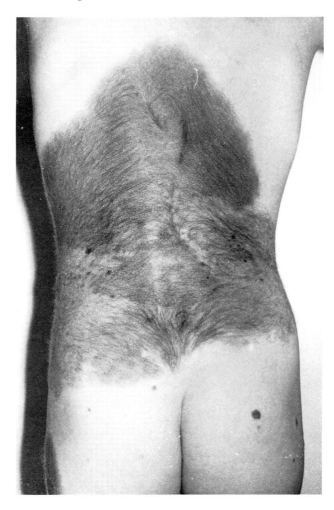

Fig. 8.1. Congenital melanocytic naevus with hypertrichosis (Addenbrooke's Hospital, Cambridge).

Clinical features (Frain-Bell & Rook 1956; Mascaro *et al.* 1970).
Becker's naevus commonly first develops between the ages of 10 and 15, but is
sometimes present in early childhood. An irregularly shaped patch of brown
pigmentation with smaller islands of pigmentation beyond its margin, slowly
extends. The main lesion coalesces with the outlying macules and new macules
appear beyond the advancing edge. Soon after puberty hypertrichosis develops,
but the pigmented and hypertrichotic areas are not precisely coextensive; some
pigmented skin is not hypertrichotic, and some coarse hairs appear in
contiguous apparently normal skin. Both pigmentation and hypertrichosis
extend irregularly for several years, but do not cross the midline. The
pigmentation is said slowly to decrease in some cases (Entwistle & Nurse 1967).
    Becker's naevus is unilateral. It occurs most commonly in the scapular

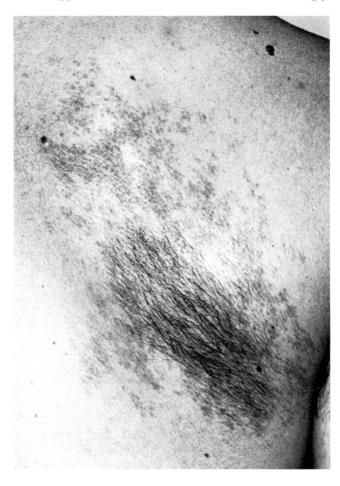

Fig. 8.2. Becker's naevus of the right scapular region (Addenbrooke's Hospital, Cambridge).

region (Fig. 8.2), extending to the shoulder and arm, but is not uncommon in the region of the pelvic girdle (Fig. 8.3). Rarely it occurs on the neck and face (Krebs 1975).

Other changes, e.g. hypoplasia of the breast (Mascaro *et al.* 1970) or morphoea (Ruffli 1972) may occur within the same extensive distribution.

Diagnosis. Hypertrichosis extending onto the face beyond the edge of the pigmented areas may cause diagnostic problems unless the characteristic pattern of the pigmentation is recognized.

Treatment. Either the hypertrichosis or the pigmentation may present the greater cosmetic problem. We have seen a good result from electrolysis in unilateral facial hypertrichosis. The pigmentation is very difficult to treat, particularly in an already highly pigmented skin in which dermabrasion gives rise to a disfiguring

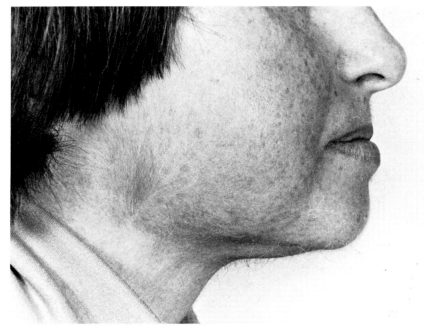

Fig. 8.3. Acquired hypertrichosis of the face associated with carcinoma of the uterus (Slade Hospital, Oxford).

mottled appearance. In a young fair-skinned Caucasoid, a small trial area was dermabraded. The patient was so satisfied with the result that he asked to have the whole naevus similarly treated. His physicians were less favourably impressed.

References

Bharvan J. & Chang W.H. (1979) Becker's melanosis: an ultrastructural study. *Dermatologica*, **159**, 221.

Copeman P.W.M. & Wilson Jones E. (1965) Pigmented hairy epidermal naevus (Becker). *Archives of Dermatology*, **92**, 249.

Entwistle B.R. & Nurse D.S. (1967) Becker's melanosis and hypertrichosis. *Australasian Journal of Dermatology*, **9**, 198.

Frain-Bell W. & Rook A. (1956) Pigmented and hypertrichotic epidermal naevus. *Transactions of the St John's Hospital Dermatological Society*, **39**, 51.

Frenk E. & Delacrétaz J. (1970) Zur Ultrastruktur der Beckerschen Melanom. *Hautarzt*, **21**, 397.

Haneke E. (1979) The dermal component in melanosis neviformis Becker. *Journal of Cutaneous Pathology*, **6**, 53.

Krebs A. (1975) Beckernevus in der Kinnregion. *Dermatologica*, **150**, 249.

Mascaro J.M., Mascaro C.G. de & Piñol Aguadé J. (1970) Historia natural del nevus de Becker. *Medicina cutanea*, **4**, 427.

Ruffli T. (1972) Melanosis Becker mit localisierter Sklerodermie. *Dermatologica*, **145**, 222.

Spinal dysraphism

Lumbosacral hypertrichosis in spinal dysraphism. Dysraphism—failure of spinal fusion—occurs four times more frequently in girls than in boys. Transfixation of the cord by a bony spicule—diastematomyelia—or tethering of cord or cauda by fibrous cords, may result in serious damage to the cord as differential growth of vertebra and cord exerts traction on the latter. The defect is usually in the sacral region but may be lumbar, thoracic or cervical. There may be no overlying cutaneous abnormality but usually there is a tuft of long soft silky hair—*a faun tail* (Fig. 8.4)—a capillary naevus, a lipoma or a dimple or sinus. In the presence

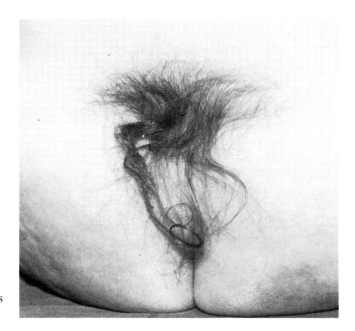

Fig. 8.4. Lumbar-sacral hypertrichosis in spinal dysraphism (Addenbrooke's Hospital, Cambridge).

of cord traction progressive neurological signs develop from early childhood: weakness of the legs, sensory loss and sphincter impairment.

In every case full neurological and radiological investigation is essential. Diastematomyelia is an indication for surgical intervention. In the absence of conclusive radiological findings prolonged observation is essential so that surgery may be undertaken at the first sign of cord damage.

References
Harris H.W. & Miller O.F. (1976) Midline cutaneous and spinal defects. *Archives of Dermatology*, 112, 1724.
James C.C.M. & Lassman L.P. (1960) Spinal dysraphism. *Archives of Disease in Childhood*, 35, 315.

Perret G. (1957) Diagnosis and treatment of diastematomyelia. *Surgery, Gynecology and Obstetrics*, 105, 69.

Thursfield W.R.R. & Ross A.A. (1961) Faun-tail (sacral hirsutism) and diastematomyelia. *British Journal of Dermatology*, 73, 328.

Naevoid hypertrichosis

Hypertrichosis of limited extent may occur as a developmental defect in the absence of any other cutaneous abnormality (Figs. 8.5, 8.6).

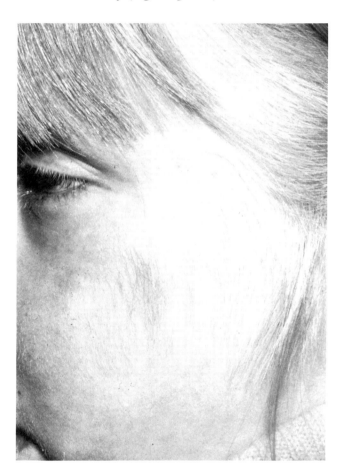

Fig. 8.5. Naevoid hypertrichosis of the cheeks without other cutaneous defect (Addenbrooke's Hospital, Cambridge).

Acquired hypertrichosis lanuginosa

History and nomenclature

The rapid growth of long, fine, downy hair over a large area of the body, replacing not only normal terminal hair but also the primary vellus of forehead and cheeks and the secondary vellus of the bald scalp, is a dramatic event. The

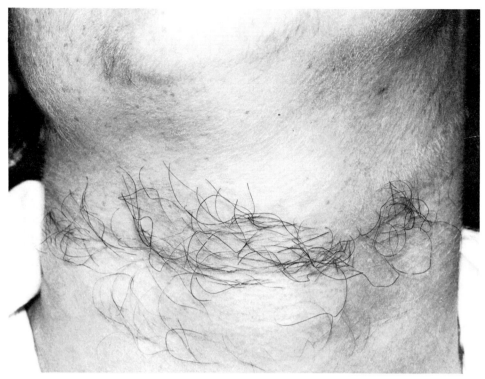

Fig. 8.6. Naevoid hypertrichosis in a linear pattern on the front of the neck in a young woman who did not have androgenetic hirsutism (Addenbrooke's Hospital, Cambridge).

illustrated account of an elderly Italian who exhibited this phenomenon after a serious illness (Le Double & Houssay 1912) is an example of the extreme and certainly very rare form. It is now becoming clear that the less conspicuous growth of lanugo, particularly on the face of patients with malignant disease is not so uncommon; Fretzin (1967) called it 'malignant down'. Since in all cases the characteristic abnormality is the replacement of hair of other types by hair with the characteristics of fetal lanugo the term acquired hypertrichosis lanuginosa is appropriate, even though in one patient (Le Marquand & Bohn 1951) the growth of hair on the previously bald scalp was apparently of terminal type.

Aetiology
In one reported case (Ormsby 1930) the patient is said to have been otherwise healthy, but no follow-up was published. The patients referred to by Morris (1894) and by Le Double & Houssay (1912) were said to have had 'influenza'.

With these inconclusive exceptions all patients with acquired hypertrichosis lanuginosa have had malignant diseases, the nature of which is shown in Table

Table 8.1. Acquired hypertrichosis lanuginosa.

F.42	Carcinoma of breast	Turner 1865
M.61	Carcinoma of bronchus	Le Marquand & Bohn 1951; Goodfellow *et al.* 1980
F.35	Carcinoma of bladder with metastasis	Lyell & Whittle 1951
F.56	Carcinoma of ovary	Dingley & Martin 1957
M.69	Carcinoma of bronchus	Fretzin 1967
M.44	Carcinoma of bronchus with metastasis	Hensley & Glynn 1969
M.65	Carcinoma of gall-bladder with metastasis	Herzberg *et al.* 1968, 1969
F.39	Carcinoma of rectum	Djajadiningrat *et al.* 1970
F.79	Carcinoma of rectum	Chadfield & Khan 1970
F.45	Carcinoma of colon	Hegedus & Schorr 1972
F.56	Carcinoma of colon	Hegedus & Schorr 1972
F.43	Carcinoma of rectum	Van der Lugt & Dudok de Wit 1973
F.73	Carcinoma of colon	Van de Lugt & Dudok de Wit 1973
F.66	Carcinoma of uterus	Samson *et al.* 1974
F.35	Lymphoma	Samson *et al.* 1974
F.54	Carcinoma of breast	Wadskof *et al.* 1976
F.46	Carcinoma of uterus	Kaiser *et al.* 1976
F.19	Carcinoma of pancreas	McLean & McCaulay 1977
F.60	Carcinoma of colon	Reinold *et al.* 1977
M.67	Carcinoma of bronchus	Ikeya *et al.* 1978
F.59	Carcinoid	Davis *et al.* 1978

8.1. The ages of the patients ranged from 19 to 79, and females have outnumbered males in a ratio of about 3:1. Endocrine investigations, carried out in some cases, have shown no consistent or apparently relevant abnormalities. Ludwig (1971) in reviewing these cases referred to the Cushing syndrome, which may occur in oat-cell carcinoma of the bronchus, but which has been conspicuously absent in these cases.

Pathology
The abnormal hair is fine, poorly pigmented, or unpigmented, long and straight. In one case papillomatosis of the skin of the trunk, with histological features somewhat similar to acanthosis nigricans (Hensley & Glynn 1969). Histological studies in another case (Hegedus & Schorr 1972) showed the lanugo follicles lying almost parallel to the surface, and apparently derived from 'mantle' hair follicles.

Clinical features
All accounts emphasize the rapidity with which the hypertrichosis develops. Dense fine white or red-black hairs replace the normal vellus hairs. The hairs are finest on the face, where they grow on forehead, eyelids, nose and ears, giving the

patient a simian appearance. Terminal hair on the scalp, beard and pubes tends not to be replaced, but lanugo up to 15 cm long may densely cover all other surfaces except the penis and the palms and soles. Long-bald scalp may show an equally dense growth, its lighter colour and firm texture contrasting with the remaining darker and coarser terminal hair. In one case the rate of growth of the lanugo on trunk and limbs was found to be about 2.5 cm per week (Le Marquand & Bohn 1951).

The extent and degree of the lanuginous transformation varies considerably. In early cases the growth of down on the forehead and temples may be the only abnormality.

The lanugo may develop a few weeks or up to 2 years before a carcinoma is diagnosed.

In one patient (Hegedus & Schorr 1972) prominent, discrete red papules were present on the distal two-thirds of the tongue: it is not yet known whether this association is significant.

The association with hypertrichosis of acquired ichthyosis, another cutaneous manifestation of systemic neoplasia, was reported in a woman with lymphatic leukaemia (Ricken 1979).

Differential diagnosis
Congenital hypertrichosis lanuginosa is excluded by the age of onset. Otherwise the condition is partially simulated only by certain drugs (p. 254).

Treatment
The diagnosis is an indication for a most intensive search for a neoplasm. There appears, however, to be no record of the successful treatment of an associated carcinoma.

References
Chadfield H.W. & Khan A.V. (1970) Acquired hypertrichosis lanuginosa. *Transactions of the St John's Hospital Dermatological Society*, **56**, 30.
Davis R.A., Newman D.M., Phillips M.J., Laidlaw J.C. & Zinman B. (1978) Acquired hypertrichosis lanuginosa as a sign of internal malignant disease. *Canadian Medical Association Journal*, **118**, 1090.
Dingley E. & Marten R.H. (1957) Adenocarcinoma of the ovary presenting as acanthosis nigrans. *Journal of Obstetrics and Gynaecology of the British Commonwealth*, **64**, 898.
Djajadiningrat A.P., Gilse H.A. van, Siddre W.J. & Lugt L. van der (1970) Acquired lanuginous hypertrichosis. *Dermatologica*, **140**, 327.
Fretzin D.F. (1967) Malignant down. *Archives of Dermatology*, **95**, 294.
Goodfellow A., Calvert H. & Bohn G. (1980) Hypertrichosis lanuginosa acquisita. *British Journal of Dermatology*, **103**, 431.
Hegedus S.I. & Schorr W.F. (1972) Acquired hypertrichosis langinosa and malignancy. *Archives of Dermatology*, **106**, 84.

Hensley G.T. & Glynn K.P. (1969) Hypertrichosis lanuginosa as a sign of internal malignancy. *Cancer*, **24**, 1051.

Herzberg J.J., Potjan K. & Gebauer D. (1968) Hypertrichosis lanuginosa (et terminalis) acquisita als paraneoplastisches Syndrom. *Archiv für klinische und experimentelle Dermatologie*, **232**, 176.

Herzberg J.J., Potjan K. & Gebauer D. (1968) Hypertrichosis lanuginosa acquise. *Annales de Dertmatologie et de Syphiligraphie*, **96**, 129.

Ikeya T., Izumi A. & Suzuki M. (1978) Acquired hypertrichosis lanuginosa. *Dermatologica*, **156**, 274.

Kaiser I.H., Perry G. & Yoonasse M. (1976) Acquired hypertrichosis lanuginosa associated with endometrial malignancy. *Obstetrics and Gynaecology*, **47**, 479.

Le Double A.-F. & Houssay F. (1912) *Les Vélus*. Paris, Vigot, p. 28.

Le Marquand H.S. & Bohn G.L. (1951) Recurrent peptic ulcer with general hypertrichosis including growth of hair on the bald scalp and later development of signs suggesting adrenal failure. *Proceedings of the Royal Society of Medicine*, **44**, 155.

Ludwig E. (1971) *Paraneoplastische Veränderungen am Haarklied und Cutane paraneoplastische Syndrom*, ed. J.J. Herzberg. Stuttgart, Fischer, p. 31.

Lugt, H. van der & Dudok de Wit, C. (1973) Hypertrichosis lanuginosa acquisita. *Dermatologica*, **146**, 46.

Lyell A. & Whittle C.H. (1951) Hypertrichosis lanuginosa. Acquired type. *Proceedings of the Royal Society of Medicine*, **44**, 576.

McLean D.I. & McCaulay J.C. (1977) Hypertrichosis lanuginosa acquisita associated with pancreatic carcinoma. *British Journal of Dermatology*, **96**, 313.

Morris M. (1894) *Medico-Chirurgical Transactions*, **77**, 305.

Ormsby O. (1930) Acute hypertrichosis. *Archives of Dermatology and Syphilology*, **21**, 663.

Reinold H.-M., Schlüter E. & Schlaak M. (1977) Hypertrichosis lanuginosa acquisita bei Kolonkarzinoma. *Innere Medizian*, **4**, 281.

Ricken K.H. (1979) Hypertrichosis lanuginosa et terminalis acquisita und pseudoichthyosis als paraneoplastische Syndrom bei chronisch lymphatische leukämie. *Zeitschrift für Hautkrankheiten*, **54**, 819.

Samson M.K., Buroker T.R., Henderson M.D., Baker M.H. and Vaitkevicius V.K. (1974) Acquired hypertrichosis lanuginosa. *Cancer*, **36**, 1519.

Turner M. (1865) Case of a woman whose face and body in two or three weeks' time became covered with a thick crop of short and white downy hair. *Medical Times and Gazette*, **2**, 507.

Wadskov S., Bro-Jorgensen A. & Sondergaard J. (1976) Acquired hypertrichosis lanuginosa. *Archives of Dermatology*, **112**, 1442.

Symptomatic hypertrichosis

Hypertrichosis occurs as a manifestation of, or as a sequel of, a wide variety of pathological states. In many the hair growth is an incidental and perhaps a transitory feature, but in others it is conspicuous and persistent, of diagnostic value and of therapeutic importance.

Unfortunately the precise mechanism by which hypertrichosis is induced is known in only a few instances. The clinical details of the type and pattern of hypertrichosis are quite inadequate in many case reports.

Head injuries and other cerebral disturbances

The development of hypertrichosis some 1–4 months after a head injury is a well-recognized phenomenon, especially in children, but occasionally reported in adults. The head injury has usually been severe but the precise localization of the lesion responsible for the hair growth has usually not been ascertained, although in one case compression injury of the midbrain leading to adrenal overactivity was suspected (Epstein 1947).

A typical case (Bartuska 1963) was a Negro boy aged 7. Six weeks after a severe head injury he developed long silky hair on the forehead, cheeks, trunk and limbs, but no pubic or axillary hair. However, in some cases a generalized hypertrichosis, more or less extensive than in this case, has been accompanied by hirsutism. A young German woman aged 17 in the 3rd month after a severe head injury, showed a strong growth of fine hair on her face, shoulders, chest and abdomen. Her eyebrows merged and vibrissae projected from her nostrils. The pattern of her pubic hair changed from horizontal to accuminate. Four months later she had regained her previous hair pattern at all sites (Tarnow 1957, 1971). A comparable case (Tarnow 1971) was a German boy aged 7 who developed a dense growth of fine hair on his limbs during the 4th month after a head injury, and also some pubic hair. All the excess hair had been lost 15 months later. A girl aged 14 (Robinson 1955) developed generalized hypertrichosis 3 months after receiving multiple injuries in a motor accident; the excess hair, which was mainly on the extensor aspects of the limbs, was lost within 6 months. These and other similar case reports make it clear that a head injury, and perhaps severe shock without physical injury, can induce either hypertrichosis or hirsutism or both. Spontaneous recovery is the rule.

Rarely cerebral damage of infective origin can cause hypertrichosis; it followed encephalitis in a child aged $2\frac{1}{2}$ (Stegagno & Vignetti 1955).

The rare hereditary globoid leucodystrophy, also known as Krabbe's disease, is usually fatal before the age of 2. Hypertrichosis has been present in some cases (Tavri *et al.* 1970).

References

Bartuska D.G. (1963) Hypertrichosis in a brain-damaged child. *Journal of the American Medical Women's Association*, **18**, 711.

Epstein E. (1947) Posttraumatisch zentragener Hirsutismus nach Commotio cerebri. *Wiener klinische Wochenschrift*, **47**, 520.

Robinson R.L.V. (1955) Temporary acquired hypertrichosis following traumatic shock. *A.M.A. Archives of Dermatology*, **71**, 401.

Stegagno G. & Vignetti P. (1955) Considerazioni su di un caso di ipertricosi con cerebropatia in una bambina di 2 e $\frac{1}{2}$ anni. *Archivio Italiano di pediatria e puericoltura*, **17**, 421.

Tarnow G. (1957) Vorübergehender Hirsutismus nach Contusio cerebri. *Nervenarzt*, **28**, 327.

Tarnow G. (1971) Haarkleidstörungen nach schweren Hirntraumen 1971. *Journal of Neuro-Visceral Relations* (Suppl.), **10**, 549.

Tavri G.M., Shalini K.C.M., Martin K.B., Bhaktavizian A. & Backharvat B.K. (1970) Globoid leucodystrophy (Krabbe's disease). *Indian Journal of Medical Research*, **58**, 993.

Lipoatrophic diabetes (syn. Berardinelli syndrome; Lawrence–Seip syndrome)
Loss of subcutaneous fat may be evident at birth. Growth is rapid until puberty.
The sunken cheeks, broad nasal root and large ears produce a distinctive facies.
Liver and spleen may be large. There may be some degree of mental retardation.
The penis or clitoris is enlarged and polycystic ovaries are common.

Hypertrichosis of face, neck, arms and legs increases from birth onwards. The
head hair is abundant and curly. Acanthosis nigricans of the axillae, wrists and
ankles is common.

Insulin-resistant diabetes begins in childhood or adolescence. There may at
first be no glycosuria. Hyperlipaemia is constant.

References

Berardinelli W. (1954) An undiagnosed endocrine-metabolic syndrome. *Journal of Endocrinology*,
    14, 193.
Janaki V.P., Premalantha S., Raghuvarta Rao N. & Thambiah A.S. (1980) Lawrence–Seip
    syndrome. *British Journal of Dermatology*, 103, 693.

Cornelia de Lange syndrome
Hypertrichosis is a constant and distinctive feature of this not excessively rare
syndrome. The cause of the syndrome is not known. Chromosomal abnormalities have been exceptional and of no consistent type (Falck *et al.* 1966). Most
cases are sporadic, but siblings have been affected, and some features of the
syndrome have been identified in other relatives (Daniel & Higgins 1971; Beck
1974).

The birth weight is low and physical and mental development are retarded.
There is abundant head hair with low frontal and nuchal margins. The bushy
eyebrows are confluent. There is also generalized hypertrichosis with fine hair on
forehead, back, shoulders and limbs. The hair on the lower back may be quite
long. The eyelashes are long and curved and the palpebral fissure has an
antimongolian slant. Marbling of the skin is conspicuous and often persistent.
One or more fingers may be short. The nose is upturned, but downturned labial
commissures result in a 'carp' mouth.

To these features, which are more or less constant, are added a wide and
variable range of other defects mainly ocular (Milot & Demay 1972) and skeletal,
but also involving other systems (Noé & Hammond 1967; Soderquist & Reed
1968; Pashayan *et al.* 1969; Jaqueti *et al.* 1973).

References

Beck B. (1974) Familial occurrence of Cornelia de Lange's syndrome. *Acta paediatrica scandinavica*,
    63, 225.
Daniel W.L. & Higgins J.V. (1971) Biochemical and genetic investigation of the de Lange
    syndrome. *American Journal of Diseases of Children*, 121, 401.
Falck A., Schmidt R. & Jervis G.A. (1966) Familial de Lange syndrome with chromosome
    abnormalities. *Pediatrics*, 37, 92.

Jaqueti G., Ledo A., Gay C., Gallego J.R., Gonzalez P. & Corripio F. (1973) Syndrome de Cornelia Lange. *Hospital General,* 13, 359.
Milot J. & Demay F. (1972) Ocular anomalies in De Lange syndrome. *American Journal of Ophthalmology,* 74, 394.
Noé O. & Hammond J. (1967) De Lange's Amsterdam dwarfism: case report and etiological considerations. *American Journal of Mental Deficiency,* 71, 991.
Pashayan H., Whelan D., Guttman S. & Fraser F.C. (1969) Variability of the de Lange syndrome: report of 3 cases and genetic analysis of 54 families. *Journal of Pediatrics,* 75, 853.
Soderquist N.A. & Reed W.B. (1968) Cornelia de Lange syndrome. *Cutis,* 4, 1335.

Rubinstein–Taybi syndrome

The main features of this complex syndrome, which is probably hereditary, but not proved to be so, are short stature, mental retardation, broad thumbs and big toes, a high arched palate and a beaked nose.

Some 50% of patients have hypertrichosis, especially of the back, and about the same proportion have a capillary naevus of the nape or of the forehead (Bartok *et al.* 1968; Filipi 1973).

References

Bartok W.R., Reed W.B. & Fish C. (1968) Rubinstein–Taybi syndrome. *Cutis,* 4, 1350.
Filipi G. (1973) The Rubinstein–Taybi syndrome. Report of 7 cases. *Clinical Genetics,* 3, 303.

Craniofacial dysostosis and patent ductus arteriosis

This syndrome was reported in two sisters (Gorlin *et al.* 1960). Craniofacial dysostosis is associated with patent ductus arteriosus, hypoplasia of the labia majora and mutiple defects of eyes and teeth. There was severe hypertrichosis, particularly of the arms and legs and on the back.

Reference

Gorlin R.J., Chanothry A.P. & Moss M.I. (1960) Craniofacial dysostosis, patent ductus arteriosus, hypertrichosis, hypoplasis of labia majora, dental and eye anomalies—a new syndrome? *Journal of Paediatrics,* 56, 778.

Gingival hyperplasia with hypertrichosis

This rather variable syndrome was first reported by Tomes & Coles in 1855 (Gorlin & Pindborg 1964). The essential abnormalities, gingival hyperplasia and hypertrichosis, are both present at birth. The gingival hyperplasia increases, but the hypertrichosis, although it remains severe, becomes relatively less conspicuous in adult life. In several patients acromegaloid features have been reported (Vontobel 1973).

Electronmicroscopic studies of the dermis show changes which suggest that there may be increased production of collagen fibrils (Vontobel 1973).

The changes induced by diphenylhydantoin may be regarded as a phenocopy of this syndrome, and must be considered in differential diagnosis, but it is characteristic of this syndrome that the hypertrichosis and gingival hyperplasia are already present at birth (Witkop 1971).

In the Zimmermann–Laband syndrome, gingival hyperplasia is combined with acromegaloid features but there is no hypertrichosis (Laband *et al.* 1961).

References

Gorlin R.J. & Pindborg J.J. (1964) *Syndromes of the Head and Neck.* New York, McGraw-Hill, p. 314.

Laband P.F., Habib O. & Humphrey G.S. (1961) Hereditary gingival fibromatosis. Report of an affected family with associated sphenomegaly and skeletal and soft tissue abnormalities. *Oral Surgery,* **17**, 339.

Vontobel F. (1973) Idiopathic gingival hyperplasia and hypertrichosis associated with acromegaloid features. *Helvetica Paediatria Acta,* **28**, 401.

Witkop C.J. (1971) Heterogeneity in gingival fibromatosis. *Birth Defects: Original Article Series,* **7**, 210.

Gingival fibromatosis and hypertrichosis

Aetiology. The inheritance of this syndrome is determined by an autosomal dominant gene.

Clinical features. During the first 2 years hypertrichosis develops. Head hair is abundant and the eyebrows are long and bushy. Hypertrichosis, often with black hair even in blonde families, affects the face and trunk.

Gingival fibromatosis also becomes evident during early childhood. About 50% of patients are mentally retarded or epileptic or both.

The condition must be differentiated from the Cowden syndrome.

Reference

Byars L.T. & Sarnat B.G. (1944) Congenital macrogingivae (fibromatosis gingivae) and hypertrichosis. *Surgery,* **15**, 964.

Mucopolysaccharidoses

At least seven distinct genetically determined disorders of mucopolysaccharide metabolism are now recognized (Rampini 1969). The syndromes show some features in common but differ in many ways both clinically and biochemically.

Hurler's syndrome (Hambrick & Scheie 1962), the most severely disabling, combines dwarfism, chondrodystrophy, mental retardation, a 'gargoyle' facies, corneal opacities and hypertrichosis. The hypertrichosis may be conspicuous with a low frontal hair line and bushy eyebrows and a vigorous growth of fine hair on the face and limbs. Inheritance is determined by an autosomal recessive gene.

Hypertrichosis is not a regular feature of the other mucopolysaccharidoses (Rampini 1969; Greaves & Inman 1969).

References

Greaves M.W. & Inman P.M. (1969) Cutaneous changes in the Morquio syndrome. *British Journal of Dermatology*, **81**, 29.

Hambrick G.W. & Scheie H.G. (1962) Studies of the skin in Hurler's syndrome. *Archives of Dermatology*, **85**, 455.

Rampini S. (1969) Der spät-Hurler. *Schweiz medizinische Wochenschrift*, **99**, 1769.

Winchester syndrome

This rare hereditary disease is probably the consequence of an abnormality of fibroblast function. Skeletal deformities are severe; dwarfism, carpal–tarsal osteolysis and destruction of small joints result in gross disability. Other features include corneal opacity and extensive areas of thickened, pigmented and hypertrichotic skin (Cohen *et al.* 1975).

Reference

Cohen A.H., Hollister D.W. & Reed W.B. (1975) The skin in the Winchester syndrome. *Archives of Dermatology*, **111**, 230.

Schinzel–Giedion syndrome

This recently recognized syndrome of multiple congenital anomalies is associated with hypertrichosis. The nasal bridge is depressed and the midface is hyperplastic and the forehead is high and protruding. There are skeletal abnormalities in the skull, ribs, hands and feet.

References

Donnai D. & Harris R. (1979) A further case of a new syndrome including midface retraction, hypertrichosis and skeletal anomalies. *Journal of Medical Genetics*, **16**, 483.

Schinzel A. & Giedion A. (1978) A syndrome of severe midface retraction, multiple skull anomalies, club feet and cardiac and renal malformations in sibs. *American Journal of Medical Genetics*, **1**, 361.

Epidermolysis bullosa

This term describes a group of genetically distinct hereditary diseases all characterized by bulla formation, with trauma, or spontaneously. Hypertrichosis has been reported as a most uncommon feature of the dystrophic form of the disease (Cofano 1955).

Reference

Cofao A.R. (1955) Su un caso di epidermolisi bollosa distrofica con accentuada ipertricosi. *Annali italiani di Dermatologia*, **10**, 195.

Leprechaunism

Aetiology. This rare syndrome is probably determined by an autosomal recessive gene.

Clinical features. Hypertrichosis, which may be extensive, has been a feature of the majority of cases of leprechaunism. Deficient subcutaneous tissue leads to a characteristic folding of redundant skin. The facies is described as elfin, with thick lips. There is motor and intellectual retardation and early death is usual.

The porphyrias

Hypertrichosis is a feature, sometimes a conspicuous one, in several of the forms of porphyria. Many of the porphyrias are genetically determined, and it is not yet clear to what extent genetic factors are important in those forms which are provoked by exogenous agents.

Erythropoietic porphyria, inherited as a recessive trait, is very rare. It is sometimes referred to as Gunther's disease, or simply as congenital porphyria. Exposure to sunlight induces bulla formation. Hypertrichosis of face and limbs is usually present (Caruso & Previti 1959; Dean 1963). It is occasionally extensive, particularly on the face (Handa 1965).

Erythropoietic protoporphyria, which is not rare, is also hereditary, inheritance being determined by an autosomal dominant gene. The most common symptom is burning of the skin after exposure to sunlight; erythema and oedema soon develop. In children, purpura, vesicles and scars may develop (Rimington *et al.* 1967). The exposed skin gradually becomes thickened and scarred, and in some children markedly hypertrichotic (Bhutani *et al.* 1972; Bhutani & Deshpande 1973).

Porphyria cutanea tarda is commonly seen in alcoholic adults; abnormal hair growth is not a conspicuous feature in Caucasoids, but may be conspicuous in Negroes in whom blistering is unusual (Zeligman 1963). In children, there is often evidence of inheritance of this hepatic defect; haemorrhagic bullae on light-exposed skin may develop during the first year (Barnes *et al.* 1957), and hypertrichosis of face and limbs may be conspicuous (Piñol Aguadé *et al.* 1973). In the form of hepatic porphyria induced by exposure to chemicals such as hexachlorobenzene, hypertrichosis may be very gross. Many of those affected in the Turkish epidemic of 1954–5 were known as 'monkey children' (Dean 1963).

Porphyria variegata, also known as mixed porphyria, is more common in South Africa and Sweden than elsewhere. Its inheritance is determined by an autosomal dominant gene of variable expressivity. Pigmentation and hypertrichosis occur on exposed skin.

The association, particularly in a child, of hypertrichosis with light sensitivity, should suggest the need for a full investigation of the patient's porphyric metabolism and a careful study of the family histories (see Dean 1963; Rimington *et al.* 1967) (Fig. 8.7).

References
Barnes H.D., Frootko J. & Parnell J.L. (1957) Unusually early manifestations of porphyria cutanea tarda. *South African Medical Journal*, 31, 342.

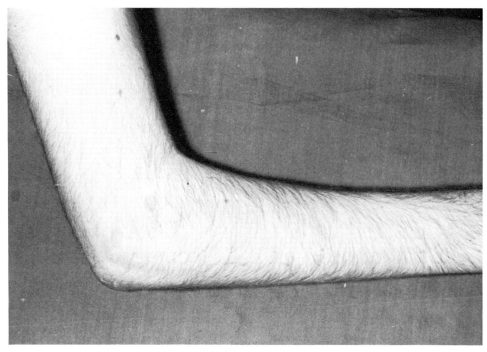

Fig. 8.7. Hypertrichosis in porphyria (Slade Hospital, Oxford).

Bhutani L.K., Deshpande S.G. & Sood S.K. (1972) Erythropoietic protoporphyria: first report in an Indian. *British Medical Journal*, **ii**, 741.

Bhutani L.K. & Deshpande S.G. (1973) Erythropoietic protoporphyria. *Dermatologica*, **147**, 263.

Caruso P. & Previti A. (1960) Contributo allo studio del la porfiria eritropoietica: dúe casi con anemia emolitica, splenomegalia. ipofunzionlita surrenalica. *Minerva pediatrica*, **12**, 250.

Dean G. (1963) *The Porphyrias*. London, Pitman.

Handa F. (1965) Congenital Porphyria. *Archives of Dermatology*, **91**, 130.

Piñol Aguadé J., Lecha M., Almeida J., Herrero C. & Gaby de Mascaro C. (1973) Porfiria cutánea tarda en niños. *Medicina cutanea*, **7**, 37.

Rimington C., Magnus I.A., Ryan E.A. & Cripps D.J. (1967) Porphyria and photosensitivity. *Quarterly Journal of Medicine*, **36**, 29.

Zeligman I. (1963) Patterns of porphyria in the American Negro. *Archives of Dermatology*, **88**, 616.

Anorexia nervosa

The patient is usually a young woman who quite suddenly restricts her diet, excluding carbohydrates in particular. Severe emaciation may result. In some patients downy hypertrichosis of the trunk and arms is a striking feature; it was present in 12 of 33 women aged 15–29 (Ryle 1936). More recent studies record a much lower incidence of hypertrichosis (Bartels 1946) or fail to mention this symptom (Williams 1958). In our experience hypertrichosis is unusual in these cases, but we agree with Ryle (1936) that some cases of long duration develop 'coarse hairs on the chin'; in fact hirsutism of mild or moderate degree may occur. Since amenorrhoea is usual, the differential diagnosis from hypopituitarism is important. The normal or even excessive pubic hair is not seen in the latter, nor is hypertrichosis.

References
Bartels E.D. (1946) Studies on hypometabolism. I. Anorexia nervosa. *Acta medica scandinavica*, **124**, 185.
Ryle J.A. (1936) Anorexia nervosa. *Lancet*, **ii**, 893.
Williams E. (1958) Anorexia nervosa: A somatic disorder. *British Medical Journal*, **ii**, 190.

Malnutrition
Changes in hair growth resulting from malnutrition are discussed on pp. 127–130. Hypertrichosis of the limbs and trunk has been observed in previously well-fed children receiving a grossly deficient diet (Castellani 1938). It has been recorded also in coeliac disease (Holzel 1951).

References
Castellani A. (1938) Note on some little known conditions of the lanugo hair. *Journal of Tropical Medicine and Hygiene*, **41**, 400.
Holzel A. (1951) Hypertrichosis in childhood. *Acta paediatrica scandinavica*, **40**, 59.

Dermatomyositis
Hypertrichosis, sometimes of marked degree may occur in dermatomyositis particularly in childhood (Fig. 8.8). The excessive hair is lost soon after recovery from the disease.

Pretibial myxoedema
Localized plaques of myxoedema of the lower legs occur in about 4% of patients with hyperthyroidism (Gimllett 1960) and in about 40% of those with malignant exophthalmos. Most have elevated levels of long-acting thyroid stimulator. In some cases lesions first appear only after the start of anti-thyroid treatment.

Flesh-coloured nodules appear on the shins; sometimes the firm non-pitting oedema of the shins and ankles is more diffuse. Hypertrichosis over the lesions is frequent. Clubbing and other features of thyroid acropachy may be associated.

Reference
Gimllett T.N.D. (1960) Pretibial myxoedema. *British Medical Journal*, **2**, 398.

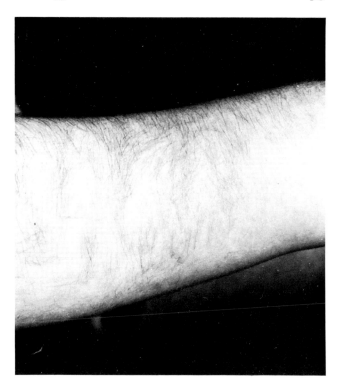

Fig. 8.8. Hypertrichosis in dermatomyositis. The hair was shed within a year (Dr K. Crow, Swindon).

Hypertrichosis in teratogenic syndromes

Fetal alcohol syndrome

The fetal alcohol syndrome is not uncommon. The infants of about 40% chronically alcoholic women are affected (Jones & Smith 1975).

Such infants are small and microcephalic with mental and physical retardation and defects of the heart and of the joints. The facies is unusual and may be distinctive with short palpebral fissures, a prominent nose and maxillary hypoplasia. Numerous other defects may include hypertrichosis, which may be very conspicuous, and capillary haemangiomatosis (Hanson *et al.*).

References

Hanson J.W., Jones K.L. & Smith D.W. (1976) Fetal alcohol syndrome: experience with 41 patients. *Journal of the American Medical Association*, **235**, 1458.
Jones K.L. & Smith D.W. (1975) The fetal alcohol syndrome. *Teratology*, **12**, 1.

Fetal hydantoin syndrome

Diphenyl hydantoin is teratogenic. There is psychomotor retardation. The broad nasal bridge is depressed and the nose is retroussé. There is ocular hypertelorism with ptosis and strabismus. The mouth is wide with prominent lips and the neck is short and may be webbed. A variety of other defects may occur. The posterior hair line is often low. Hypertrichosis is common and may be marked (Hanson & Smith 1975).

Reference
Hanson J.W. & Smith D.W. (1975) The fetal hydantoin syndrome. *Journal of Paediatrics*, **87**, 285.

Iatrogenic hypertrichosis

Nomenclature
A clear distinction should be drawn between iatrogenic hirsutism, in which hair growth is increased in part or all of the male sexual pattern, and iatrogenic hypertrichosis, in which the growth of fine hair is increased over extensive areas of the trunk, hands or face.

Aetiology
The mode of action of the offending drugs on the hair follicles is not known; the same mechanism is certainly not involved in all cases. Cortisone, diphenylhydantoin and penicillamine are all known to affect collagen, but in different ways. Psoralens presumably induce hypertrichosis in predisposed subjects by accentuating the tendency of sunlight to induce this temporary change.

Clinical features
Existing vellus hairs increase in length and less so in diameter. The hairs are seldom more than 3 cm in length and are considerably finer than terminal hair. The increased growth is seldom noticed until the drug responsible has been taken for several weeks, and often for considerably longer. The hair growth is often first noticed on the back and the extensor aspects of the limbs, but later involves the rest of the trunk and the face. The hair usually reverts to the normal for the sex, age and site, within a year after the drug is discontinued.

It is not clear whether possible differences in the pattern of hypertrichosis are significantly related to any particular drug, since racial and other genetic factors must be taken into account.

Diphenylhydantoin induces hypertrichosis after 2–3 months, more in girls than in boys. It affects the extensor aspects of the limbs, then the face and trunk (Livingstone *et al.* 1955; Hamblen 1963).

Diazoxide causes hypertrichosis in about 50% of children, but rarely in adults (Koblenzer & Baker 1968, 1969; Burton *et al.* 1975) (Figs. 8.9, 8.10).

Minoxidil, a piperidino-pyrimidine derivative used in the treatment of hypertension, quite commonly induces hypertrichosis (Burton & Marshall 1979) (Fig. 8.11), which may disappear although treatment is continued (Ryckmanns 1980).

Streptomycin caused hypertrichosis in 22 of 27 children who had received 1 g

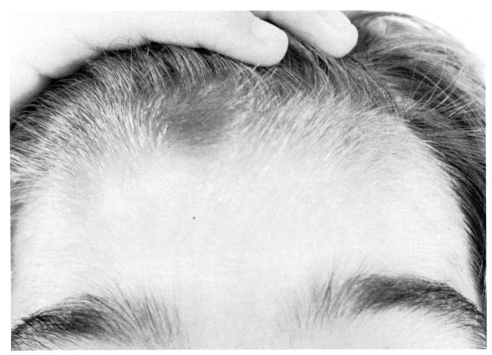

Fig. 8.9. Hypertrichosis caused by diazoxide (Dr J.L. Burton).

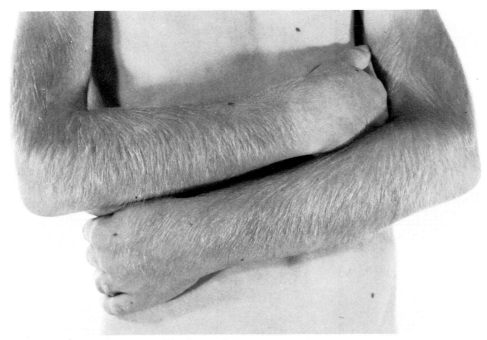

Fig. 8.10. Hypertrichosis caused by diazoxide (Dr J.L. Burton).

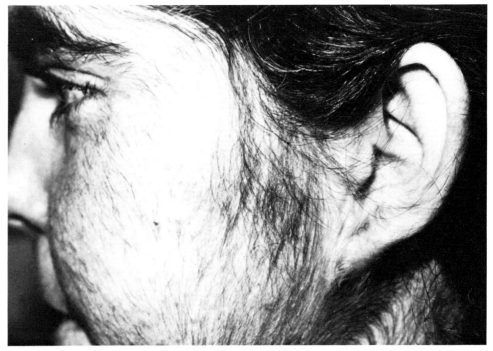

Fig. 8.11. Hypertrichosis caused by minoxidil (Dr J.L. Burton).

daily for miliary tuberculosis meningitis (Fono 1950). Buffoni (1951), who observed hypertrichosis in about 66% of cases of meningitis so treated, postulated that the streptomycin did not act directly on the follicles.

Cortisone. Prolonged administration of cortisone may induce hypertrichosis, most marked on the forehead, the temples and the sides of the cheeks, but also on the back and the extensor aspects of the limbs.

Penicillamine appears to cause lengthening and coarsening of hair on the trunk and limbs.

Psoralens, used in the treatment of vitiligo and psoriasis, may induce temporary hypertrichosis of light-exposed skin (Singh & Lal 1967).

References

Buffoni L. (1951) Streptomicina e ipertricosi. *Minerva paediatrica*, **3**, 710.

Burton J.L. & Marshall A. (1979) Hypertrichosis due to minoxidil. *British Journal of Dermatology*, **101**, 593.

Burton J.L., Schutt W.H. & Caldwell I.W. (1975) Hypertrichosis due to diazoxide. *British Journal of Dermatology*, **93**, 707.

Fono R. (1950) Appearance of hypertrichosis during streptomycin treatment. *Annali paediatrici*, **174**, 389.

Hamblen E.C. (1963) Iatric hirsutism. In *The Hirsute Female*, ed. R.B. Greenblatt. Springfield, Thomas, p. 269.

Koblenzer P.J. & Baker, L. (1968) Hypertrichosis lanuginosa associated with diazoxide therapy in prepubertal children. A clinico-pathologic study. *Annals of the New York Academy of Medicine*, **150**, 373.

Koblenzer P.J. & Baker L. (1969) (1) Hypertrichosis lanuginosa acquisita. (2) Congenital leucine-sensitive hypoglycaemia. *Archives of Dermatology*, **99**, 776.

Livingstone S., Peterson D. & Bohs L.L. (1955) Hypertrichosis occurring in association with dilantin therapy. *Journal of Pediatrics*, **47**, 351.

Ryckmanns F. (1980) Hypertrichosis durch minoxidil. *Hautarzt*, **31**, 205.

Singh G. & Lal S. (1967) Hypertrichosis and hyperpigmentation with systemic psoralen treatment. *British Journal of Dermatology*, **79**, 501.

Acquired circumscribed hypertrichosis

Cutting or shaving hair influences neither its rate of growth nor the calibre of the hair shaft. However, repeated or long-continued inflammatory changes involving the dermis, whether or not clinically evident scarring is produced, may result in the growth of long and coarse hair at this site. Although rarely reported the phenomenon is of common occurrence. The cause of the hair growth is usually obvious but may be overlooked when the trauma is occupational; for example, circumscribed patches of hypertrichosis on the left shoulder in men frequently carrying heavy sacks (Csillag 1921). A patch of hypertrichosis on one forearm is sometimes seen in mental defectives who have acquired the habit of chewing this site (Ressmann & Butterworth 1952). Sometimes the hypertrichosis, which may involve too few follicles to have attracted the patient's attention, develops at the site of an accidental wound or a vaccination scar (Linser 1926). It has developed on the back of the hand and fingers 3 months after the excision of warts; the coarse dark hairs, 3–5 cm in length, were shed after 2 months (Friederich & Gloor 1970). We have seen it surrounding a meniscectomy scar. It has been reported also in irregular pattern on the legs in chronic venous insufficiency (Schraibman 1967), around the edges of a burn (Shafir & Psur 1979), and at the site of multiple clusters of excoriated insect bites (Tisocco *et al.* 1981).

Long-continued cutaneous hyperaemia without permanent dermal change can also induce increased hair growth which is usually reversible. Hypertrichosis of this type may occur in the neighbourhood of inflamed joints and has been reported particularly in association with gonococcal arthritis (Heidemann 1934) and in the skin overlying chronic osteomyelitis of the tibia (Schuller & Frost 1956). Very exceptionally inflammatory dermatoses, especially in children, may induce a temporary overgrowth of hair. It has been observed after eczema (Edel 1938), and after variella (Naveh & Friedman 1972).

Children have developed itching eczema and local hypertrichosis at the site of injection of diphtheria/tetanus vaccine adsorbed on aluminium chloride (Pembroke & Marten 1979). We have observed similar changes at the site of BCG vaccination.

Unexplained hypertrichosis was present on the limbs at birth in a full-term male infant. The hairy skin appeared somewhat thickened and parchment-like. The hair had been shed after 4 months and the texture of the skin had returned to normal (Van der Meiren *et al.* 1960).

Hypertrichosis may occur in the indurated skin in melorheostotic sclero-derma. The diagnosis is established by radiological examination (Miyachi *et al.* 1979).

Hypertrichosis of one leg after a prolonged period of occlusion by plaster of Paris is a phenomenon well known to orthopaedic surgeons. It occurs mainly in children. The hypertrichosis must presumably be attributed to protection of the skin by the plaster from normal weathering. The hair returns to normal within a few weeks of removal of the plaster (Fig. 8.12a and b).

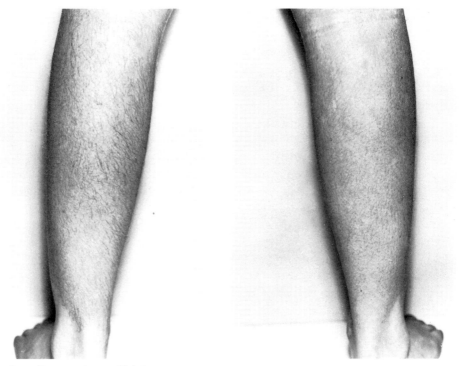

Fig. 8.12. Hypertrichosis of left leg (a) and after six weeks' occlusion by plaster of Paris in a girl aged 12. Right leg (b) not in plaster (Addenbrooke's Hospital, Cambridge).

References

Csillag J. (1921) Uber Berufshypertrichose. *Archiv für Dermatologie und Syphilologie,* **134,** 147.

Edel K. (1938) Hypertrichosis als verwikkeling bej eczeem. Nederlandische Tijdschrift vor Geneeskunde **82,** 2466.

Friederich H.C. & Gloor M. (1970) Postoperativ 'irritative' Hypertrichose. *Zeitschrift für Haut und Geschlectskrankheiten,* **45,** 10.

Heidemann H. (1934) Et Tilfaelde af Hypertrichose opstaalt i Tilkuytning til en gonorrhoisk ledaffektion. *Ugeskrift vor Laeger*, **96**, 553.

Linser, —. (1926) Demonstrationen: Patient mit einer hypertrichosis irritativa. *Klinische Wochenschrift*, **5**, 1490.

Miyachi Y., Hori T., Yamada A. & Ueo T. (1979) Linear melorheostotic scleroderma and hypertrichosis. *Archives of Dermatology*, **115**, 1233.

Naveh Y. & Friedman A. (1972) Transient circumscribed hypertrichosis following chickenpox. *Pediatrics*, **50**, 487.

Pembroke H.C. & Marten R.H. (1979) Unusual cutaneous reactions following diphtheria and tetanus immunization. *Clinical and Experimental Dermatology*, **4**, 345.

Ressmann A.C. & Butterworth T. (1952) Localized acquired hypertrichosis (as result of biting in mentally deficient). *Archives of Dermatology and Syphilology*, **65**, 458.

Schraibman I.G. (1967) Localized hirsutism. *Postgraduate Medical Journal*, **43**, 545.

Schuller P.A. & Frost J.A. (1956) Osteomilitis cronica de perone e hipertrichosis localizada. *Medicina (Madrid)*, **24**, 360.

Shafir R. & Tsur H. (1979) Local hirsutism at the periphery of burned skin. *British Journal of Plastic Surgery*, **32**, 93.

Tisocco L.A., Del Campo D.V., Bennin B. & Barsky S. (1981) Acquired localised hypertrichosis. *Archives of Dermatology*, **117**, 129.

Van der Meiren L., Achten G. & Piérard P. (1960) Hypertrichose chez un nouveau-né. *Archives Belges de Dermatologie and et Syphiligraphie*. **16**, 206.

Chapter 9
Traumatic Alopecia

Introduction

The term traumatic alopecia is applied to alopecia induced by physical trauma. These cases fall into three main categories:

(1) Alopecia resulting from the deliberate though at times unconscious efforts of the patient, who is under tension or is psychologically disturbed—trichotillomania.
(2) Alopecia resulting from cosmetic procedures applied incorrectly or with misguided and excessive vigour or frequency—cosmetic alopecia.
(3) Alopecia resulting from accidental trauma—accidental alopecia.

Trichotillomania
(References p. 266)

History and nomenclature
The term trichotillomania was suggested by Hallopeau in 1889 for the compulsive habit which induces an individual repeatedly to pluck his own hair. There are obvious objections to this overdramatic term for what is often a trivial problem, but its use has been generally preferred to 'trichomania' proposed by Besnier, or to 'autodépilation', proposed by Coppola (cit. Galewsky 1928). The term 'tic d'épilation', used by Raymond, is particularly appropriate for the condition commonly seen in young children, but has not found favour.

Pathology (Lachapelle & Pierard 1977) (Figs. 9.1, 9.2)
The histological changes vary according to the severity and duration of the hair plucking. Numerous empty hair canals are the most consistent feature. Some follicles are severely damaged; there are clefts in the hair matrix, the follicular epithelium is separated from the connective tissue sheath, and there are intraepithelial and perifollicular haemorrhages (Mehregan 1970). Injured follicles may form only soft, twisted hairs—a process which has been described as a separate entity under the name of trichomalacia (Mehregan 1970; Sanderson & Hall-Smith 1970). Many follicles are in catagen and some in early anagen.

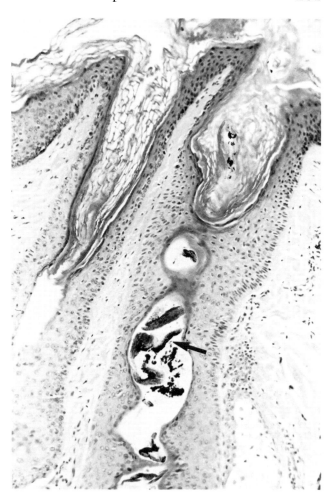

Fig. 9.1. Trichotillomania; biopsy of scalp, showing empty hair follicles. The empty follicle assumes a corkscrew shape and contains melanin casts (arrow) (Professor J.M. Lachapelle, Louvain).

There are few or no follicles in telogen (Steck 1979). Some dilated follicular infundibula contain horny plugs (Muller & Winkelmann 1972).

Experimental studies in sheep (Lyne & Jolly 1969) showed that tension on the wool fibres leads to an increase in growth rate, but a decrease in diameter and in overall volume. The surrounding epidermis becomes thickened, with a well-defined granular layer.

Aetiology and psychopathology

Trichotillomania occurs more than twice as frequently in females as in males but below the age of 6 boys outnumber girls by 3:2, and the peak incidence in boys is in the 2–6 age group (Muller 1980). The child develops the habit of twisting hair round its fingers and pulling it whilst in bed, or in class or watching television. The act is only partially conscious and may replace the habit of thumb-sucking.

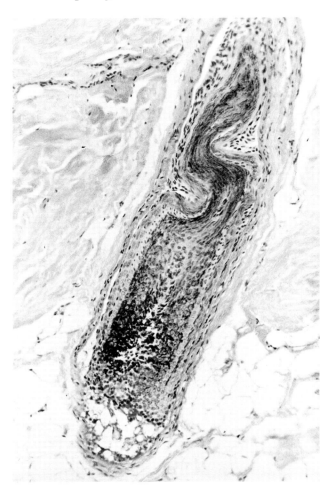

Fig. 9.2. A hair bulb has been
partially plucked. Serous exudate fills the space between
bulbar cells and the sur-
rounding connective tissue
sheaths. Clefts have formed
between the cells of the hair
matrix. Trichomalacia, the
distortion of a fully developed
anagen hair, is diagnostic of
trichotillomania. Note the
absence of inflammatory
reaction.

Various psychiatric studies (Schachter 1961; Monroe & Abse 1963; Greenberg &
Sarner 1965; Mannino & Delgado 1969) are not in complete agreement but
emotional deprivation in the maternal relationship is considered important in
initiating the habit. Others believe that the habit develops in the presence of
repressed aggression (Meirs *et al.* 1973). The habit is perhaps more common in
children of low intelligence, but also occurs in those of average or high
intelligence (Bartsch 1956).

   The rarer and more severe form occurs predominantly in females of any age
from early adolescence onwards, and most are aged 11–40; the peak incidence in
females is between 11 and 17 (Muller 1980). The hair pulling begins in a
provocative social situation in a subject who is often greatly disturbed
psychologically (Sanderson & Hall-Smith 1970). Exceptionally severe forms may
be seen in young patients and the minor forms in older patients.

Clinical features

In the younger patients the hair pulling tic develops gradually and unconsciously but is not usually denied by the patient. Hair is plucked most frequently from one frontoparietal region. There results an ill-defined patch on which the hairs are twisted and broken at various distances from the clinically normal scalp (Figs. 9.3–9.6). The texture and colour of the broken hairs are of course unaffected. Sometimes other parts of the scalp are attacked. More than one member of a family may be found to have acquired the habit, or even several members of a community such as a school (Davis 1922). One young child plucked the hair or her contemporaries as well as her own (Reuter 1951).

In the more severe form the patient usually consistently denies that she is touching her hair, but in a few cases admits it and complains that uncomfortable sensations, described in bizarre terms, are relieved by plucking the hair (Blaisdell 1916). The patient presents with an extensive area of scalp on which the hair has been reduced to a coarse stubble uniformly 2.5–3 mm long; the length is dictated by the impossibility of manually plucking shorter hairs. Most characteristically the plucked area covers the entire scalp apart from the margin, hence the

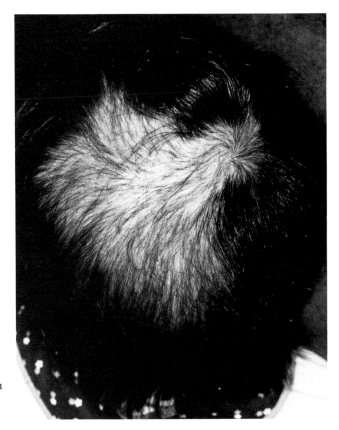

Fig. 9.3. Trichotillomania. Circumscribed but irregular pattern of alopecia, with numerous twisted and broken hairs (Professor J.M. Lachapelle, Louvain).

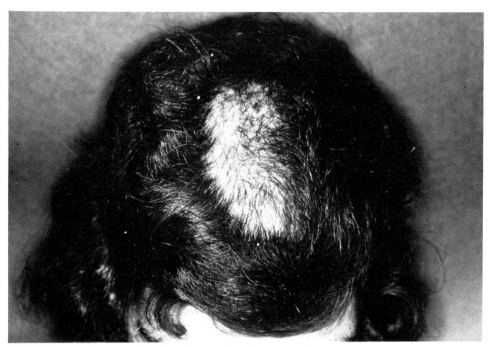

Fig. 9.4. Trichotillomania (Professor J.M. Lachapelle, Louvain).

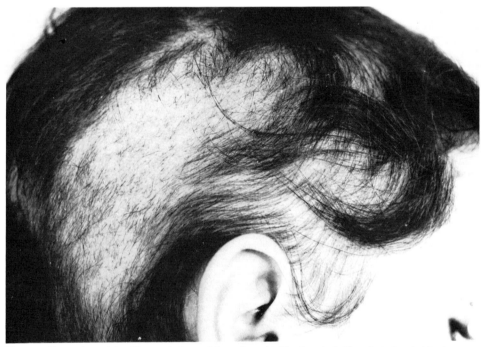

Fig. 9.5. Extensive trichotillomania in a girl aged 17 (Addenbrooke's Hospital, Cambridge).

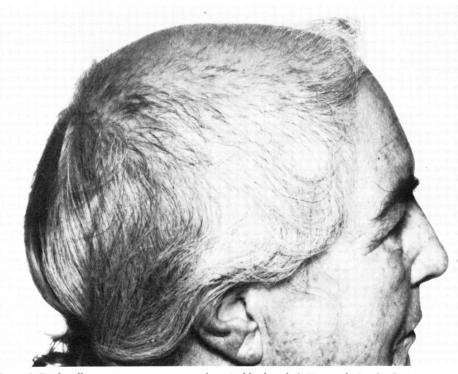

Fig. 9.6. Trichotillomania in a woman aged 72 (Addenbrooke's Hospital, Cambridge).

validity of the term 'tonsure alopecia' (Sanderson & Hall-Smith 1970). The hair-plucking may be continued for years and the disfiguring baldness is held by the patient to be responsible for her psychological problems. A mother and daughter have been affected at the same time (Hall-Smith 1966).

Much more unusual is the habit of plucking the eyelashes (Sonck 1958; Rohrback 1963).

Very exceptionally the patient may pluck hair also, or only, from other regions of the body, such as the mons pubis and perianal region (Galewsky 1928). Rare cases are reported in which the hair is cut with scissors, as in a strange case reported by Meiers (1971); he used the term trichotemnomania for this activity.

Differential diagnosis

The minor form in young children is often confused with ringworm or with alopecia areata. In ringworm the texture of the infected hairs is abnormal and the scalp surface may be scaly. It is wise to examine all cases under Wood's light and also to examine broken hairs under the microscope. Alopecia areata may be difficult to exclude with certainty at the first examination, but the course of the

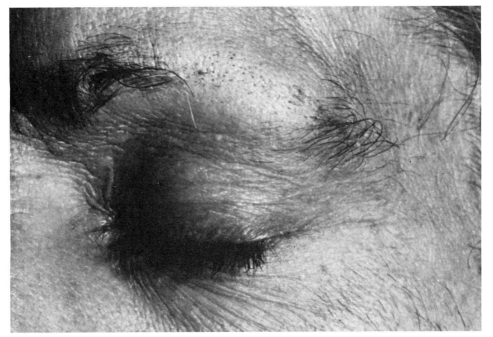

Fig. 9.7. Traumatic alopecia of the eyebrow in atopic dermatitis (Slade Hospital, Oxford).

condition soon establishes the correct diagnosis. We have known the hair-pulling tic develop in a child recovering from typical alopecia areata.

The severe form presents no real problem if the diagnosis is once considered. In the face of the patient's persistent denials, biopsy may be useful and conclusive. The almost complete lack of telogen hairs may provide a helpful clue.

Treatment and prognosis
The habit tic in young children is usually readily eradicated, except in the mentally retarded. The child's problem should be discussed with him and with his parents.

Tonsure trichotillomania is a very different proposition. Some patients recover, but many fail to do so, despite skilled psychiatric care.

References
Bartsch E. (1956) Beitrag zur Ätiologie der Trichotillomanie im Kindesalter. *Psychiatrie, Neurologie und Medizinische Psychologie,* **8,** 173.
Blaisdell J.H. (1916) Trichotillomania: a report of two cases of this rare neurodermatosis. *Journal of Cutaneous and Genitourinary Diseases,* **34,** 363.
Davis H. (1922) Pseudo-alopecia areata. *British Journal of Dermatology,* **34,** 162.
Galewsky E. (1928) Uber Trichotillomania. *Dermatologische Zeitschrift,* **53,** 208.
Greenberg H. & Sarner C.A. (1965) Trichotillomania. *Archives of General Psychiatry,* **12,** 482.

Hallopeau H. (1889) Alopécie par grattage (Trichomanie ou Trichotillomanie). *Annales de Dermatologie et de Syphiligraphie*, **10**, 440.

Hall-Smith S.P. (1966) Familial trichotillomania. *Transactions of the St John's Hospital Dermatological Society*, **52**, 135.

Lachapelle J-M. & Pierard G.E. (1977) Traumatic alopecia in trichotillomania: a pathologic interpretation of histologic lesions in the pilosebaceous unit. *Journal of Cutaneous Pathology*, **4**, 57.

Monroe J.T., Jr & Abse D.W. (1963) The psychopathology of trichotillomania and trichophagy. *Psychiatry*, **26**, 95.

Muller S.A. (1980) Trichotillomania. In *Hair, Trace Elements and Human Illness*, eds. A.C. Brown & R.G. Crounse. New York, Praeger, p. 306.

Muller S.A. & Winkelmann R.K. (1972) Trichotillomania. *Archives of Dermatology*, **105**, 535.

Reuter K. (1951) Ein besonderer Fall von Trichotillomanie. *Zeitschrift für Haut und Geschlechtskrankheiten*, **10**, 287.

Rohrbach D. (1963) Zwei Fälle von Trichotillomanie im Bereich der Cilien. *Hautarzt*, **114**, 122.

Sanderson K.V. & Hall-Smith P. (1970) Tonsure trichotillomania. *British Journal of Dermatology*, **82**, 343.

Schachter M. (1961) Zum Problem der Kindlichen Trichotillomanie. *Praxis der Kinderpsychologie*, **10**, 120.

Sonck C.E. (1958) Ein seltene Abart von Trichotillomanie. *Hautarzt*, **9**, 183.

Steck W.D. (1979) The clinical evaluation of pathologic hair loss with a diagnostic sign of trichotillomania. *Cutis*, **24**, 293.

Cosmetic traumatic alopecia
(References p. 270)

History and nomenclature

The dictates of religion, of custom and of fashion have imposed an immense variety of physical stresses on human hair. The nomenclature of the resulting patterns of baldness inevitably lacks any consistency. It is possible only to list the clinical syndromes most widely reported; any new hairdressing technique may give rise to new patterns. The 'chignon alopecia' of our grandmothers' days may yet return.

Pathology

Two processes are responsible for most of the pathological changes observed. Hair, sometimes already weakened by chemical applications, may be broken by friction or by tension. Prolonged tension may induce follicular inflammatory changes which may eventually lead to scarring. Traction alopecia is induced particularly readily in subjects with incipient common baldness, for the telogen hairs, which make up a higher proportion of the total, are more readily extracted than anagen hairs (Ikeda & Yamada 1967).

Clinical features

Traumatic marginal alopecia. The essential changes in the many variants of this syndrome are the presence of short broken hairs, folliculitis and some scarring in circumscribed patches at the scalp margins.

In one form which is caused by the tension imposed by procedures intended to straighten kinky hair (Costa 1946) alopecia commonly begins in triangular areas in front of and above the ears, but may involve other parts of the scalp margin, or even linear areas in other parts of the scalp (Fig. 9.8). Sabouraud (1931) had described as alopecia linearis frontalis (Fig. 9.9), a similar process in young French girls, beginning with inflammatory papules and broken hairs in front of the ears, and extending anteriorly as a band 1–3 cm wide. Itching and crusting were sometimes severe. The so-called 'pony-tail' hair style, traditional in the women of Greenland, but enjoying intermittent popularity elsewhere, may cause similar changes in the frontal hair margin (Hjorth 1957; Slepyan 1958). Keratin cylinders—'hair casts'—may surround many hairs just above the scalp surface (Rolins 1961).

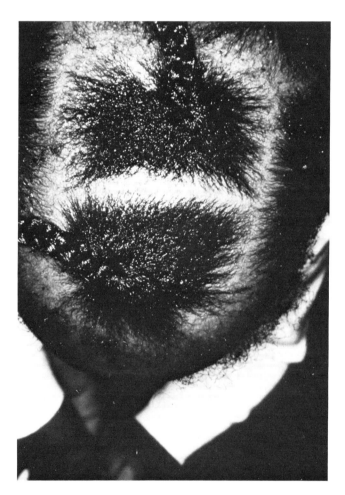

Fig. 9.8. Traction alopecia (Slade Hospital, Oxford).

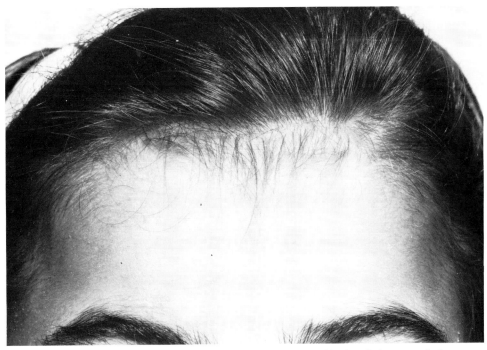

Fig. 9.9. Traumatic alopecia—mild alopecia linearis frontalis (Addenbrooke's Hospital, Cambridge).

Frontal and parietal traction alopecia may occur in young Sikh boys as a result of twisting their uncut hair tightly on top of the head (Singh 1975), and tight braiding and wooden combs produce traction alopecia in the Sudan (Morgan 1960); frontal loss is reported in Libyan women as a result of traction from a tight scarf (Malhotra & Kanwar 1980). Parietal patches have been produced by the traction exerted by clips holding a nurse's cap in place (Renna & Freedberg 1973).

Brush roller alopecia. The popular brush rollers, if applied frequently and with too much vigour, may cause irregular patches of more or less complete alopecia, surrounded by a zone of erythema with broken hairs (Lipnik 1961).

Hot-comb alopecia. Negro women who use hot combs to straighten the hair, may develop a progressive cicatricial alopecia, slowly extending centrifugally from the vertex (Lo Presti *et al.* 1968).

Massage alopecia. The overenthusiastic application of medication to the scalp, with firm massage, may cause baldness (Bowers 1950); one of these six patients had trichorrhexis nodosa.

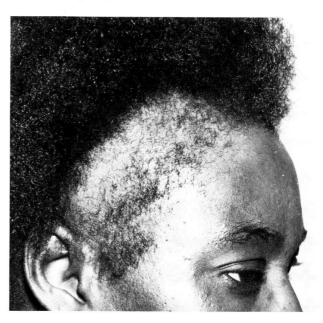

Fig. 9.10. Traumatic alopecia from the use of hair straighteners (Addenbrooke's Hospital, Cambridge).

Brush alopecia. Vigorous brushing may cause significant damage to hair that is already fragile as the result of a developmental defect. The 'bristles' with a square or otherwise angular tips, present in some brushes made of synthetic fibres, may prove particularly traumatic (Savill 1958).

Alopecia secondary to hair weaving. Patchy traction alopecia has been reported to result from the cosmetic procedure of weaving additional hair into persistent terminal hair in order to camouflage common baldness (Perlstein 1969).

Diagnosis

The traumatic cosmetic alopecias do not present any diagnostic difficulties, provided the possibility is considered. Their cause is rarely recognized by the patient, and is often accepted with suspicion.

References

Bowers R.E. (1950) Massage alopecia. *British Journal of Dermatology*, **62**, 262.

Costa O.G. (1946) Traumatic Negroid alopecia. *British Journal of Dermatology*, **58**, 280.

Hjorth N. (1957) Traumatic marginal alopecia. A special type—alopecia Greenlandica. *British Journal of Dermatology*, **69**, 317.

Ikeda T. & Yamada M. (1967) Both telogen effluvium and traction alopecia mainly occur in patients with a condition of alopecia prematura. *Acta Dermatologica (Kyoto)*, **62**, 47.

Lipnik M.J. (1961) Traction alopecia from brush rollers. *Archives of Dermatology*, **84**, 493.

Lo Presti P., Papa C.M. & Kligman A.M. (1968) Hot comb alopecia. *Archives of Dermatology*, **98**, 234.

Malhotra Y.K. & Kanwar A.J. (1980) Traumatic alopecia among Libyan women. *Archives of Dermatology*, **116**, 987.

Morgan H.V. (1960) Traction alopecia. *British Medical Journal*, **ii**, 115.

Perlstein H.H. (1969) Traction alopecia due to hair weaving. *Cutis*, **5**, 440.

Renna F.G. & Freedberg I.M. (1973) Traction alopecia in nurses. *Archives of Dermatology*, **108**, 684.

Rollins T.G. (1961) Traction folliculitis with hair casts and alopecia. *American Journal of Diseases of Children*, **101**, 609.

Sabouraud R. (1931) De l'alopécie liminaire frontale. *Annales de Dermatologie et de Syphiligraphie*, **2**, 446.

Saville A. (1958) The nylon brush. *British Journal of Dermatology*, **70**, 296.

Singh G. (1975) Traction alopecia in Sikh boys. *British Journal of Dermatology*, **92**, 232.

Slepyan A.H. (1958) Traction alopecia. *Archives of Dermatology*, **78**, 395.

Accidental traumatic alopecia

Alopecia secondary to accidental mechanical trauma to the scalp is usually no diagnostic problem (Friederich 1950) but in some circumstances the trauma may be unperceived and the cause of the hair loss undetected.

Women who had undergone prolonged pelvic operations in the Trendelenburg position, developed 12 to 26 days later a vertical patch of alopecia, which was preceded by oedema, exudation and crusting. Pressure ischaemia during the operation was considered to be the cause of the alopecia (Abel & Lewis 1960; Abel 1964).

In one large clinic 60 cases of occipital pressure alopecia were observed after open-heart surgery over a period of 3 years (Lawson *et al.* 1976). In 29 of these cases the hair loss was permanent. To prevent the development of alopecia under these conditions prolonged pressure ichaemia must be avoided.

Temporary alopecia followed prolonged pressure on the scalp of a foam rubber ring, used to prevent such an occurrence (Patel & Henschel 1980).

Permanent alopecia followed constant pressure during more than 6 hours of an operation by the head strap securing a face mask (Gormley & Sokoll 1967).

References

Abel R.R. & Lewis G.M. (1960) Postoperative (pressure) alopecia. *Archives of Dermatology*, **81**, 34.

Abel R.R. (1964) Postoperative (pressure) alopecia. *Anesthesiology*, **25**, 870.

Friederich H.-C. (1950) Ein Beitrag zu dem mechanischen Schädigungen des Haares und des Haarbodens. *Dermatologische Wochenschrift*, **121**, 344.

Gormley T. & Sokoll M.D. (1967) Permanent alopecia from pressure of headstrap. *Journal of the American Medical Association*, **199**, 157.

Lawson N.W., Mills N.L. & Ochsner N.L. (1976) Occipital alopecia following cardiopulmonary bypass. *Journal of Thoracic and Cardiovascular Surgery*, **71**, 342.

Patel K.D. & Henschel E.O. (1980) Postoperative alopecia. *Anaesthesia and Analgesia*, **59**, 311.

Chapter 10
Alopecia Areata

History and nomenclature
(References p. 274)

The distinctive but variable syndrome or syndromes commonly known as alopecia areata (AA) (pelade in France) have suffered many changes in nomenclature which have added to diagnostic confusion and a bewildering multiplicity of aetiological hypotheses.

Cornelius Celsus, landowner and encyclopaedist, who flourished in Rome *c.* AD 14–37, has been credited with the first description of AA, which even now is sometimes referred to as 'area celsi'. The term 'alopecia areata' was first used by Sauvages (1706–67) in his *Nosologia medica*, published in Lyons in 1760. Robert Willan gave a fuller description of the condition but named it 'porrigo decalvans', and Thomas Bateman used the same term in his atlas. Alibert, Willan's rival as a classifier of the dermatoses, regarded what he called 'porrigo tonsurans' as the same as 'porrigo decalvans'. It was therefore inevitable that when Gruby in 1843 found a fungus in 'porrigo decalvans' the parasitic theory of AA was firmly launched on its misleading course. In 1851 Hebra clearly separated AA from herpes tonsurans, but at first still accepted that AA was of fungous origin. He later revised his opinion (Hebra & Kaposi 1874).

The period from 1850 to 1900 saw the rapid development of microbiology, at a time when the need for controls in clinical and laboratory investigations had yet to be appreciated. There were few diseases for which one or more 'causative organisms' were not described. At first it was incorrect terminology which associated AA with a parasite, but even after sound diagnostic criteria were established a battle raged between the 'parasitic' school, which included both Hutchinson and Radcliffe Crocker (1903) in Britain and Bazin in France, and their opponents, most of whom favoured the fashionable 'trophoneurotic' hypothesis put forward originally by von Bärensprung of Berlin in 1858. The dictatorial Erasmus Wilson held this view, but before he is given credit for denying the parasitic origin of AA it must be recalled that he also denied that ringworm was an infection. The earlier protagonists of the parasitic origin of AA believed that a fungus was the organism concerned. Later, bacteria were suspected. A paper by the dermatologist George Thin, presented by Thomas Huxley, described to the Royal Society his *Bacterium decalvans* (Thin 1882). Many other bacteria were incriminated for a time; Sabouraud in 1896 blamed the microbacillus which he held responsible also for seborrhoea (p. 90) but later admitted his error. These claims may seem fanciful, but as late as 1913 Jackson and MacMurtry of New York felt that the parasitic theory 'cannot be wholly rejected'. Outbreaks of AA in closed communities (p. 316) are still unexplained.

The trophoneurotic theory, with some modifications in emphasis, is still held by some authorities. The theory is highly adaptable and, if it cannot be proved, is difficult to disprove. The alleged production of AA in cats by nerve section (Joseph 1886) and the many clinical observations relating the onset of alopecia to emotional stress (p. 282) or to head injury could be taken to support this rather vaguely formulated hypothesis. Vitiligo, scleroderma and hypothyroidism, which were known to be significantly associated with AA, were considered to be 'trophic' or 'nervous' disorders. The trophoneurotic hypothesis could be modified and elaborated to admit the concept of 'irritation'. Some dozens of papers claimed significant associations between AA and dental defects or errors of refraction. The most extravagant claims were those of the 'dystrophic theory' of Jacquet (1902) of Paris who found a dental 'cause' in almost every case; he appears not to have been disconcerted when his countryman Bailly of Lyons showed (Bailly 1910) that dental defects were equally common in those without AA.

With the development of endocrinology late in the nineteenth century another tangled strand had to be woven into the working hypothesis. AA was demonstrably sometimes associated with disorders of endocrine glands, notably the thyroid. These disorders, themselves 'trophic', were treated and the fortuitous regrowth of the bald patches was accepted as proof that the endocrine disorder had 'caused' the alopecia.

By the 1920s most dermatologists had abandoned the parasitic theory of AA and put forward hypotheses which blended the trophoneurotic and the endocrine in theories appropriate to each national temperament. Then came the ogre of 'focal sepsis', which found favour in many countries since it offered and justified a vigorous therapeutic approach.

Even the most conservative of clinicians claimed that focal sepsis, usually of teeth or upper respiratory tract, but occasionally gastrointestinal, was the cause of almost all cases of alopecia areata.

In the past 20 years the growing volume of reliable clinical observations have been reviewed in the light of new immunological data—and theories. New hypotheses have been propounded, but the historically minded cynic cannot fail to wonder whether their factual basis is any more solid than that of von Bärensprung's trophoneurotic theory. The account of AA which follows endeavours to separate fact from speculation.

References
Bailly (1910) *L'Origine Gingivodentaire de la Pelade.* Lyons, publisher unknown.
Hebra F. & Kaposi M. (1974) *On Diseases of the Skin*, vol. 3. Trans. and ed., W. Tay. London, New Sydenham Society, p. 209.
Jackson G.T. & McMurtry C.W. (1913) *A Treatise on Diseases of the Hair.* London, Kimpton, p. 107.
Jacquet L. (1902) Nature et traitement de la pelade—la pelade d'origine dentaire. *Annales de Dermatologie et de Syphiligraphie*, **3**, 97, 180.
Joseph M. (1886) Experimentelle Untersuchungen über die Ätiologie der Alopecia areata. *Monatshefte für praktischer Dermatologie*, **5**, 483.
Radcliffe Crocker H. (1903) *Diseases of the Skin*, 3rd edn. London, Lewis, p. 1138.
Thin G. (1882) On bacterium decalvans, an organism associated with the destruction of the hair in alopecia areata. *Proceedings of the Royal Society*, **33**, 247.

Aetiology
(References p. 279)

It is not at present possible to attribute all or indeed any cases of AA to any single cause. Among the many factors which appear to be implicated in at least a proportion of cases are the patient's genetic constitution, the atopic state, organ-specific autoimmune reactions, and emotional stress. The different degrees to which these factors appear to be concerned in patients from different parts of the world serve to emphasize the importance of the genetic background, since this largely influences both the atopic state and the predisposition to organ-specific autoimmune disorders.

Heredity

Cockayne (1933), reviewing the older literature, concluded that AA was due to two factors, one inherited and one environmental. He said also that all authorities are agreed that AA almost always occurs in the dark haired. There are striking differences in the percentage of cases of AA giving a family history of the same condition. Sabouraud (1929) in Paris obtained a positive family history in 22% of his cases; Brown (1929) in Scotland, in 20%. Muller & Winkelman (1963) in USA reported a figure of 10% in their entire series, but of 18% of their adult cases. In contrast Bastos Araujo and Poiares Baptista (1967) in Portugal found a positive family history in only 6.3%, Olivetti (1965) of Milan, Italy in 4% and Saenz (1963) in Spain found no evidence of any hereditary factor.

There were certainly differences in the diligence with which a family history was sought, but there is no reason to doubt that real differences may exist. The most recent investigation, carried out at the Cleveland Clinic, USA (Sander *et al.* 1980) revealed a positive family history in 27% of cases, and these authors suggested that there was autosomal dominant inheritance with variable penetrance.

The association with dark hair so confidently asserted by Cockayne (1933) could not be confirmed by Anderson (1950) of Sheffield, England, or in an unpublished investigation in Cambridge, England (Rook 1976). If there is a significant association between AA and dark hair in some countries, then racial differences in the prevalence of AA are probable, but evidence that they occur is inconclusive; hospital attendance statistics show AA accounting for from less than 1% to over 3% of new patients in departments of dermatology, but the factors influencing hospital attendance with any particular disease vary widely from one country to another. However, Arnold found AA disproportionately common among the Japanese in Hawaii (Arnold 1952) and other figures suggest but do not prove that there may be considerable racial variations.

Other evidence of a genetic factor predisposing to AA is provided by a number of case reports of which the following are representative. A man aged 25 with AA which became total; his father and the latter's brother and sister were similarly affected (Noble 1933). Twin brothers aged 20 both had AA of scalp and eyebrows (Omens & Omens 1946). More difficult to explain was the occurrence of AA in the same site on the same day in identical twin boys aged 11 (Hendren 1949); the same phenomenon was later reported in another pair of identical twin boys aged 8 (Weidmann *et al.* 1956). There are many further reports of the occurrence of AA in twins, though not simultaneously (Bereston & Robinson 1951; Fischer 1953).

Too few HL antigen studies in AA have been reported to justify any conclusions. In a Finnish population (Kiantu *et al.* 1977) AA but not alopecia universalis, was associated with HLA–B12.

The atopic state

Cases of AA associated with atopic dermatitis have been reported with emphasis on supposed common emotional factors (Robinson & Tasker 1948). The appreciation that the association between AA and the atopic state is frequent in some populations has been stressed only relatively recently. In a large North American series eczema or asthma or both were present in 18% of children with AA and in 9% of adults; no fewer than 23% of children with alopecia totalis were atopic subjects (Muller & Winkelmann 1963). In Japan, Ikeda (1965) found 10% of AA patients to be atopic, whilst in Holland (Penders 1968) 52.4% were atopic. In a Danish study the incidence of atopic dermatitis in association with AA was only 1% (Gip *et al.* 1969). There were doubtless differences in diagnostic criteria, but these figures may indicate real differences worthy of detailed study.

Autoimmune reactions

The association of AA with a number of endocrine disorders has long been recognized by clinicians. Recent investigations have tended to assume that the basis of such associations is the formation of organ-specific autoantibodies which may play a pathogenetic role in both disorders. The evidence is, however, far too contradictory to allow any generalization.

At the clinical level there are wide differences in the frequency of the association of AA and thyroid disease. In Spain, Grona & Requena (1955) found that the association occurred frequently. Muller & Winkelmann (1963) in North America found thyroid disease in 8% of their patients with AA, and considered this association to be significant. In Newcastle, England (Cunliffe *et al.* 1969), the incidence of thyroid disease in patients with AA was 28%, significantly higher than in control subjects with psoriasis. In Aberdeen, Scotland (Main *et al.* 1975), no such association was demonstrable. Salamon in Jugoslavia (Salamon *et al.* 1971) found no evidence of thyroid dysfunction in 47 patients with AA. Reliable statistics based on the prospective study of large numbers of patients are lacking, but there are reports of cases (e.g. Klein *et al.* 1974) in which Hashimoto's thyroiditis and AA have co-existed and Kern (1974) has found a statistically significant association between AA and Hashimoto's disease and pernicious anaemia and Addison's disease.

Recently Brown (1980) has studied the association between AA and autoimmune testicular disease; he claims that the complaint of sterility or infertility is frequent in AA and vitiligo. He investigated 33 males. Six had depressed morning testosterone levels, and semen analysis in two of three patients in whom this was carried out, showed oligospermia. Four other patients with low to normal testosterone levels also showed oligospermia. Brown noted that of the patients whose first AA lesions occurred in the scalp 44% had developed their lesions during puberty. The association of AA with autoimmune gonadal disease is clearly worthy of further investigation.

The association of vitiligo with AA is accepted by most authors. Vitiligo was present in 4% of one series of cases (Muller & Winkelmann 1963) as compared with less than 1% of the population concerned. In an investigation in Sheffield,

England (Anderson 1950), the incidence was also 4%. Perinaevoid vitiligo (Sutton's halo naevus) is familiar to the dermatologist, and perinaevoid alopecia also occurs (Pecoraro 1963). The special interest of the association of AA with vitiligo lies in the fact that vitiligo is itself significantly associated with thyroid disease, Addison's disease, diabetes mellitus and pernicious anaemia, although, as in the case of AA, there are striking differences in the frequency of such associations in different series of cases (Fig. 10.1).

The association of AA with lupus erythematosus has been reported on a number of occasions (Muller & Winkelmann 1963; Lerchin & Schwimmer (1975), as has the association with ulcerative colitis (Allen & Moschella 1974). More unusual associations have been reported between AA, lichen schlerosus and polymyalgia rheumatica (Faergemann 1979) and between AA, vitiligo, morphoea, nail dystrophy and lichen planus (Brown *et al.* 1979), and between AA and Sjogren's syndrome (Todd *et al.* 1977).

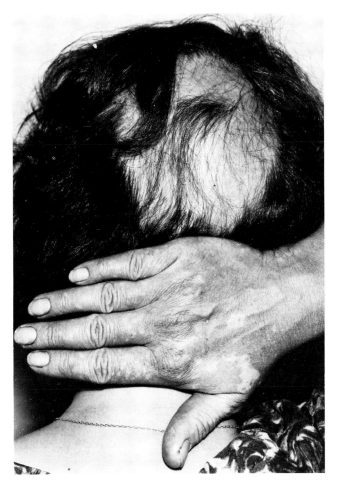

Fig. 10.1. Alopecia areata and vitiligo in the same patient (Addenbrookes Hospital, Cambridge).

AA in Down's syndrome

The observation that AA is unusually frequent in Down's syndrome made by Wunderlich & Braun-Falco (1965), who found 13 cases of AA among 1000 mongols, has recently been confirmed by Du Vivier & Munro (1975) who found 60 cases among 1000 patients with Down's syndrome but only 1 in 1000 mentally retarded controls. In 25 of the 60 cases the alopecia was total or universal. Of the mongols with AA 14 had fluorescent antibodies. Of the 14, 10 were female and of these 8 had thyroid antibodies, 1 had gastric parietal cell antibodies and 1 had antinuclear factor. The 4 male patients who had antibodies gave only weakly positive results, no more than would be expected in a control population. As 8 of the 23 female mongols with AA had antithyroid antibodies these were sought in 23 age-matched female mongols without AA, and were found to be present in only 2; 2 had antinuclear antibodies.

Mongolism is a chromosomal defect. Thyroid antibodies occur more frequently in mongols than in normal subjects and this increased incidence has been reported also in two other chromosomal defects, Klinefelter's syndrome and Turner's syndrome. The incidence of thyroid antibodies in mongols with AA is significantly higher than in mongols without AA and in normal subjects. In 18 of 19 patients with Down's syndrome and AA, T-cell levels in the peripheral blood were depressed (Brown *et al.* 1977).

These interesting findings cannot yet be reliably interpreted. Mongols and their mothers are abnormally susceptible to thyroid disease (Fialkow 1966). The incidence of AA in the parents of mongols has not been studied. However, an unusual mongol child with webbed neck and other defects also had AA, as did the child's father (Korting & Holzman 1962).

Immunological investigations

Autoantibody studies have yielded inconsistent findings. In Newcastle (Cunliffe *et al.* 1969) there was no increase in the incidence of thyroglobulin and thyroid complement-fixing antibodies as compared with control subjects. Main *et al.* (1975) in Aberdeen likewise found no increase in thyroid autoantibodies, but antibodies to smooth muscle were significantly increased. In contrast Kern *et al.* (1973) in North America, in 44 patients found a significant association between AA and the presence of autoantibodies against thyroglobulin, cytoplasm of parietal cells and of thyroid and adrenal, but no antibodies to hair follicle cells. Betterle *et al.* (1975) in Italy examined their AA patients for a wide range of autoantibodies—not including smooth muscle—and found no differences from control subjects. Klaber & Munro (1978) and Muller *et al.* (1980) found no antibodies to epidermal elements and hair follicles within the patients' sera or bound in vivo in the scalp biopsies. They also found no increase in thyroid or other autoantibodies.

In a more recent investigation (Schenk *et al.* 1980) 202 patients were studied, including 150 with AA, 21 with alopecia universalis and 31 with vitiligo. Circulating autoantibodies were demonstrated by indirect immuno-fluorescence. The findings were as follows:

	AA	A. universalis	Vitiligo
Antinuclear antibodies	28%	14%	26%
Antithyroid antibodies	14%		16%
Antibodies to testicular tissue	11%		10%

Direct immunofluorescence studies of biopsy material from 12 patients with AA showed abnormal deposits of C3 and sometimes of IgG and IgM especially in the lower part of the hair follicle. Similar changes were found in 21% of patients with androgenetic alopecia but not in 4 patients with alopecia totalis (Bystryn *et al.* 1979).

An investigation in Japan (Igarashi *et al.* 1980) also showed deposits of C3 in the connective tissue sheath of the lower part of the hair follicle in AA and also in the normal scalp. In neither the normal nor AA scalps could immunoglobulins be demonstrated.

The investigation of T-cell numbers in 13 cases showed a reduction from $75.2 \pm 5.3\%$ to $50.36 \pm 17.1\%$ (Sander *et al.* 1980). Taking into account the conflicting immunological evidence, the histological changes and the regrowth of many cases on treatment with induced contact allergy (see p. 304) it has been suggested that AA results from a defect in immunoregulation. A suppressor cell defect resulting in a failure to suppress T-cell function, affects first the B cells, leading to autoantibody formation. Unchecked T-effector cells then attack the follicle. The lymphocytic infiltrate probably indicates (Happle 1980) a cell-mediated reaction to some hair-associated antigen. Contact allergy (e.g. to DNCB) produces a new allergen at the same site. The infiltrate of the allergic contact dermatitis contains suppressor T cells and suppressor macrophages which exert a non-specific inhibitory effect on the immune response against hair follicles. Decreased numbers of T cells were found also by Nunzi *et al.* (1980) in 6 of 8 patients with AA. The two with normal T cell levels had AA confined to the beard. These same investigators found in all eight cases antibodies specifically directed against the endothelial cells in the capillary network of the hair bulb.

References

Allen H.B. & Moschella S.L. (1974) Ulcerative colitis associated with skin and hair changes. *Cutis*, 14, 85

Anderson I. (1950) Alopecia areata: a clinical study. *British Medical Journal*, ii, 1250.

Arnold H.L. (1952) Alopecia areata. Prevalence in Japanese and prognosis after reassurance. *A.M.A. Archives of Dermatology and Syphilology*, 66, 191.

Bastos Araujo A. & Poiares Baptista A. (1967) Algunas consideracions sobre 300 casos de pelada. *Traballos da Sociedad Portugesa de Dermatologia e Venereologia*, **25**, 135.

Bereston E.S. & Robinson H.M. (1951) Alopecia areata in two brothers and two sisters. *A.M.A. Archives of Dermatology and Syphilology*, **64**, 204.

Betterle C., Peserico A., Dal Prete G. & Trisotto A. (1975) Autoantibodies in alopecia areata. *Archives of Dermatology*, **111**, 927.

Brenner W., Diem E. & Gschnait F. (1979) Coincidence of vitiligo, alopecia areata, onychodystrophy, localised scleroderma and lichen planus. *Dermatologica*, **159**, 356.

Brown A.C., Olkowski Z.L., McLaren J.R. & Kutner M.H. (1971) Alopecia areata and vitiligo associated with Down's syndrome. *Archives of Dermatology*, **113**, 1296.

Brown A.C. (1980) Autoimmune gonadal disease. In *Trace Elements, Hair and Human Illness*. Eds. A.C. Brown & R.G. Crounse. New York, Praeger, p. 313.

Brown W.H. (1929) The aetiology of alopecia areata and its relationship to vitiligo and possibly schlerodermia. *British Journal of Dermatology*, **41**, 299.

Bystryn J.C., Orentreich N. & Shezel F. (1979) Direct immunofluorescence studies in alopecia areata and male pattern alopecia. *Journal of Investigative Dermatology*, **73**, 317.

Cockayne E.A. (1933) Inherited abnormalities of the skin and appendages. Oxford, Oxford University Press, p. 354.

Cunliffe W.C., Hall R., Stevenson C.F. & Weightman D. (1969) Alopecia areata, thyroid disease and autoimmunity. *British Journal of Dermatology*, **81**, 879.

Du Vivier A. & Munro D.D. (1975) Alopecia areata, autoimmunity and Down's syndrome. *British Medical Journal*, **i**, 191.

Faergemann T. (1979) Lichen scherosus and atropicus generalisata, alopecia areata and polymyalgia rheumatica found in the same patient. *Cutis*, **23**, 757.

Fialkow P.J. (1966) Autoimmunity and chromosomal aberrations. *American Journal of Human Genetics*, **18**, 93.

Fischer H.R. (1953) Alopecia areata bei eneiigen Zwillingen. *Zeitschrift für Haut und Geschlechtskrankheiten*, **15**, 178.

Gip L., Lodin A. & Molin L. (1969) Alopecia areata. *Acta Dermatovenereologica*, **49**, 180.

Grona M.B. & Requena J.E. (1955) Nuestra experiencia con el tratamiento de las peladas con disfuncion tiroidea. *Medicina Española*, **34**, 483.

Hendren O.S. (1949) Identical alopecia areata in identical twins. *Archives of Dermatology and Syphilology*, **60**, 793.

Igarashi A., Takeuchi S. & Seto Y. (1980) Immunofluorescence studies of complement C3 in hair follicles of normal scalp and of scalp affected by alopecia areata. *Acta Dermatologica Venereologica*, **60**, 33.

Ikeda T. (1965) A new classification of alopecia areata. *Dermatologica*, **131**, 421.

Kern F., Hoffmann W.H., Hambrick G.W. & Blizzard R.M. (1973) Alopecia areata: immunologic studies and treatment with prednisone. *Archives of Dermatology*, **107**, 407.

Kern F. (1974) Laboratory evaluation of patients with alopecia areata. *First Human Hair Symposium*, ed. A.C. Brown. New York, Medcom, p. 222.

Kiantu U., Reumaia T., Karvonen J., Lassus A. & Tiilikainen A. (1977) HLAB12 in alopecia areata. *Archives of Dermatology*, **113**, 1716.

Klaber M.R. & Munro B.D. (1978) Alopecia areata: immunofluorescence and other studies. *British Journal of Dermatology*, **99**, 383.

Klein V., Weissheimer B. & Zaun H. (1974) Simultaneous occurrence of alopecia areata and immunothyroiditis. *International Journal of Dermatology*, **13**, 116.

Korting G.W. & Holzmann H. (1962) Uber eine mongoloide Abartung mit Flügelfellbildung und (familiäre) Alopecia areata. *Dermatologische Wochenschrift*, **145**, 505.

Lerchin E. & Schwimmer B. (1975) Alopecia areata associated with discoid lupus erythematosus. *Cutis*, **15**, 87.

Main R.A., Robbie R.B., Gray E.S., Donald D. & Horne C.H.W. (1975) Smooth muscle antibodies and alopecia areata. *British Journal of Dermatology*, **92**, 389.

Muller H.K., Rook A.J. & Kubba R. (1980) Immunohistology and autoantibody studies in alopecia areata. *British Journal of Dermatology*, **102**, 609.

Muller S.A. & Winkelmann R.K. (1963) Alopecia areata. *Archives of Dermatology*, **88**, 290.

Noble G. (1933) Familiäre universelle Alopecie: Spontanheilung nach fünf Jahren. *Weiner klinische Wochenschrift*, **46**, 90.

Nunzi E., Hamarlinck F. & Cormane R.H. (1980) Immunopathological studies in alopecia areata. *Archives of Dermatological Research*, **269**, 1.

Olivetti L. & Bubola D. (1965) Osservazioni cliniche su 160 Casi de Area Celsi. *Giornale Italiano de Dermatologia*, **106**, 376.

Omens D.V. & Omens H.D. (1946) Alopecia areata in twins. *Archives of Dermatology and Syphilology*, **53**, 193.

Pecoraro V. (1963) Relaciones etiologicas entre la pelada y el vitiligo. *Archivos Argentinos de Dermatologia*, **13**, 297.

Penders A.J.M. (1968) Alopecia areata and atopy. *Dermatologica*, **136**, 395.

Robinson S.S. & Tasker S. (1948) Alopecia areata associated with neurodermatitis. *Urological and Cutaneous Review*, **52**, 468.

Sabouraud R. (1929) Sur l'étiologie de la pelade. *Archives de Dermato-Syphiligraphiques de la Clinique de l'Hôpital Saint-Louis*, **1**, 31.

Saenz H. (1963) Nuevo contribucion al estudio de la alopecia areata en España. *Actas Dermo-Sifiliograficas*, **54**, 357.

Salamon T., Musafija A. & Miličerić M. (1971) Alopecia Areata und Erkrankungen der Thyreoidea. *Dermatologica*, **142**, 62.

Sander D.N., Bergfeld W.F. & Krakauer R.S. (1980) Alopecia areata: An inherited autoimmune disease. In *Hair, Trace Elements and Human Illness*, eds. A.C. Brown & R.G. Crounse. New York, Praeger, p. 343.

Schenk E.A., Schneider P. & Brown A.C. (1980) Autoantibodies in alopecia and vitiligo. In *Hair, Trace Elements and Human Illness*, eds. A.C. Brown & R.G. Crounse. New York, Praeger, p. 334.

Torok M., Kincses E. & Bohatka L. (1977) Common incidence of the alopecia totalis maligna and Sjogren syndrome. *Szemeszet*, **114**, 49 (Hungarian).

Weidmann A.I., Zion L.S. & Mamelok A.E. (1956) Alopecia areata occurring simultaneously in identical twins. *A.M.A. Archives of Dermatology*, **74**, 424.

Wunderlich C. & Braun-Falco O. (1965) Mongolism and alopecia areata. *Medizinische Wochenschrift*, **10**, 477.

Emotional stress

The old trophoneurotic concept did not imply any more than a disturbance of follicular nutrition mediated by nerves; 'Neurotic' did not imply psychosomatic. However, the concept was sufficiently imprecise to accommodate any advance in psychiatric knowledge or change in nomenclature.

Opinions expressed on the role of emotional stress in AA have been widely divergent. Most authors consider that at least some cases are induced by stress, but they rarely give the criteria on which this assement is based. Attempts at objective evaluation using standard psychiatric procedures such as the Ror-schach test showed over 90% of patients with AA to be psychologically abnormal (Panconesi & Mantellassi 1955, 1956). On the other hand Macalpine (1958), a psychiatrist, studied 125 patients with AA and came to the conclusion that emotional factors did not play a significant role in this disorder. The incidence of AA appeared to be the same in refugees coming to Israel in 1947, and after resettlement in 1958 (Spitzner 1962). However, despite Macalpine's authoritative opinion, doubts still remain. There are many reports of individual cases in which emotional stress appeared to precipitate the initial attack of AA, or subsequent recurrences (Peck 1948; Kaplan & Reisch 1952; Ledo-Dunipe 1952; Reinhold 1960; Swift 1961; Greenberg 1955; Degossely 1965; Feldman & Rondón Lugo 1973). Experienced clinicians (e.g. Obermayer & Bowen 1956) wrote 'the perpetuating role of emotional tension states . . . is well authenticated'; and it is indeed true that most authorities express similar views. Alleged cures by suggestion (Bonjour 1932) or sleep therapy (Martin *et al.* 1959) have been claimed to support the stress hypothesis. A very prolonged and intensive investigation of twins with AA was inconclusive (Hommes & Prick 1968).

It is the opinion of the authors that stress is an important precipitating factor in some cases of AA. In many cases it appears to play no part, except when it arises secondarily as a result of the cosmetic disfigurement (Lubowe 1959), when it may be important in perpetuating the condition. The findings of Ferraro (1979) using the Bernereuter personality index showed 'feelings of inferiority, introspection and a need for encouragement'. Surely such features are commonly secondary to the AA.

The role of organic nervous disease in AA is unknown. The claim that the EEG showed that abnormalities in the region of the brain stem were present in 70% of 50 patients awaits confirmation (Haas & Lehnert 1971). An earlier study of the EEG in 45 patients (Parisis *et al.* 1968) has shown an apparent association between AA particularly in acute forms in postmenopausal women, and EEG abnormalities.

The 'reflex-irritation' extension of the trophoneurotic theory is revived from time to time either in association with errors of refraction (Haynes & Parry 1949), with intraocular foreign bodies (McGrath 1951) or with dental lesions (Grace 1942). No evidence suggesting that such occurrences are more than fortuitous has been reported. The significance of the observation that 67% of 428 bald patches in 134 patients were within the distribution of C2 is uncertain (Hönemann & Höfer 1970). The radiological examination of the cervical region of the spine showed no relevant abnormalities (Höfer *et al.* 1969).

References

Bonjour J. (1932) Observations on alopecia areata. *Urological and Cutaneous Review,* **36**, 674.
Degossely M. (1965) L'Interêt de l'etude psychosomatique dans quelques cas de pelade totale. *Archives Belges de Dermatologie et Syphiligraphie,* **21**, 257.

Feldman M. & Rondón Lugo A.J. (1973) Consideracions psicosomaticas en la alopecia areata. *Medicina Cutanea*, **7**, 95.

Ferraro S. (1979) Il Bernereuter Personality Inventory in ammelati di area Celsi. *Clinica Dermatologica*, **10**, 51.

Grace J.D. (1942) Extensive alopecia areata of dental origin. *Archives of Dermatology and Syphilology*, **45**, 349.

Greenberg S.I. (1955) Alopecia areata. A psychiatric survey. *A.M.A. Archives of Dermatology*, **72**, 454.

Haas W. & Lehnert W. (1971) Elektroenzephalographisch nachgewissene Funktionstörungen des oralen Hirnstammes bei der Alopecia areata. *Dermatologische Wochenschrift*, **157**, 855.

Haynes H.A. Jr. & Parry T.L. (1949) Alopecia areata associated with refractive errors. *Archives of Dermatology and Syphilology*, **59**, 340.

Höfer W., Hönemann W. & Sierke M.L. (1969) Haufigkeit und Bedeutung degenerativer Veränderungen der Halswirbelsäule bei der Alopecia areata. *Hautarzt*, **20**, 276.

Hommes O.P. & Prick J.J.G. (1968) *Alopecia Maligna*. Amsterdam, North-Holland Publishing Company.

Hönemann W. & Höfer W. (1970) Bestehen Beziehungen zwischen der Lokalisation der Alopecia-areata-Herde und der nervalen Versorgung des Kopfes? *Dermatolegische Monatschrift*, **156**, 683.

Kaplan H. & Reisch M. (1952) Universal alopecia: a psychosomatic appraisal. *New York State Journal of Medicine*, **52**, 1144.

Ledo-Dunipe E. (1952) Emocion y alopecias en areas. *Actas Dermo-Sifiliograficas*, **44**, 139.

Lubowe I.I. (1959) The clinical aspects of alopecia areata, totalis and universalis. *Annals of the New York Academy of Science*, **83**, 458.

Macalpine I. (1958) Is alopecia areata psychosomatic? *British Journal of Dermatology*, **70**, 117.

McGrath H. (1951) Alopecia associated with an intraocular foreign body. *Archives of Ophthalmology*, **46**, 319.

Martin P., Levy A., Minvielle J., Risacher D. & Birouste M.-J. (1959) Application de la médicine psychosomatique à la dermatologie. *Presse médicale*, **67**, 461.

Obermayer M.E. & Bowen E.T. (1956) Trichotillomania and alopecia areata. *Pediatric Clinics of North America*, **3**, 639.

Panconesi E. & Mantellassi G. (1955) Fattori psichici nella etiopatogenesi dess' area celsi. *Rassegna di Dermatologia e Sifilografia*, **8**, 121.

Panconesi E. & Mantellassi G. (1956) Ulteriori risultati di indageni psicodiagnostiche nella alopecia areata. *Rassegna di Dermatologia e Sifilografia*, **8**, 205.

Parisis N.G., Fabry H. & Muller E. (1968) Neue Aspekte der Pathogenese des Alopecia areata in Zusammenhang mit elektroencephalographische Untersuchungen. *Aesthetische Medizin*, **17**, 277.

Peck, R.E. (1948) Alpoecia [sic] areata as conversion symptom. *Journal of the Medical Association of Georgia*, **37**, 226.

Reinhold M. (1960) Relationship of stress to the development of symptoms in alopecia areata and chronic urticaria. *British Medical Journal*, **i**, 846.

Spitzner R. (1962) Alopecia areata und psychische Spannung. *Hautarzt*, **13**, 257.

Swift S. (1961) Folie à deux. *Archives of Dermatology*, **84**, 932.

Experimental induction of alopecia areata

Since the classical experiments of Max Joseph of Berlin in 1886, there have been numerous attempts to induce AA in man and in other mammals. The methods employed have been determined by the pathogenetic concept fashionable at the time. For example, Joseph used nerve section and produced alopecia, but not AA, in cats. Ikeda (1967), accepting the possible relevance of focal infection and stress, used noradrenalin and a staphylococcal vaccine in human volunteers; she succeeded in producing a bald patch which had only some of the features of AA. Among many other such experiments, those of Thiers & Klaschka (1970) in guinea-pigs also failed to produce lesions acceptable as AA.

References

Ikeda T. (1967) Produced alopecia areata based on the focal infection theory and mental motion theory. *Dermatologica*, **134**, 1.

Joseph M. (1886) Experimentele Untersuchungen über die Atiologie der Alopecia areata. *Monatshefte für praktischer Dermatologie*, **5**, 483.

Thiers W. & Klaschka F. (1970) Tierexperimentelle Sensibilisings studien als Beitrag zur Pathogenese der Alopecia areata. *Archiv für klinische und experimentelle Dermatologie*, **237**, 51.

Pathology
(References p. 286)

The earliest histological changes are a combination of degenerative changes in connective tissue around vessels leading to the papilla, and a perivascular inflammatory infiltrate, mainly lymphocytic, around the bulb. It does not invade the papilla but may involve the internal root sheath (Van Scott 1959). There may be spongiosis of the epidermis and lymphocytic infiltration around the openings of the follicles (Goos 1971). The follicles are much reduced in size as the disease becomes established, and the volume of the matrix is disproportionately decreased in relation to that of the papilla (Van Scott & Ekel 1958). These small follicles are in a phase comparable to Anagen IV, beyond which they appear to be restrained from proceeding (Van Scott 1958). Melanin granules may be seen in the papilla. In well-established lesions the inflammatory infiltration is less in evidence (Vilanova & Moragas 1963).

Degenerative connective changes in the papilla have been emphasized by some authors (Tagliavini & Dal Pozzo 1964). An inconclusive claim has been made on the basis of studies of serial sections that the degeneration of the matrix may be attributed to a cell-mediated reaction against matrix cells (Thies 1966). The number of mast cells in involved skin is no greater than normal (Späth & Steigleder 1970), although the bald patches were the first to develop weals when a histamine liberator was administered (Juhlin 1963).

The changes of AA may be more extensive than is clinically evident. Around the edge of a patch the proportion of telogen hairs and of dystrophic anagen hairs is increased, and similar but less severe changes may be found in the contralateral clinically normal scalp (Braun-Falco & Zaun 1962; Kostanecki & Kwiatkowska 1966). The presence of dystrophic hair in clinically normal scalp is, however, not a constant finding (Eckert *et al.* 1968). It has been claimed that in some patients with AA of the scalp, the clinically normal skin of the upper arm shows an intense cellular infiltrate around follicles and between the lobes of sebaceous glands (Lazovic-Tepavac & Salamon 1970).

Changes in the capillaries of affected follicles are regarded as secondary to the follicular changes and a response to the reduced circulatory requirements of the follicles (Uchiyama 1967). Alkaline phosphatase activity is diminished or absent in the papillae in early AA but as anagen becomes re-established in the miniature follicles alkaline phosphatase activity becomes intense (Kopf & Orentreich 1957). Investigations using Na^{131} suggested, however, that in chronic cases there may be some reduction in blood flow (Mian 1966).

In attempts to find anatomical support for the neurotrophic theory there have been many studies of the nerve supply of affected follicles. Most authorities find no abnormality using the light microscope (Winkelmann & Jaffe 1960; Gomez Orbaneja & Torres 1963). However, degenerative changes are said to occur in the vegetative nervous system, but this observation requires confirmation (Gohlke & Holtschmidt 1950). With the electronmicroscope degenerative changes in nerve fibres have been found in six cases of AA, but they may be a secondary phenomenon (Gay Prieto *et al.* 1974).

In prolonged AA the secretory activity of sebaceous glands declines with the duration of the disease (Schweikert 1967).

The abnormalities in the structure of the hair shaft characteristic of AA have been recognized for over a century. Pathognomonic are the exclamation-mark hairs (Fig. 10.2), which are, however, not invariably present. These hairs average about 3 mm in length (Eckert *et al.* 1968). They are club hairs the distal ends of which are ragged and frayed but of normal calibre and pigmentation. Below their broken tips they taper towards a small but otherwise normal club. Dystrophic anagen hairs are several centimetres long, but of reduced calibre and misshapen.

Electronmicroscopic studies of exclamation-mark hairs (Carteaud 1969; Jackson *et al.* 1971) show that the imbricated pattern of cuticular scales is well maintained up to the point of fracture; beyond this point strands of cortical and medullary tissue are evident.

Pathodynamics

Many attempts have been made to establish the sequence of follicular events in the development of AA. Eckert *et al.* (1968) studied hairs plucked from a series of concentric zones. Their results confirm earlier suggestions that an attack of AA begins with the premature entry of follicles into telogen at a focal point from which this process spreads outwards in a wave-like manner. However, the variations observed in the numbers of normal telogen hairs, dystrophic hairs and

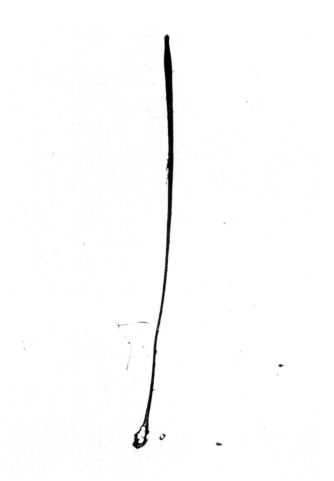

Fig. 10.2. Exclamation-mark
hair (Slade Hospital, Oxford).

exclamation-mark hairs can best be interpreted if it is postulated that the follicles
can respond in three different ways to the pathological trauma, depending on the
latter's severity. At its greatest severity it damages and weakens the hair in the
keratogenous zone, and at the same time precipitates the follicle into catagen.
Such hairs break when the keratogenous zone reaches the surface of the scalp,
and are later extruded as exclamation-marks. Alternatively a follicle may simply
be precipitated into normal catagen and subsequently be shed as a club hair.
Such follicles may then produce dystrophic anagen hairs. Finally it is possible
that some follicles are injured just sufficiently to induce dystrophic changes,
whilst they continue to grow in the anagen phase.

References

Braun-Falco O. & Zaun H. (1962) Uber die Beteiligung des gesamten Capilitiums bei Alopecia
areata. *Hautarzt*, 13, 342.

Carteaud J.-P. (1969) Cheveux de plaques peladiques examinés en microscope électronique par balayage. *Bulletin de la Société française de Dermatologie et de Syphilographie*, **76**, 660.

Eckert J., Church R.E. & Ebling F.J. (1968) The pathogenesis of alopecia areata. *British Journal of Dermatology*, **80**, 203.

Gay Prieto J., Gonzalez G. & Urio-Roco A. (1974) Inervación del folículo piloso de las alopecias universales. *Actas Dermo-Sifiliográficas*, **65**, 477.

Gohlke & Holtschmidt (1950) Neurohistologische Studien bei Alopecia areata. *Archiv für Dermatologie und Syphilologie*, **191**, 527.

Gomez Orbaneja J. & Torres A. de C. (1963) Inervación del folículo pilosebacea en la alopecia areata. *Actas Dermo-Sifiliográficas*, **54**, 387.

Goos M. (1971) Zur Histopathologie der Alopecia areata. *Archiv für Dermatologische Forschung*, **240**, 160.

Jackson D., Church R.E. & Ebling F.J. (1971) Alopecia areata hairs. A scanning electron microscopic study. *British Journal of Dermatology*, **85**, 242.

Juhlin L. (1963) Reactions to infusion of a histamine liberator. *Archives of Dermatology*, **88**, 771.

Kopf A.W. & Orentreich N. (1957) Alkaline phosphatases in alopecia areata. *Archives of Dermatology*, **76**, 288.

Kostanecki W. & Kwiatkowska E. (1966) Uber Wachstums und Melanogenese-Störungen der Haare bei Alopecia areata. *Archiv für klinische und experimentelle Dermatologie*, **226**, 21.

Lazovic-Tepavac O. & Salamon T. (1970) Uber die Histopathologie der Alopecia areata. *Dermatologische Monatschrift*, **156**, 665.

Mian E.U. (1966) Sull'irrorazione del cuoro capelluto nell'alopecia areata. *Giornale Italiano di Dermatologia*, **107**, 919.

Schweikert H.U. (1967) Quantitative Untersuchungen über die Telgdrüsenfunktion bei Alopecia areata. *Archiv für klinische und experimentelle Dermatologie*, **230**, 96.

Späth U. & Steigleder G.K. (1970) Zahl der Mastzellen bei Alopecia areata. *Zeitschrift für Haut und Geschlechtskrankheiten*, **45**, 435.

Tagliavini R. & Dal Pozzo V. (1964) Osservazioni istochemische in alcuni casi di area Celsi. *Giornale Italiano di Dermatologia*, **105**, 195.

Thies W. (1966) Vergleichende histologische Untersuchungen bei Alopecia areata und narbig-atrophierenden Alopecia. *Archiv für klinische und experimentelle Dermatologie*, **227**, 541.

Uchiyama M. (1967) Histological and histochemical studies of alopecia areata. *Japanese Journal of Dermatology*, **72**, 281.

Van Scott E.J. (1958) Morphologic changes in pilosebaceous units and anagen hairs in alopecia areata. *Journal of Investigative Dermatology*, **31**, 35.

Van Scott E.J. (1959) Evaluation of disturbed hair growth in alopecia areata and other alopecias. *Annals of the New York Academy of Science*, **83**, 480.

Van Scott E.J. & Ekel T.M. (1958) Geometric relationships between the matrix of the hair bulb and its dermal papilla in normal and alopecic scalp. *Journal of Investigative Dermatology*, **31**, 281.

Vilanova X. & de Moragas J.M. (1963) Alopecia areata (injertos e histologia) *Actas Dermo-Sifiliográficas*, **54**, 337.

Winkelmann R.K. & Jaffe M.O. (1960) Nerve network of the hair follicles in alopecia areata. *Archives of Dermatology*, **82**, 750.

Heterogeneity

(References p. 288)

Most authorities have regarded AA as a clinicopathological entity but the bewildering variety of its associated diseases and the unpredictability of its course are more readily explained if AA is in fact a heterogeneous clinical syndrome.

Ikeda (1965) proposed a classification which took into account other clinical features in addition to the alopecia itself. Studies in Nijmegen (Penders 1967; Mali 1975) and in Cambridge (Rook 1977) have supported Ikeda's hypothesis and are providing evidence which suggests that there may be considerable geographical variation in the relative incidence of the various types of AA.

Ikeda's four types may be categorized as follows—the incidence figures are those she recorded in Japan.

Type I. The common type accounted for 83% of patients. It occurred mainly between the ages of 20 and 40, and usually ran a total course of less than 3 years. Individual patches tended to regrow in less than 6 months, and alopecia totalis developed in only 6%.

Type II. The atopic type accounted for 10% of patients. The onset was usually in childhood and the disease ran a lengthy course in excess of 10 years. Individual patches tended to persist for over a year and alopecia totalis developed in 75%.

Type III. The prehypertensive type (4%) occurred mainly in young adults and ran a rapid course with an incidence of alopecia totalis of 39%.

Type IV. The 'combined' type (5%) occurred mainly in patients over 40 and ran a prolonged course, but resulted in alopecia totalis in only 10%.

Almost all published work on AA has been based on the assumption that AA is a single entity. The clinical description below follows this convention since Ikeda's approach to the disease has not yet been applied sufficiently widely for its validity to be established.

References

Ikeda T. (1965) A new classification of alopecia areata. *Dermatologica*, **131**, 421.

Mali J.W.H. (1975) Alopecia areata. *British Journal of Dermatology*, **93**, 605.

Penders A.J.M. (1967) Alopecia areata and atopy. *Dermatologica*, **136**, 395.

Rook A.J. (1977) Common baldness and alopecia areata. In *Recent Advances in Dermatology*, vol. 4, ed. A.J. Rook. Edinburgh, Churchill Livingstone, p. 223.

Age and sex incidence

The available statistics are all based on hospital attendance figures and may therefore not reflect the true incidence of AA. It is certain that financial status, accessibility and customs influence outpatient attendance in different ways in different countries and that therefore apparent geographical differences cannot be accepted without further evidence.

In 164 cases of AA in Sheffield, England (Anderson 1950), the onset was before the age of 21 in 44% and over the age of 40 in 19.5%. The sexes were

equally affected. In Portugal (Bastos Araujo & Poiares Baptista 1967) the onset
was before the age of 20 in 32.5% and over the age of 40 in about 20%. Males
accounted for 60% of all cases and between the ages of 20 and 39 outnumbered
females 3:1. In Sweden (Gip *et al.* 1969) 35% of cases began under the age of 21
and 25% over the age of 40. Figures from Cadiz, Spain (Lopez 1951) show 35%
under 20 and 20% over 40, with a significant predominance of males. In North
America (Muller & Winkelmann 1963) about 27% of cases began before the age
of 20 and about 30% after the age of 40. Many other series of cases show
apparently the same age incidence with minor variations, the significance of
which cannot be evaluated.

Onset in the first year is unusual, but has been recorded in the 4th month of
life (Switzer 1947). In an investigation in Italy confined to children with AA
(Bessone 1965), only 0.93% of 213 cases began in the 1st year, and the peak
incidence was in the 4th and 5th years. Onset before the age of 2 was recorded in
under 2% of 736 cases in North America (Muller & Winkelmann 1963).

In summary, if all clinical variants of AA are grouped together the hospital
statistics of most countries show the sexes to be equally affected, and the onset to
occur at any age, with a peak decade lying at some point between the ages of 20
and 50.

References
Anderson I. (1950) Alopecia areata: a clinical study. *British Medical Journal*, **ii**, 1250.
Bastos Araujo A. & Poiares Baptista A. (1967) Algunas consideracons sobre 300 casos de pelada. *Traballos da Sociedade Portugesa de Dermatologia e Venereologia*, **15**, 135.
Bessone L. (1965) Rilievi statistici sull'alopecia areata nell'infanzia. *Aggiornamento Pediatrico*, **16**, 1.
Gip L., Lodin A. & Molin L. (1969) Alopecia areata. *Acta Dermatovenereologica*, **49**, 180.
Lopez B. (1951) Contribucion al conocimiento de la etiopatogenia y tratamiento de la pelada. *Actas Dermo-Sifiliograficas*, **42**, 589.
Muller S.A. & Winkelmann R.K. (1963) Alopecia areata. *Archives of Dermatology*, **88**, 290.
Switzer S.E. (1947) Alopecia areata in an infant. *Archives of Dermatology and Syphilology*, **55**, 143.

Clinical features
(References p. 298)

The initial lesion of AA is most characteristically a circumscribed totally bald
smooth patch, asymptomatic and noticed by chance by a parent, hairdresser or
friend (Fig. 10.3). The surface of the patch is white and without scale.
Exclamation-mark hairs (Fig. 10.4) may be present at its margin, in which
region hairs which appear normal may also be very readily extracted. Subjective
symptoms are commonly lacking, but some few patients complain of irritation,
tenderness or paraesthesiae immediately preceding the development of a new
patch.

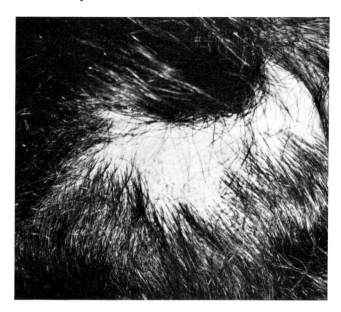

Fig. 10.3. Alopecia areata: circumscribed patches in a man aged 20 (Addenbrooke's Hospital, Cambridge).

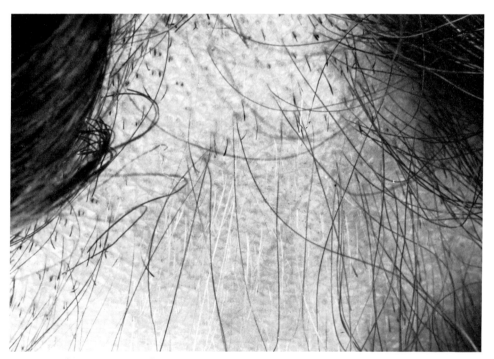

Fig. 10.4. Alopecia areata with numerous exclamation-mark hairs (Addenbrooke's Hospital, Cambridge).

The initial patch may regrow within a few months, or further patches may appear after an interval of 3–6 weeks and then still more patches after a similar interval (Figs. 10.5, 10.6). These intervals are of no constant duration. A succession of discrete patches may rapidly become confluent by the diffuse loss of the remaining hair (Fig. 10.7). In some cases, however, the initial hair loss is diffuse and total denudation of the scalp may occur within 48 hours. When regrowth takes place it is often at first fine and unpigmented, but the hairs gradually resume their normal calibre and colour. Regrowth in one region of the scalp may occur whilst the alopecia is extending in others (Fig. 10.8).

Although it is sometimes claimed that, in over 60% of cases, the scalp is the first site to be affected, this figure may be totally inaccurate: in children and in fair-haired adults, small patches of AA on the limbs or face may be difficult to detect even when they are deliberately sought. In dark-haired men patches in the beard are conspicuous, and in such individuals are often the first to be noticed.

The eyebrows and eyelashes are lost in many cases of AA and at times only the lashes or only the eyebrows may be affected by the disease (Fig. 10.9).

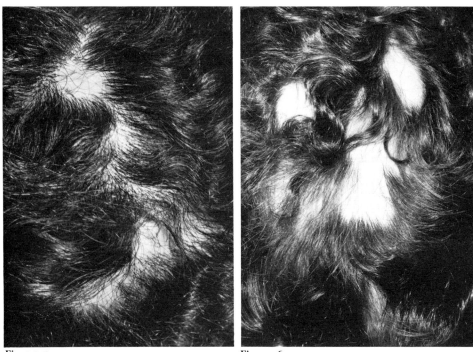

Fig. 10.5   Fig. 10.6

Fig. 10.5. The reticular pattern of AA at an early stage; often seen in atopic subjects (Addenbrooke's Hospital, Cambridge).

Fig. 10.6. A more advanced stage of the same clinical form, not in the same patient. This form, in which there is a network of irregularly linked patches, has a less good prognosis than the commoner form with multiple discrete patches.

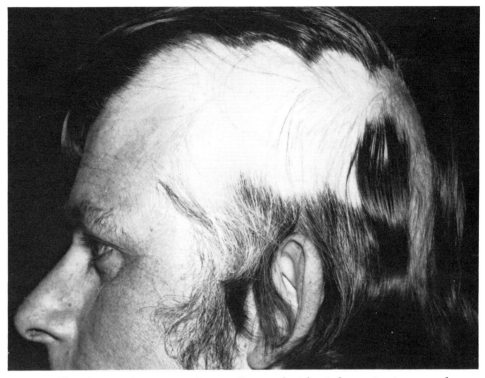

Fig. 10.7. Alopecia areata in a man aged 43: confluence of patches to form extensive areas of baldness (Addenbrooke's Hospital, Cambridge).

The term alopecia totalis is applied to total or almost total loss of scalp hair (Fig. 10.10), and alopecia universalis is the loss also of all body hair. The extension of alopecia along the scalp margin is known as ophiasis (Fig. 10.11). AA strictly confined to one half of the body is very rarely seen. It has been reported after a head injury (Klingmüller 1958).

Several investigators have recorded the site of the initial patch in the scalp and it has been claimed (Anderson 1950) that the occiput is favoured in the male (35%, cf. female 15%) and the frontovertical region in the female (31%, cf. male 15%). However, the site of the initial patch, whether in the scalp or not, appears to have no prognostic significance. AA may remain confined to a single patch in the scalp, or in the beard, or on an extremity, or to the lashes or brows of one eye only (Kile 1960). Equally, however, the onset in any of these sites does not preclude subsequent generalization.

The course of AA, considered as a single entity, is unpredictable. Statistics published from different countries show significant differences in prognosis. Such differences are readily explained if, as may be the case, the different types of AA as defined by Ikeda (p. 288) differ in their relative incidence. In Chicago (Walker &

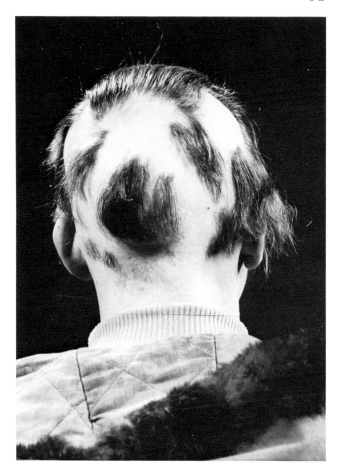

Fig. 10.8. Alopecia areata in a male adolescent. Hair of normal calibre regrows but further patches develop simultaneously and the pattern changes over a period of weeks. This variant of the reticular pattern of Alopecia areata tends to run a long course (Addenbrooke's Hospital, Cambridge).

Rothman 1950) the duration of the initial attack was less than 6 months in 33%, and less than 1 year in 50%, but 33% never recovered from the initial attack. The incidence of relapses in the whole series of 230 patients was 86%, but in those followed up for over 20 years it was 100%. Of those developing AA before puberty 50% became totally bald and none recovered. In contrast only 25% of those developing AA after puberty became totally bald and 5.3% recovered. In the Mayo Clinic series (Muller & Winkelmann 1963) only 1% of the children and 10% of adults with alopecia totalis showed complete regrowth. The course in 140 cases in Madrid (Gomez Orbaneja 1963) was apparently less unfavourable, since the AA ran a short course in 49% and became total in 3.4% and universal in 6.7%. In Sweden (Gip *et al.* 1969) a 10–15-year follow-up showed complete recovery in 34% of males and 37% of females and a tendency for regrowth to begin earlier in females (54% within 6 months) than in males (34% within 6 months). A study of 50 patients with alopecia universalis (Schmitt 1953)

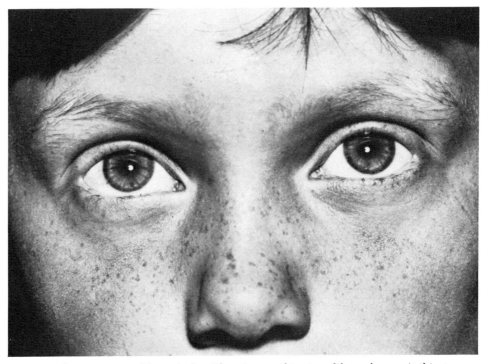

Fig. 10.9. Alopecia areata of the eyelashes. There is some thinning of the eyebrows. At this stage no other site was affected (Addenbrooke's Hospital, Cambridge).

showed complete recovery in only 20% with a worse prognosis in cases of prepubertal onset.

These diverse and not strictly comparable findings are difficult to interpret intelligently. Our findings in Cambridge emphasize the importance of associated disorders. AA in the atopic state has a poor prognosis, and if total before puberty is unlikely to regrow permanently. AA at any age, in a nonatopic subject, may be given a reasonably good prognosis, if it has remained circumscribed for over 6 months. It has been stated that the prognosis is less good in patients with a family history of AA, but this has not been our experience. The ophiasic pattern of AA has, in our material, been associated with atopy, and deserves its traditional bad reputation. The same pattern of AA occurs in sickle-cell anaemia, when it again suggests a poor prognosis (El Nasr & Roaiyah 1954) (Figs. 10.12, 10.13).

Pregnancy is sometimes associated with the regrowth of long-standing severe AA, but the recovery is usually only temporary (Sulen *et al.* 1956). In no case of AA is a completely confident prognosis justifiable; one woman lost all her hair at 16, failed to regrow it despite eight pregnancies, but recovered it almost completely at the age of 50 (Freeman 1952).

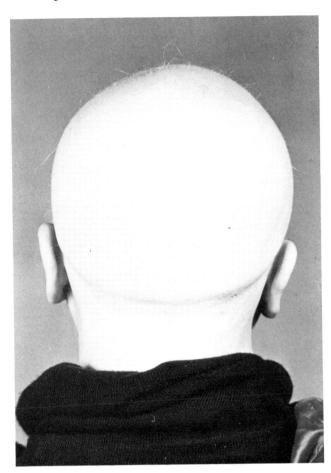

Fig. 10.10. Alopecia totalis.
There is a sparse regrowth of
unpigmented vellus hair
(Slade Hospital, Oxford).

White hair in alopecia areata

If the patient has some white hairs at the time of onset of AA, these are usually
spared by the disease process (Klingmüller 1958). If, therefore, the white hairs
are numerous the sudden diffuse onset of AA may result in the patient's shedding
only his pigmented hairs, and they appearing to 'go white' over the course of a
few days (Helm & Milgrom 1970). This phenomenon has taken place in dramatic
circumstances where severe stress has induced AA in some celebrated personali-
ties of history (Jellinek 1972).

Associated clinical changes

Nails. The reported incidence of nail dystrophy in AA ranged from over 33%
(Demis & Weiner 1963) to 2–3%, and clearly depends on the diligence with
which such changes are sought, but it also depends on the severity of the AA. In

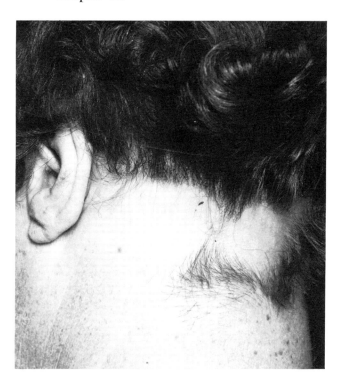

Fig. 10.11. Alopecia areata: ophiasic form. This patient also had extensive vitiligo of which one small patch can be seen here (Addenbrooke's Hospital, Cambridge).

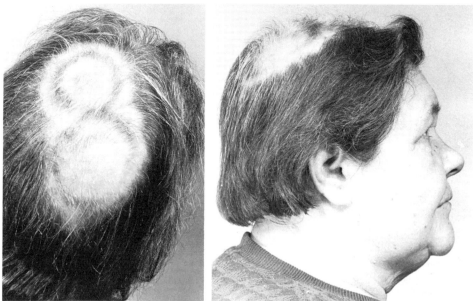

Figs. 10.12 and 10.13. Alopecia areata in a patient with myxoedema. The annular pattern of regrowth is occasionally seen in any patient with AA treated with topical corticosteroids (Staffordshire Hospital Centre, Stoke-on-Trent).

some 50% of cases of total or universal alopecia the nails are opaque and longitudinally ridged, with a serrated free edge (Anderson 1950). In such cases the dystrophy may be severe and conspicuous (Arutjunow 1971). Irregular pitting was found in 66% of 62 cases of AA in Germany, as compared with 8.6% of school children (Klingmüller & Reeh 1955). In another series of 123 cases in North America (Tobias 1954) nail changes were noted in 10%; pitting in 4%, longitudinal ridging in 5% and onychorrhexis in 3%. Our experience confirms the frequency of ridging and opacity of the nails in alopecia totalis, but we found pitting in only 10% of cases of ordinary AA. However, ridging, pitting and opacity may occur in typical AA and may persist long after the hair has regrown (Horn & Odom 1980) (Fig. 10.14).

Eyes. The conflicting reports on the incidence of lens opacities in AA once again reflect the heterogeneity of this disorder. Symptomless punctate lens opacities were no more frequent in 58 patients with AA than in normal controls (Summerly *et al.* 1966). There are, however, many reports of cataracts in association with alopecia totalis (Muller & Brunsting 1963), and in two of five adults so affected rapid impairment of vision coincided with episodes of sudden and widespread alopecia.

Other ocular abnormalities have been found in AA, e.g. Horner's syndrome, ectopias of the pupil, iris atrophy or tortuosity of the fundal vessels (Langhof & Lenke 1962), but these findings require confirmation in a larger series of patients with appropriate controls. The presence of optic atrophy and pigmentary

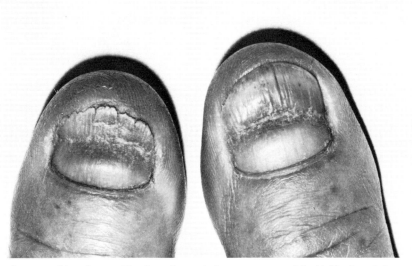

Fig. 10.14. Severe nail involvement in alopecia areata in a woman aged 62 (Addenbrooke's Hospital, Cambridge).

changes in the retina in a girl with alopecia totalis may have been fortuitous (Pisatsky & Kozinn 1942).

Other associations. The association of AA with atopy, vitiligo and various endocrine disorders has been discussed above. Such associations in the patient and his family should always be sought.

Many other associations have been reported, which may not be significant, e.g. retarded development and undescended testes (Schirren 1964); hypogonadism (Pozzo 1964); acute polyneuritis—the diagnosis of AA in these two cases is not beyond doubt (Radermecker 1944); left facial hemiatrophy and hypochromia of the iris (Collin 1960).

AA is one component of the Vogt–Koyanagi syndrome.

Diagnosis

The diagnosis of AA in the typical circumscribed form usually presents no difficulties, and can be confirmed microscopically by the presence of exclamation-mark and dystrophic hairs. Occasionally lupus erythematosus may simulate AA, and must be differentiated by biopsy (Borda *et al.* 1965). In the absence of exclamation-mark hairs or in the presence of scaling, ringworm must be excluded by examination under Wood's lamp, and by microscopy and culture. A traumatic alopecia, self-inflicted as a result of a hair pulling tic, may cause difficulties and can indeed be associated with AA which has drawn the child's attention to his scalp.

The presence of numerous small irregular patches should suggest the possibility of secondary syphilis; other clinical evidence of this disease should be sought and serological tests for syphilis should be carried out. Such tests are advisable in all cases of apparently atypical AA in which the diagnosis is in some doubt.

The diffuse onset of AA cannot be differentiated clinically from post-febrile and other disturbances of the hair cycle, but dystrophic hairs should be sought since they are readily distinguished from the normal club hairs of the latter.

In chronic circumscribed lesions it is sometimes difficult to exclude scarring with certainty. After a period of observation if doubt still remains a biopsy may be desirable.

The rare congenital triangular alopecia (p.   ) is often not noted until the age of 5 or 6 or even later. It is diagnosed by its characteristic shape and site.

References

Anderson I. (1950) Alopecia areata: a clinical study. *British Medical Journal*, **i**, 1250.
Arutjunow W.J. (1971) Hochgradige Alopecia areata mit Nageldystrophie. *Dermatologische Monatschrift*, **157**, 789.

Borda J.M., Abulafia J. & Brechsbaum E. (1965) Lupus eritematoso peladoide de cuero canelludo. *Archives Argentinos de Dermatologia*, **15**, 129.

Collin M. (1960) Un cas de pelade avec alopécie temporale symétrique résiduelle chez un malade atteint d'hémiatrophie progressive de la face associée à une hypochromie irienne avec cataracte. *Journal de Génétique humaine*, **9**, 118.

Demis D.J. & Weiner M.A. (1963) Alopecia universalis, onychodystrophy and total vitiligo. *A.M.A. Archives of Dermatology*, **88**, 195.

El Nasr H.S. & Roaiyah M.F.A. (1954) Prognosis of alopecia areata. *Journal of the Egyptian Medical Association*, **37**, 476.

Freeman K.I. (1952) Alopecia areata. *Canadian Medical Association Journal*, **67**, 6.

Gómez Orbaneja J. (1963) Modalidades clínicas evolutivas de la alopecia areata. *Actas Dermo-Sifilográficas*, **54**, 353.

Gip L., Lodin A. & Molin L. (1969) Alopecia areata. *Acta Dermatovenereologica*, **49**, 180.

Helm F. & Milgrom H. (1970) Can scalp hair suddenly turn white? *A.M.A. Archives of Dermatology*, **102**, 162.

Horn R.T. & Odom R.E. (1980) Twenty-nail dystrophy of alopecia areata. *Archives of Dermatology*, **116**, 573.

Jellinek J.E. (1972) Sudden whitening of the hair. *Bulletin of the New York Academy of Medicine*, **48**, 1003.

Kile R.L. (1960) Alopecia of the eyelashes. *A.M.A. Archives of Dermatology*, **81**, 959.

Klingmüller G. (1958) Uber 'plötzliches Weissworden' und psychische Traumen bei der Alopecia areata. *Dermatologica*, **117**, 84.

Klingmüller G. (1958) Alopecia areata—Alopecia traumatica diffusa. *Dermatologische Wochenschrift*, **138**, 1053.

Klingmüller G. & Rech E. (1955) Nagelgrübchen und deren familiäre Häufungen bei der Alopecia areata. *Archiv für klinische und experimentelle Dermatologie*, **201**, 574.

Langhof H. & Lenke L. (1962) Ophthalmologische Befunde bei Alopecia areata. *Dermatologische Wochenschrift*, **146**, 585.

Muller S.A. & Brunsting L.A. (1963) Cataracts in alopecia areata. *A.M.A. Archives of Dermatology*, **88**, 202.

Muller S.A. & Winkelmann R.K. (1963) Alopecia areata. *A.M.A. Archives of Dermatology*, **88**, 290.

Pisetski J.E. & Kozinn P.J. (1942) Total alopecia associated with ocular disorders. *American Journal of Diseases of Children*, **64**, 80.

Pozzo G. (1964) Alopecia areata e impuberismo ipofisaria ipogonadotrofico maschile. *Giornale Italiano di Dermatologia*, **105**, 431.

Radermecker M.A. (1944) Alopécies et troubles endocrino-végétatifs au cours de la polyradiculonévrite avec dissociation albuminocytologique. *Dermatologica*, **90**, 248.

Schirren C. (1964) Allgemeine Entwicklungsretardierung bei Hodenhochstand, Vitiligo und Alopecia areata. *Zeitschrift für Haut und Geschlectskrankheiten*, **37**, 14.

Schmitt C.L. (1953) Trauma as a factor in the production of alopecia universalis. (Preliminary Report.) *Pennsylvania Medical Journal*, **56**, 975.

Sulen J.C., Stolte L.A.M., Bakker J.A.J. & Verboom E. (1956) Alopecia areata. *Acta Endocrinologica*, **23**, 60.

Summerly R., Watson D.M. & Copeman P.W.M. (1966) Alopecia areata and cataracts. *A.M.A. Archives of Dermatology*, **93**, 411.

Tobias N. (1954) Alopecia areata. *Postgraduate Medicine*, **15**, 50.

Walker S.A. & Rothman S. (1950) Alopecia areata. A statistical study and consideration of endocrine influences. *Journal of Investigative Dermatology*, **14**, 403.

Treatment

The variable and unpredictable course in the untreated patient with AA accounts for the multiplicity of uncritical claims for a variety of therapeutic procedures. Variations from country to country in the relative proportion of different types of AA may partly explain some striking differences between the benefits claimed by different authors for the same treatment. For example Arnold (1952) noted the excellent prognosis, without treatment, of AA in the Japanese of Hawaii. A high proportion of cases of Ikeda's Type 1 would account for this benign course and also for the claims in some other series such as that (Robinson & Robinson 1954) in which benzoyl benzoate gave 90% and phenol 80% of good results.

Many counter-irritants have been employed in AA, and some are still prescribed. There is no evidence from controlled trials, but they do, perhaps, stimulate regrowth in a proportion of cases. The same may be said of ultraviolet light which, however, remains popular. Grenz rays are said to have been beneficial (Keller-Podhrazky 1949) and so is the Kromayer lamp (Krook 1961), but once again controlled trials are lacking.

Applications of Thorium X still enjoy some waning support, although Wilson (1952) noted significantly that no 'refractory' case was cured.

Systemic corticosteroids will in most cases restore normal hair growth in AA. The hairs show abrupt repigmentation and thickening without discontinuity of the shaft (Berger & Orentreich 1960). There is still controversy, however, as to the justification for prescribing these potentially hazardous drugs, and as to the route by which they should be administered.

The efficacy of cortisone in all but a few cases of long duration and early onset was reported by Dillaha & Rothman (1952a, b) who emphasized that the hair was lost when the steroid was discontinued and that the treatment could not be recommended for general use. Regrowth of alopecia universalis of 18 years' duration was obtained with methyl prednisolone 12 mg daily (Lubowe 1959) and in another case of 9 years' duration by triamcinolone in a dose not less than 6 mg daily (Shelley *et al.* 1959). The problem of recurrence on cessation of treatment was again noted. Another trial (Alexander & Schmidt 1961) used prednisone in doses up to 100 mg daily; the response was good in 21 of 26 patients, and the tendency to early recurrence was greatest in cases of long duration. The problem of recurrence and the risks of maintenance treatment have continued to tax the ingenuity of dermatologists. Alternate day administration of oral triamcinolone was thought to minimize side effects (Reichling & Kligman 1961). In occasional cases of alopecia totalis the necessary maintenance dose may be acceptably small (Darvill 1963). It is likely that most of the patients whose hair is not lost when the steroids are discontinued would have recovered without their use, though perhaps more slowly (Duchková *et al.* 1971).

In attempts to reduce the hazards of systemic steroids both topical applications and intralesional injections have been advocated. The topical application under polythene of 0.025% fluocinolone was said to be effective (Gill & Baxter 1963) but subsequent experience with this and many other corticosteroids has not been encouraging. Persistent regrowth occurs in those cases in which it could be expected to occur spontaneously. In other cases the patient obtains no benefit and may suffer a troublesome folliculitis.

Intralesional steroids have proved more helpful but the positive indications for their use remain limited. Intralesional hydrocortisone was first shown to stimulate regrowth by Rony & Cohen (1955). In many cases of AA regrowth occurs 3–4 months after intralesional injection, but the hair is often lost again after a few months (Orentreich *et al.* 1960) (Fig. 10.15). Kalkoff & Macher (1958) had also shown that the regrowth was only temporary. However, in some cases, presumably those in which spontaneous regrowth would have taken place, the recovery is more persistent (Gombiner & Malkinson 1961). The

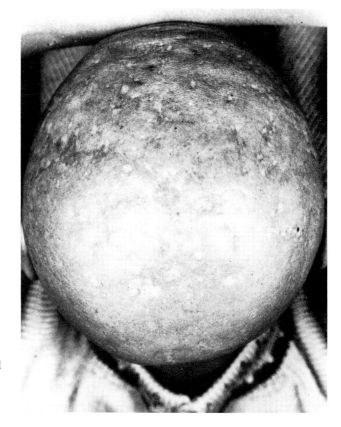

Fig. 10.15. Total alopecia areata with extensive scarring, the result of intralesional injection of cortiscosteroids (Addenbrooke's Hospital, Cambridge).

response to intralesional triamcinolone acetonide or hexacetonide has been described as 'all or nothing'; if it occurs it is maintained for about 9 months (Porter & Burton 1971).

Intralesional corticosteroids have a small but useful role in the management of AA. They can be used to accelerate regrowth in a circumscribed patch of AA which is cosmetically disfiguring and difficult to conceal. We have not found them to be of practical value in more extensive AA of the scalp. They can, however, be valuable even in alopecia totalis, for maintaining regrowth of the eyebrows (Berger 1961). Atrophy may be an unsightly complication of intralesional corticosteroids; it is usually confined to the injection sites, but sometimes following in linear pattern the direction of lymphatic flow over the forehead (Kikuchi & Horikawa 1975).

The treatment of AA by means of allergic contact dermatitis to dinitrochlor-benzene (DNCB) was at first reported with some enthusiasm. The technique employed has shown some variation. Sensitization is induced by painting the skin with a 2% solution of DNCB. The application 10 days later of a 0.1% solution will provoke a reaction in those patients (and they are the great majority), who

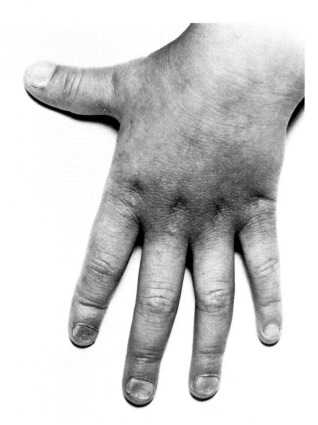

Fig. 10.16. Alopecia areata: severe dystrophy of all finger nails in a girl aged 5 (Addenbrooke's Hospital, Cambridge).

become sensitized. Weekly applications are then made to the bald areas using a concentration which may be as low as 0.0001% which is just sufficient to induce mild inflammatory changes. Regrowth is reported in a high proportion of cases (Happle *et al.* 1978).

Happle & Echtenecht (1977) treated only one half of the scalp with DNCB in 46 patients with AA. Some response was observed in 36. In 26 regrowth occurred only on the treated side but in another 14 it was faster and denser on the treated side. In 8 patients there was no response and in 2 the response was equal on both sides. In a later report Happle (1979) was able to claim complete regrowth in 78% of 227 patients treated. Promising results are reported by Gutschmidt (1979) and by Nagy *et al.* (1979).

The extent rather than the duration of alopecia appears to be important in determining response to treatment (Zisiades *et al.* 1980). All of three cases of patchy AA and all of three of almost total AA regrew with DNCB, but only 2 of 9

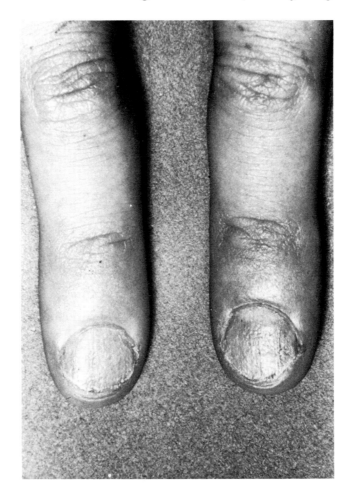

Fig. 10.17. Alopecia areata: nail pitting and longitudinal striation (Slade Hospital, Oxford).

with total AA. These findings are in general agreement with Damian & Rosenberg (1978). They found that if only refractory cases are treated, the response is much less good and in some 20% of these developing dermatitis there is no regrowth. De Prost *et al.* (1979) obtained a good result in only 25% of cases. Allavato *et al.* (1979) noted that control areas sometimes regrew as well as the treated areas. Warin's (1979) experience has been shared by many other dermatologists. He obtained only one excellent response in 9 cases. In 5 cases there was no regrowth after 17–32 weeks of treatment. The patient who gave an excellent response lost her hair again despite continued treatment. If this treatment is to be attempted it should be borne in mind that it may be uncomfortable and that DNCB may cross-sensitize to chloramphenicol and to chemicals used in laboratories and in agriculture. DNCB is mutagenic and some workers have therefore preferred to substitute squaric acid dibutyl ester, which is also a potent contact sensitizer but is not mutagenic (Happle *et al.* 1980). They used a 2% solution in acetone to induce sensitization and then a 0.1% solution to maintain a mild dermatitis. Only one side of the head was treated; a persistent regrowth was obtained in about 70%.

It has been questioned whether the induction of an allergic dermatitis has any special virtues. A primary irritant dermatitis caused by anthralin stimulated regrowth in 18 out of 24 patients (Schmoeckel *et al.* 1979). However, a recent comparative trial of an irritant—croton oil—and DNCB showed the latter to be very much more effective (Swanson *et al.* 1981).

It is probably too early to assess reliably the place of contact sensitization in the treatment of AA. The rate of response of alopecia totalis seems in general to be so disappointing that it is doubtful if it is worthwhile subjecting the patient to the discomfort of this treatment. However, in alopecia which is almost total and in which the patient has occasional tufts of hair, it may well be worth attempting treatment. It may also be worth trying this method of treatment in persistent patchy alopecia areata. If the lowest effective concentration of the allergen is used the discomfort is slight.

PUVA treatment has been used with success in some cases (Weismann *et al.* 1978; Claudy & Gagnaire 1980) but the treatment cannot be maintained as the growth of the hair tends to make further treatment ineffective. Nevertheless it has a place in the management of some cases. Lassus *et al.* (1980) used with equal success oral 8-methoxypsoralen 0.6 mg/kg of body weight 2 hours before exposure to UVA or 1% methoxypsoralen ointment 1 hour before light exposure. In 20% of patients there was no growth after 20 treatments and in a further 8 patients there was less than 30% recovery after 40 treatments. These cases, 37% of the total, were regarded as failures. Alopecia of prepubertal origin and of long duration in general responded less well than alopecia of late onset. Alopecia in atopic subjects showed as good an initial response to treatment as in nonatopics but there were fewer 'excellent' results in atopics.

The decision whether or not to treat AA should be made at an early stage. Nothing can justify the prolonged use of expensive placebos. If the prognosis is poor, e.g. if alopecia is total in a prepubertal atopic, full explanation and help in adjusting to the problems of wearing a wig will be of far greater value to a child than the false raising of unwarranted hopes. However, in the majority of cases in which the prognosis is good, reassurance, aided if necessary by topical or intralesional corticosteroids, can be advised. Systemic corticosteroids are justifiable only in exceptional circumstances. Treatment with DNCB probably has a place as mentioned above in some resistant cases.

References

Alexander L. & Schmidt G. (1961) Behandlungsergebnisse fortgeschrittener Fälle von Alopecia areata mit Prednison. *Dermatologische Wochenschrift,* **144,** 1342.

Allevato M.A., Chavarria G.M., Cordero A.A., Alonso A., Donatti C.B. & Del Aguila P.N. (1979) Empleo del dinitroclorobencena (DNCB) an ciertes tipos de alopecia areata. *Archivos Argentinos de Dermatologia,* **29,** 121.

Arnold H.L. (1952) Alopecia areata. Prevalence in Japanese and prognosis after reassurance. *A.M.A. Archives of Dermatology and Syphilology,* **66,** 191.

Berger R.A. (1961) Alopecia areata of eyebrows—corticosteroids. *A.M.A. Archives of Dermatology,* **83,** 151.

Berger R.A. & Orentreich N. (1960) Abrupt changes in hair morphology following corticosteroid therapy in alopecia areata. *A.M.A. Archives of Dermatology,* **82,** 408.

Claudy A.L. & Gagnaire D. (1980) Photochemotherapy in alopecia areata. *Actadermovenereologica* **60,** 171.

Daman L.A. & Rosenberg E.W. (1978) Treatment of alopecia areata with DNCB. *Archives of Dermatology,* **114,** 1036.

Darvill F.T. (1963) Steroid therapy in alopecia universalis. *A.M.A. Archives of Dermatology,* **87,** 706.

De Prost Y., Paquez F.-R. & Touraine R. (1979) Traitement de la pelade par application locale de DNCB. *Annales de Dermatologie et Venereologie,* **106,** 437.

Dillaha C.J. & Rothman S. (1952a) Therapeutic experiments in alopecia areata with orally administered cortisone. *Journal of the American Medical Association,* **150,** 546.

Dillaha C.J. & Rothman S. (1952b) Treatment of alopecia areata totalis and universalis with cortisone acetate. *Journal of Investigative Dermatology,* **18,** 5.

Duchková H., Horáková E. & Kulanda Z. (1971) Alopecia areata; its therapy and results of some biochemical tests. *Ceskoslovenská Dermatologie,* **46,** 203.

Gill K.A. & Baxter D.L. (1963) Alopecia totalis. *A.M.A. Archives of Dermatology,* **87,** 384.

Gombiner A. & Malkinson F.D. (1961) Triamcinolone suspension in alopecia areata. *A.M.A. Archives of Dermatology,* **83,** 1004.

Gutschmidt E. (1979) Beitrug zur DNCB Therapie der Alopecia areata. *Laryngologie, Rhinologie, Otologie und der Grenzgebiete,* **58,** 430.

Happle R. (1979) DNCB Therapie de Alopecia Areata. *Laryngologie, Rhinologie, Otologie und der Grenzgebiete,* **58,** 426.

Happle R., Cebulla K. & Echtnecht-Happle K. (1978) Dinitroclorobenzene therapy for alopecia areata. *Archives of Dermatology,* **110,** 1629.

Happle R. & Echternacht K. (1977) Alopecia areata: erfolgreich Halbseitenbehandlung mit DNCB. *Zeitschrift fur Hautkrankheiten,* **52,** 1129.

Happle R., Kalvaran K.J., Buchner U., Echternecht-Happle K., Goggelmann W., Summer J.H. (1980) Contact allergy as a therapeutic tool for alopecia areata: application of squaric acid dibutylester. *Dermatologica*, **161**, 289.

Kalkoff K.W. & Macher E. (1958) Uber des Nachwachsen der Haare bei der Alopecia areata und maligna nach intracutane Hydrocortisoninjektion. *Hautarzt*, **9**, 441.

Keller-Podhrazky H. (1949) Die Behandlung der Alopecia areata mit Grenzstrahlen. *Klinische Medizin (Vienna)*, **4**, 152.

Kikuchi I. & Horikawa S. (1975) Perilymphatic atrophy of the skin. *Archives of Dermatology*, **111**, 795.

Krook G. (1961) Treatment of alopecia areata with Kromayer's ultraviolet lamp. *Acta Dermato-venereologica*, **41**, 178.

Lassus A., Kiantu W., Johansson E. & Jurokoski T. (1980) PUVA treatment for alopecia areata. *Dermatologica*, **161**, 298.

Lubowe I.I. (1959) The treatment of alopecia universalis with methyl prednisolone (Medrol) associated with vitiligo, involving arms, forearms, neck and thigh. *A.M.A. Archives of Dermatology*, **79**, 665.

Nagy E., Torek E., Meszeros C. & Szekely I. (1979) DNCB Behandlung von Alopecia. *Zeitschrift für Hautkrankheiten*, **54**, 533.

Orentreich N., Sturm H.M., Weidman A.I. & Polzig A. (1960) Local injection of steroids and hair regrowth in alopecias. *A.M.A. Archives of Dermatology*, **82**, 894.

Porter D. & Burton J.L. (1971) A comparison of intralesional triamcinolone hexacetonide and triamcinolone acetonide in alopecia areata. *British Journal of Dermatology*, **85**, 272.

Reichling G.H. & Kligman A.M. (1961) Alternate day corticosteroid therapy. *A.M.A. Archives of Dermatology*, **83**, 980.

Rony H.R. & Cohen D.M. (1955) The effect of cortisone in alopecia areata. *Journal of Investigative Dermatology*, **25**, 285.

Schmoeckel C., Weissmann I., Pleurig G. & Braun-Falco O. (1979) Treatment of alopecia areata by artificially induced dermatitis. *Archives of Dermatology*, **115**, 1254.

Shelley W.B., Harun J.S. & Lehmann J.M. (1959) Long-term triamcinolone therapy of alopecia universalis. *A.M.A. Archives of Dermatology*, **80**, 433.

Swanson N.A., Mitchell A.J., Leahy N.S., Haddington J.T. & Diaz L.A. (1981) Topical treatment of Alopecia Areata. *Archives of Dermatology*, **117**, 384.

Warin A.P., Hehir M.E. & Du Vivier A. (1979). Alopecia areata treated with DNCB. *Clinical and Experimental Dermatology*, **4**, 385.

Weissmann I., Hoffmann C., Wagner G., Plewig G. & Braun-Falco O. (1978) PUVA therapy for alopecia areata. *Archives of Dermatological Research*, **262**, 333.

Wilson H.T.H. (1952) Thorium X in the treatment of alopecia areata. *Archives of the Middlesex Hospital*, **2**, 239.

Zisiadis S., Wuthrich B. & Schnyder U.W. (1980) Zur DNCB-Lokalbehandlung der alopecia areata. *Dermatologica*, **161**, 365.

Chapter 11
Cicatricial Alopecia

Introduction

Cicatricial alopecia is the generic term applied to alopecia which accompanies or follows the destruction of hair follicles, whether by a disease affecting the follicles themselves, or by some process external to them. The follicles may be absent as the result of a developmental defect or may be irretrievably injured by trauma, as in burns or radiodermatitis. They may be destroyed by a specific and identifiable infection—favus, tuberculosis or syphilis, for example—or by the encroachment of a benign or malignant tumour. In other cases their destruction can be reliably attributed to a named, though still mysterious disease process such as lichen planus or lupus erythematosus or sarcoidosis. When all the clinically and histologically acceptable causes have been eliminated, two named syndromes of cutaneous origin remain, pseudopelade and the less well defined foliculitis decalvans. Once these too have been excluded, there still remain cases in which any greater precision of diagnosis than 'cicatricial alopecia' may be unwarranted.

The clinical recognition of an area of scarring in the scalp should initiate a detailed investigation. Scarring is not always easy to identify with complete confidence, even with a hand lens if the scarred area is small, and it may be desirable to re-examine the patient after an interval, or to take a biopsy. Once the preliminary diagnosis of cicatricial alopecia has been made, the scalp should be searched for other changes—folliculitis, follicular plugging, telangiectasia or

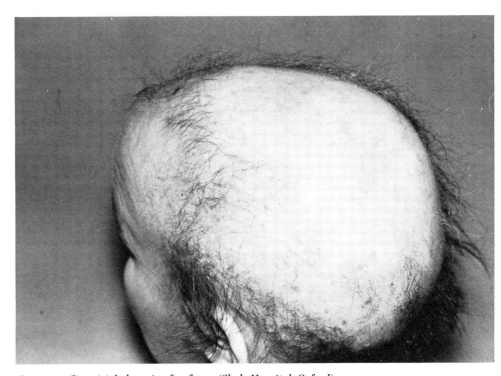

Fig. 11.1. Cicatricial alopecia after favus (Slade Hospital, Oxford).

broken hairs—and hairs, even if grossly normal in appearance, should be extracted from the edge of the bald area for microscopy and culture. If no satisfactory progress has been made towards a firm diagnosis, the patient's whole skin surface should be examined and a general physical examination also may be essential.

If the decision is made to take a biopsy, its site must be carefully selected and an early lesion should be preferred; late lesions may have lost all evidence of their origin.

Classification of causes
(Reference p. 310)

The causes of cicatricial alopecia are here classified into broad groups, and the individual causes are then considered in greater detail (classification modified from Ebling and Rook 1968).

1. *Developmental defects and hereditary disorders*
   Aplasia cutis (p. 55)
   Facial hemiatrophy (p. 336)
   Epidermal naevi (p. 500)
   Hair follicle hamartomas (p. 340)
   Incontinentia pigmenti (p. 339)
   Porokeratosis of Mibelli (p. 338)
   Scarring follicular keratosis (p. 324)
   Ichthyosis (p. 489)
   Darier's disease (p. 489)
   Epidermolysis bullosa (p. 340)
   Polyostotic fibrous dysplasia (p. 341)

2. *Physical injuries*
   Mechanical trauma (p. 330)
   Burns (p. 330)
   Radiodermatitis (p. 331)

3. *Fungous infections*
   Kerion (p. 380)
   Trichophyton violaceum (p. 378)
   T. sulphureum (p. 378)
   Favus (p. 378 and Fig. 11.1)

4. *Bacterial infections*
   Tuberculosis (p. 430)
   Syphilis (p. 430)

5. *Pyogenic infections*
   Carbuncle (p. 402)
   Furuncle (p. 401)
   Folliculitis (p. 476)
   Acne necrotica (p. 476)

6. *Protozoal infections*
   Leishmaniasis (p. 432)

7. *Virus infections*
   Herpes zoster (p. 435)
   Varicella (p. 435)

8. *Neoplasms*
   Basal cell epithelioma (p. 515)
   Squamous cell epithelioma (p. 518)
   Syringoma (p. 515)
   Metastatic tumours (p. 538)
   Reticuloses (p. 446)

9. *Dermatoses of uncertain origin*
   Lichen planus (p. 317)
   Graham-Little syndrome (p. 322)
   Dermatomyositis (p. 439)
   Lupus erythematosus (p. 438)
   Scleroderma (p. 336)
   Necrobiosis lipoidica (p. 334)
   Lichen sclerosus (p. 337)
   Sarcoidosis (p. 435)
   Cicatricial pemphigoid (p. 328)
   Follicular mucinosis (p. 496)
   Erosive pustular dermatosis (p. 329)

10. *Clinical syndromes*
    Pseudopelade (p. 311)
    Folliculitis decalvans (p. 314)
    Alopecia parvimacularis (p. 315)

Small irregular areas of scarring, together with broken hairs, may occur as the only defects as the result of the continued abuse of hair dyes and other cosmetics (p. 415 *et seq*). However, such changes may complicate other forms of alopecia as a result of the patient's misguided efforts to improve her appearance.

Reference
Ebling F.J. & Rook A.J. (1968) In *Textbook of Dermatology*, eds. A.J. Rook, D.S. Wilkinson and F.J.
    Ebling. Oxford, Blackwell Scientific Publications.

The clinical syndromes

History and nomenclature

In the literature of a hundred years ago and earlier there are descriptions of cases of cicatricial alopecia probably conforming to these three clinical syndromes, but although the cause of favus was discovered in the fifth decade of the last century such influential authorities as Erasmus Wilson continued for several decades to deny that the structures observed were anything other than 'phytiform degeneration'. The routine exclusion of bacterial and fungous infection in all cases of scarring alopecia was certainly not widely practised until the turn of the century. The earlier case reports cannot, therefore, be assessed with any confidence.

In 1885 Brocq of Paris described what later became known as *pseudopelade*, but as he himself subsequently admitted (Brocq 1907) it continues to confuse the nomenclature. Pseudopelade, studied in detail by Photinos (1930) is now regarded as a syndrome in which destruction of follicles leading to permanent patchy baldness is not accompanied by any clinically evident folliculitis.

Quinquaud (1888–9) described a form of scarring alopecia in which pustular folliculitis of the advancing margin was a conspicuous feature. To this condition the term *folliculitis devalvans* is now commonly applied. Unfortunately Lailler described similar cases as acne decalvans. Folliculitis decalvans affecting areas other than the scalp has been separately described by Arnozan (1892). Differing in degree from folliculitis decalvans is lupoid sycosis, so called by Milton (1865) and by Brocq et al. (1905). The follicles are destroyed by a granulomatous inflammatory process simulating lupus vulgaris. Unna (1889) applied the term ulerythema sycosiforme to the same condition.

Alopecia parvimaculata as described by Dreuw (1910) is a questionable entity. It has been regarded as pseudopelade occurring in childhood, but it differs from that syndrome in several respects.

Pinkus (1978), using acid alcoholic orcein stain, studied the distribution of elastic fibres around the hair follicles in many sections from biopsies in cicatricial alopecia of a variety of types. He found that the fibrous strands which replaced destroyed follicles in lichen planus and lupus erythematosus consist of collagen without elastic-like bodies or elastic fibres. In lupus erythematosus there is, in addition, widespread destruction of elastic fibres in the interfollicular dermis. The cases included 180 which satisfied the diagnostic criteria of pseudopelade: absence of sebaceous glands, more or less normal epidermis, no significant follicular plugging, small areas of subepidermal loss of elastic fibres, collagenous and elastic fibrosis at sites of destroyed follicles. Of these 180 cases, 106 showed additional features, which led Pinkus to differentiate them provisionally as 'fibrosing alopecia'. The most striking of these features is the development of elastic fibres around the lower part of the follicle, even at an early stage in the process. The features of fibrosing alopecia were a general hyperplasia of elastic fibres in the interfollicular dermis and the presence of less perifollicular cellular infiltrate than in pseudopelade. The age and sex incidence of the two conditions did not differ significantly. It remains to be established whether there are clinical differences.

References

Arnozan H. (1892) Folliculites dépilantes des parties glabres. *Annales de Dermatologie et de Syphiligraphie,* **3,** 491.

Brocq L. (1885) Alopecia. *Journal of Cutaneous and Venereal Diseases,* **3,** 49.

Brocq L., Lenglet E. & Ayrignac J. (1905) Recherches sur l'alopécie atrophiante, variété pseudopelade. *Annales de Dermatologie et de Syphiligraphie,* **6,** 1, 97, 209.

Brocq L. (1907) Pseudopelade. In *Traité élémentaire de Dermatologie pratique,* vol. 2. Paris, Doin, p. 648.

Dreuw H. (1910) Uber epidemische Alopecie. *Monatshefte für practische Dermatologie,* **51,** 18.

Milton J.L. (1865) cit. Jackson G.T. & McMurtry C.W. (1913) *A Treatise of Diseases of the Hair.* London, Kimpton, p. 182.

Photinos P. (1930) *La Pseudopelade de Brocq.* Paris, Maloine.

Pinkus H. (1978) Differential patterns of elastic fibres in scarring and non-scarring alopecias. *Journal of Cutaneous Pathology,* **5,** 93.

Quinquaud E. (1888) Folliculite destructive des regions vélues. *Bulletin et Mémoires de la Société médicale des Hôpitaux de Paris,* **5,** 395.

Quinquaud E. (1889) Folliculite épilante décalvante. *Annales de Dermatologie et de Syphiligraphie,* **10,** 99.

Unna P.G. (1889) Uber Ulerythema sycosiforme. *Monatshefte für practische Dermatologie,* **9,** 134.

Pseudopelade (references p. 312)

Nomenclature and aetiology. The term pseudopelade is used here to designate a slowly progressive cicatricial alopecia, without clinically evident folliculitis. There is no doubt that lichen planus can produce this clinical picture and there are some authorities who maintain on the basis of associated skin lesions and histopathological findings that 90% of cases of 'pseudopelade' are caused by lichen planus (Kaminsky *et al.* 1967). In another series of 35 cases lichen planus was diagnosed in only about 15% (Gay Prieto 1955). At a later stage lupus erythematosus also can cause similar changes. However, some patients with pseudopelade never show any clinical or histological evidence of lichen planus (Ronchese 1960). Pseudopelade is best regarded as a clinical syndrome which may be the end result of any one of a number of different pathological processes (known and unknown) (Degos *et al.* 1954).

Pathology (Laymon 1947; Lopez & Cardenas 1948; Degos *et al.* 1954). If clinically normal scalp at the edge of a plaque of pseudopelade is examined, numerous lymphocytes are seen around the upper two-thirds of the follicles. Later the follicles are destroyed and the epidermis becomes thin and atrophic, and the dermis densely sclerotic.

Clinical features (Van der Meiren 1933; Laymon 1947; Degos *et al.* 1954). Although both sexes may be affected, and the condition has occurred in childhood (Reinertson 1958), the patient is usually a woman and usually over 40. She may complain of slight irritation at first, but more often a small bald patch, discovered by chance by the patient or by her hairdresser, is the first evidence of the disease. The initial patch is most often on the vertex, but may occur anywhere on the scalp. The course thereafter is extremely variable. In a majority of cases extension of the process takes place only very slowly; indeed after 15 or 20 years the patient may still be able to arrange her hair to conceal the patches effectively. In some cases extension occurs more rapidly, and exceptionally there may be almost total baldness after 2 or 3 years.

On examination the affected patches are smooth, soft and slightly depressed. At an early stage in the development of any individual patch there may be some erythema, diffuse or perifollicular (Miescher & Lenggenhager 1947). The patches tend to be small and round or oval, but irregular bald patches may be formed by confluence of many lesions. The hair in uninvolved scalp is normal, but if the process is active the hairs at the edges of each patch are very easily extracted (Figs 11.2, 11.3).

Diagnosis. The characteristic feature is the development of small patches of cicatricial alopecia in the absence of any other clinical change, with the possible exception of transitory erythema.

Treatment. If the pseudopelade can be shown to be secondary to lichen planus or lupus erythematosus, then the treatment appropriate for these conditions may be prescribed. However, whether the baldness is of known or unknown origin it is irreversible. If the disfigurement is considerable and no active inflammatory changes are present, autografting from unaffected to scarred scalp may be considered (Stough *et al.* 1968; Curban & Gollman 1973).

The intradermal injection of corticosteroids has seemed not to influence the extension of the disease process in cases of unknown origin.

References

Curban G.V. & Gollman B. (1973) Pseudopelade de Brocq. *Medicina Cutanea*, **7**, 65.
Degos R., Rabut R., Duperrat B. & Leclerq R. (1954) L'état pseudopeladique. *Annales de Dermatologie et de Syphiligraphie*, **81**, 5.

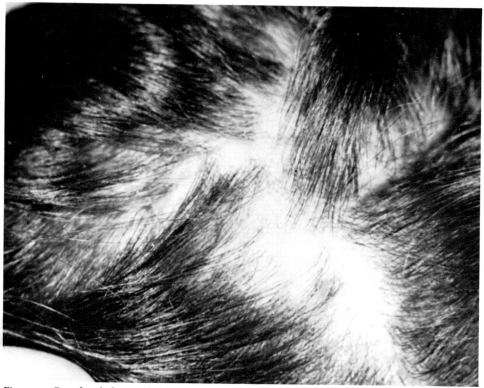

Fig. 11.2. Pseudopelade—early lesions (Addenbrooke's Hospital, Cambridge).

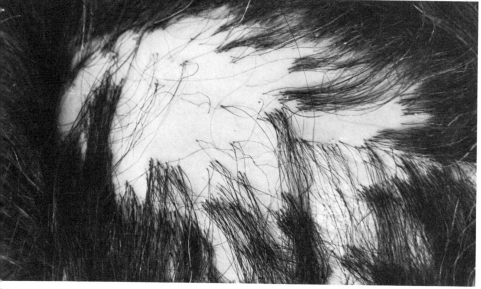

Fig. 11.3. Pseudopelade—advanced (North Staffordshire Hospital Centre, Stoke-on-Trent).

Gay Prieto J. (1955) Pseudopelade of Brocq: its relationship to some forms of cicatricial alopecia
    and to lichen planus. *Journal of Investigative Dermatology*, **24**, 323.
Kaminsky A., Kaminsky C.A., de Kaminsky A.R. & Abulafia J. (1967) Liquen folicular alopeciante.
    Medicina Cutanea, **2**, 135.
Laymon C.W. (1947) The cicatricial alopecias. *Journal of Investigative Dermatology*, **8**, 99.
Lopez B. & Cardenas M. (1948) Contribucion al estudio de la pseudopelade de Brocq. *Actas
    Dermo-Sifiliográficas*, **39**, 478.
Miescher G. & Lenggenhager R. (1947) Uber Pseudopelade, Brocq. *Dermatologica*, **94**, 122.
Reinertson R.P. (1958) Pseudopelade with nail dystrophy. *Archives of Dermatology*, **78**, 282.
Ronchese F. (1960) Pseudopelade. *Archives of Dermatology*, **82**, 336.
Stough D.B., Berger R.A. & Orentreich N. (1968) Surgical improvement of cicatricial alopecia of
    diverse etiology. *Archives of Dermatology*, **97**, 331.
Van der Meiren L. (1933) Contribution à l'étude de la pseudopelade. *Annales de Dermatologie et de
    Syphiligraphie*, **4**, 928.

Folliculitis decalvans

History and nomenclature. The history of the complex cicatricial alopecia
syndromes has been briefly summarized above (p. 307). Under the general term
folliculitis decalvans we group together the various syndromes in which
clinically evident chronic folliculitis leads to progressive scarring. The 'foliculite
dépilante' of Arnozan differs from Quinquaud's folliculitis decalvans in that the
latter affects the scalp, and the former other regions of the body; but they may
coexist. Similarly lupoid sycosis, with its many synonymns, is a scarring
folliculitis affecting predominantly the beard.

Aetiology. The cause of folliculitis decalvans is still uncertain. *Staphylococcus
aureus* may be grown from the pustules but, more often, only ordinarily
non-pathogenic organisms are isolated. Some abnormality of the host must be
postulated. Some authors have emphasized the possible role of the seborrhoeic
state and some have used the term 'cicatrizing seborrhoeic eczema' (Laymon
1947), but folliculitis decalvans is rare and the seborrhoeic state is common, so
the association probably has no special significance.

   Shitara *et al.* (1947) reported severe folliculitis devalvans in two siblings who
also had chronic oral candidiasis; defective cell-mediated immunity was
demonstrated. It seems probable that a failure in the immune response or in
leucocyte function may be the essential abnormality in most cases, perhaps in
all.

   Folliculitis decalvans of the scalp occurs in both sexes. It affects women aged
30–60 and men from adolescence onwards; rarely it may be present from
infancy (Loewenthal 1957). In other sites it affects mainly adult males.

Pathology. Follicular abscesses with a polymorphonuclear infiltrate are directly
succeeded by scarring, or there may be a prolonged intermediate stage of
granulomatous folliculitis with numerous lymphocytes, and some plasma cells

and giant cells. Eventually only the remains of follicles can be detected in areas of scar tissue.

Clinical features. Any or all hairy regions may be involved, and in the syndrome sometimes referred to as 'atrophic folliculitis in seborrhoeic dermatitis' as described by Hallopeau, the beard, pubes, axillae and inner thighs may be involved, and less often the scalp as well. The severity of the inflammatory changes fluctuates, but the course is prolonged.

The scalp alone may be involved or the scalp together with pubes and axillae. There are multiple rounded or oval patches each surrounded by crops of follicular pustules. There may be no other changes, but successive crops of pustules, each followed by destruction of the affected follicles, produce slow extension of the alopecia. In some cases the folliculitis spreads along the scalp margin in a coronal distribution (Bogg 1963).

When the face is affected the area in front of the ears is often the first to be involved. Large pustules or reddish-brown lupoid papules are succeeded by dense scarring. The process tends to remain unilateral and if it spreads to the scalp, is usually confined to the temple, although it may extend along the frontal hair line (Binazzi 1954).

In the clinical syndrome in which the so-called 'glabrous' skin is principally involved (Miller 1961) the lesions, on thighs, legs and arms, tend to be symmetrical.

Diagnosis. See p. 309.

Treatment. All patients should be investigated for underlying defects of immune response and of leucocyte function, as a possible guide to effective treatment.

Systematic antibiotics will often prevent further extension of the disease, but only for as long as they are administered.

References
Binazzi M. (1954) In tema di folliculiti decalvanti. *Annali italiani di Dermatologia e di Sifiligrafi*, **9**, 325.
Bogg, A. (1963) Folliculitis decalvans. *Acta dermatovenereologica*, **43**, 14.
Laymon C.W. (1947) The cicatricial alopecias. *Journal of Investigative Dermatology*, **8**, 99.
Loewenthal L.J.A. (1957) A case of lupoid sycosis or ulerythema sycosiforme, beginning in infancy. *British Journal of Dermatology*, **69**, 443.
Miller R.F. (1961) Epilating folliculitis of the glabrous skin. *Archives of Dermatology*, **83**, 115.
Shitara A., Igareshi R. & Morohashi M. (1974) Folliculitis decalvans and cellular immunity—two brothers with oral candidiasis. (In Japanese). *Japanese Journal of Dermatology*, **28**, 133.

Alopecia parvimaculata

History and nomenclature. Dreuw in Germany in 1910 reported an outbreak of alopecia affecting 60 of the 85 boys in two schools. The patches of alopecia were small, irregularly round or angular, and appeared atrophic, but in 90% the hair regrew satisfactorily, permanent scarring alopecia developing in the remaining 10%. There were no inflammatory changes and no fungus or other organisms could be discovered.

Bowen (1899) of Boston, USA, had reported two outbreaks of a similar clinical entity. Four of 26 girls affected in the second outbreak had some residual atrophy. Bowen later (1915) expressed the opinion that his cases had been similar to those reported by Dreuw, and not alopecia areata.

At intervals other outbreaks have been reported. Each report arouses the same heated controversy as have earlier publications on epidemic alopecia areata. Some critics insist that a fungus infection must have been overlooked; other critics are more concerned in establishing whether or not the condition is 'true' alopecia areata. The mystery is at present unresolved, but there is sufficient evidence that outbreaks of alopecia, distinct from alopecia areata and not of mycotic origin, do occur. It is not yet clear whether they constitute a single aetiological entity (Davis 1914).

Pathology. Few histological studies have been recorded. Sabouraud (1932) mentions non-specific inflammatory changes involving some follicles, whilst sparing others. The degree of scarring depends on the number of contiguous follicles destroyed. In some cases the pathological changes eventually resemble those of pseudopelade (Loewenthal & Lurie 1956).

Clinical features (Semon 1923; Hoffmann & Martin 1925; Heermann 1930; Höfer 1964). All reported cases have been children. The patches of alopecia are of rapid onset, quickly reaching their greatest extent, and are usually numerous. They seldom exceed 1–2 cm in diameter, and are characteristically irregularly angular in shape. Over the course of a few weeks the hair regrows in most cases, to leave no clinically evident alopecia, but in some patches in some patients cicatricial alopecia results.

Diagnosis. Mycotic infection must be excluded by microscopy and by culture. The multiple bites of insects, scratched and secondarily infected, can give rise to small patches of alopecia, but the history should exclude this diagnosis.

References

Bowen J.T. (1899) Two epidemics of alopecia areata in an asylum for girls. *Journal of Cutaneous Diseases,* **17,** 1899.

Bowen J.T. (1915) Epidemic alopecia in small areas. *Journal of Cutaneous Diseases,* **33,** 343.

Davis H. (1914) Epidemic alopecia areata. *British Journal of Dermatology,* **26,** 207.

Dreuw, H. (1910) Klinische Brobachtungen bei 101 haarkranken Schulknaber. *Monatsheft für practische Dermatologie,* **51,** 103.

Heermann (1930) Uber Alopecia parvimaculata. *Zentralblatt für Dermatologie*, **32**, 174.

Höfer W. (1964) Sporadisches Auftreten von Alopecia parvimacularis. *Dermatologische Wochenschrift*, **149**, 381.

Hofmann E. & Martin H. (1925) Ueber epidemisch auftretenden klein-fleckigen haarausfall (Alopecia parvimaculata) *Deutsche Medizinsche Wochenschrift*, **51**, 1153.

Loewenthal L.J.A. & Lurie H.I. (1956) An outbreak of linear scarring alopecia. *British Journal of Dermatology*, **68**, 88.

Sabouraud R. (1932) Diagnostic et traitement des affections du cuir chevelu. Paris, Masson, p. 404.

Semon H.C. (1923) Epidemic alopecia in small areas. *Archives of Dermatology and Syphilology*, **8**, 785.

Lichen planus

Aetiology

Lichen planus is a disease or, more probably, a pattern of reaction, of unknown origin. It accounts for about 1% of new cases referred to departments of dermatology in Europe. It occurs throughout the world, but there are marked regional variations in its incidence and in its clinical manifestations. These variations probably result from relative differences in the importance of various aetiological agents.

A lichenoid eruption with all or most of the pathological and clinical features of lichen planus can be induced by a wide range of drugs (Almeyda & Levantine 1971), including gold, mepacrine (syn. atebrin), para-aminosalicylic acid, aminophenazole, and phenothiazine derivatives. Since only a small proportion of individuals exposed to any of these drugs develop a reaction of this type, it has been suggested that the afflicted are predisposed, perhaps by a congenital deficiency in the epidermis of glucose-6-phosphate dehydrogenase (Cotton *et al.* 1972). The familial incidence of ordinary lichen planus, though unusual, is well recognized (Jadassohn 1953; Depaoli 1970). It is possible that immunological mechanisms will prove to be implicated in some of the many cases without discoverable cause; claims that a virus has been incriminated have not been confirmed.

Pathology

The initial abnormality is in the epidermis: fibrillar changes in the basal cells lead to the formation of colloid bodies, and at an early stage these, and macrophages containing pigment, may be seen in the dermis. By immunofluorescence fibrin and IgM may be detected in the upper dermis, and various components of complement in the basement zone (Baart de la Faille Kuyper & Baart de la Faille 1974). The wounded basal cells are continually replaced by the migration of cells from neighbouring normal epidermis (Presbury & Marks 1974).

In the established lesion (Ellis 1967) the horny layer and granular layer are thickened and there is irregular acanthosis. Flattening of the rete pegs gives rise to a saw-tooth configuration. There is liquefaction degeneration of the basal cells. Close up against the epidermis is a dense infiltrate of lymphocytes and some histiocytes. In many sections some colloid bodies can be seen. If the process involves hair follicles the infiltrate extends around them and the hairs are replaced by keratin plugs. The follicles may ultimately be totally destroyed.

Clinical features

Lichen planus occurs at any age, but in over 80% of cases the onset is between 30 and 70 (Altman & Perry 1961). Significant involvement of the scalp is relatively infrequent—only 10 of 807 patients in one series (Altman and Perry 1961)—but the incidence is probably rather higher than such figures suggest since they tend to exclude those patients in whom alopecia, classified as pseudopelade, was the only manifestation of the disease. Scalp involvement occurs in over 40% of patients with either of two unusual variants of lichen planus, the bullous or erosive form and lichen planopilaris (Fig. 11.4). Most

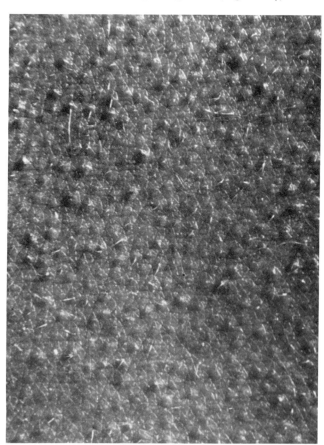

Fig. 11.4. Lichen planopilaris. Alopecia occurs in 40% of cases of this unusual form of lichen planus (Slade Hospital, Oxford).

patients seen with scalp lesions are middle-aged women, but a girl aged 13 with scarring and follicular keratosis has been reported (Borda *et al.* 1961).

Recent scalp lesions may show violaceous papules, erythema and scaling (Borda *et al.* 1961; Sannicandro 1954), but before long follicular plugs become conspicuous and scarring replaces all other changes (Figs. 11.5, 11.6). Eventually the plugs are shed from the scarred areas which remain white and smooth. If the patch is extending horny plugs may still be present in follicles around its margins.

More often the scalp lesions are well established by the time the patient attends hospital and the irregular white patches are not clinically diagnostic and may indeed not show any distinctive histological features. This is the clinical picture known as pseudopelade (see p. 311). The diagnosis of lichen planus can be made only in the presence of unquestionable lesions elsewhere. These may take the form of bullous lichen planus with shedding of nails (Cram *et al.* 1966), of bullous lesions associated with typical lichen planus of the skin and mucous membranes (Ebner 1973) or of lichen planus of very limited extent involving for example only the nails (Corsi 1937). In some cases of lichen planus of the scalp a presumptive diagnosis has to be based on a history of lichen planus in other sites.

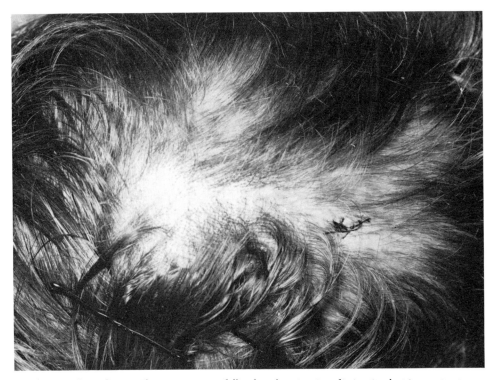

Fig. 11.5. Lichen planus. The conspicuous follicular plugging is a distinctive but inconstant feature (Addenbrooke's Hospital, Cambridge).

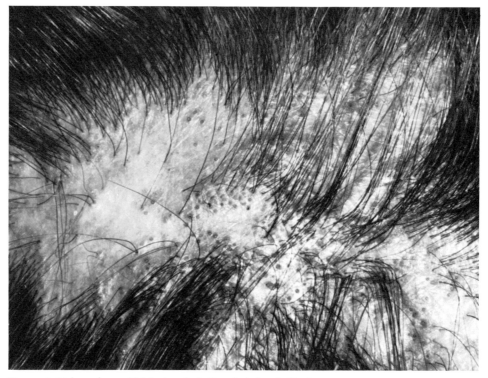

Fig. 11.6. Lichen planus (Addenbrooke's Hospital, Cambridge).

In a clinical syndrome which has caused much controversy (see Graham-Little syndrome, p. 322) groups of horny follicular papules on the trunk and limbs either precede or follow the development of scarring alopecia. The evidence that this syndrome is at least in many cases a manifestation of lichen planus is based on its occasional association with typical lichen planus (Sachs & de Oreo 1942; Silver *et al.* 1953) and the presence in early lesions of histological changes acceptable as lichen planus (Ellis & Kirby-Smith 1941; Sachs & de Oreo 1942; Spicer & Keilig 1953; Waldorf 1966).

The scalp may be involved also in lichenoid eruptions of chemical origin. For example when the hypertrophic plaques of a lichenoid reaction to gold involve the scalp, they are liable to leave permanent scars (Woods 1968) and the scalp is affected in a proportion of lichenoid reactions to mepacrine (Feder 1949).

Prognosis
In some patients the course of lichen planus of the scalp is slow and only a few inconspicuous patches are present after many years. However, particularly if the skin lesions are of bullous or planopilaris type, they may rapidly result in extensive and permanent baldness.

Diagnosis

Except in the rare cases in which classical papular lesions occur in the scalp, the diagnosis is based on the presence of typical lichen planus elsewhere. It follows that in all cases of cicatricial alopecia the whole skin surface and the oral mucosa must be examined. Histological examination may provide confirmatory evidence if the lesions are not of long duration.

The differential diagnosis of cicatricial alopecia is considered on p. 309.

Treatment

Drugs or other chemicals causing the reaction must be diligently sought and excluded, with greater hope of success in 'atypical' lichenoid eruptions. In such cases a short course of systemic treatment with a corticosteroid may be desirable. In other cases intralesional corticosteroids are helpful but only at a stage when active inflammatory changes are still present.

References

Almeyda J. & Levantine A. (1971) Drug reactions. XVI. Lichenoid drug eruptions. *British Journal of Dermatology*, **85**, 604.

Altman J. & Perry H.O. (1961) The variations and course of lichen planus. *Archives of Dermatology*, **84**, 179.

Baart de la Faille Kuyper E.H. & Bart de la Faille H. (1974) An immunofluorescence study of lichen planus. *British Journal of Dermatology*, **90**, 365.

Black M.M. & Wilson Jones E. (1972) The role of the epidermis in the histopathogenesis of lichen planus. *Archives of Dermatology*, **105**, 81.

Borda J.M., Mazzini R.H.E. & Ruiz D.A. (1961) Liquen del cuero cabelludo. *Archivos argentinos de Dermatologia*, **11**, 257.

Corsi H. (1937) Atrophy of hair follicle and nail matrix in lichen planus. *British Journal of Dermatology*, **49**, 376.

Cotton D.W.K., Van den Hurk J.J.M.A. & van der Staak W.B.J.M. (1972) Lichen planus: an inborn error of metabolism. *British Journal of Dermatology*, **87**, 341.

Cram D.L., Kierland R.R. & Winkelmann R.K. (1966) Ulcerative lichen planus of the feet. *Archives of Dermatology*, **93**, 692.

Depaoli M. (1970) Lichen ruber planus familiare. *Giornale italiano di Dermatologia*, **45**, 1.

Ebner H. (1973) Lichen ruber planus mit Onychatrophie und narbiger Alopezie. *Dermatologica*, **147**, 219.

Ellis F.A. & Kirby-Smith H. (1941) Lichen planus et acuminatus atrophicans (Feldman). *Archives of Dermatology and Syphilology*, **43**, 628.

Ellis F.A. (1967) Histopathology of lichen planus based on analysis of one hundred biopsy specimens. *Journal of Investigative Dermatology*, **48**, 143.

Feder A. (1949) Clinical observations on atypical lichen planus and related dermatoses presumably due to atabrine toxicity. *Annals of Internal Medicine*, **31**, 1078.

Jadassohn W. (1953) Lichen ruber planus familiaris. *Journal de Génétique humaine*, **2**, 153.

Presbury D.G.C. & Marks R. (1974) The epidermal disorder in lichen planus: an *in vitro* study. *British Journal of Dermatology*, **90**, 373.

Sachs W. & de Oreo W. (1942) Lichen planopilaris. *Archives of Dermatology and Syphilology*, **45**, 1081.

Sannicandro, G. (1954) Etudes sur le lichen ruber planus typique et atypique: ulcéro-érosif, ulcero-hémorragique, scléro-cicatriciel, alopécique et sur ses rapports avec les modifications de la protidopoièse. *Annales de Dermatologie et de Syphiligraphie*, **81**, 380.

Silver H., Chargin L. & Sachs P.M. (1953) Follicular lichen planus (lichen planopilaris). *Archives of Dermatology and Syphilology*, **67**, 346.

Spier H.W. & Keilig W. (1953) Lichen ruber follicularis decalvans (Graham-Little Syndrom) und seine Beziehungen zur Pseudopelade Brocq. *Hautarzt*, **4**, 457.

Waldorf D.S. (1966) Lichen planopilaris. *Archives of Dermatology*, **93**, 684.

Woods B. (1968) Lichen post-aurique. *Transactions of the St John's Hospital Dermatological Society*, **54**, 118.

Graham-Little syndrome

History and nomenclature

In 1915 Graham-Little of London reported the case of a woman aged 55, who had been referred to him by Lassueur of Lausanne. She had suffered for 10 years from slowly progressive cicatricial alopecia and for 5 months from groups of horny papules. Piccardi (1914) had reported a similar case the previous year. Since then many further cases have been reported but the discussion as to whether or not this syndrome is or is not a form of lichen planus is still unresolved after 60 years. However, whatever its cause or causes the syndrome is distinctive. It is known eponymously and variously as the Graham-Little, Lassueur–Graham-Little, or Piccardi–Lassueur–Little syndrome.

Pathology

In the scalp the mouths of affected follicles are filled by large horny plugs. The underlying follicle is progressively destroyed and eventually an atrophic epidermis covers sclerotic dermis. In the axillae and pubic region the follicles are likewise destroyed, although the skin does not appear clinically to be atrophic.

Clinical features

Most patients have been women between the ages of 30 and 70. The essential features of the syndrome are progressive cicatricial alopecia of the scalp, loss of pubic and axillary hair without clinically evident scarring, and the rapid development of keratosis pilaris. The sequence of events and their relative severity differ widely from case to case.

In most patients the earliest change has been patchy cicatricial alopecia of the scalp. In Graham-Little's (1915) patient, aged 55, the scalp had been affected for about 10 years by what is described as 'an inflammatory process' resulting in bald patches, before she suddenly developed a widespread irritable eruption consisting of horny papules with spine-like projections grouped in well defined plaques on trunk and limbs. In several other patients (e.g. Dore 1915; Beatty & Speares 1915; Pagès *et al.* 1961; McCafferty 1928) the scalp alopecia has preceded the widespread keratosis pilaris by months or years. In Senear's (1920) patient alopecia was present from the age of 9: grouped horny papules of the back and arms developed at 22, then cleared, but recurred at 30. In some patients, however (e.g. Reiss *et al.* 1958; Valentino *et al.* 174) the alopecia and the keratosis pilaris appear to have developed more or less simultaneously, or the keratosis pilaris has preceded the discovery of the alopecia (e.g. Alessi & Dal Pozzo 1968).

The scalp changes are commonly described simply as patches of cicatricial alopecia. Some authors specifically mention associated follicular plugging of the scalp (Reiss *et al.* 1958) and others refer to 'scaly red patches' (Alessi & Dal Pozzo 1968).

The keratosis pilaris is referred to in early case reports of lichen spinulosus, which emphasize that the horny papules are prolonged into conspicuous spines. In most cases they have developed progressively over a period of weeks or months and have been grouped into plaques, often on the trunk, or on the trunk and limbs, but occasionally involving the eyebrows and the sides of the face. Such a distribution has been noted in a woman aged 69 (Reiss *et al.* 1958), in a man aged 46 (Ormsby 1920) and also in a man aged 22, in whom cicatricial alopecia had been present since the age of 10 (Pagès *et al.* 1961) Pruritus is an inconstant symptom; it was noted in several reported cases and was troublesome in a patient under the author's care (Kubba & Rook 1975).

Thinning and ultimately total loss of pubic and axillary hair has been noted in many cases; other reports fail to mention it.

Treatment
None is known. Autografting may be considered as in other cicatricial alopecias.

References
Alessi E. & Dal Pozzo V. (1968) Sindrome di Piccardi–Little–Lassueur. *Giornale Italiano di Dermatologia*, **109**, 493.
Arnozan X. (1892) Folliulite dépilantes des partier glabres. *Bulletin de la Societé Français de Dermatologie et Syphiligraphie*, **3**, 187.
Beatty W. & Speares J. (1915) A Case of Folliculosis (? Folliculitis) decalvans and lichen spinulosus. *British Journal of Dermatology*, **27**, 331.
Brocq L., Langlet & Agrinac (1905) Recherches sur alopécie atrophisante, variété pseudo-pelade. *Annales de Dermatologie*, **6**, 1, 97, 209.
Dore S.E. (1915) Lichen spinulosus and folliculitis decalvans. *British Journal of Dermatology*, **27**, 295.
Graham-Little E.G. (1915) Folliculitis decalvans et atrophicans. *British Journal of Dermatology*, **27**, 183.
Kubba R. & Rook A. (1975) The Graham-Little syndrome. *British Journal of Dermatology*, **93**, Suppl. 11, 53.
McCafferty L.K. (1928) Folliculitis decalvans et atrophicans (Little). *Archives of Dermatology and Syphilology*, **18**, 514.

Ormsby O. (1920) Folliculitis decalvans and lichen spinulosus. *Archives of Dermatology and Syphilology*, **1**, 471.

Pagès F., Lapeyre J. & Misson R. (1961) Syndrome de Lassueur–Graham-Little. *Annales de Dermatologie et de Syphiligraphie*, **88**, 272.

Piccardi G. (1914) Cheratosi spinulosa del capillizio a suoi rapporti con al pseudo-pelade di Brocq. *Giornale Italiano della Malattie Veneree e della Pelle.*, **49**, 416.

Reiss F., Reisch M. & Buncke C.M. (1958) Keratodermatitis folliculitis decalvans. *Archives of Dermatology*, **78**, 616.

Senear F.E. (1920) Folliculitis decalvans and lichen spinulosus. *Archives of Dermatology and Syphilology*, **2**, 198.

Valentino A., Andreassi L. & Sbano E. (1974) Sindrome de Piccardi–Little–Lassueur. *Giornale e Minerva Dermatologica*, **109**, 588.

Scarring follicular keratosis

History and nomenclature

Numerous syndromes have been described and elaborately named, all of them characterized by keratosis pilaris, associated with some degree of inflammatory change leading to destruction of the affected follicles.

Only detailed clinical and genetic studies can provide the essential facts to allow reliable differentiation of syndromes which some authorities regard as forms or degrees of a single state and others accept as distinct entities. The reported cases can be temporarily but conveniently classified in three groups, in addition to which certain apparently well-defined entities can be recognized.

(1) Atrophoderma vermiculata syn. acne vermiculata syn. folliculitis ulerythematosa reticulata: there is honeycomb atrophy of the cheeks. Scarring alopecia may occur, but rarely.

(2) Keratosis pilaris atrophicans faciei syn. ulerythema oophryogenes: the process is more or less confined to the eyebrow region.

(3) Keratosis pilaris decalvans syn. keratosis follicularis spinulosa decalvans syn. follicular ichthyosis. Keratosis pilaris of variable extent is associated with cicatricial alopecia.

Aetiology

All these conditions are assumed to be genetically determined although many cases occur sporadically. Such genetic data as are available are considered under the individual forms.

Pathology

The follicles are initially distended by horney plugs, the dermis is oedematous and there is some lymphocytic infiltration around follicles and vessels. Later the follicles are destroyed. Small epithelial cysts may be numerous, particularly in keratosis pilaris atrophicans faciei.

Clinical features

Atrophoderma vermiculata usually begins in childhood. Follicular plugs, often in the pre-auricular regions, are gradually shed to leave reticulate atrophy. The extent of the process on the face is variable. Exceptionally cicatricial alopecia of the scalp may be associated (Fisher 1957).

Keratosis pilaris atrophicans facieri is present from early infancy. Erythema and horny plugs begin in the outer halves of the eyebrows which they eventually destroy, and then advance medially and to a variable extent on to the cheeks. Involvement of the scalp has apparently not been reported in cases in which the eyebrows are predominantly involved, but there are case histories to which this diagnosis has been applied but which appear to be more rationally classified in one of the other categories in which alopecia has occurred. Such cases emphasize the need for improved diagnostic criteria.

Autosomal dominant inheritance has been reported on several occasions (e.g. Mertens 1968).

Keratosis pilaris decalvans is also such a variable syndrome that several genotypes must be considered. Keratosis pilaris begins in infancy or childhood, often on the face. Its ultimate extent may be confined to the face or to face and limbs, or be more or less universal. It is often succeeded by atrophy on the face, but rarely on the limbs or trunk. Cicatricial alopecia is noted from early childhood or later, and may be localized or extensive.

A brother and sister (Barber 1928) had follicular scars on cheeks and temples, numerous epithelial cysts, keratosis pilaris of limbs and trunk with atrophy in some sites, and cicatricial alopecia of the vertex.

A girl aged 17 with cicatricial alopecia since 3 (Degos & Delzant 1961) had extensive keratosis pilaris of limbs and trunk.

Three members of one family developed keratosis pilaris of the face in early childhood (MacLeod 1909) and then extensively on the back and limbs, and on the scalp where horny papules replaced hairs. Somewhat similar changes were noted in two boys by Zeligman & Fleisher (1959). A similar syndrome was recently reported (Kubba *et al.* 1975) in a young man who had keratosis pilaris and severe cicatricial alopecia; recurrent attacks of folliculitis of the scalp were controlled by systemic antibiotics. Cockayne (1938) in his notable review of the existing literature attempted to impose some order on the incomplete published case reports. The occurrence of cases similar to those reported by MacLeod (1909) in other siblings, born of normal parents, suggested recessive inheritance but the evidence was incomplete. Other case reports with several of these features are those of Oliver & Gilbert (1926) and of Hadida (1948). The former described two American boys with sparse hair and keratosis pilaris of the scalp. Hadida's patient was an Algerian girl who lost all her hair at the age of 2 months and then grew sparse black, short brittle hair; she had keratosis pilaris of face, scalp, trunk and limbs. Her eyebrows and eyelashes were normal.

The pattern of hair loss in the family reported by Ullmo (1944) was in the distribution of the Marie-Unna type of congenital alopecia apart from the presence of keratosis pilaris on the face, and mildly on the back and limbs.

Five individuals in three generations of a Finnish family (Kuokkanen 1971) showed in varying degree keratosis pilaris of face, trunk and limbs, cicatricial alopecia, keratoderma of the distal third of palms and soles and corneal dystrophy. The full syndrome was present only in one of the two affected males. In a pedigree reported by Lamaris (cited by Cockayne 1938) in which keratosis follicularis decalvans was associated with corneal dystrophy, sex-linked recessive inheritance was demonstrated. Franceschetti *et al.* (1956) reported a sporadic instance of this association, also in a boy. In a pedigree (Greither 1960) 7 of 13 females in three generations had scalp alopecia progressing from puberty to menopause; complete loss of axillary and pubic hair; prominent keratosis pilaris of scalp and axillae; slight palmoplantar keratoderma, brittle small nails; centrofacial lentiginosis and reduced sweat gland function.

What may be another distinct syndrome associates extremely severe keratosis pilaris—'closely woven keratotic bristles'—with almost complete alopecia, reduced sweating and deafness (Morris *et al.* 1969). An infant which died on the 7th day had the same syndrome (Myers *et al.* 1971).

Also distinct is a sex-linked recessive syndrome (Cantu *et al.* 1974) reported from Mexico in which almost complete absence of hair, eyebrows and eyelashes, and generalized keratosis pilaris are associated with congenital proportionate dwarfism, microcephaly and cerebral atrophy.

Diagnosis

Although the scalp may be involved in Darier's disease (p. 489), gross loss of hair is exceptional. The Graham-Little syndrome (p. 322) commonly affects middle-aged women. Cicatricial alopecia is associated with follicular horny papules which are usually in well-defined groups and do not develop until after the alopecia has become established. The histological findings will exclude the rare generalized follicular hamartoma.

Treatment

Only symptomatic measures are available. Retinoic acid deserves a trial.

References

Barber H.W. (1928) Folliculitis erythematosa reticulata combined with lichen spinulosus, epidermal cysts and folliculitis decalvans. *British Journal of Dermatology*, **40**, 24.

Cantu J.-M., Hernandez A., Larracilla J., Trejo A. & Macotela-Ruiz E. (1974) A new X-linked recessive disorder with dwarfism, cerebral atrophy, and generalized keratosis follicularis. *Journal of Pediatrics*, **84**, 564.

Cockayne E.A. (1938) *Inherited Abnormalities of the Skin and its Appendages.* Oxford, Oxford University Press, p. 140.

Degos R. & Delzant O. (1961) Keratose pilaire rouge avec large plaque d'alopécie atrophiante. *Bulletin de la Société française de Dermatologie et de Syphiligraphie*, **68**, 688.

Fisher A.A. (1957) Keratosis pilaris rubra atrophicans faciei with diffuse alopecia of the scalp. *Archives of Dermatology*, **75**, 283.

Franceschetti A., Rossano R., Jadassohn W. & Paillard R. (1956) Keratosis follicularis spinulosa decalvans. *Dermatologica*, **112**, 512.

Greither A. (1960) Über drei Generationen vererbte, auf Frauen beschränkte Keratosis follicularis mit Alopecie, Hypidrose und abortiven Palmar-Plantar-Keratosen in ihren Beziehungen zur Hypotrichosis congenita hereditaria. *Archiv für klinische und experimentelle Dermatologie*, **210**, 123.

Hadida E. (1948) Hypoplasie congénitale des cheveux. *L'Algérie médicale*, **51**, 115.

Kubba R., Mitchell J.N.S. & Rook A. (1975) Keratosis pilaris with recurrent folliculitis decalvans. *British Journal of Dermatology*, **93**, Suppl. 11, 55.

Kuokkanen K. (1971) Keratosis follicularis spinulosa decalvans, in a family from northern Finland. *Acta Dermatovenereologica*, **51**, 146.

MacLeod J.M.H. (1909) Three cases of 'Ichthyosis follicularis' associated with baldness. *British Journal of Dermatology*, **21**, 165.

Mertens R.L.J. (1968) Ulerythema ophryogenes and atopy. *Archives of Dermatology*, **97**, 662.

Morris J., Ackerman A.B. & Koblenzer P.J. (1969) Generalized spiny hyperkeratosis, universal alopecia and deafness. *Archives of Dermatology*, **100**, 692.

Myers E.N., Stool S.E. & Koblenzer P.J. (1971) Congenital deafness, spiny hyperkeratosis and universal alopecia. *Archives of Otolaryngology (Chicago)*, **93**, 68.

Oliver E.A. & Gilbert N.C. (1926) Congenital alopecia. *Archives of Dermatology and Syphilology*, **13**, 359.

Ullmo A. (1944) Un nouveau type d'agénésie et de dystrophie pilaire familiale et héréditaire. *Dermatologica*, **90**, 74.

Zeligman I. & Fleisher T.C. (1959) Ichthyosis follicularis. *A.M.A. Archives of Dermatology*, **80**, 413.

Cicatricial pemphigoid
(syn. benign mucosal pemphigoid/ocular pemphigus)

Aetiology
Cicatricial pemphigoid affects predominantly the elderly, and women more than men.

Pathology
Bullae are formed beneath the intact epidermis (Susi & Sklar 1971). Linear deposits of IgG, IgA, C3 and C4 are found in the basement membrane zone, but circulating basement membrane zone antibodies are not always demonstrable (Bean & Michel 1973; Holubar *et al.* 1973).

Clinical features
The skin is involved in 40–50% of cases, and the disease affects predominantly the ocular and/or genital mucous membrane. However, the skin lesions may precede the mucosal lesions by months or years.

The skin lesions are usually confined to a limited area within which bullae repeatedly recur, leaving a dense scar. The favoured sites are the face, and in particular the scalp (Slepyan *et al.* 1961; Honeyman *et al.* 1980).

Diagnosis
The bullae and the frequently associated mucosal lesions differentiate the scalp lesions from other forms of cicatricial alopecia. Immunofluorescence histology is helpful.

Treatment
Management will often be dictated by the need to control mucosal lesions. If recurrent bullae in a localized area of skin are troublesome, excision and grafting may be successful (Slepyan *et al.* 1961).

References
Bean S.F. & Michel B. (1973) Cicatricial pemphigoid. In *Immunopathology of the Skin. Labeled Antibody Studies*, eds. E.H. Beutner, T.P. Chorzelski, S.F. Bean & R.G. Jordon. Stroudsburg, Dowde Hutchings & Rees, p. 55.

Holubar K., Hönigsmann H. & Wolff K. (1973) Cicatricial pemphigoid. *Archives of Dermatology*, **108**, 50.

Honeyman J., Navarrette W., De le Parra M.A. & Pinto, A. (1980) Pemfigoid cicatricial cutaneo localizado en cabeza y cuello (Brunsting-Perez). *Archivos Argentinos de Dermatologia*, **30**, 135.

Slepyan A.H., Burks J.W. & Fox J. (1961) Persistent denudation of the scalp in cicatricial pemphigoid. Treatment by skin grafting. *Archives of Dermatology*, **84**, 444.

Susi F.R. & Sklar G. (1971) Histochemistry and fine structure of oral lesions of mucous membrane pemphigoid. *Archives of Dermatology*, **104**, 244.

Erosive pustular dermatosis of the scalp

Aetiology
This recently recognized clinical entity (Pye *et al.* 1979) has so far been reported only in women over 70 years of age. Its cause is unknown but there is no evidence that it is primarily infective in origin.

Pathology
Histological examination shows atrophy, some parakeratosis, and areas of epidermal erosion. A chronic inflammatory infiltration in the dermis consists predominantly of lymphocytes and plasma cells. Small foci of foreign body giant cells may be seen where hair follicles have been destroyed.

Clinical features
Initially a small area of scalp becomes red and crusted and may be irritable. On examination crusting and superficial pustulation overlie a moist eroded surface

(Fig. 11.7). As the condition extends areas of activity coexist with areas of cicatricial alopecia. There is little or no tendency to spontaneous cure. Squamous carcinoma has developed in the scars (Lovell *et al.* 1980).

Differential diagnosis
Pyogenic infection is excluded by bacteriological examination and the lack of response to antibacterial agents. Biopsy may be necessary to exclude pustular psoriasis and cicatricial pemphigoid.

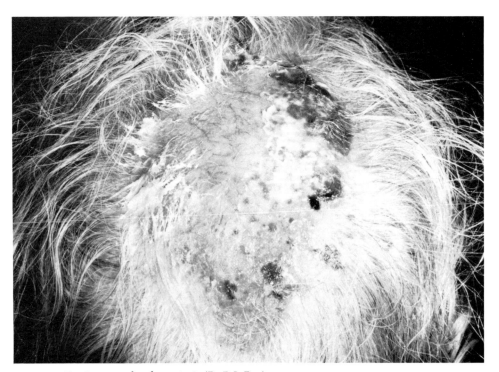

Fig. 11.7. Erosive pustular dermatosis (Dr R.J. Pye).

Treatment
The stronger topical corticosteroids such as 0·05% clobetasol propionate will temporarily suppress the inflammatory changes.

References
Lovell C.R., Harman R.R.M. & Bradfield J.W.B. (1980) Cutaneous carcinoma arising in erosive pustular dermatosis of the scalp. *British Journal of Dermatology*, **102**, 325.
Pye R.J., Peachey R.D.G. & Burton J.L. (1979) Erosive pustular dermatosis of the scalp. *British Journal of Dermatology*, **100**, 559.

Cicatricial alopecia resulting from physical trauma

The diagnosis and treatment of the consequences of physical injuries of the scalp will seldom confront the dermatologist, but he may be consulted as to the cause of an apparent physical injury, for example aplasia cutis may be falsely attributed to a forceps injury at childbirth.

The attachment of an electrode to the scalp for monitoring the fetal heart-beat during labour may occasionally cause some superficial damage to the scalp and, particularly if secondary infection supervenes, this may be followed by a small scar. Aplasia cutis has sometimes been mistaken for such a lesion (Brown *et al.* 1977).

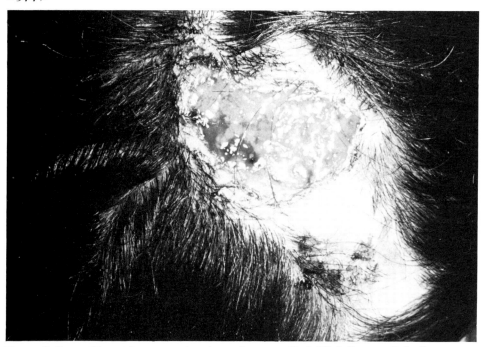

Fig. 11.8. Dermatitis artefacta—erosions becoming scars (Radcliffe Infirmary, Oxford).

An unusual case of cicatricial alopecia in a boy aged 13 was due to injury to the scalp by an intravenous infusion given in infancy for gastroenteritis (Strong 1979).

Exceptionally, self-inflicted injuries may involve the scalp and may leave scars (Fig. 11.8).

See also Chapter 9.

References

Brown Z.A., Jung A.L. & Stenehuver M.A. (1977) Aplasia cutis congenita and the fetal scalp electrode. *American Journal of Obstetrics and Gynaecology,* **129,** 351.

Strong A.M.M.M. (1979) Extensive cicatricial alopecia following a scalp vein infusion. *Clinical and Experimental Dermatology*, 4, 197.

Chronic radiodermatitis
(References p. 334)

History (Albert & Omran 1968; Getzrow 1976)

Roentgen discovered X-rays in 1895. Seven years later the first carcinoma of the skin attributable to X-rays was reported. X-ray epilation of the face for hirsutism was frequently employed during the first two decades of the twentieth century, and although Schultz, an international authority, condemned this treatment as early as 1912, it continued to be used irresponsibly to such an extent that in 1947 Cipollaro & Einhorn entitled their paper on this subject 'The use of X-rays for the treatment of hypertrichosis is dangerous'.

X-ray epilation for the treatment of scalp ringworm was introduced by Sabouraud in 1904 and the technique was improved and standardized by Kienbock and by Adamson. The discovery of griseofulvin in 1958 gradually made X-ray epilation unnecessary, but it has been estimated that between 1904 and 1959 some 300,000 children throughout the world were treated with X-rays for ringworm of the scalp. The Kienbock–Adamson technique, strictly followed, did not cause clinically evident chronic cutaneous damage. However, technical errors were frequent, particularly in the early days, from inadequate and poorly calibrated apparatus. The object of the technique was to divide the scalp into five fields and give to each 300–400 rads at 75–100 kV. This produced complete epilation in about 3 weeks, and regrowth after 2 months. The most frequent mistake to be made in carrying out X-ray epilation was to allow overlap of the fields so that certain areas of the scalp received double the intended dose. The follow-up of 2,043 patients treated in childhood, showed a higher incidence of cancer and of mental illness in the patients than in a control group (Albert & Omran 1968).

Radiodermatitis of the scalp may occur also as an unavoidable consequence of skin damage during the treatment of internal malignant disease and also inevitably occurs when malignant disease of the skin is treated.

Pathology

The use of X-rays for epilation depends on the high susceptibility of anagen hairs to radiation. Epilating and sub-epilating doses produced dystrophic changes in human hairs as early as the 4th day after exposure (Van Scott & Reinertson 1959). Unfortunately the dose required to produce permanent epilation inevitably produces atrophy and telangiectasia. Doses of 500–800 rads produced in 20% of subjects a generalized reduction of the follicle population of the scalp and a reduction in follicle size (Albert *et al.* 1968).

Chronic radiodermatitis may follow acute radiodermatitis but may develop only slowly as degenerative changes induced by sun-exposure and ageing are superimposed on those directly due to the ionizing radiation.

In chronic radiodermatitis the epidermis is generally atrophic with loss of hair follicles and sebaceous glands but there are also irregular areas of acanthosis. Degenerative changes and nuclear abnormalities are frequent in the epidermis. Dermal collagen stains irregularly. Superficial small vessels are telangiectatic but deeper vessels are partially or completely occluded by fibrosis. The unstable anaplastic epidermis readily gives rise to keratoses and to squamous or basal cell carcinomas. The occlusive vascular changes may result in necrosis.

Clinical features (Fig. 11.9)
Chronic radiodermatitis of the scalp may present clinically in a number of different ways. The development of a basal cell carcinoma in middle age or later in a still hairy area of the scalp should lead the dermatologist to enquire about X-ray epilation for ringworm in childhood (Anderson & Anderson 1951; Ridley 1962). Patients sometimes refer to this as 'light treatment'. Sometimes the area of the scalp around the lesion may show sparser and finer hairs than the rest of the scalp, and there may be evident atrophy and telangiectasia.

In other cases the patient complains of ordinary baldness which is apparently

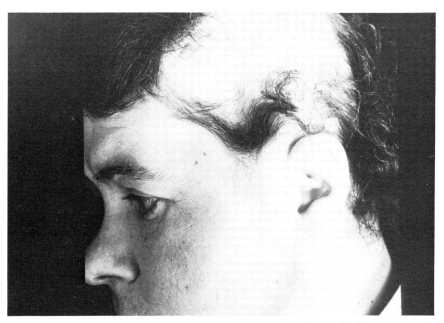

Fig. 11.9. Cicatricial alopecia as a sequel to X-ray epilation of the scalp for ringworm (Slade Hospital, Oxford).

accentuated in certain areas and these areas are found to show both common baldness and reduction of follicle population as a result of the earlier radiation. If the initial dose of radiation was large enough to produce acute radiodermatitis this is rapidly followed by chronic radiodermatitis.

Chronic radiodermatitis produced by radiation therapy of a malignant tumour of the scalp presents a circumscribed area of cicatricial alopecia.

In chronic radiodermatitis of any region, but particularly when the dosage was high, as in the treatment of a malignant tumour, late radiation necrosis may occur (Traenkle & Mulay 1960). Exposure to sunlight and to cold may precipitate necrosis in an area of skin with a blood supply already precarious. Radiation necrosis is an important condition for it may simulate a recurrence of carcinoma but the edges of the necrotic ulcer are not raised. The diagnosis should be confirmed by a biopsy.

Treatment

For alopecia of chronic radiodermatitis there is no treatment unless the affected area is small enough to be covered by a graft. Malignant tumours arising in radiodermatitis should be excised, preferably by a plastic surgeon (Conway & Hugo 1976).

References

Albert R.E. & Omran A.R. (1968) Follow-up study of patients treated by X-ray epilation for tinea capitis. I. Population characteristics, posttreatment illnesses and mortality experience. *Archives of Environmental Health*, **17**, 899.

Albert R.E., Omran A.R., Brauer E.W., Cohen N.C., Schmidt H., Dove D.C., Becker M., Baumring R. & Baer R.L. (1968) II. Results of Clinical and Laboratory Examinations. *Archives of Environmental Health*, **17**, 919.

Anderson N.P. & Anderson H.P. (1951) Development of basal cell epithelioma as a consequence of radiodermatitis. *Archives of Dermatology and Syphilology*, **63**, 586.

Cipollaro A.C. & Einhorn M.B. (1947) The use of X-rays for the treatment of hypertrichosis is dangerous. *Journal of the American Medical Association*, **135**, 349.

Conway H. & Hugo N.E. (1966) Radiation dermatitis and malignancy. *Plastic and Reconstructive Surgery*, **38**, 255.

Getzrow P.L. (1976) Chronic radiodermatitis and skin cancer. In *Cancer of the Skin*, eds. R. Andrade, S.L. Gumport, G.L. Popkin & T.D. Rees. Philadelphia, Saunders, p. 458.

Ridley C.M. (1962) Basal-cell carcinoma following X-ray epilation of the scalp. *British Journal of Dermatology*, **74**, 222.

Schultz F. (1912) *The X-ray Treatment of Skin Diseases*. London, Rebman, p. 139.

Traenkle H.L. & Mulay D. (1960) Further observations on late radiation necrosis folowing therapy of skin cancer. *Archives of Dermatology*, **81**, 988.

Van Scott E.J. & Reinertson R.P. (1957) Detection of radiation effects on hair roots of the human scalp. *Journal of Investigative Dermatology*, **29**, 205.

Necrobiosis lipoidica
(References p. 336)

Necrobiosis occurs in 2 or 3 per 1000 cases of diabetes mellitus, and approximately 70% of patients with necrobiosis have diabetes. The diabetic cases begin in childhood or early adult life and the non-diabetic cases rather later and usually in women.

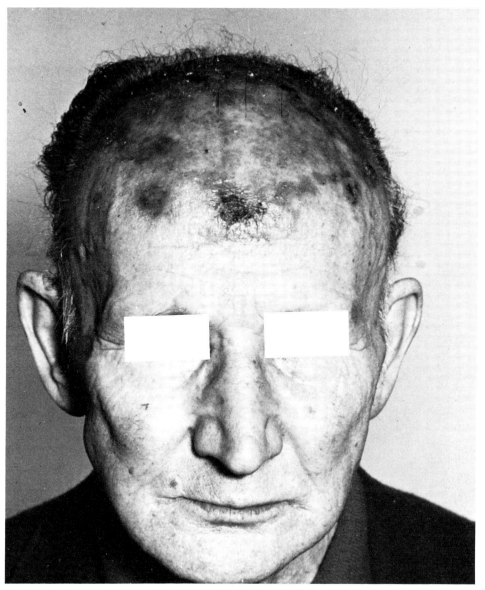

Fig. 11.10. Necrobiosis lipoidica of forehead and anterior scalp margin (Slade Hospital, Oxford).

The oval atrophic plaques classically occur on the shins but may be seen in other parts of the body including the scalp. The patches are glazed and yellowish, often with conspicuous telangiectases. Scarring may be dense. The clinical features in the scalp have varied from large plaques of cicatricial alopecia (Gaethe 1964) to multiple small areas of scarring resembling the clinical entity described as 'alopecia parvimaculata' (Gartmann & Dickmans-Burmeister 1969).

An atrophic form affecting predominantly the forehead and the scalp has been described (Wilson Jones 1971; Navaratnan & Hodgson 1973). It occurs mainly in women and in middle age. The earliest onset was at 25. Round or oval lesions appear on the forehead and the scalp margins: when they invade the scalp there may be little or no alopecia. There may be similar patches in other parts of the body. The degree of atrophy is slight. The edge is slightly raised; the centre is at first red but becomes brown or depigmented (Fig. 11.10).

References

Gaethe G. (1964) Necrobiosis lipoidica diabeticorum of the scalp. *Archiv für Dermatologie und Syphilologie*, **89**, 865.

Gertmann H. & Dickmans-Burmeister D. (1969) Ungewöhnliche Hautveränderungen bei einem 4 jahrigen Kinde mit Diabetes mellitus, 'Nekrobiosis diabetica acute parvimaculata'. *Hautarzt*, **20**, 265.

Navaratnan A. & Hodgson G.A. (1973) Necrobiosis lipoidica presenting on the face and scalp. *British Journal of Dermatology*, **89**, Suppl. 9, 100.

Wilson Jones E. (1971) Necrobiosis lipoidica presenting on the face and scalp. *Transactions of the St John's Hospital Dermatological Society*, **57**, 202.

Circumscribed scleroderma

Circumscribed scleroderma, commonly known as morphoea, is rare in the scalp, but may occur there as the only lesion or as one of many. Females are affected almost three times more frequently than males, and the peak age of onset is from 10–30.

The early stages of morphoea are rarely seen in the scalp unless a bald area is affected. Morphoea appears as a lilac macule which slowly extends centrifugally. The centre becomes pearly or ivory white, smooth and shinning and attached to deeper structures. A lilac ring persists as long as active extension is taking place. Morphosa tends to regress spontaneously after 3–5 years, but the plaque may continue to enlarge for much longer periods. The hair is shed at an early stage to leave a cicatricial alopecia (Fig. 11.11), which may show no distinctive features, but the diagnosis may be suggested by the presence of morphoea in other parts of the body (Fig. 11.12). The diagnosis must be confirmed histologically.

Linear circumscribed morphoea in the frontal region—'en coup de sabre' from its fancied resemblance to the scar of a sabre cut—may be associated with facial hemiatrophy, but not in all cases. Paramedian greying or loss of hairs may be the

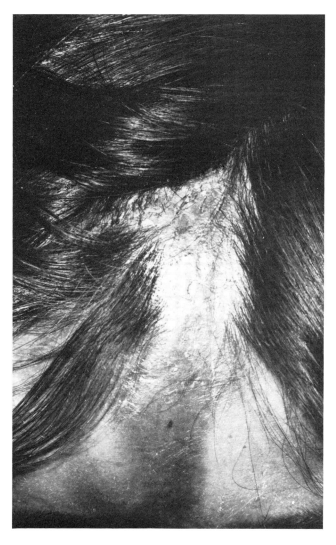

Fig. 11.11. Cicatricial alopecia at an early stage of facial hemiatrophy (Addenbrooke's Hospital, Cambridge).

earliest sign; soon the lesion's scar-like structure is apparent (Fig. 11.13). If hemiatrophy is to supervene facial asymmetry is usually apparent within a year.

Lichen sclerosus et atrophicus

This relatively uncommon disease affects females ten times more often than males. It involves the vulva only, or the vulva and perineum in a high proportion of women (Wallace 1972), but lesions may also be present on the trunk or limbs, and in some cases such sites may be affected in the absence of genital lesions.

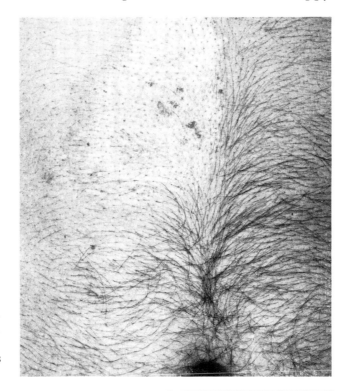

Fig. 11.12. A plaque of morphoea of the abdominal wall showing loss of hair in the affected area (Addenbrooke's Hospital, Cambridge).

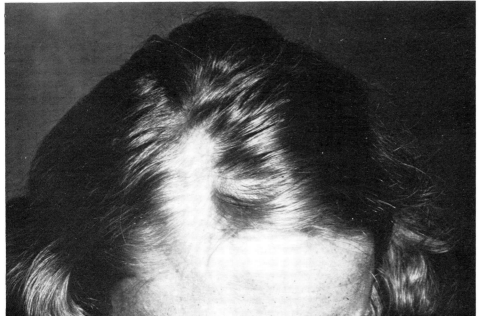

Fig. 11.13. Paramedian circumscribed scleroderma (Slade Hospital, Oxford).

Lichen sclerosus of the scalp appears to be rare. In one case (Foulds 1980) in an elderly woman, it caused extensive cicatricial alopecia (Fig. 11.14). The scalp lesions were pruritic. There were also lesions of the trunk and of the vulva.

The diagnosis must be established histologically.

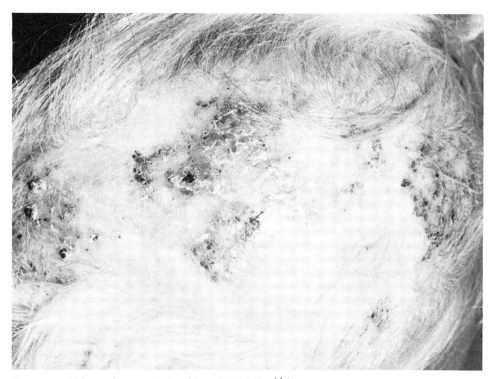

Fig. 11.14. Lichen sclerosus et atrophicus (Dr I.S. Foulds).

References

Foulds I.S. (1980) Lichen sclerosus et atrophicus of the scalp. *British Journal of Dermatology,* **103,** 197.

Wallace H.J. (1972) Lichen sclerosus et atrophicus. *Transactions of the St John's Hospital Dermatological Society,* **57,** 148.

Porokeratosis of Mibelli

This is a rare disorder of keratinization characterized by extending plaques of hyperkeratosis succeeded by atrophy. The rapid extension of a previously minimal lesion in a patient receiving immunosuppressive agents, suggested that in porokeratosis there is a mutant clone of cells in the epidermis, the proliferation of which is normally controlled by immune processes (Macmillan & Roberts 1974). There is also evidence of chromosomal instability of fibroblasts from affected areas of skin (Taylor *et al.* 1978). Most cases are sporadic but some pedigrees show autosomal dominant inheritance.

Histologically the lesion shows hyperkeratosis and irregular acanthosis, penetrated by a furrow filled by a dense horny plug with a column of parakeratotic cells in its centre. Serial sections may be needed to identify this diagnostic feature, the cornoid lamella.

Porokeratosis of Mibelli commonly begins in childhood (Saunders 1961) but may first appear at any age. It is most frequent in limbs, particularly the hands and feet, the neck, the shoulders and the face but may occur anywhere including the scalp (Savage & Lederer 1951; Sehgal & Dube 1967). The initial lesion is a crateriform horny papule which gradually extends to form a circinate or irregular atrophic plaque with a raised horny margin which may be surmounted by a furrow from which the lamina of horn projects. In the scalp there is loss of hair in the atrophic phase. Squamous carcinoma (Court & Abdel-Aziz 1972) may occur in porokeratosis as early as the third decade and these patients should therefore be kept under regular supervision if excision and grafting are not practicable.

References

Cort D.F. & Abdel-Aziz A.H.M. (1972) Epithelioma arising in porokeratosis of Mibelli. *British Journal of Plastic Surgery,* **25**, 318.

Macmillan A.L. & Roberts S.O.B. (1974) Porokeratosis of Mibelli. *British Journal of Dermatology,* **90**, 45.

Saunders T.S. (1961) Porokeratosis. *Archives of Dermatology,* **84**, 98.

Savage J. & Lederer H. (1952) Porokeratosis (Mibelli). *British Journal of Dermatology,* **63**, 187.

Sehgal V.M. & Dube B. (1967) Porokeratosis (Mibelli) in a family. *Dermatologica,* **134**, 269.

Taylor A.M.R., Harnden D.G., Fairburn E.A. (1973) Chromosomal instability associated with susceptibility to malignant disease in patients with porokeratosis of Mibelli. *Journal of the National Cancer Institute,* **51**, 371.

Cicatricial alopecia in hereditary syndromes

Incontinentia pigmenti (references p. 342)

This rare syndrome occurs almost exclusively in females; its inheritance is probably determined by an X-linked gene, usually lethal in the male (Carney & Carney 1970; Gordon & Gordon 1970).

Cicatricial alopecia has been present in at least 25% of reported cases; it appears in early infancy and ceases to extend after a variable period of up to 2 years, but the loss of hair is of course permanent. Other hair defects present in some cases have been hypoplasia of the eyebrows and eyelashes and woolly-hair naevus of the scalp (Wiklund & Weston 1980).

The diagnosis is based on the skin lesions which occur in three overlapping phases. The first phase, which begins soon after birth, consists of erythema and bullae; after 3–5 months these are succeeded by hypertrophic warty papules which may be present for several months, to be succeeded in turn by a bizarre pattern of pigmentation which gives the syndrome its name, and which eventually fades. Dental and ocular anomalies are frequent.

Confusion in diagnosis is largely terminological. The name incontinentia pigmenti is best reserved for the present syndrome, associated with the names of Bloch and Sulzberger. It is sometimes applied also to the two different pigmentary syndromes associated respectively with the names of Naegele and of Ito.

References
Carney R.G. & Carney R.G. Jr. (1970) Incontinentia pigmenti. *Archives of Dermatology*, **102**, 157.
Gordon H. & Gordon W. (1970) Incontinentia pigmenti: clinical and genetical studies of two familial cases. *Dermatologica*, **140**, 150.
Wiklund D.A. & Weston W.L. (1960) Incontinentia pigmenti. *Archives of Dermatology*, **115**, 701.

Generalized follicular hamartoma

Cicatricial alopecia, beginning in childhood, was a feature of a syndrome described by Mehregan & Hardin (1973).

Their patient was a woman aged 23. From infancy she had widespread horny plugs over the trunk and limbs and small pits on the palms and soles. She later developed cicatricial alopecia, in which, from the age of 8, appeared follicular tumours.

The tumours of the scalp were proliferating tricholemmal cysts. The lesions of palms and soles showed funnel-shaped dilatation of sweat ducts, which were plugged with parakeratotic material containing acid mucopolysaccharide.

Reference
Mehregan A.H. & Hardin I. (1973) Generalized follicular hamartoma. *Archives of Dermatology*, **107**, 435.

Epidermolysis bullosa

History and nomenclature
The term epidermolysis bullosa is applied to a group of distinct genetically determined disorders characterized by the formation of bullae of skin, and often also of mucous membranes, in response to trauma or spontaneously. Only one of these diseases is accompanied by abnormalities of scalp or hair; this disease is known as recessive dystrophic epidermolysis bullosa.

Histopathology
Bullae form beneath the epidermis and fragments of dermis may adhere to the roof.

Clinical features.

The inexorable blistering of skin and mucous membranes dominates the picture. The blisters are followed by atrophic scarring. This may give rise to more or less extensive cicatricial alopecia of the scalp (Wagner 1956). In addition the hair generally may be fine and sparse (Vuorinen 1970).

In many case reports the state of the hair is not mentioned. Of 30 cases studied by Videl (1974) 3 had cicatricial alopecia.

References

Videl J. (1974) Epidermolisis ampollares. *Actas Dermo-Sifiliograficas*, **65**, 3.

Vuorinen E. (1970) Uber ein Zwillingspaar mit Epidermolysis bullosa dystrophica polydysplastica. *Dermatologica*, **140**, Suppl. II, 3.

Wagner W. (1956) Alopezia und Nagelveränderungen bei Epidermolysis bullosa hereditaria. *Zeitschrift für Haut und Geschlectskrankheiten*, **20**, 278.

Cleft lip–palate, ectodermal dysplasia and syndactyly

Aetiology

This rare, or rarely recognized syndrome is probably hereditary, and determined by an autosomal recessive gene.

Clinical features

The constant features of the syndrome are mental retardation, cleft palate, genital hypoplasia, cicatricial alopecia and defective teeth. Other features include syndactyly.

Reference

Brown P. & Armstrong H.B. (1976) Ectodermal dysplasia, mental retardation, cleft lip/palate and other anomalies in three sibs. *Clinical Genetics*, **9**, 35.

Polyostotic fibrous dysplasia

The progressive enlargement over a period of 10 years of a bald patch present since childhood was shown histologically to be due to the replacement of the follicles by coils of fibrous tissue. The patient had polyostotic fibrous dysplasia (Shelley & Wood 1976).

Reference

Shelley L.B. & Wood M.G. (1976) Alopecia with fibrous dysplasia and osteoma of the skin. *Archives of Dermatology*, **112**, 715.

Chapter 12
The Colour of the Hair

Normal hair colour
(References p. 352)

Melanin literally means black, but scientists have long used the term to describe a range of pigments from yellow to black (Robin, 1873). Animal biologists usually define melanin as a pigment derived from melanocytes. The superficial structures of most vertebrates contain such melanin pigments—skin, hair, scales and feathers.

In man, hair pigmentation depends entirely on the presence of melanin from melanocytes but the actual colour perceived may sometimes also depend on physical phenomena (p. 349). The range of colours produced by melanins is limited to shades of grey, yellow, brown, red and black. In contrast, many lower animals display brighter colours due to such pigments as porphyrins and carotenoids in addition to melanins (Munro Fox & Vevers 1960).

Melanin chemistry

Many problems remain to be resolved regarding the structure of natural melanins. They usually exist bound to protein and cannot be solubilized without degradation. They bind various other substances avidly thus making purification and exact chemical analysis impossible at present; and X-ray diffraction patterns cannot be obtained. This implies that melanins do not form crystal structures and furthermore suggests that they are mixtures of related but dissimilar molecules which are likely to result at least partly from a chemical condensation rather than from a purely enzyme-catalysed reaction (Mier and Cotton, 1976).

The whole range of human hair colour is due to two types of melanin, eumelanins, which are mainly black but give black and brown hair, and phaeomelanins, which are yellow or red and give auburn and blond hair. Fig. 12.1 shows their suggested sub-unit structure (Riley, 1974):

Eumelanins
These appear to be polymers of irregular structure often occurring conjugated to proteins. They are insoluble in almost all solvents, resist chemical treatment and lack well-defined spectral and other physical characteristics. Eumelanins are derived from tyrosine, dopa and perhaps, dopamine (Fig. 12.2).

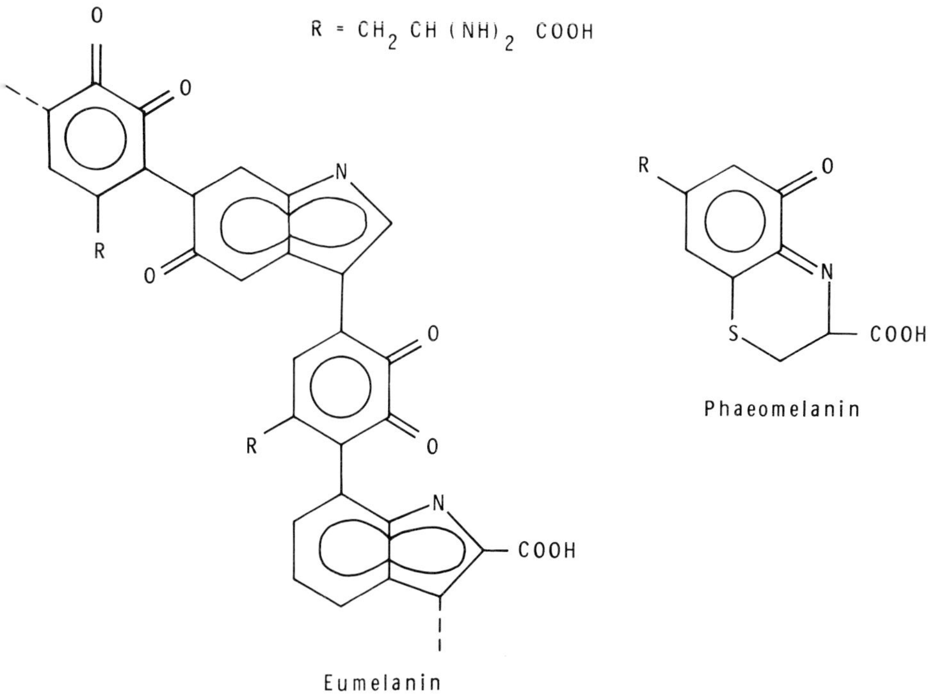

Fig. 12.1. The suggested sub-unit structure of eumelanins and phaeomelanins.

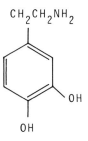

$$CH_2CH(NH)_2COOH \qquad CH_2CH(NH)_2\ COOH \qquad CH_2CH_2NH_2$$

Tyrosine   Dopa   Dopamine

Fig. 12.2. Eumelanins.

In the presence of the enzyme tyrosinase and molecular oxygen, via various intermediates, melanin is produced (Roper 1928; Mason 1948; Lerner & Fitzpatrick 1950). The exact status of tyrosinase in man remains controversial (Jimbow *et al.* 1976). There seems little doubt that the hair bulb produces eumelanin similar to that found in other sites (Nicolaus *et al.* 1964).

Phaeomelanins
These are formed in nature by a modification of the eumelanin pathway (Prota 1972) which involves an interaction of dopaquinone with cysteine (Fig. 12.3).

Early workers used acid treatment for isolation of pigments from red hair or feathers. This is now known to be unsuitable since it gives only minor fragments, the so-called trichosiderins, and even these may be structurally modified. Prota *et al.* (1970) using an alkaline extraction procedure from the feathers of New Hampshire chickens produced a red–brown precipitate and a yellow–orange supernatant. Chromatographic analysis of the dialysed precipitate gave rise to four gallophaeomelanin fractions which have not yet been structurally

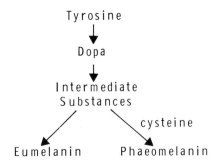

Tyrosine

Dopa

Intermediate
Substances

cysteine

Eumelanin   Phaeomelanin

Pathways of Melanin Production

Fig. 12.3. Phaeomelanins.

characterized, but they are probably based on the sub-unit structure shown in Fig 12.1; they were polymeric and contained sulphur; some also contained protein. Further treatment of the orange–yellow supernatant yielded a number of pigments; one group of these, the acid-soluble fraction, was considered to be that fraction previously regarded as trichosiderins. They did not contain iron as had previously been suggested (Flesch 1968). The structure shown in Fig. 12.4 has been proposed for three of these pigments (Prota *et al.* 1971).

In support of melanin structures obtained from work based on degradation fractions of natural melanins, both eu- and phaeomelanins have been produced *in vitro* (Cleftman 1963).

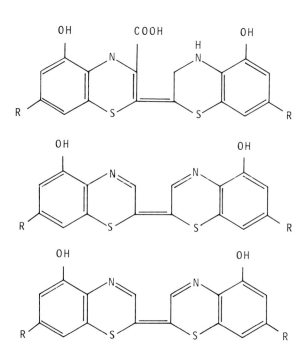

Fig. 12.4. Suggested structures of three acid soluble pigments (formerly called Trichosiderins).

Melanocytes

Functional melanocytes are situated in the hair bulb at the apex of the dermal papilla among the germinative cells of the hair matrix, the main body of the cell being in contact with the basement membrane (Fig. 12.5). Melanocytes are also present in the external root sheath and other parts of the follicle (Montagna & Chase 1956; Starrico 1960). Prior to the work of Rawle (1948) melanocytes were considered by many authorities to derive from the local cell population (Bloch 1927); Rawle showed them to be of neural crest origin. Transmission electronmicroscope studies (Birbeck *et al.* 1956) later established clearly the secretory nature of the melanocyte and the structure of its product, the melanosome. The presence of developing melanosomes and the scarcity of tonofilaments in the cytoplasm, together with the absence of desmosomal attachments, easily differentiates melanocytes from adjacent matrix cells.

Biochemical, histochemical, electronmicroscopic and autoradiographic studies have shown that melanosome formation proceeds in an orderly fashion. The process involves the construction of four basic components that include structural proteins, tyrosinase, 'membranes' and possibly also certain auxiliary enzymes. The process has been well reviewed (Jimbow *et al.* 1976). The main constructional theory (Birbeck 1963; Seiji & Twashita 1965) states that tyrosinase is synthesized on membrane-bound ribosomes and transported via endoplasmic reticulum to the Golgi region where it accumulates in small, round, membrane-limiting vesicles. These increase in size either by enlargement or fusion, become oval and acquire a characteristic patterned internal structure consisting of an ordered arrangement of tyrosinase molecules on a protein matrix. Alternative theories to this sequence of events have been proposed

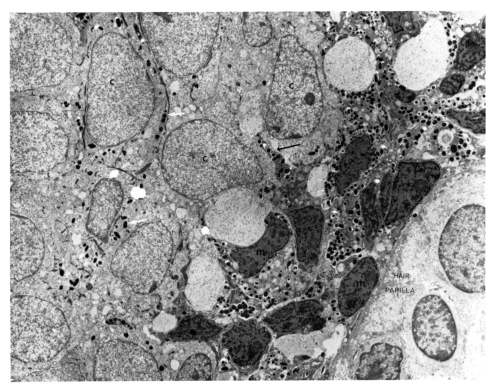

Fig. 12.5. A melanocyte (M) is present adjacent to the dermal papilloma: the dark staining nucleus (M) is surrounded by large numbers of cytoplasmic melanosomes in the melanocyte (black arrows) and matrix cells (white arrows). Many paler staining matrix cells are present (C).

(Wellings & Siegel 1963; Overbeck & Philipp 1968; Jimbow *et al.* 1971), but all lead to the stage one melanosome (unmelanized) containing inactive tyrosinase. Subsequent stages involve the activation of tyrosinase and increasing deposition of electron-dense melanin within the melanosomes. The complete development of melanosomes has been divided into four stages (Zelickson & Mottaz 1974). Stage four is the fully mature melanosome; in the past many studies have intimated that this electron-dense, melanin-laden structure is amorphous. However, Jimbow & Kukita (1971) have shown that completely mature melanosomes contain spherical translucent structures of unknown function called vesicoglobular bodies; they are present throughout all stages of melano-some development and increase in number as the melanosomes mature (Jimbow & Fitzpatrick 1974).

Within the cytoplasm of melanocytes, early melanosomes are distributed close to the nucleus in the Golgi region. With increasing maturity the melanosomes enlarge (Zelickson & Mottaz 1974), move away from the nuclear region and enter the dendritic processes (Jimbow & Kukita 1971).

In black hair follicles deposition of melanin within melanosomes continues until the whole unit is uniformly dense. Lighter coloured hair shows less melanin deposition and blonde hair follicles show melanosomes with a moth-eaten appearance. Red and blonde hair follicles have spherical melanosomes; those in brown and black hair are ellipsoidal (Montagna & Parakkal 1974).

Melanocytes in the hair bulb (and epidermis) differ from those found in internal structures in donating pigment to receptor cells, i.e. the hair matrix cells that ultimately differentiate to produce the hair cortex. No pigment is donated to presumptive cuticular and internal root sheath cells (Orfanos & Ruska 1968) though pigment granules have been detected in the cuticle of human nostril hair and in the coat of many animals (Swift 1977). In the epidermis each melanocyte has a relationship to a determined pool of adjacent keratinocytes to which, under suitable conditions, it donates melanosomes usually via dendritic processes; under certain circumstances melanocytes without dendrites may transfer pigment (Fitzpatrick & Breathnach 1963; Hadley & Quevedo 1966). At present there is no evidence to show whether a similar defined pool of receptor cells exists for each melanocyte in the hair follicle but it remains a probability.

Much speculation has arisen regarding the mechanism of transfer of melanosomes. Melanocytes were thought to inject pigment into recipient cells, the so-called 'cytocrine' activity (Masson 1948). It has become evident that receptor cells actively phagocytose melanin-laden dendritic fragments (Fitz-patrick & Breathnach 1968; Mottaz & Zelickson 1967). Within the matrix cells the engulfed dendritic tips undergo partial lysosomal digestion releasing some pigment granules into the cytoplasm. As the presumptive cortical cells differentiate they harden prior to keratinization, thus fixing the position of the melanin granules between keratin fibrils.

Melanocytes are functionally active only during the anagen phase of the hair cycle. They were formerly thought to disappear during telogen but it is now known that they remain at the surface of the papilla in a shrunken adendritic form. Jimbow *et al.* (1974) found melanocytes with mature melanosomes in resting feather follicles, whilst other workers detected aggregated pigment granules in clear cells of telogen hair follicles (Silver *et al.* 1969). It is possible that the full complement of melanocytes present during successive anagen phases is the result not only of reactivation of 'dormant' cells but also new cells due to melanocyte replication (Jimbow *et al.* 1975).

Definitive hair pigmentation

Melanin granules are distributed throughout the hair cortex (Fig. 12.6) but in greater concentration towards the periphery. Paracortex is thought to contain more granules than the less-dense orthocortex (Laxer *et al.* 1954). The pigment granules of black and brunette hair have oval pigment grains with a more or less homogeneous inner structure and sharp boundaries; the surface is finely grained

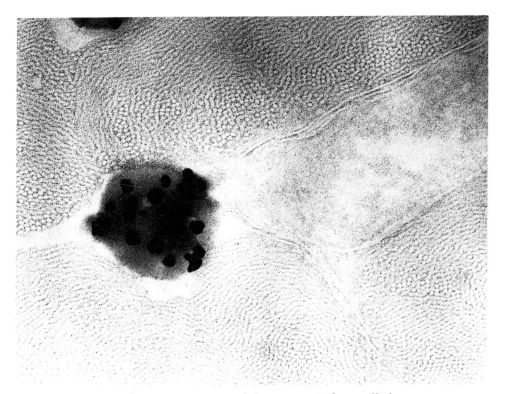

Fig. 12.6. Hair cortex, showing pigment granule between cortical macrofibrils.

with a thin surrounding membrane-like layer of osmophilic material (Orfanos & Ruska 1968). Black hair granules are also relatively hard as judged from ultramicrotome sectioning, have a high refractive index (Swift 1977) and a greater absolute number of such granules are present in dark hair compared to lighter shades. Blonde hair granules are smaller, partly ellipsoid and partly rod-shaped in longitutinal section and frequently have a rough, irregular and pitted surface.

Hair colour due to physical phenomena

The white colour of hair seen when melanin is absent is an optical effect due to reflection and refraction of incident light from various interfaces at which zones of different refractive index are in contact (Fig. 12.7).

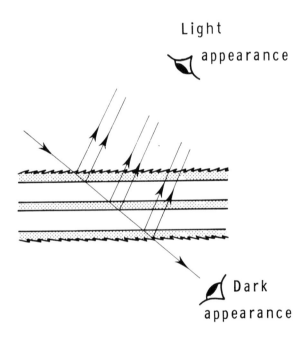

Fig. 12.7. Diagrammatic view of main hair structure interfaces which reflect and refract light.

Thus, in general non-pigmented hair with a broad medulla appears paler than non-medullated hair. Many arctic animals have such broadly medullated hair which contributes to the whiteness necessary for camouflage. Normal 'weathering' of hair along its length may lead to the terminal part appearing lighter than the rest due to a similar mechanism—the cortex and cuticle become disrupted and form numerous interfaces for internal reflection and refraction of light. This also applies in trichorrhexis nodosa (excessive 'weathering') in which patients often note a lightening in colour of the brittle hair, and in the white bands of pili annulati (Dawber 1972).

Since these optical whitening effects are due to reflection and refraction of incident light, when such hairs are viewed by transmitted light microscopy, they appear dark.

Newly formed unpigmented hair with no medulla appears yellowish rather than white. This is probably the intrinsic colour of dense keratin as orientated in hair fibres.

Function of hair colour

In lower animals, coat colour and patterning are important as camouflage, for sexual attraction, in releasing certain behaviour patterns and for protection against sunlight (Cott 1956; Lorenz 1970). Hair colour in man is purely decorative and has no essential biological function. The racial and genetic colour differences that have evolved are probably related to the u.v.r. protective colours seen in the skin, i.e. dark-skinned races have dark hair. Hair pigment, however, is not important in protection against the effects of sunlight. The decorative function of hair colour thus appears to be a matter of serendipity.

Colour variation

Lanugo hair present in utero is unpigmented. Vellus hair is also typically unpigmented but, in men in particular, some vellus fibres may pigment slightly after puberty. Hair colour varies according to body site in most people (Wasserman 1974). Eyelashes are usually the darkest. Scalp hair is generally lighter than genital hair which often has a reddish tint even in subjects having essentially brown hair. Grobbelaar (1952) showed that hair on the lower and lateral scrotal surfaces is lighter than on the pubes. He also noted the frequent presence of a red tint in axillary hairs even in the absence of auburn hair on other body sites; this change was not seen in Rehoboth coloureds. Apart from individuals with red scalp hair, a red tint to axillary hair is commonest in brown-haired individuals.

Hair on exposed parts may be bleached by sunlight. Very dark hair first lightens to a brownish-red colour but rarely becomes blonde even after strong sunlight exposure; brown hair, however, may be bleached white.

Slow oxidation of hair melanin occurs after death with consequent colour lightening (Brothwell and Spearman, 1963).

Control of hair colour

Hair colour is primarily under close genetic supervision. However, the exact hormonal and cellular mechanisms controlling melanocyte function are not clearly worked out. An intimate relationship must exist between the factors controlling melanocyte and matrix cell activity since melanocyte mitosis and melanosome production and transfer occur only during the anagen phase of the hair cycle. A negative feedback system has been postulated. Enzyme degradation products of melanosomes within matrix cells may cross cell membranes to melanocytes and control further melanin production or transfer (Jimbow *et al.* 1975). Melanosome degradation within melanocytes may also have an inhibitory effect on melanogenesis and even destroy melanocytes. A melanocyte specific 'chalone' acting within a negative feedback system may well exist for follicular melanocytes (Bullough 1975). Voorhees *et al.* (1973) have proposed that such control mechanisms utilize the 'second messenger' adenyl cyclase–cyclic AMP system (Sunderland 1970). Lerner (1971) suggested that cAMP controls hormonal and neural regulation of melanosome movement and stimulates tyrosinase synthesis prior to increased melanogenesis. Follicular melanocytes are known to respond like epidermal melanocytes to melanocyte stimulating hormone (α-MSH) which can darken light-coloured hair. α-MSH may act on tyrosinase by converting it to an active form by inactivation of an inhibitor (Wong & Pawelek 1975). cAMP may also control replication of melanocytes which show mitosis during the anagen phase (Jimbow *et al.* 1975); whether cGMP is active in controlling matrix cell division is not clear. The effect of hormones other than MSH on hair pigmentation has yet to be clearly elucidated. Oestrogens and progestogens may increase hair colour in view of their effect on the epidermis during pregnancy.

References

Birbeck M.S.C., Mercer E.H. & Barnicot N.A. (1956) The structure and formation of pigment granules in human hair. *Experimental Cell Research*, **10**, 505.

Birkbeck M.S.C. (1963) Electron microscopy of melanocytes: the fine structure of hair bulb premelanosomes. *Annals of the New York Academy of Sciences*, **100**, 540.

Bloch B. (1927) Das Pigment Anatomie der Haut, eds. B. Bloch, F. Pinkus & W. Spalteholz. Berlin, Springer, p. 434.

Bullough W.S. (1975) Chalone control mechanisms. *Life Science*, **16**, 323.

Brothwell D. & Spearman R.I.C. (1963) The hair of earlier people. In *Science in Archaelogy* 1st edn., eds. D. Brothwell & E. Higgs. London, Thames & Hudson, ch. 41.

Cleffman G. (1963) Agouti pigment cells *in situ* and *in vitro*. *Annals of the New York Academy of Sciences*, **100**, 749.

Cott H.B. (1956) *Adaptive Coloration in Animals*. London, Methuen.

Dawber R.P.R. (1972) Investigations of a family with pili annulati associated with blue naevi. *Transactions of the St John's Hospital Dermatology Society*, **58**, 51.

Fitzpatrick T.B. & Breathnach A.S. (1963) Das epidermale melanin einheit system. *Dermatologie Wochenschrift*, **147**, 481.

Fletch P. (1968) Inhibitory action of extracts of mammalian skin on pigment formation. *Proceedings of the Society of Experimental Biological Medicine*, **70**, 136.

Grobbelaar C.S. (1952) The distribution of, and correlation between eye, hair and skin colour in male students at the University of Stellenbosch. *Annals of the University of Stellenbosch*, **28**, Sect. A/1.

Hadley M.E. & Quevado W.C. Jnr (1966) Vertebrate epidermal melanin unit. *Nature (London)*, **209**, 1334.

Jimbow K. & Kukita A. (1971) In *Biology of Normal and Abnormal Melanocytes*, eds. T. Kawamura, T.B. Fitzpatrick & M. Seiji. Baltimore, University Park Press.

Jimbow K., Takahashi M., Sato S. & Kukita A. (1971) Ultrastructural and cytochemical studies on melanogenesis in melanocytes of normal human hair matrix. *Journal of Electron Microscopy (Tokyo)*, **20**, 87.

Jimbow K. & Fitzpatrick T.B. (1974) The characterization of a new melanosomal body—the vesiculo-globular body—by conventional transmission, high voltage and scanning electron microscopy. *Journal of Ultrastructural Research*, **48**, 269.

Jimbo K., Szabo G. & Fitzpatrick T.B. (1974) Ultrastructural investigation of autophagocytosis of melanosomes and programmed death of melanocytes in white Leghorn feathers. *Developmental Biology*, **36**, 8.

Jimbo K., Roth S., Fitzpatrick T.B. & Szabo G. (1975) Mitotic activity in non-neoplastic melanocytes in vivo as determined by histo-chemical autoradiographic and electron microscopic studies. *Journal of Cell Biology*, **66**, 663.

Laxer G., Sikorski J., Whewell C.S. & Woods H.J. (1954) The electron microscopy of melanin granules isolated from pigmented mammalian fibres. *Biochemie Biophysics Acta*, **15**, 174.

Lerner A.B. (1971) Neural control of pigment cells. In *Biology of Normal and Abnormal Melanocytes*, eds. T. Kawamura, T.B. Fitzpatrick & M. Seiji. Tokyo, University of Tokyo Press.

Lerner A.B. & Fitzpatrick T.B. (1950) Biochemistry of melanin formation. *Physiology Review*, **30**, 91.

Lorenz K. (1970) Studies in animal and human behaviour, vol. 1. London, Methuen.

Mason H.S. (1948) The chemistry of melanins. *Journal of Biological Chemistry*, **172**, 83.

Masson P. (1948) Pigment cells in man. In *The Biology of Melanosomes*, eds. R.W. Miner & M. Gordon. Special Publication of New York Academy of Sciences, p. 15.

Mier P.D. & Cotton D.W.K. (1976) *The Molecular Biology of Skin*, 1st edn. Oxford, Blackwell Scientific Publications.

Montagna W. & Chase H.B. (1956) Histology and cytochemistry of human skin. X. X-irradiation of the scalp. *American Journal of Anatomy*, **99**, 415.

Montagna W. & Parakkal P.F. (1974) In *The Structure and Function of Skin*, 3rd edn. New York, Academic Press, p. 232.

Mottaz J.H. & Zelickson A.S. (1967) Melanin transfer: A possible phagocytic process. *Journal of Investigative Dermatology*, **49**, 605.

Munro Fox H. & Vevers G. (1960) *The Nature of Animal Colours*. London, Sidgwick & Jackson.

Nicolaus R.A., Piattelli M. & Fattorusso E. (1964) The structure of melanins and melanogenesis. IV. On some natural melanins. *Tetrahedron*, **20**, 1163.

Orfanos C. & Ruska H. (1968) Die Feinstruktur des Menschlichen Haares. III. Das Haarpigment. *Archiv für klinische und experimentelle Dermatologie*, **231**, 279.

Overbeck L. & Philipp E. (1968) Zur Melanogenese in Menschlichen Tumorzellen. *Naturwissenschaften*, **55**, 232.

Prota G., Crescenzi S., Miscuraca G. & Nicolaus R.A. (1970) New intermediates in phaeomelanogenesis *in vitro*. *Experientia*, **26**, 1058.

Prota G., Suarato A. & Nicolaus R.A. (1971) The isolation and structure of trichosiderin B. *Experientia*, **27**, 1381.

Prota G. (1972) Structure and biogenesis of phaeomelanins. In *Pigmentation, its Genesis and Biological Control*, ed. V. Riley. New York, Appleton-Century-Crofts, p. 615.

Raper H.S. (1928) The aerobin oxidases. *Physiology Review*, **8**, 245.

Rawle M.E. (1948) Origin of melanophores and their role in development of color patterns in vertebrates. (Review) *Physiology*, **28**, 383.

Riley P.A. (1974) The nature of melanins. In *The Physiology and Pathophysiology of Skin*, vol. 3, ed. A. Jarrett. London, Academic Press, p. 1102.

Robin C.P. (1873) *Anatomie et Physiologie Cellulaire*. Paris, Baillière et Fils.

Seiji M. & Iwashita S. (1965) Intracellular localisation of tyrosinase and site of melanin formation in the melanocyte. *Journal of Investigative Dermatology*, **45**, 305.

Silver A.F., Chase H.B. & Potten C.F. (1969) Melanocyte precursor cells in the hair follicle germ during the dormant stage (telogen). *Experientia*, **25**, 209.

Staricco R.G. (1960) The melanocyte and the hair follicle. *Journal of Investigative Dermatology*, **35**, 185.

Sunderland W.E. (1970) On the biological role of cyclic AMP. *Journal of the American Medical Association*, **214**, 1281.

Swift J.A. (1977) The histology of keratin fibres. In *Chemistry of Natural Protein Fibres*, 1st edn., ed. R.S. Asquith. New York, Plenum Press, p. 114.

Voorhees J.J., Duell E.G., Bass L.J. & Harrell E.R. (1973) Role of cyclic AMP in the control of epidermal cell growths and differentiation. In *Chalones: Concept and Current Researchers*, eds. B.K. Forscher & J.C. Houck. National Cancer Institute Monograms, **38**, 47.

Wassermann H.P. (1974) *Ethnic pigmentation*. Amsterdam, Excerpta Medica.

Welling S.R. & Siegal B.V. (1963) Electron microscopic studies on the subcellular origin and ultrastructure of melanin granules in mammalian melanosomes. *Annals of the New York Academy of Sciences*, **100**, 548.

Wong G. & Pawelek J. (1975) Melanocyte-stimulating hormone promotes activation of pre-existing tyrosinase molecules in Cloudeman 591 melanoma cells. *Nature (London)*, **255**, 644.

Zelickson A.S. & Mottaz J.H. (1974) In *The First Human Hair Symposium*, ed. A.C. Brown. New York, Medcom Press, p. 277.

Variations in hair colour
(References p. 363)

Genetic and racial aspects (Baker 1974)

Mammalian hair colour has long been a subject of considerable interest to geneticists and in a variety of species, including man, a number of genetic variants have been described. Most of the large studies have been in species which provide many hair colour mutations, e.g. the house mouse; in such animals the required stocks demonstrating the mutations are available and easily produced in view of the large number of inbred strains in existence (Silvers 1968). Genetic studies of hair colour do not only provide us with knowledge of gene function; they also give insight into the mechanism of hair pigmentation (Takeuchi 1975). From laboratory and animal studies a general conformity has been shown in the complement of genes affecting hair colour (Fitzpatrick *et al.* 1958; Rife 1967) and it is reasonable to assume that an essentially similar complex of genes may be involved in man. Human hair (and skin) colour is influenced by at least four gene loci which are probably allelic (Harrison & Owen 1965; Livingstone 1969; Stern 1970; Harrison 1973); several of the allelic series of other mammals (Deol 1963) are probably present in man but the agouti allele is not. The chief obstacle to more detailed studies of hair colour inheritance in man is the absence of clear data on crosses between individuals with 'pure' caucasoid, negroid and mongoloid skin. Much has been read into crosses between American Negroids and Caucasoids but such studies do not provide clear answers since American blacks are not a pure race. Stern (1953) estimated the Caucasoid alleles in the American Negroid at 30%; Reed (1969) suggested 20%.

Ethnic differences in hair colour are very conspicuous, as are the differences in hair morphology, though colour and hair form are inherited separately (Trotter & Duggins 1950). Many early studies on ethnic hair colour differences are difficult to relate since they did not compare like with like, using different descriptive terms of hair colour (Wassermann 1974). Verbal description has been used widely for general studies: blond hair colour is considered with 'bamboo' and 'flax'. Other terms often used are flaxen, platinum blonde, dark blonde, golden brown and hairbrown. Grey variations of hair include ash blond, golden grey and ash grey. Golden or reddish variations are: golden blond, reddish blond, red-haired, golden, golden yellow, reddish golden, titian (red) and henna (Kornerup & Wanscher 1963). Colour matching is the usual method now used for describing hair colour more specifically, e.g. the Fischer–Saller Hair Colour Scale (Sunderland 1965). When sufficient hair is available reflectance spectro-photometry may be usefully used (Reed 1952; Sunderland 1956; Barnicott 1956); Hanna (1956) used colorimetric estimation of extracted pigment.

Dark hair predominates in the world. Among Caucasoids there is wide variation in colour within geographical regions (Sunderland 1956). Blond hair is most frequent in northern Europe and black hair in southern and eastern Europe; foci of blondness are to be found even in North Africa, the Middle East and in some Australoids. Congoid, Capoid, Mongoloid and Australoid hair is mainly black. Previous description (p. 346) has shown that melanin pigment is synthesized in the melanocyte and deposited in the melanosomes; the chemical nature of the melanin and the shape, number and final position of pigment granules in the hair cortex determine the exact colour. Density of cortical pigment shows greater variation between, rather than within races. In dark-haired populations there is marked variation in the quantity of pigment and, as hair tends towards black, differentiations of shades becomes more difficult. In specific countries variations in hair colour may be found associated with eye colour changes. Blond hair is often linked with blue eyes.

Red hair (syn. rutilism)

This has attracted more attention than other colours because it is less common and because it is so distinctive. The melanin pigment is phaeomelanin, not eumelanin—the differences of melanin distribution and melanosome structures are described on p. 344. In the United Kingdom and Italy the distribution of red hair is similar to that of blood group O, excluding East Anglia (Harrison *et al.* 1964). The incidence of red hair varies from 0.3% in northern Germany, 1.6% in Paris to 3.7% in England; it is as high at 11% in parts of Scotland. Red-hair inheritance is dominant to non-red but hypostatic to brown and black (Rife 1967). This contrasts with earlier reports that it is recessive to non-red (Singleton & Ellis 1964). Reddish hair may occur as an isolated abnormality or in association with xanthism in certain areas (Barnicott 1952). Like hair of many other colours, red hair often darkens with age from red through brown to sandy or auburn in the adult. The skin of red-heads is generally pale, burns easily in sunlight and pigments very little even after prolonged and frequent sun exposure; there is also poor resistance to skin irritants, e.g. red-haired psoriatic patients receiving topical dithranol will tolerate only relatively low strengths without burning. The evidence for the widely held view that red-haired individuals are more susceptible to tuberculosis and rheumatic fever is only anecdotal.

Heterochromia

This implies the growth of hair of two distinct colours in the same individual. A colour difference between scalp and moustache is not uncommon. In fair-haired individuals pubic and axillary hair, eyebrows and eyelashes are much darker than scalp hair. In humans, eyelashes are generally the most darkly pigmented hairs. Black- and brown-haired subjects often have red or auburn sideburns. In other than the fair-haired, genital hair is usually lighter than scalp hair and it may have a reddish tint even in those with brown pubic hair: 33% of a series of South African whites had red axillary hair whilst this was only occasionally seen in coloureds; also hair on the lower and lateral aspect of the scrotum was lighter than on the pubes (Grobbelaar 1952). In brown-haired individuals a reddish tint is more common in axillary hair than on the scalp.

In general scalp hair darkens with age (Sunderland 1956). May fair-haired children have brown hair by adult life; in a Polish population, blond-haired children between 13 and 24 months of age changed to dark colouring by the age of 15 years (Miszkiewicz 1965).

Rarely a circumscribed patch or patches of hair occur of different colour. This generally has a genetic basis though the type of inheritance is not known in man. In the mouse, haphazard colour patterns may be due to somatic mutations during embryonic life; clones of altered melanocytes, or keratinocytes with changed inductive effects, form a mosaic in the skin (Russell 1946). Patchy differences of hair colour are of five types:

(a) Tufts of very dark, coarse hair growing from a melanocytic naevus.

(b) Hereditary, usually autosomal dominant heterochromia, e.g. tufts of red hair at the temples in a black-haired subject or a single black patch in a blond.

(c) Perhaps as a result of somatic mosaicism partial asymmetry of hair and eye colour may occur sporadically.

(d) The white forelock of piebaldism (p. 360).

(e) The 'flag' sign in kwashiorkor.

Greying of hair (syn. canities)

Greying of hair is usually a manifestation of the ageing process and is due to a progressive reduction in melanocyte function. The larger medullary spaces of older people may contribute to the process. There is no gross change in the cuticle or cortex with age but it has been suggested that increased reflection of light may occur on cell interfaces and islets of interfibrillary matrix (Orfanos *et al.* 1970).

There is a gradual dilution of pigment in greying hairs, i.e. the full range of colour from normal to white can be seen both along individual hairs and from hair to hair. Loss of hair shaft colour is associated with decrease and eventual cessation of tyrosine activity in the lower bulb (Kukita & Fitzpatrick 1955). Transmission electronmicroscopic studies (Orfanos *et al.* 1970) have shown that many melanocytes are still present in their normal anatomical position in grey hairs; however, many contain large cytoplasmic vacuoles and others, normal looking but incompletely melanized melanosomes. In white hairs melanocytes are infrequent or absent (Herzberg & Gusek 1970) or possibly dormant (Fitzpatrick *et al.* 1966). It has been suggested that auto-immunity plays a part in the pathogenesis of greying: grey hair certainly has an association with the auto-immune disease pernicious anaemia; Dawber (1970) found that 55% of patients with pernicious anaemia were grey before 50 years of age compared with only 30% in a matched control group. Altered nerve supply may also be relevant (Lerner, 1966); compared to the normal side the sympathectomized scalp shows fewer grey hairs. In this respect it is interesting that there have been reports of pilocarpine taken orally darkening white hair (Savill 1944). True canities is probably never associated with pathological processes such as malabsorption syndrome and vitamin B deficiencies (Savill 1944; Klaus 1980).

The age of onset of canities is primarily dependent on the genotype of the individual though acquired factors may play a part. The visual impression of greyness is more obvious (seen earlier) in dark-haired individuals but complete greying may appear to be earlier in the fair-haired. In Caucasoid races white hair first appears at the age of 34.2 ± 9.6 years, and by the age of 50 years, 50% of the population have at least 50% grey hairs (Keogh & Walsh 1965). The onset in negroes is 43.9 ± 10.3 years, and in Japanese between 30 and 34 years in men and 35 and 39 years in women (Wassermann 1974). The beard and moustache areas commonly become grey before scalp or body hair. On the scalp, the temples usually show greying first, followed by a wave of greyness spreading to the crown and later the occipital area.

Rapid onset, allegedly 'overnight' greying of hair, has excited the literary, medical and anthropological worlds for centuries (Jelinek 1972). Many reports have been over-dramatized but it certainly occurs. Historical examples often quoted include Sir Thomas More and Marie Antoinette whose hair became grey over the night preceding their execution. Henry de Navarre showed white hair in his moustache within hours of hearing that the edict of Nemours had been conceded. Brown-Séquard (1869) studied the rate of hair whitening on his own beard. He pulled out all the white hairs and carefully observed the remainder. Two days later, apart from many hairs which were grey near the root, five were white long their entire length. Further similar observations over several weeks confirmed this finding: unfortunately no microscopical studies were carried out and the length of affected hairs was not stated. The probable mechanism for rapid greying is the selective shedding of pigmented hairs in diffuse elopecia areata, the non-pigmented hairs being retained. Most grey-haired individuals have both grey and pigmented hair and the visual impression of greyness may not be obvious until the dark hairs are lost. The flaw in his hypothesis is the frequent absence of hair loss associated with rapid whitening, though often as much as 50% of scalp hair may need to be lost before alopecia is noted.

Despite occasional reports to the contrary, in general greying of hair is progressive and permanent. Most of the reports of the return of normal hair colour from grey are examples of a pigmented regrowth following alopecia areata, which eventually repigments in many cases. The reported repigmentation of grey hair in association with Addisonian hypoadrenalism may result from a mechanism similar to that in alopecia areata or vitiligo, in view of the known association between these diseases (Addison 1855; Dunlop 1963; Cunliffe *et al.* 1968; Main *et al.* 1975). Darkening of grey hair may occur following large doses of p-aminobenzoic acid; Sieve (1941) gave 100 mg three times per day by mouth to 460 grey-haired people and noted a response in 82%. Pigmentation was obvious within 2–4 months of starting treatment. The hairs became grey again 2–4 weeks after stopping the therapy.

Premature greying of hair

Premature greying of hair (Fig. 12.8) has been defined as onset of greying before 20 years of age in Caucasoids and 30 years of age in Negroids. It probably has a genetic basis and occasionally occurs as an isolated autosomal dominant condition. The association between premature greying and certain organ-specific auto-immune diseases is well documented. The relationship is probably not one of common pathogenesis but on the basis of genetic linkage. It is often stated that premature greying may be an early sign of pernicious anaemia, hyperthyroidism and less commonly hypothyroidism, all auto-immune diseases which individually have a genetic predisposition. In a controlled study of the integumentary associations of pernicious anaemia, 11% had premature greying (Dawber 1970). It has been suggested that coronary artery disease, hypertension and left bundle branch block are significantly associated with premature greying but the evidence is largely anecdotal and the relationship remains unproven.

In Böök's syndrome, an autosomal dominant trait, premature greying is associated with premolar hypodontia and palmoplantar hyperhidrosis (Böök, 1950).

The premature ageing syndromes, progeria and Werner's syndrome (pangeria), may have very early greying as a prominent feature. It does not occur in metageria, acrogeria or total lipodystrophy (Gilkes *et al.* 1974). In progeria it is associated with marked loss of scalp hair as early as 2 years of age. Werner's syndrome is inherited as an autosomal recessive condition. Temporal greying usually commences in adolescence, rarely as early as 8 years of age. Further

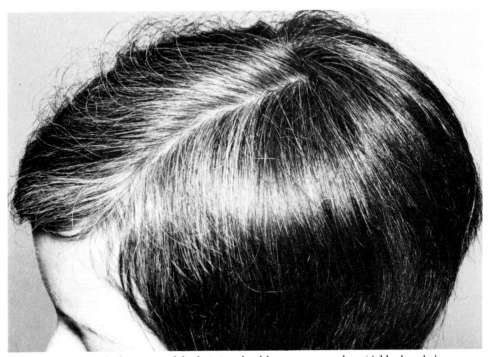

Fig. 12.8. Well-marked greying of the hair in a healthy woman aged 22 (Addenbrooke's Hospital, Cambridge).

spread of grey hair on the scalp is followed by progressive baldness by 25 years of age in association with other manifestation of premature ageing in many tissues (Fleischmajer & Nedwich 1973).

In dystrophia myotonica the onset of grey hair may preceed the myotonia and muscle wasting.

Premature canities is an inconstant feature of the Rothmund–Thomson syndrome; when present it typically commences in adolescence.

Waardenburg's syndrome (p. 360) may include early greying of hair as a feature (Rugel & Keats 1965).

One-third of adult patients with chromosome five p-syndrome (cri du chat syndrome) have prematurely grey hair (Breg 1975).

Poliosis

Poliosis is defined as the presence of a localised patch of white hair due to the absence or deficiency of melanin in a group of neighbouring follicles. Essentially the changes in melanogenesis are the same in the hair follicle as in the affected epidermis.

Hereditary defects

Piebaldism (syn. white spotting or partial albinism) is an autosomal dominant abnormality with patches of skin totally devoid of pigment, which remain unchanged throughout life (Comings & Odland 1966). Most commonly a frontal white patch occurs—the white forelock—which may be the only sign. Melanocytes are decreased in number, but are morphologically abnormal and contain normal non-melanized pre-melanosomes, and also pre-melanosomes and melanosomes of abnormal appearance (Grupper *et al.* 1970). Similar pathological changes are seen in Tietz's syndrome of generalized 'white spot' loss of skin and hair pigment, complete deaf mutism and eyebrow hypoplasia (Witkop 1971).

Waardenburg's syndrome (Waardenburg 1951) shows skin changes so similar to piebaldism that they are presumed to have a similar pathogenesis. Symptoms and signs are present from birth and include dystopia cantharum with lateral displacement of the medial canthi, hypertrophy of the nasal root and hyperplasia of the inner third of the eyebrows with confluent brows. Total or partial iridal heterochromia may occur as may perceptive deafness. The white forelock is present in 20% of cases. Premature greying may develop with or without the white forelock (Rugel & Keats 1965; Pantke & Cohen 1971); a minority have piebaldism and congenital nerve deafness but no other overt signs of Waardenburg's syndrome, suggesting that this association may be genetically distinct.

Vitiligo is an acquired cutaneous achromia probably determined by an autosomal gene, in which the white patches of skin frequently have white hairs within them. The histological changes are consistent with an 'auto-immune injury' to the melanocytes.

The Vogt–Koyanagi–Harada syndrome (Vogt 1906; Harada 1926; Koyanagi 1929) consists of a post-febrile illness comprising bilateral uveitis, labrynthine deafness, tinnitus, and vitiligo, poliosis and alopecia areata (Rosen 1945; Howsden 1973). Alezzandrini's syndrome combines unilateral facial vitiligo, retinitis and poliosis of eyebrows and eyelashes (Alezzandrini 1964); perceptive deafness is rarely associated.

In alopecia areata (p. 295) regrowing hair is frequently white. It may remain so, particularly in cases of late onset. Though absent hair pigment is only evident at this stage of resolution, melanocytes are lost from the hair bulb quite early and migrate to the dermal papilla. The last formed hair above the catagen root in 'exclamation mark' hairs is poorly pigmented, indicating impaired melanization of keratinocytes before matrix cell division ceases.

Poliosis occurs in 60% of cases of tuberose sclerosis (Nickel & Read 1962); depigmented hair may be the earliest sign (McWilliam & Stephenson 1978).

The pathognomonic signs of Von Recklinghausen's multiple neurofibromatosis (Canale & Bebin 1972) relate to hyperpigmented areas—café au lait macules and axillary and perineal freckling. Scalp neurofibromas may have a patch of poliosis overlying them; this must not be mistaken for vitiliginous changes, though the latter may occur as a halo around neurofibromata since they are neuroectodermal in origin.

Acquired defects

Permanent pigmentary loss may be induced by inflammatory processes which damage melanocytes, e.g. herpes zoster. X-irradiation often causes permanent hair loss but less intense treatment leads to hypopigmented and, rarely, hyperpigmented hair. Patchy white hair may develop on the beard area after dental treatment.

Albinism

In autosomal recessive oculocutaneous albinism (syn: complete, perfect, or generalized albinism) similar changes are found in the hair bulb melanocytes as in the epidermis (Witkop 1971). This applies to tyrosine positive and negative types. Melanocytes are structurally normal and active in producing melanosomes of grades I and II (p. 346). They are, however, enzymically inactive. The melanocyte system is never completely devoid of melanin. In Caucasoids the hair is typically yellowish-white though it may be cream, yellow, yellowish-red or vibrant red. This range of colours parallels those seen in normal blond

Caucasoids. In Negroid albinos the hair colour is white or yellowish brown (Barnicott 1952).

Chediak–Higashi syndrome

This syndrome is basically an autosomal recessive defect of the membrane-bound organelles of several cell types. It combines oculocutaneous hypopigmentation with a lethal defect of leucocytes (Clawson *et al.* 1979; White & Clawson 1979). Most patients die of recurrent infections by 10 years of age. Melanocytes contain very large melanosomes derived from defective pre-melanosomes. Continued growth and fusion of the latter give rise to the giant melanosomes which eventually degenerate (Zelickson & Mottaz 1974). The hair is silvery grey or light blond and may be sparse (Stegmaier & Schneider 1965; Bedoya 1971).

Colour changes induced by drugs and other chemicals (Rook 1965)

Some topical agents temporarily change hair colour. Dithranol and chrysarobin stain light-coloured or grey hair mahogany brown. Resorcin, formerly used a great deal in a variety of skin diseases, colours black or white hair, yellow or yellowish-brown.

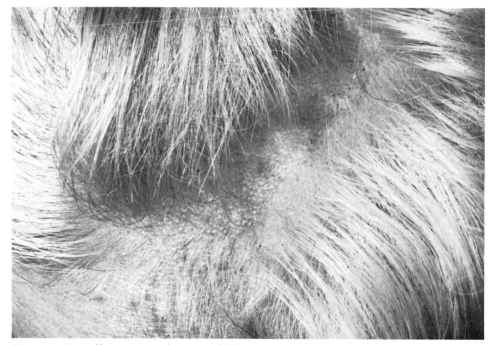

Fig. 12.9. Loss of hair pigment from use of chloroquine (Addenbrooke's Hospital, Cambridge).

Some systemic drugs alter hair colour by interfering with the eumelanin or phaeomelanin pathway; in others, the mechanism is not known. Chloroquine interferes with phaeomelanin synthesis (Saunders *et al.* 1959), i.e. it only affects blond- and red-haired individuals. After 3–4 months' treatment, hair becomes increasingly silvery or white; it is usually patchy and first affects the temples or eyebrows (Fig. 12.9). The changes are completely reversible. Mephenesin, a glycerol ether used for diseases with muscle spasms, causes pigmentary loss in dark-haired people (Spillane *et al.* 1963). Triparanol, an anti-cholesterolaemic drug, and fluorobutyrophenone, an anti-psychotic drug, both interfere with keratinization and cause hypopigmented and sparse hair; the altered colour may be due to impaired phagocytosis of melanosomes by presumptive cortical cells or an optical effect due to micropathological changes in the definitive cuticle or cortex. Minoxidil and diazoxide (Burton & Marshall 1979; Ridgley & Kassassieh 1979), two potent anti-hypertensive agents, both cause hypertrichosis and darkening of hair. The colour produced by diazoxide is reddish, whilst minoxidil darkens hair mainly by converting vellus hair to terminal hair, i.e. the increased colour equates with other body hair of the affected individual. Hydroquinone and phenylthiourea interfere with tyrosine activity causing hypopigmentation of skin and hair (Dieke 1947).

Colour changes due to nutritional deficiencies

Because specific dietary deficiencies are rare in man, most clinical knowledge of their effects is derived from laboratory and animal studies. Copper deficiency in cattle causes achromotrichia since it is the prosthetic group of tyrosinase. Loss of hair colour from this mechanism occurs in humans as Menkes' kinky hair syndrome (p. 195). In protein malnutrition, exemplified by kwashiorkor (p. 127), hair colour changes are a prominent feature; normal black hair becomes brown or reddish, and brown hair becomes blond (Bradfield 1974). Intermittent protein malnutrition leads to the 'flag' sign of kwashiorkor (signe de la bandera)—alternating white (abnormal) and dark bands occur along individual hairs (Fitzpatrick *et al.* 1979). Similar changes to kwashiorkor have been described in severe ulcerative colitis and after extensive bowel resection.

The lightening of hair colour from black to brown described in severe iron-deficiency anaemia may be an effect on keratinization rather than melanocytic function.

Hair colour in metabolic disorders

Phenylketonuria is an autosomal recessive disorder in which the tissues are unable to metabolize phenylalanine to tyrosine because of phenylalanine hydroxylase deficiency (Scriver & Rosenberg 1973). Mental retardation, fits and decreased pigmentation of skin, eyes and hair occur with eczema and dermographism. Black hair may become brown whilst older institutionalized phenyletonurias may have pale blond or grey hair. Tyrosine treatment causes darkening towards normal colour within 1–2 months.

The paling of hair seen in homocystinuria is probably due to keratinization changes in view of the error in methionine metabolism (Fitzpatrick *et al.* 1979).

Light, almost white hair and recurrent oedema are the surface manifestations of the rare condition, oast-house disease. Methionine concentration in the blood is raised.

Accidental hair discoloration

Hair avidly binds many inorganic elements and thus hair colour changes are occasionally seen after exposure to certain substances.

Exposure to high concentration of copper in industry or from inadvertently high concentrations in tap water (Nordlund *et al.* 1977; Goldschmidt 1979) or in swimming pools (Goette 1978), may cause green hair, particularly visible in blond-haired subjects. Cobalt workers get bright blue hair whilst a deep blue tint may be seen in indigo handlers (Beigel 1965). A yellow hair colour is not uncommon in white or grey-haired heavy smokers due to tar in cigarette smoke; yellow staining may also occur from picric acid. Trinitrotoluene (TNT) workers sometimes develop yellow skin and reddish-brown hair.

References

Addison T. (1855) *On the Constitutional and Local Effects of the Diseases of the Supra-renal Capsule*. London, Highly.

Alezzandrini A.A. (1964) Manifestations unilaterales de degenerescence tapetoretinienne de vitiligo, de poliose, de cheveux blancs et hypoacousie. *Ophthalmoligica*, **147**, 409.

Baker J.R. (1974) *Race*, 1st edn. London, Oxford University Press.

Barnicott N.A. (1952) Albinism in south western Nigeria. *Annals of Eugenics (London)*, **17**, 38.

Barnicott N.A. (1956) The relation of the pigment trichosiderin in hair colour. *Annals of Human Genetics*, **21**, 31.

Biegel H. (1867) Blue hair in indigo handlers. *Archives of Pathology, Anatomy and Physiology*, **83**, 324.

Böök J.A. (1950) Clinical and genetic studies of hypodontia. I. Premolar aplasia, hyperhidrosis and canites prematura: a new hereditary syndrome in man. *American Journal of Human Genetics*, **2**, 240.

Bradfield R.B. (1974) Hair tissue as a medium for the differential diagnosis of protein-calorie malnutrition: a commentary. *Journal of Paediatrics*, **84**, 294.

Breg W.R. (1975) Abnormalities of chromosomes 4 and 5. In *Endocrine and Genetic Diseases of Childhood and Adolescence*, ed. L.I. Gardner. Philadelphia, Saunders.

Brown-Sequard C. (1869) Rapid hair whitening. *Archives de Physiologie*, **2**, 442.

Burton J.L. & Marshall A. (1979) Hypertrichosis due to minoxidil. *British Journal of Dermatology*, **101**, 593.

Canale D. & Bebin J. (1972) Von Recklinghausen's multiple neurofibromatosis. In *Handbook of Clinical Neurology*. Amsterdam, North-Holland, p. 132.

Clawson C.C., Repine J.E. & White J.G. (1979) The Chediak–Higashi syndrome: quantitation of a deficiency in maximum bacterial capacity. *American Journal of Pathology*, **94**, 539.

Comings D.E. & Odland G.F. (1966) Partial albinism. *Journal of the American Medical Association*, **195**, 519.

Cunliffe W.J., Hall R., Newell D.J. & Stevenson C.J. (1968) Vitiligo, thyroid disease and auto-immunity. *British Journal of Dermatology*, **80**, 135.

Dawber R.P.R. (1970) Integumentary associations of pernicious anaemia. *British Journal of Dermatology*, **82**, 221.

Ded M.S. (1963) Inheritance of coat colour in laboratory rodents. In *Animals for Research*, ed. W. Lane-Petter. London, Academic Press.

Dieke S.H. (1947) Pigmentation and hair growth in black rats as modified by the chronic administration of thiourea, phenyl thiourea and alpha-naphthyl thiourea. *Endocrinology*, **40**, 123.

Dunlop D. (1963) Eighty-six cases of Addison's disease. *British Medical Journal*, ii, 887.

Fitzpatrick T.B., Brunet P. & Kukita A. (1958) The nature of hair pigmentation. In *Biology of Hair Growth*, eds. W. Montagna & R.A. Ellis. New York, Academic Press.

Fitzpatrick T.B., Quevedo W.C., Levene A.L., McGovern V.J., Mishima Y. & Oettle A.C. (1966) Terminology of vertebrate melanin-containing cells. *Science*, **152**, 88.

Fitzpatrick T.B., Eisen A.Z., Wolff K., Freedberg I.M. & Austen F. (1979) *Dermatology in General Medicine*, 2nd edn. New York, McGraw-Hill.

Fleischmajer R. & Nedwich A. (1973) Werner's syndrome. *American Journal of Medicine*, **54**, 111.

Gilkes J.J.H., Sharvill D. & Wells R.S. (1974) The premature ageing syndrome. *British Journal of Dermatology*, **91**, 243.

Goette D.K. (1978) Swimmers' green hair. *Archives of Dermatology*, **114**, 127.

Goldschmidt H. (1979) Green hair. *Archives of Dermatology*, **115**, 1288.

Grobbelaar C.S. (1952) The distribution of and correlation between eye, hair and skin colour in male students at the University of Stellenbosch. *Annals of University of Stellenbosch*, **28**, sect. A/1.

Grupper C., Brunieras M., Hincky, M. & Garelly E. (1970) Albinisme partiel familial; étude ultrastructurale. *Annales de Dermatologie et Syphilologie*, **97**, 267.

Hanna B.L. (1956) Colorimetric estimation of the pigment concentration in hair of various color grades. *American Journal of Physiological Anthropology*, **14**, 153.

Harada Y. (1926) Fruhzeitiges Ergrauen der Cillen und Bemerkungen uber den sogenannten plotzlicher Einstritt dieser Veranderung. *Klinische Monatsblatt für Augenheilkunde*, **44**, 228.

Harrison G.A., Weiner, J.S., Tanner J.M. & Barnicott, N.A. (1964) *Human Biology, An introduction to Human Evolution, Variation and Growth*. London, Oxford University Press.

Harrison G.A. & Owen J.J.T. (1964) Studies on the inheritance of human skin colour. *Annals of Human Genetics*, **28**, 27.

Harrison G.A. (1973) Differences in human pigmentation: measurement, geographical variation and causes. *Journal of Investigative Dermatology*, **60**, 418.

Herzberg J. & Gusck W. (1970) Das Ergrauen des Kopfhaares. Eine histo- und fermentshemische sowie elektronen-mikroskopische Studie. *Archiv für klinische und experimentelle Dermatologie*, **236**, 368.

Howsden H.M. (1973) Vogt–Koyanagi–Harada syndrome and psoriasis. *Archives of Dermatology*, **108**, 395.

Jelinek J.E. (1972) Sudden whitening of hair. *Bulletin of the New York Academy of Medicine*, **48**, 1003.

Keogh E.V. & Walsh R.J. (1965) Rate of greying of human hair. *Nature (London)*, **207**, 877.

Klaus S.N. (1980) Acquired pigment dilution of the skin and hair; a sign of pancreatic disease in the tropics. *International Journal of Dermatology*, **19**, 508.

Kligman A.M. (1961) Pathological dynamics of human hair loss. *Archives of Dermatology*, **83**, 175.

Kornerup A. & Wanscher J.H. (1963) *Methuen's Handbook of Colour*. London, Methuen.

Koyanagi Y. (1929) Dysacusis, alopecia, und poliosis bei schwerer uveitis nicht traumatischen ursprunges. *Klin Monatabl. Augenheilkd*, **82**, 194.

Kukita A. & Fitzpatrick T.B. (1955) The demonstration of tyrosinase in melanocytes of the human hair matrix by autoradiography. *Science*, **121**, 893.

Lerner A.B. (1966) *Archives of Dermatology*, **93**, 235.

Livingstone F.B. (1969) Polygenic models for the evolution of human skin colour differences. *Human Biology*, **41**, 480.

McWilliam T.S. & Stephenson J.B.P. (1978) Depigmented hair: The earliest sign of tuberose sclerosis. *Archives of Diseases of Childhood*, **53**, 961.

Main R.A., Robbie R.B., Gray E.S., Donald D. & Horne C.H.W. (1975) Smooth muscle antibodies and alopecia areata. *British Journal of Dermatology* **92**, 389.

Nickel W.R. & Reed W.B. (1962) Tuberose sclerosis: special reference to the microscopic alterations in the cutaneous haematomas. *Archives of Dermatology*, **85**, 209.

Orfanos C., Ruska H. & Mahle G. (1970) White hair of older people. *Archiv für klinische und experimentelle Dermatologie*, **236**, 395.

Pantke O.A. & Cohen M.M. Jr (1971) The Waardenburg syndrome. In Part XI, *Orafacial Structures*, ed. D. Bergsma. *Birth Defects. Original Article Series*, vol. VII, No. 7. Baltimore, Williams and Wilkins.

Reed T.W. (1952) Red hair colour as a genetic character. *Annals of Eugenics*, **17**, 115.

Reed T.E. (1969) Caucasian genes in American Negroes. *Science*, **165**, 762.

Ridgley G.V. & Kassassieh S.D. (1979) Minoxidil. *Lahey Clinic Foundation Bulletin*, **28**, 80.

Rife D.E. (1967) The inheritance of red hair. *Acta Genetica Medica (Roma)*, **16**, 342.

Rosen E. (1945) Uveitis with poliosis, vitiligo, alopecia and dysacousia. *Archives of Ophthalmology*, **33**, 281.

Rugel S.J. & Keats E.U. (1965) Waardenburg's syndrome in six generations of one family. *American Journal of Diseases of Childhood*, **109**, 579.

Russell L.B. (1964) Genetic and functional mosaicism in the mouse. In *Role of Chromosomes in Development*, ed. M. Locke. New York, Academic Press.

Savill S. (1944) *The Hair and Scalp*, 3rd edn. London, Edward Arnold.

Saunders T.S., Fitzpatrick T.B., Seiji M., Brunet P. & Rosenbaum E.E. Decrease in human hair colour and feather pigment of fowl following chloroquine diphosphate. *Journal of Investigative Dermatology*, **33**, 87.

Scriver C.R. & Rosenberg L.E. (1973) Phenylketoneuria. In *Amino acid Metabolism and its Disorders*, vol. X, *Major Problems in Clinical Paediatrics*. Philadelphia, Saunders, p. 290.

Sieve, B.F. (1941) Darkening of grey hair following para-aminobenzoic acid. *Science*, **94**, 257.

Singleton W.R. & Ellis B. (1964) Inheritance of red hair for six generations. *Journal of Heredity*, **55**, 261.

Silvers W.K. (1968) Genes and the pigment cells of mammals. *Science*, **134**, 368.

Spillane J.D. (1963) Brunette to Blond. Depigmentation of hair during treatment with oral mephenesin. *British Medical Journal*, **1**, 997.

Stern C. (1953) Model estimates of the frequency of white and near white segregants in the American Negro. *Acta Genetica (Basel)*, **4**, 281.

Stern C. (1970) Model estimates of the number of gene pairs involved in pigment variability of the Negro American. *Human Heredity*, **20**, 165.

Sunderland E. (1956) Hair colour variation in the United Kingdom. *Annals of Human Genetics,* **20,** 312.

Takeuchi T. (1975) Genetic control of mammalian hair colour. In: *Biology and Diseases of the Hair,* eds. T. Kobori & W. Montagna. Baltimore, University Park Press.

Trotter M. and Duggins O.H. (1950) Age changes in head hair from birth to maturity. *American Journal of Physiological Anthropology,* **8,** 467.

Waardenburg P.J. (1951) New syndrome combining developmental abnormalities of the eyelids, eyebrows, nose root with pigmentary defects of the iris and head hair and with congenital deafness. *American Journal of Human Genetics,* **3,** 195.

Wassermann H.P. (1974) *Ethnic Pigmentation: Historical, Physiological and Clinical Aspects,* 1st edn. Amsterdam, Excerpta Medica.

White J.G. & Clawson C.C. (1979) The Chediak–Higashi syndrome: Ring-shaped lysosomes in circulating monocytes. *American Journal of Pathology,* **96,** 781.

Witkop C.J. Jr (1971) Albinism. In *Advances in Human Genetics,* eds. H. Harris & K. Hirschorn. New York, Plenum Press.

Zelickson A.S. & Mottaz J.H. (1974) Ultrastructure of hair melanosomes. In *The First Human Hair Symposium,* ed. A.C. Brown. New York, Medcom Press.

Zelickson A.S. & Mottaz J.H. (1974) In *First Human Hair Symposium,* ed. A.C. Brown. New York, Medcom Press, p. 277.

Chapter 13
Infections and Infestations

Ringworm of the scalp

History and nomenclature (references p. 369)

Scalp ringworm is an infection of the scalp by a ringworm fungus or dermatophyte. The disease has been known for many centuries, and had become a worldwide public health problem until the last two decades; it remains a problem in those parts of the world where the antibiotic griseofulvin is not freely available.

Although the disease has long been recognized, its diagnostic features were poorly defined until the causative fungi were isolated and identified, and non-infective disorders such as alopecia areata were frequently confused with it. The discovery of the ringworm fungi occupies an important, often unacknowledged place in the development of knowledge of the microbial causes of disease.

The old nomenclature of skin diseases was devastatingly simple. All skin diseases affecting the scalp were called porrigo, which was then qualified by a descriptive adjective. Tinea was an old word used by the Arab physicians, and it too was applicable to any disease of the scalp. All skin diseases affecting any other part of the body were tetters (dartres in France). Herpes, which had had a more precise meaning in antiquity, had come to be a more scientific sounding synonym for a tetter. Ringworm was the popular term for any annular or expanding lesion. Scalled head was the usual English term for scaling of the scalp and hair loss in children. At the end of the eighteenth century Plenck of Vienna introduced a classification of skin diseases based on morphology, and his classification was later modified by Willan. Both authors used the old terms with new meanings. The porrigos were classified with the pustular eruptions and came to include porrigo scutulata and lupinosa, which were different stages of favus, porrigo tonsurans and porrigo decalvans. Very gradually tinea replaced porrigo to leave tinea favosa (favus), tinea tonsurans and tinea decalvans, the last including what we now call alopecia areata. This classification contained the seeds of future controversies.

The improvement in and increased availability of microscopes in the 1830s led to the discovery by Agostino Bassi in 1834 of a fungus as the cause of the disease muscardin in silkworms. J.L. Schoenlein, later professor of medicine in Berlin, repeated Bassi's observations which led him to discover a fungus in a patient with favus (Schoenlein 1839). Between 1841 and 1844 David Gruby, born in Austro-Hungary, but working in Paris, independently discovered a fungus in favus, and also in what is now called scalp ringworm. Gruby's discoveries were soon widely known, but it was many years before fungi were universally accepted as the cause of ringworm. Erasmus Wilson (1809–84), the most influential British dermatologist of his day, believed that the granules visible with the microscope were merely degenerative products. Jabez Hogg (1817–99), a leading microscopist, accepted that fungi were present in the lesions, but did not accept them as their cause. Opinion in other countries was equally divided (see Rook 1978). The controversy was long and often bitter. Microscopes were still regarded with suspicion, the concept of vegetable parasites causing contagious disease was too revolutionary, and clinical definitions were inadequate, so that alopecia areata was often still confused with ringworm. Gradually the microbial origin of fungous and other diseases was recognized and the conceptual barrier was surmounted.

The acceptance of fungi as the cause of ringworm brought further controversy, because of the inadequacy of mycological techniques. The contamination of cultures by *Aspergillus* and other common airborne mould fungi led many authors to suggest that the ringworm fungi and the moulds were forms of a single organism. After this problem had been resolved there was still no agreement concerning the interrelationship of the ringworm fungi themselves. Was there a single variable species, or were there numerous distinct species? The French dermatologist Raymond Sabouraud (1864–1938) played a very large part in establishing the status and characteristics of dermatophyte species. Since his time further taxonomic studies have clarified the classification of these organisms.

The greatest therapeutic advance has been the discovery of griseofulvin.

References

Rook A.J. (1978) Early concepts of the host–parasite relationship in mycology. *International Journal of Dermatology*, 17, 371.

Schoenlein J.L. (1839) Zur Pathogenese der Impetigines. *Archiv für Anatomie, Physiologie und wissenschaftliche Medizin*, p. 82.

The dermatophytes (references p. 372)

The dermatophytes are a group of fungi which colonize and parasitize keratinized structures in man and other animals. Some related species have been isolated from the soil, where they play a part in the degradation of keratinous debris. The pathogenic dermatophytes are classified in three genera, *Microsporum*, *Trichophyton* and *Epidermophyton*. Most of the many species in the first two genera can invade in varying degree the horny layer, the nails and the hair. The single species of *Epidermophyton* does not invade hair and will not be further discussed. The genera *Microsporum* and *Trichophyton* both include species whose natural host is man, and others which occur naturally in one or more other animal species, and parasitize man only accidentally. The distinction between the former, anthropophilic, species, and the latter, zoophilic species, is important from the epidemiological and clinical points of view, as the natural history of the two groups of infections differs in important respects. In Western Europe before 1945 zoophilic fungi accounted for only a very small proportion of cases of scalp ringworm, e.g. 2.4% of cases in Rome in 1910 (Caprilli *et al.* 1979, 1980). Now scalp ringworm of any kind is rare in most of Europe, and zoophilic species account for the majority, e.g. *Microsporum canis* for 87.9% in Rome 1972–7.

Microsporum gypseum

At least one species, *M. gypseum*, normally occurs in the soil, from which man and other animals may acquire the infection. Table 13.1 lists all the important known causes of scalp ringworm and, in the case of the zoophilic species, the animals from which human infections are usually contracted. The geographical distribution of the various dermatophytes indicated in Table 13.1 is necessarily incomplete. Movements of population are introducing tropical species to temperate regions. A further source of error is introduced by the uneven world distribution of mycologists.

Whenever it is practicable the infecting species should be reliably identified by culture, for without an identification reliable epidemiological surveys and preventive measures are impossible.

Pathogenesis

The type of tissue response induced in a given individual by parasitization by a

Table 13.1. Fungi causing scalp ringworm

Anthropophilic		Zoophilic			Geophilic	
Microsporum audouini	Worldwide	*Microsporum canis*	Cats and dogs	Worldwide		
M. ferrugineum	China, Japan, parts of Russia, Central and E. Africa*	*M. equinum*	Horses	W. Europe		
		M. nanum	Pigs	Worldwide		
Trichophyton rubrum (rarely affects the scalp)	Widespread endemic. Extension from Asia	*M. persicolor*	Field-vole	Widespread		
		Trichophyton mentagrophytes	Many species. Reservoirs in rodents	Widespread		
T. schoenleini	Widespread. but uncommon in most areas. Common in the Middle East, N. Africa	*T. verrucosum*	Cattle	Widespread		
		T. equinum	Horses	Widespread		
		T. erinacei	Hedgehogs	Europe, New Zealand		
T. tonsurans	Widespread. Common in parts of Latin America	*T. quinckeanum*	Mice (may be transmitted to man by cats and dogs)	Widespread. but generally rare		
T. violaceum	Dominant in many parts of Africa*, Central and S. Europe, Middle East†	*T. simii*	Monkeys	India		
T. gourvilii	W. Africa				*Microsporum gypseum*	Soil. Man infected by contact with soil or from infected animals	Widespread
T. megninii	S. Europe, Africa					
T. soudanense	Central Africa					
T. yaoundi	Africa					

* Verhagen B.A. (1976) Distribution of dermatophytes causing tinea capitis in Africa. *Tropical and Geographical Medicine.* **26**, 101.
† Asgari M. & Satevi H. (1973) Common mycoses in Bandon Abbas, Iran. 2. Scalp ringworm. *Iran Journal of Public Health.* **2**, 65.

dermatophyte depends on a multitude of variables which determine the inherent mode of growth of the species concerned in relation to the hair shaft, and the immune response of the host. Thus with some species in some patients scalp ringworm may be acutely inflammatory and rapidly self-limiting, whilst with other species, or in other patients, extensive scaling and broken hairs may persist for months or years, but eventually resolve without scarring. In other cases, usually but not invariably induced by species different from those associated with the syndromes already mentioned, there may be a prolonged course and permanent residual scarring.

Our knowledge of the pathogenesis of scalp ringworm is derived largely from the experimental studies of A.M. Kligman with *M. audouini* (Fig. 13.1) (Kligman

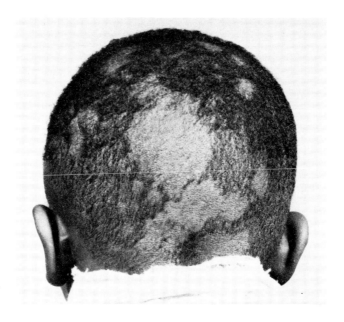

Fig. 13.1. *Microsporum audouini* ringworm of the scalp (Addenbrooke' Hospital, Cambridge).

1955). Minor trauma favours the successful inoculation of a child's scalp. From the point of inoculation the fungal hyphae grow centrifugally in the stratum corneum. By the 6th or 7th day a narrow band of fluorescence can be detected with Wood's light 1 mm above the hair bulb; only hairs in the growing phase (anagen—see p. 11) are attacked. The fungus grows downwards, invading keratin as it is formed, so that the zone of fluorescence extends upwards at the rate at which the hair grows, and is visible above the surface by the 12th–14th days. The infected hair is brittle, and by the 3rd week broken hairs are evident. The infection continues to spread in the stratum corneum to involve other hairs for 8–10 weeks, by which time the infected area is usually about 3.5 cm, but may be up to 7 cm in diameter. In some cases only a few scattered hairs around the inoculated site become infected. In the usual centrifugally spreading infection, the period of extension is followed up by a refractory period, during which host–parasite equilibrium is maintained in the infected follicles, but mycelium is no longer present in the horn of the scalp surface. Inoculation of another area of scalp during this period usually fails, but may produce a trivial infection which rapidly resolves. The primary experimental infection tended to resolve spontaneously in under 7 months, even in the absence of inflammatory changes, but occasionally persisted for over a year; spontaneous infections tended to last still longer. Even in the absence of clinically apparent inflammation, histological examination shows that intense inflammatory changes are in fact present (Graham *et al.* 1964). Adult scalps showed relative immunity to experimental inoculation. The spontaneous cure of naturally occurring infection at puberty is a familiar clinical observation, but the precise mechanism is not fully understood (Kligman & Ginsberg 1950).

The experimental inoculation of *M. canis* in children showed essentially the same sequence of events, but the hairs were invaded more rapidly, and resolution, frequently accompanied by inflammatory changes, usually occurred within 3 months.

Equally detailed studies of the pathodynamics of infection with other species have not been published but it is highly probable that with most species the various stages of infection differ only in detail and in duration, according to the degree of inflammatory response evoked in the host. There are, however, differences in mode of growth in relation to the hair shaft. The *Microsporum* species form an irregular mosaic of small spores outside the hair shaft. This ectothrix mode of growth is shown also by *Trichophyton mentagrophytes*, but with this species the spores which ensheath the shaft are arranged in chains; polymorphic mycelia within the hair are broken up into large quadrangular elements. *Trichophyton tonsurans*, *T. rubrum* and *T. violaceum* produce longitudinal chains of large spores within the shaft (endothrix); *T. schönleini* does likewise, and the combination of chains of large spores, narrow flat budding mycelium and scattered air bubbles is sometimes distinctive.

The favus fungi (*T. schönleini* and *T. quinckeanum*) give rise to additional pathological changes. They cause spongiosis and acanthosis of the epidermis and form *scutula*, which consist of spores and cellular debris in a dense feltwork of mycelium.

References

Graham J.H., Johnson W.C., Burgoon C.F. & Helwig E.B. (1964) Tinea capitis. *Archives of Dermatology*, **89**, 528.

Kligman A.M. (1955) Tinea capitis due to *Microsporum audouini* and *Microsporum canis. Archives of Dermatology*, **71**, 313.

Kligman A.M. & Ginsberg D. (1950) Immunity of the adult scalp to infection with *Microsporum audouini. Journal of Investigative Dermatology*, **14**, 345.

Epidemiology (references p. 374)

Microsporum audouini and *M. ferrugineum*, the two most important anthropophilic *Microsporum* species, are spread directly or indirectly from child to child. *Microsporum audouini* infection has occurred in dogs (Kaplan & Georg 1957) but the rare animal infections are seldom of epidemiological significance. The spores remain viable in shed human hairs for a year or more (Glass 1948), and allow the transmission of the disease by brushes, combs, hats or caps, or the seats of cinemas and public vehicles. In some children there may be only a few infected hairs, undetectable without Wood's light, and it is the difficulty of identifying such cases and the ease with which spores are disseminated in the hair (Alexander *et al.* 1965; Friedman *et al.* 1960; Gip 1966) which explain the very high incidence of the infection in susceptible age groups during the epidemics which occur periodically in so many populations. In a Nigerian school about 10% of children were shown to be asymptomatic carriers of *M. audouini* (Ive 1966). When treatment facilities are poor the endemic rate may remain constantly high.

Infectivity varies; at the height of an epidemic all or almost all children in a family or an institution may be infected. Far more commonly only some 30–50% of those exposed are infected, and the disease is rare in older children or adults. In most school epidemics the peak age of incidence is 6 or 7 and boys are affected more often than girls (Curry & Daniels 1958) but in one epidemic in a mixed residential school boys and girls appeared to be equally susceptible and the greatest incidence was in younger children, aged 2 and 3 (Walby 1952).

Microsporum canis ringworm is particularly a disease of kittens and puppies and its incidence in humans reflects the incidence in the small animal population, and the size of the latter. The spores remain viable in infected hair for a shorter period than those of *M. audouini* (Glass 1948) and almost all human infections are acquired by direct contact with animals. Child to child transmission occurs only to a very limited extent. Boys and girls are equally affected and, although the age in children has varied in different epidemics, the cases are usually fairly evenly distributed throughout the various ages (Curry & Daniels 1958); infants may be affected, though rarely (Hubener 1957). In some outbreaks the infectivity has been very high, up to 93% of all children exposed developing the infection (Lawson & McLeod 1957).

Microsporum equinum rarely infects man, even where it is prevalent in horses, but it is occasionally acquired by direct contact with their associates, and has been reported in children, and in an adult (O'Grady *et al.* 1972). The other zoophilic *Microsporum* species also are rare causes of scalp ringworm, and are acquired by contact with their primary hosts.

Microsporum gypseum is primarily a soil saprophyte and most human infections result from direct contact with soil (e.g. Meinhof 1964). This fungus was isolated from 4% of samples of soil from children's playgrounds in Mannheim, Germany (Bojanovsky *et al.* 1979). However, infections are not rare in cats (Kaplan *et al.* 1957), dogs (Menges & George 1957), and other animals, and human infections may be acquired by contact with them.

The *anthropophilic trichophyton* infections (see Table 13.1) are spread by direct or mediate contact. Adults are susceptible to infection, and although there is some tendency for males and for many females to develop a resistance to infection, some females fail to do so (Seal & Richardson 1960). Spontaneous cures occur, but are unpredictable in the individual patient. Lesions may be insignificant and be overlooked for years, and many members of a household may acquire the infection from adult carriers, usually women (Raubitschek 1959). Immigrants may introduce infections which, unsuspected, cause outbreaks in hospitals, schools and homes (Rosenthal *et al.* 1958; Putkonen & Blomqvist 1959). In parts of the United States, notably the South, *Trichophyton tonsurans* has replaced *Microsporum* as the predominant cause of scalp ringworm (Prevost 1979). As these infections show no fluorescence under Wood's light the diagnosis is readily overlooked. Similar diagnostic problems are reported from Benghazi, Libya (Malhotra *et al.* 1979) while 4.5% of school-children have tinea capitis caused by *Trichophyton schoenleini* or *T. violaceum* and these infections tend to simulate seborrhoeic dermatitis. The mode of spread of human favus is essentially similar; reserves of infection are maintained in backward communities (Hannell & Partridge 1955). 'Witkop', relatively frequent among Bantu children in Africa, is a severe form of favus; poor nutrition is probably a factor in its wide extension (Murray *et al.* 1957).

The *zoophilic trichophyton* species (see Table 13.1) may be contracted by direct contact with the host species, but mediate transmission is very frequent. *Trichophyton verrucosum* for example, is acquired from stalls or fences against which infected cattle have rubbed their lesions. *Trichophyton mentagrophytes* often follows a minor abrasion in the region of farm buildings, but may also be contracted from cats or dogs. Similarly *T. quinckeanum* infection may result from direct contact with infected mice, or with a dog as intermediate host (Schneider 1954).

References

Alexander S., Clayton Y.M. & Noth W.C. (1965) Tinea capitis in a primary school. *British Journal of Dermatology*, **77**, 373.

Bojanovsky A., Mueller H. & Freigang K. (1979) Zur Vorkemmen von Dermatophyten und anderen Keratophilen Pitze auf Kinderspeilplatzen. *Mykosen*, **22**, 149.

Caprilli F., Marcantini R., Farotti E. *et al.* (1979) Etiologia delle dermatofitosi in Roma. *Bolletino del'Instituto San Gallicano*, **10**, 123.

Caprilli F., Marcantini R., Marsella R. & Farotti E. (1980) Etiology of ringworm of the scalp, beard and body in Rome, Italy. *Sabouraudia*, **18**, 129.

Curry J. & Daniels G. (1958) Ringworm of the scalp in school children in the Manchester region. *Medical Officer*, **93**, 165.

Friedman L., Derbes V.J., Hodges E.P. & Gimshi J.T. (1960) The isolation of dermatophytes from the air. *Journal of Investigative Dermatology*, **35**, 3.

Gip L. (1966) Investigation of the occurrence of dermatophytes on the floor and in the air of indoor environments. *Acta Dermato-venereologica*, **46**, Suppl. 58.

Glass F.A. (1948) Viability of fungus in hairs from patients with tinea capitis and *Microsporum audouini*. *Archives of Dermatology and Syphilology*, **57**, 122.

Hannell J. & Partridge B.M. (1955) Favus: a report of some selected cases. *British Medical Journal*, i, 1509.

Hubener L.F. (1957) Tinea capitis (*M. canis*) in a thirty day old infant. *Archives of Dermatology*, **76**, 242.

Ive F.A. (1966) The carrier stage of tinea capitis in Nigeria. *British Journal of Dermatology*, **78**, 219.

Kaplan W. & Georg L.K. (1957) Isolation of *M. audouini* from a dog. *Journal of Investigative Dermatology*, **28**, 313.

Kaplan W., Georg L.K. & Bronley C.L. (1957) Ringworm of cats caused by *Microsporum gypseum*. *Veterinary Medicine*, **52**, 374.

Lawson G.T.N. & McLeod W.J. (1957) *Microsporum canis*—an intensive outbreak. *British Medical Journal*, ii, 1159.

Malhotra V.K., Gang M.D. & Kanwar A.J. (1979) A school survey of tinea capitis in Benghazi. *Journal of Tropical Medicine and Hygiene*, **82**, 59.

Meinhof W. (1964) Endogene und exogene Faktoren der Entstellung von *Microsporum gypseum* Infektionen. *Hautarzt*, **15**, 352.

Menges R.W. & Georg L.K. (1957) Canine ringworm caused by *Microsporum gypseum*. *Cornell Veterinarian*, **47**, 1.

Murray J.F., Freedman M.L., Lurie H.I. & Merriweather A.M. (1957) Witkop: a synonym for favus. *South African Medical Journal*, **31**, 657.

O'Grady K.J., English M.P. & Warin R.P. (1972) *Microsporum equum* infection of the scalp in an adult. *British Journal of Dermatology*, **86**, 175.

Prevost E. (1974) Nonfluorescent tinea capitis in Charleston S.C.: a diagnostic problem. *Journal of the American Medical Association*, **242**, 1765.

Putkonen T. & Blomqvist K. (1959) *Trichophyton violaceum* infection in a home for mental defectives in Finland. *Acta Dermato-venereologica*, **39**, 310.

Raubitschek F. (1959) Infectivity and family incidence of black-dot tinea capitis. *Archives of Dermatology*, **79**, 477.

Rosenthal S.A., Fisher D. & Farneri D. (1958) A localized outbreak in New York City of tinea capitis due to *Trichophyton violaceum*. *Archives of Dermatology*, **78**, 689.

Schneider W. (1954) Favusepidemie durch Feldmäuse. *Hautarzt*, **5**, 348.

Seale E.R. & Richardson J.B. (1960) *Trichophyton tonsurans*. *Archives of Dermatology*, **81**, 87.

Walby A.L. (1952) Tinea capitis (*M. audouini*) in a residential school. *British Medical Journal*, i, 1114.

Wood's light in diagnosis (references p. 376)

Wood's light, named after the American physicist R.W. Wood, is ultraviolet light passed through glass containing 9% nickel oxide. It was first used in dermatology by Margarot & Deveze in 1925.

The fungi of the genus *Microsporum*, and also *Trichophyton schoenleini*, when growing in hair, give a green fluorescence in Wood's light. Non-fluorescent variants of *Microsporum audouini* and *M. canis* have been reported, but are rare

(Beare & Walker 1955). Non-fluorescent *M. gypseum* has also been reported (Wilson & Plunkett 1951; Funt 1959). In *Microsporum* infections the light-green fluorescence may be limited to a narrow band just above the scalp. Hairs infected by *Trichophyton schoenleini* show a duller fluorescence, but along the whole length of the hair.

The effective use of Wood's light requires some experience. The examination must be made in a fully darkened room. The reflected light from white coats or uniforms may make occasional lesions difficult to detect. If the scalp has been smeared with ointment, this must be washed off with a detergent shampoo. The actinic fluorescence of scales and exudates soon becomes familiar and can then be ignored.

References
Beare J.M. & Walker J. (1955) Non-fluorescent *Microsporum audouini* and *canis* ringworm of the scalp. *British Journal of Dermatology*, **67**, 101.
Funt T.R. (1959) Nonfluorescent *Microsporum* in tinea capitis. *Journal of the Florida Medical Association*, **45**, 1021.
Margarot J. & Deveze P. (1925) Aspect de quelques dermatoses en lumiere ultraviolette; note preliminaire. *Bulletin de la Société des Sciences Médicales et Biologiques de Montpellier et du Languedoc Méditerranéen*, **6**, 375.
Wilson J.W. & Plunkett O.A. (1951) Lack of fluorescence of scalp hairs infected with *Microsporum gypseum*. *Journal of Investigative Dermatology*, **16**, 119.

Clinical features (references p. 384)

The patient's immune responses, their modification by medication, whether prescribed for the infection, or for concomitant disease, the nutritional status of the patient, and the special properties of the strain of fungus concerned, introduce such a multiplicity of variables that almost any species of dermatophyte can be associated with any of the ringworm syndromes. Nevertheless each group of species produces a reasonably consistent clinical picture, in the majority of cases.

Anthropophilic microsporum species
Infections with *M. audouini* have been extensively studied. The less comprehensive literature on *M. ferugineum* infections suggests that the behaviour of the two species is similar. Most patients present with single or multiple rounded or irregular patches in which the hairs are broken off a few millimetres above the scalp; the stumps are twisted and brittle and are often greyish-white. The individual patch seldom exceeds 5 cm in diameter, but by confluence of neighbouring patches large areas may be involved. Less commonly only scattered hairs are infected, and clinical diagnosis without Wood's light is impossible. During the earliest stages of infection, the scalp may be reddened, but the redness soon fades to leave superficial scaling. Persistent inflammatory

changes with kerion formation occur in 2–3% of cases. Associated lesions of the glabrous skin occur rather uncommonly.

If inflammatory changes occur, spontaneous cure takes only a few weeks. Even in the absence of clinically obvious inflammation the infection rarely extends for more than 10 weeks, but it may then persist, apparently unchanged for many months, even for 3 or 4 years. Almost all infections resolve at puberty and the many non-inflammatory infections in younger children are self-limiting within a few months (Rivalier 1950; Whittle 1953); in a small proportion of cases the natural duration, without treatment, is about 3 years (Friedman *et al.* 1964).

It seems probable that cases of very long duration are unusual except in the presence of malnutrition or of other factors impairing the immune response. *Microsporum audouini* has been isolated from a young adult with cicatricial alopecia since childhood (Avram & Porojan 1962); such exceptional cases require immunological investigation.

Zoophilic and geophilic Microsporum *species*

Although there are probably significant differences between the reactions to species within this group, the characteristic clinical features as compared with infections with anthropophilic species are the greater incidence of grossly inflammatory lesions, with kerion formation in over 40% of cases in some outbreaks (Sonck 1965) and the frequent presence of associated lesions on glabrous skin. However, there are racial differences in the response to *M. canis*, which causes little evident inflammation in Australian aboriginals (Donald *et al.* 1965) (Fig. 13.2).

Anthropophilic Trichophyton *species*

(i) *Favus. Trichophyton schoenleini* classically gives rise to distinctive, readily recognizable lesions. In fact such lesions occur in a minority of infections in individuals of good nutritional status and the less-striking changes which are commonly present are readily overlooked. The classical lesion is the scutulum; a yellowish concretion at the orifice of a hair follicle, enlarges to form a concave disc 1 cm or more in diameter, firmly attached at its centre to the underlying scalp. The coalescence of large scutula may give rise to crumbling asbestos-like masses. The less-distinctive changes, now more often seen, vary greatly in morphology and extent (Jung 1955; Hakendorf *et al.* 1965). The concretions may be small and plug-like but otherwise typical, or they may be replaced by patchy pityriasiform scaling or crusting. Rarely there may be marked inflammatory changes and even kerion formation. The hairs in the affected regions become opaque, and later sparse, but broken hairs are not a common finding. In long-standing cases there may be widespread cicatricial alopecia. Under Wood's light affected hairs give a dull greenish fluorescence along their entire length.

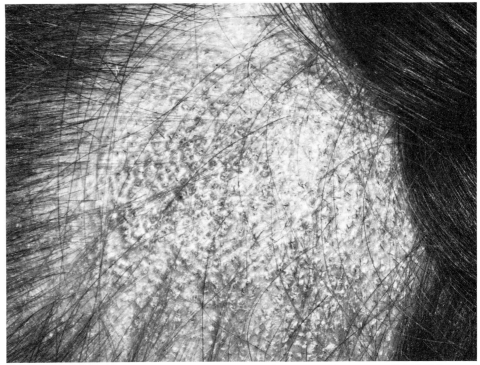

Fig. 13.2. *Microsporum canis* infection. Inflammatory changes in this case are slight (Addenbrooke's Hospital, Cambridge).

Lesions of the glabrous skin are sometimes associated; they may be of tinea circinata or herpetiform type or may consist of scattered or grouped scutula. Rarely the nails are involved (Jung 1955).

Favus of the scalp, contracted as it often is in early childhood, shows some tendency to spontaneous cure between the ages of 8 and 14 (Catanei 1950) but many infections persist long into adult life, particularly in women (Fig. 13.3). Up to four generations have been found to be infected (Blank 1962). Lesions of the glabrous skin commonly clear without treatment.

(ii) *Trichophyton tonsurans (formerly T. sulphureum), T. violaceum, T. gourvilii, T. megninii, T. soudanense and T. yaoundi.* The lesions produced by these species have many features in common and it is difficult to determine whether such differences as have been noted are inherent, or result from genetic variation in the host, or environmental factors.

The classical lesion produced by these species is 'black-dot' ringworm, in which numerous small plaques of irregular shape are studded with black

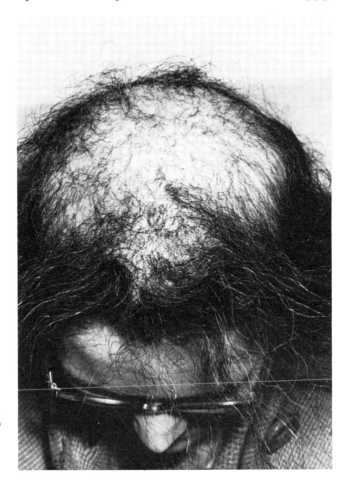

Fig. 13.3. Favus with extensive scarring. In such a scalp foci of active infection may still be present (Slade Hospital, Oxford).

dots—hairs broken off at scalp level. Long healthy hairs in groups of three or four may persist within the plaques. In most outbreaks, however, such cases form a minority, and the clinical manifestations are very variable. To some extent the type of lesions may be correlated with the duration of the infection (Howell *et al.* 1952). Scaling without loss of hair (Putkonen & Blomquist 1959) or with occasional broken hairs (Joseph & Hulde 1955; Beare 1956; Mackenzie *et al.* 1960) provides the only clinical evidence of infection in many cases. In very long-standing infections large areas of cicatricial alopecia dominate the picture, and scaling or broken hairs are found only with difficulty. The nails are sometimes infected (Calnan *et al.* 1962).

Although an inflammatory phase is not uncommon, trichophytides are not often recorded. They tend to be follicular but may take the form of erythema nodosum (Franks *et al.* 1952).

While active inflammatory changes lead often to spontaneous cure, this failed to occur in a generalized vegetating granulomatous infection with *T. tonsurans* (Beirana & Novales 1959). Those cases in which inflammatory changes are neither conspicuous nor prolonged tend eventually to clear spontaneously, but may take many years to do so, and may persist indefinitely in some adult women (Kamalam & Thambiah 1976). Adult carriers are apparently exclusively women (Raubitschek 1959).

(iii) *Trichophyton rubrum.* This species is considered apart from those in the above group because unlike them it is in many areas an extremely common cause of tinea of glabrous skin and nails, but very rarely causes scalp ringworm (Borda 1969). In the majority of cases in which infection extends far beyond the hands, feet and genitocrural region it is probable that cell-mediated immunity is impaired. It may well be so in all patients with scalp involvement. One such patient was an elderly diabetic in whom impaired cellular immunity was demonstrated (Kind *et al.* 1974). She had pustules, erythema, scaling, and loss of hair. Some patients have developed black-dot tinea (Price *et al.* 1963); others breaking of hairs at different levels, and still others kerion formation (Bazex *et al.* 1963).

Zoophilic Trichophyton *species*
(i) The species listed in Table 13.1 (excluding *T. quinckeanum*) usually cause severely inflammatory lesions, leading to kerion formation in the scalp, and spontaneous cure in a matter of months. The morphology and the course of infections with *T. verrucosum* and *T. mentagraphytes* are identical (Rook & Frain-Bell 1954; Rook 1954). Reported differences between the lesions induced by other species must be assessed in the light of possible genetic and nutritional variations in the hosts, and of the site involved (Fig. 13.4).

These infections tend to show marked inflammatory changes from the first appearance of the lesions: after an interval of 7–10 days severe pustulation develops, as a reaction to the fungus, and not as a result of secondary bacterial infection (Birt & Wilt 1954; Even-Paz & Raubitschek 1960). Immunological defects modify the course of the infection. *Trichophyton verrucosum* (Fig. 13.5) caused chronic lesions in a boy with a reticulosis (Hval 1936). Black-dot ringworm with scarring persisted for over 50 years in a patient infected with this same species (Alteras 1962).

The normal course of a scalp infection, however, is the rapid development of a plaque of erythema, which becomes increasingly oedematous and studded with large follicular pustules, the so-called agminate folliculitis, which in most cases is succeeded by a kerion, a raised boggy mass of pustules. Less often, firm inflammatory nodules are formed—Majocchi's granuloma. Scalp involvement may be very extensive, when malaise and low fever may occur. Spontaneous

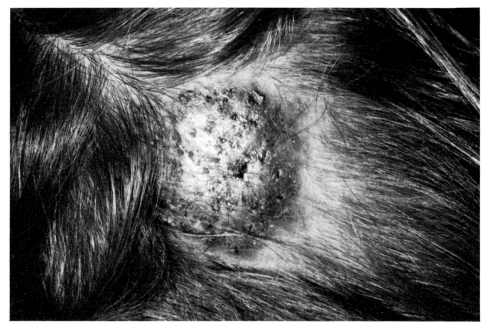

Fig. 13.4. Kerion caused by *Trichophyton mentagrophytes* (Addenbrooke's Hospital, Cambridge).

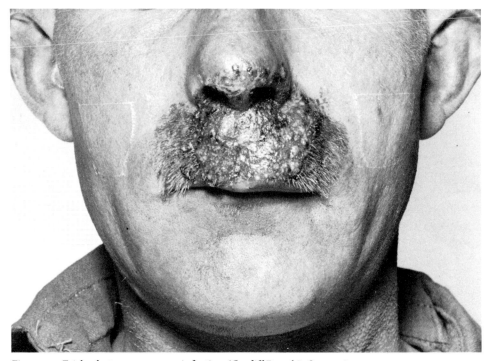

Fig. 13.5. *Trichophyton verrucosum* infection (Cardiff Royal Infirmary).

healing is the rule and although scarring is inevitable the degree of regrowth of hair is often greater than the severity of the reaction leads the inexperienced to expect.

(ii) *Mouse favus*. The lesions produced by *T. quinckeanum* are seldom immediately recognizable as such. Most distinctive is an inflammatory infiltrated plaque, with small sulphur-yellow scutula (Blank *et al.* 1961). More often there are erythematous patches with scaling and hair loss (Christmas & Clayton 1966), or kerion formation (Alteras 1959; Kabur & Plötz 1962). There may be only impetigo-like crusting.
    The infection is self-limiting.

Diagnosis of scalp ringworm (references p. 384)

The possibility of ringworm must be considered in the presence of alopecia, scaling, broken hairs or folliculitis, singly or in any combination. Since, throughout this book, the need to exclude a ringworm infection is stressed in the discussion of each of the conditions which ringworm may simulate, differential diagnosis will not be considered in detail in this chapter.
    In the child the commonest sources of error are traumatic alopecia, alopecia areata, pityriasis simplex and pityriasis amiantacea (Honig & Smith 1979). In the common form of traumatic alopecia as a habit tic (p. 263) hairs are twisted and broken, but of normal texture. In alopecia areata (p. 289) the scalp is not scaly. In pityriasis amiantacea (p. 455) the masses of sticky scale may cover a moist red area of scalp from which the hair readily falls, but the hair is not broken or abnormal in texture.
    Pyrogenic infections of the scalp are rare in childhood, except impetigo complicating head louse infestation. A history of trauma is often given by patients with zoophilic ringworm infections, and the diagnosis of 'infected abrasion' of the scalp is suspect.
    In the older child or adult scarring alopecia without evident cause is ringworm until proved not to be so.
    Where the diagnosis of ringworm is under consideration the scalp should be examined under Wood's light (see p. 375). If fluorescent hairs are present, some should be removed for microscopy and culture. If no fluorescent hairs are detected, but the lesions are otherwise suggestive of *Microsporum* infections, hairs which appear abnormal in texture or length when viewed in ordinary light should be extracted, to exclude the rare non-fluorescent strains. If there is no fluorescence and ringworm canot be excluded on clinical grounds any broken or abnormal hairs, scale or crust must be examined by microscopy and culture.
    Microscopy of infected hairs may provide immediate confirmation of the diagnosis of ringworm, and will also establish whether the fungus is small or large spore, ectothrix or endothrix.

Culture should always be carried out, since precise identification of the species is essential for epidemiological purposes.

Treatment (references p. 384)

The choice of treatment will be determined by the species of fungus concerned, the degree of inflammatory reaction, and of course by the facilities available. In some cases the immunological and nutritional status of the patient may have to be taken into account. A severe agminate folliculitis or kerion caused by a zoophilic species will usually resolve spontaneously. A kerion caused by an anthropophilic species may well resolve but coexisting non-inflammatory lesions in other regions of the scalp may persist. Totally non-inflammatory lesions run a long course, though the anthropophilic *Microsporum* infections tend to clear at puberty. If, for economic or other reasons, griseofulvin is in short supply or unobtainable, it is reasonable to leave untreated those cases which can be expected to resolve, but if it is available it is the treatment of choice in all ringworm of the scalp. Given late in inflammatory infections it may have little influence on the course of existing lesions, but it will prevent the development of new ones.

Griseofulvin*

Griseofulvin is a product of several species of *Penicillium*. It is active against the dermatophytes, but not against yeasts or bacteria. Resistant strains of dermatophytes are unusual. Griseofulvin, particularly in its fine-particle form, is readily absorbed from the gut, but absorption is enhanced if fatty food is taken simultaneously. Griseofulvin accumulates in the keratin of the horny layer, hair and nails, rendering them resistant to invasion by the fungus. Treatment must therefore be continued long enough for the infected keratin to be replaced by resistant keratin.

Griseofulvin has proved to be remarkably non-toxic but side effects such as nausea, fatigue or transient rashes are occasionally reported.

A single 500 mg capsule daily is the standard dose for adults, or 250 mg for children. The hair in and around the infected areas of scalp should be cut short and tolnaftate cream or Whitfield's ointment should be applied daily. Treatment should be continued until clinical and mycological cure has been achieved, usually some 4–6 weeks. Progress must be monitored by regular clinical examination (with the aid of Wood's light for fluorescent species). In the inflammatory lesions compresses are often needed to remove pus and scale.

---

* Ketoconazole is proving acceptable as an alternative to griseofulvin but the latter is at present to be preferred because of its exceptional freedom from significant side effects over many years and on grounds of cost.

Public health measures

The diagnosis of ringworm of the scalp imposes the obligation to determine the source of infection so that action may be taken to prevent its further dissemination. The infecting species must therefore be identified.

If the species is anthropophilic, family and school contacts must be examined, using Wood's light where this is appropriate. In the control of an outbreak caused by *Microsporum audouini* the use of a plastic scalp massager proved more reliable than Wood's light in identifying carriers with minimal sub-clinical infection (Dixon 1968). Three of eight cases thus detected had shown no abnormality under Wood's light. All infected individuals must be isolated until they have been successfully treated.

The source of infection with some zoophilic species is often difficult to trace. Outbreaks of *M. canis* infection can be very large. Patients' cats and dogs must be inspected under Wood's light, and referred for treatment. In some cases the help of the police may be required in rounding up stray dogs and cats. *Trichophyton mentagrophytes* may follow known contact with rodents, but often no source can be traced.

References

Altéras M.I. (1959) Kérion de celse du cuir chevelu dû à l'*Achorion quinckeanum*. *Annales de Dermatologie et de Syphiligraphie*, **86**, 518.

Altéras M.I. (1962) A propos d'un cas de trichophytie chronique du cuir chevelu, à type de pseudopelade, dû au *Trichophyton violaceum*. *Dermatologica*, **125**, 382.

Avram A. & Porojan I. (1962) Un cas insolite de microsporose chronique de l'adulte simulant le favus. *Dermatologica*, **125**, 259.

Bazex A., Salvador B. & Dupré A. (1963) Sur le polymorphism clinique réalisé par le *Trichophyton rubrum*. *Annales de Dermatologie et de Syphiligraphie*, **90**, 361.

Beare J.M. (1956) Tinea capitis due to *Trichophyton sulphureum*. *British Journal of Dermatology*, **68**, 193.

Beirana L. & Novales J. (1959) Tiña universal y granulomatose por *Trichophyton tonsurans*. *Dermatologia Revista Mexicana*, **3**, 4.

Birt A.R. & Wilt J.C. (1954) Mycology, bacteriology and histopathology of suppurative ringworm. *Archives of Dermatology and Syphilology*, **69**, 441.

Blank F. (1962) Human favus in Quebec. *Dermatologica*, **125**, 369.

Blank F., Tech S., Leclerc G. & Telner P. (1961) Clinical manifestations of mouse favus in man. *Archives of Dermatology*, **83**, 587.

Borda J.M. (1969) El *Trichophyton rubrum* en dermatologia. *Archivos Argentinos de Dermatologia*, **19**, 1.

Calnan C.D., Djavahiszwili N. & Hodgson C.J. (1962) *Trichophyton soudanense* in Britain. *British Journal of Dermatology*, **74**, 144.

Catanei A. (1950) Les teignes en Afrique du Nord. *Maroc Médical*, **29**, 955.

Christmas R.J. & Clayton Y.M. (1966) Studies in mycology. I. *T. quinckeanum*. *Transactions of the St John's Hospital Dermatological Society*, **52**, 241.

Dixon P.N. (1968) The mycological control of an epidemic of tinea capitis due to *Microsporum audouini*. *Medical Officer*, **120**, 59.

Donald G.F., Brown G.W. & Sheppard A.A.W. (1965) The dermatophytic flora of South Australia.

A survey of 1819 cases of tinea studied between 1954 and 1964. *Australian Journal of Dermatology*, **8**, 78.

Even-Paz Z. & Raubitschek F. (1960) Epidemics of tinea capitis due to *Trichophyton verrucosum* contracted from cattle or sheep. *Dermatologica*, **120**, 74.

Franks A.G., Rosenbaum E.M. & Mandel E.H. (1952) *Trichophyton sulphureum* causing erythema nodosum and multiple kerion formation. *A.M.A. Archives of Dermatology and Syphilology*, **65**, 95.

Friedman L., Derbes V.J. & Hodges E.P. (1964) The course of untreated tinea capitis in Negro children. *Journal of Investigative Dermatology*, **42**, 237.

Hakendorf A.J., Donald G.F. & Linn H.W. (1965) Favus. *Australian Journal of Dermatology*, **8**, 22.

Honig P.J. & Smith L.R. (1979) Tinea capitis masquerading as atopic or seborrhoeic dermatitis. *Journal of Paediatrics*, **94**, 604.

Howell J.B., Wilson J.W. & Caro M.R. (1952) Tinea capitis caused by *Trichophyton tonsurans* (sulfureum or crateriforme). *A.M.A. Archives of Dermatology and Syphilology*, **65**, 194.

Hval E. (1936) A case of reticulosis of the regional lymph glands in association with a chronic skin affection. *Acta Dermato-venereologica*, **17**, 402.

Joseph H.L. & Halde C. (1955) Tinea capitis due to *Trichophyton tonsurans*. *California Medicine*, **83**, 371.

Jung H.-D. (1955) Zur Diagnose und Therapie des Favus. *Hautarzt*, **6**, 12.

Kabur U. & Plötz W.-D. (1962) Mäusefavus im Bereich des behaarten Kopfes. *Dermatologische Wochenschrift*, **146**, 270.

Kamalam A. & Thambiah A.S. (1976) *Trichophyton violaceum* infection in an Indian school. *International Journal of Dermatology*, **15**, 136.

Kind R., Hornstein O.P., Meinhof W. & Weidner F. (1974) Tinea capitis durch *Trichophyton rubrum* und multimorbidität im Senium, mit partiellem Defekt der zellularem Immunität. *Hautarzt*. **25**, 606.

Mackenzie D.W.R., Burrows D. & Walby A.L. (1960) *Trichophyton sulphurum* in a residential school. *British Medical Journal*, **ii**, 1055.

Price V.H., Rosenthal S.A. & Villafane J. (1963) Black dot tinea capitis caused by *Trichophyton rubrum*. *Archives of Dermatology*, **87**, 487.

Putkonen T. & Blomquist K. (1959) *Trichophyton violaceum* infection in a home for mental defectives in Helsinki. *Acta Dermato-venereologica*, **39**, 310.

Raubitschek F. (1959) Infectivity and family incidence of black-dot tinea capitis. *Archives of Dermatology*, **79**, 477.

Rivalier, E. (1950) Les microspories spontanément curables. *Annales de Dermatologie et de Syphiligraphie*, **10**, 518.

Rook A.J. (1954) Cattle ringworm in man. *Medical Illustration*, **8**, 12.

Rook A.J. & Frain-Bell W. (1954) Cattle ringworm. *British Medical Journal*, **ii**, 1198.

Sonck C.E. (1965) Mikrospori i Finland. *Nordisk Medicin*, **60**, 1100.

Whittle C.H. (1953) Is scalp ringworm a self-limiting disease? *Lancet*, **ii**, 10.

Mycetoma of the scalp

An uncommon manifestation of dermatophytosis of the scalp is the formation of a mycetoma. This lesion has been reported in this site apparently exclusively in Africans. It has been suggested that trauma is responsible for the extension of the fungus from keratin to the dermis. *Trichophyton rubrum*, *T. verrucosum* and *Microsporum ferrugineum* have been isolated from such cases.

The mycetoma presents a smooth, firm mobile nodule with or without discharging sinuses. Untreated it may persist for many years.

Reference

Strobel M., Ndiaye B., Marchaund J.-P., Ravisse P. & Basset M. (1980) Mycétome à dermatophyte du cuir chevulu. *Annales de Dermatologie et de Vénéréologie*, **107**, 1181.

Ringworm of the beard

Aetiology

Ringworm of the beard is necessarily confined to adult males. Most cases are caused by zoophilic species, especially *Trichophyton mentagrophytes*, *T. verrucosum* and *Microsporum canis* (Loewenthal 1965), but some are caused by anthropophilic fungi such as *Trichophyton rubrum* (Avram 1963). In Western Australia *T. rubrum* was the most frequent species in urban cases, followed by *T. mentagrophytes* and *Microsporum canis*, whilst in rural areas all the cases were caused by *Trichophyton mentagrophytes* (McAleer 1980). Such cases are occasionally inappropriately treated with corticosteroids, which profoundly modify the course of the infection.

Clinical features

Plaques of large follicular pustules or fully developed kerions are usually seen. However, in some cases there is a diffuse area of erythema and scaling with irregularly distributed pustules. Cases treated with corticosteroids are particularly liable to show this appearance. Such lesions may slowly extent over months. Untreated agminate folliculitis too may persist for long periods, but tends eventually to resolve (Fig. 13.5).

Diagnosis

Hairs from the follicular pustules should be extracted for microscopy and culture.

Treatment

See p. 383.

References

Avram A. (1963) Sur les pilomycoses déterminées par le *Trichophyton rubrum*. *Dermatologica*, **126**, 354.

Loewenthal K. (1965) Tinea barbae due to *Microsporum canis*. *Archives of Dermatology*, **91**, 60.

McAleer R. (1980) Fungal infections as a cause of skin diseases in Western Australia. III. Tinea barbae. *Australian Journal of Dermatology*, **21**, 40.

Pediculosis capitis
(References p. 391)

History
Lice have been man's frequent companions for millennia (Essig 1931) and no race is known to be spared their attentions. Two species of louse infest man, *Pediculus humanus* and *Phthirus pubis*. *Pediculus humanus* occurs in two distinct populations, *P. humanus capitis* the head louse, and *P. humanus corporis*, the body louse. It seems probable that the body louse evolved from the head louse when man began to wear clothes. The two races, which can interbreed, show marked physiological, and some inconstant anatomical differences. The head louse is occasionally found on the body, but the body louse is rarely seen in the scalp (Buxton 1947).

Pediculus humanus capitis (Orkin *et al.* 1977)
The female head louse is 3–4 mm long; the male is slightly smaller. Its colour ranges from greyish-white to brown according to the skin colour of the human population it habitually parasitizes (Ferris 1935). The female lays 7–10 eggs each day during her life span of about a month. The eggs, which are oval-lidded white capsules (Fig. 13.6), each firmly cemented to a hair shaft, hatch in about a week. The larvae, more correctly termed nymphs, resemble small adults. They undergo three moults over a period of 8 or 9 days to reach maturity.

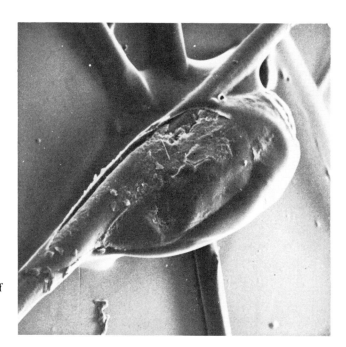

Fig. 13.6. Egg capsule (nit) of the head louse in the scanning electron microscope (Slade Hospital, Oxford).

The factors which regulate the larval population in the individual scalp are not fully understood. In most established infestations there are fewer than ten adult lice (Mellanby 1942), but Buxton (1947) found 1286 adults and nymphs in one head in West Africa and 774 adults on one head in Colombo; in general counts of over 100 are uncommon, and those of over 1000 are rare. The population tends to be related to the total weight of hair, and seasonal climatic changes appear not to be relevant. Nor is there reliable evidence that the nutritional status of the host influences the population (Buxton 1947). However, 67 refugees from Burma, who had suffered severe deprivations, showed average counts of 130 adults and 418 nymphs (Roy & Ghosh 1944). When the population is large the ratio of males to females is high and the mortality of young females is increased (Buxton 1937).

Lice and their eggs are most numerous in the occipital and post-auricular regions of the scalp (Fig. 13.7).

Epidemiology and incidence
The head louse occurs throughout the world. It is transmitted by direct contact, or by shared hats, caps, brushes or combs. The louse can travel directly from one head to another on a pillow or a chair or may be transferred as eggs on shed hairs. Long fine hair and poor hygiene favour the establishment of infestation. Girls of low intelligence showed a higher incidence than others living under the same conditions (Rollin 1943). Members of large families have greater opportunities of exposure (Mellanby 1942) as do members of schools or other communities.

Mellanby's (1941) detailed studies in a large industrial city showed up to 50% of girls infested at all ages between 2 and 13, over 20% between 14 and 18 and some 40% aged 1. The incidence in boys was lower in all age groups, and reached a peak of about 45% in those aged 2–4. During the school years the percentage of boys infested fell rapidly. Other statistics show similar age and sex differences, but no age is immune. The usually low incidence in adults, and particularly in adult males, has been said to be related to their lower total weight of hair, but this cannot be the sole explanation (Askew 1971). In some communities where living conditions are crowded and hygienic standards are low the prevalence in adults of both sexes may remain high (Davis *et al.* 1944).

The importance of social conditions in determining the prevalence of head lice was emphasized by a study of school children in Kassel in Germany (Letz 1980). Infestation was most frequent among the children of foreign workers and in children who were physically or mentally handicapped.

The prevalence of head lice in Britain was high in 1940 and the years that followed, but by 1960 was relatively uncommon, especially in rural areas. In the past 5 years the infestation has again become more common. In Glasgow in 1969 nearly 10% of girls and 4% of boys had lice (Wilson 1969). The relatively greater increase in the infestation rate of boys, which has been noted also in other recent surveys has been attributed to changes in hairdressing styles but in one survey the prevalence was highest in children with short hair (Juranek 1977). On Teesside (Coates 1971) about 12% of children returning to school after the summer holidays were infested. The incidence continued to rise (Department of Education and Science 1974), partly no doubt because some lice are becoming resistant to DDT and gammexane (Maunder 1971a). Davidson (1975) estimated the national prevalence at 2.4% since when it has fallen. The prevalence in some other parts of the world is discussed by Gretz (1977). An interesting observation, which is not fully explained, is that the prevalence of head lice is more than thirty times greater in American whites than in blacks attending the same school classes (Juranek 1977). The incidence is high in some villages in India, reaching about 18% (Hati *et al.* 1980).

Pathology

Nymphs and adults of both sexes suck blood, and in doing so inject their saliva. The pruritus which leads to scratching and hence to the secondary bacterial infection which may dominate the clinical picture, is a manifestation of hypersensitivity to antigenic constituents of the saliva. There have been few investigations in man of the immunological response to lice. Peck *et al.* (1943) used human volunteers. Experimental feeding at first produced pinpoint areas of erythema without pruritus. After about a week pruritus was first experienced. Thereafter bites provoked an immediate irritable weal followed by a persistent papule. There was wide individual variation in response and some subjects showed little or no reaction after months of daily exposure. In the investigation of home contacts of our patients we have seen very heavily infested subjects with no symptoms.

Clinical features

The clinical features of pediculosis are surprisingly variable. Pruritus, which may be intense, depends on the immune response to the salivary antigens of the louse and on the host's threshold of perception. It is seldom completely absent. Characteristically it is most severe in the occipital region where the infestation is usually most heavy. Scratching introduces secondary bacterial infection, leading to impetiginous crusts and cervical adenitis. In severe cases a child may be pale, listless and febrile. A generalized erythematous dermatitis has been reported (Ronchese 1946).

If the infestation is of long duration and secondary infection is severe and persistent the hair may become densely matted by malodorous pus and exudate to give rise to the state formerly known as 'plica polonica'.

In those individuals in whom pruritus is slight or absent, the infestation may not be recognized until it is deliberately sought.

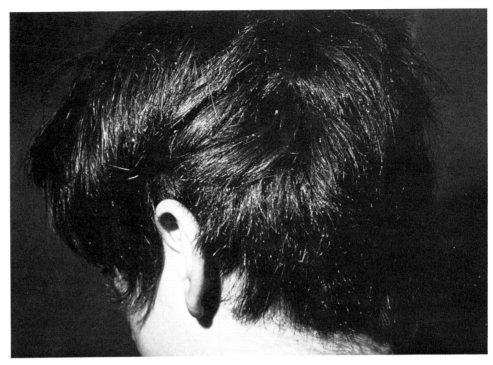

Fig. 13.7. Pediculosis capitis. Numerous egg capsules are present

Except in those few cases in which the population of lice, as nymphs or adults, is high, there is no 'mechanized dandruff' to be seen. The diagnostic feature is the presence of oval egg-capsules, popularly known as nits, firmly cemented to the hair shafts. They are most easily confused with hair casts (p. 480) but the latter slide freely along the shaft and are annular. Other foreign bodies (Kutz 1969; Gemrich 1974) have been responsible for misdiagnoses, which may have embarrassing consequences for public health administrators. With a hand-lens the distinctive shape of the egg is easy to identify. It is particularly easy to see under Wood's light, which is useful if a large school population has to be screened.

Impetigo of the scalp is never an acceptable diagnosis until pediculosis has been reliably excluded.

Treatment

If secondary infection is severe, and particularly in the presence of adenitis or toxaemia, an antibiotic should be administered systemically. If the hair is densely matted it may be necessary to cut it.

In most cases, however, treatment with a parasiticide is sufficient provided it is carried out thoroughly. Preparations of gammexan or a 5% emulsion of DDT have been widely used for some years and one or other is still the treatment of choice. The chosen application is rubbed into the scalp once daily for 5 days, and thoroughly washed off a week later. The hair is then carefully examined and any remaining eggs are removed with a fine-toothed comb.

Where lice are resistant to gammexane and to DDT (Maunder 1971a) Malathion 0.5% in spirit has been successfully used (Maunder 1971b). This lotion is applied liberally and allowed to dry. After 24 hours the hair is washed and combed.

In one investigation of school-children (Maguire & McNally 1972) 20% of treated children were reinfested within 2 months. This experience emphasizes the need to examine and treat all school and home contacts, including of course those who are allegedly symptom-free.

References

Askew R.R. (1971) *Parasitic Insects*. London, Heinemann.

Buxton P.A. (1937) The numbers of males and females in natural populations of head lice. *Proceedings of the Royal Entomological Society (London)*, A, **12**, 12.

Buxton P.A. (1947) *The Louse*, 2nd edn. London, Arnold.

Coates K.G. (1971) Control of head infestation in schoolchildren. *Community Medicine*, **126**, 148.

Davis W.A., Juvera F.M. & Lira P.H. (1944) Studies on louse control in a civilian population. *American Journal of Hygiene*, **39**, 177.

Department of Education and Science (1974) *The Health of the School Child 1971–2*. London, HMSO.

Donaldson R.J. (1975) *The Head Louse in England*. Health Education Council, U.K.

Essig E.O. (1931) *A History of Entomology—Report 1965*. New York, Hafner, p. 18.

Ferris G.F. (1935) *Contributions toward a Monograph of the Sucking Lice*. Part VIII. Stanford University, *Publications in the Biological Sciences*, **2**, No. 5.

Gemrich E.G., Brady J.G., Lee B.L. & Parham P.H. (1974) Outbreak of head lice in Michigan misdiagnosed. *American Journal of Public Health*, **64**, 805.

Gratz N.G. (1977) Epidemiology of louse infestations. In Orkin *et al., loc cit.*, p. 157.

Hati A.K., Bhetkolapyya L, Chakerobody A.K., Choudhuri A.K., Chowdhury B.J.R. (1980) The incidence and extent of head louse infestation in a West Bengal village. *Indian Journal of Dermatology*, **24/25**, 4.

Juranek B.D. (1977) Epidemiologic investigation of pediculosis capitis in school children. In Orkin *et al., loc. cit.*, p. 168.

Kutz F.W. (1969) Problem with diagnosis of head lice. *Entomological News*, **80**, 27.

Letz A. (1980) Verbreitung von Kopflausbefall in Kasseler Schulen. *Offentleche Gesundheitswesen*, **42**, 228.

Maguire J. & McNally A.J. (1972) Head infestation in school-children: extent of the problem and treatment. *Community Medicine*, **128**, 374.

Maunder J.W. (1971a) Resistance to organochlorine insecticides in head lice and trials using alternative compounds. *Community Medicine*, **125**, 27.

Maunder J.W. (1971b) Using malathion in the treatment of louse infestation. *Community Medicine*, **126**, 145.

Mellanby K. (1941) The incidence of head lice in England. *Medical Officer*, **65**, 39.

Mellanby K. (1942) Relation between family size and incidence of head lice. *Public Health*, **56**, 31.

Ministry of Education (1951) *Report of the Chief Medical Officer for the Years 1950–51.* London, HMSO, p. 36.

Orkin M., Maibach H.C., Parish L.C. & Schwartzman R.M. (1977) *Scabies and Pediculosis.* Philadelphia, Lippincott.

Peck S.M., Wright W.H. & Gant J.U. (1943) Cutaneous reactions due to the body louse (*Pediculus humanus*). *Journal of the American Medical Association,* **123,** 821.

Rollin H.R. (1943) *Pediculosis capitis* and intelligence in WAAF recruits. *British Medical Journal,* **1,** 475.

Ronchese F. (1946) Generalized dermatitis from *Pediculosis capitis. New England Journal of Medicine,* **234,** 605.

Roy D.N. & Ghosh S.M. (1944) Studies on the population of head lice—*Pediculus humanus var capitis. Parasitology,* **36,** 69.

Wilson T.S. (1969) Scabies and pediculosis: a study of the incidence in Glasgow from the early nineteen twenties. *Medical Officer,* **122,** 125.

Phthiriasis pubis
(References p. 394)

History and nomenclature

The pubic louse belongs to a different genus from the body and head lice, and is correctly termed *Phthirus pubis.* Infestation with this louse is often loosely referred to as pubic pediculosis, but the somewhat pedantic phthiriasis is preferable as this louse differs structurally and ecologically from the body louse, and as its activities are by no means confined to the pubic region.

Phthirus pubis

The descriptive term crab-louse effectively draws attention to the distinctive shape of this parasite, which is 1.5–2 mm long, and about as broad (Herms & James 1961). The middle and hind pairs of legs are armed with very short claws. The female attaches her eggs to coarse hairs; they hatch in 6–8 days, and maturity is reached in 15–17 days after hatching. The lice tend to be stationary in their habits and may remain attached to the skin at one point for days. When the infestation is heavy the lice may roam over all the hair regions of the body, including the axillae, eyebrows and lashes and the scalp. However, the width of the louse prevents it from colonizing more than the scalp margins. The colonization of all areas of the body in a hirsute patient was a consequence of prolonged application of topical corticosteroids (Nielsen & Secker 1980).

Epidemiology

The louse is usually transmitted by sexual contact, or by shed hairs in borrowed clothing, towels or sleeping bags. Eyelash infestation of infants has been derived from the breast hairs of their mothers (Ronchese 1953).

Among the promiscuous the incidence may be high. Sylvest (1951) found 30% of Copenhagen prostitutes to be infested in winter but only 15% in summer, and suggested that the seasonal difference might be explained by less frequent bathing in the cold northern winter. In Britain the incidence is rising and tends to parallel that of gonorrhoea in that it occurs predominantly in the same age groups and often in the same individuals (Fisher & Morton 1970).

Pathology
The immunological reactions to the salivary antigens of the pubic louse appear not to have been investigated. On clinical evidence the variation in host response would seem to be comparable to that to the head louse, in that in some subjects intense irritation can be present with a small louse population, whilst in others there are few or no nymphs although lice are very numerous.

Clinical features
The classical symptom is intense irritation of the pubic region, but it may extend, as may the lice, to the entire anogenital region, the abdominal wall and the axillae. On examination the lice are easily detected, unless self treatment has produced eczematization, or scratching has introduced gross secondary infection.

In many cases blue-grey macules, known as maculae caeruleae, are present on the abdominal wall and thighs. They are probably due to altered blood pigments at the sites of bites. In massive infestations (Safdi & Farrington 1947) there may also be lymphadenopathy, fever and malaise. Phthiriasis of the scalp is rare and is perhaps commoner in children than in adults (Heilesen & Lindgren 1946; Gartmann & Dickmans-Bermeister 1970). The eyebrows and lashes may also be infested. In such cases maculae caeruleae may be found on the shoulders, upper arms or trunk.

Infestation confined to the eyelashes (Korting 1967) usually occurs in infants, but is occasionally reported in older children (Bose 1955).

Exceptionally a bullous reaction to the bites has occurred (Kern 1952).

Diagnosis
Difficulties in diagnosis arise mainly where overtreatment has caused eczematous dermatitis.

Lice in the anterior scalp margin in a child, particularly if no eggs can be discovered, should raise the suspicion that pubic rather than head lice are present. The distinction is readily made under the low power of the microscope.

Parasitophobia is common and a diagnosis of pubic louse infestation should not be accepted unless lice or their eggs have been positively identified.

Treatment
A 5% emulsion of DDT applied once and washed off after 24 hours is usually effective. If resistant strains emerge it may be necessary to use 0.1% malathion in

spirit. The possible coexistence of other sexually transmitted diseases should be remembered.

Lice should be removed manually from eyelashes or eyebrows.

References

Bose J. (1955) Phthiriasis palpebrarum. *American Journal of Ophthalmology*, **39**, 211.

Fisher I. & Morton R.S. (1970) Phthirus pubis infestation. *British Journal of Venereal Diseases*, **46**, 326.

Gartmann H. & Dickmans-Bermeister D. (1970) Phthiri im Bereia der Kopfhaare, Augerbrauen und Wimpern bei einem 2½ jährigen Mädehn. *Hautarzt*, **21**, 279.

Heilesen B. & Lindgren I. (1946) *Phthirus pubis* in capillitum, cilia et supercilia. *Acta Dermato-venereologica*, **26**, 533.

Herms W.B. & James M.T. (1961) *Medical Entomology*, 5th edn., p. 106.

Kern A.B. (1952) Bullous eruption due to pediculosis pubis. *A.M.A. Archives of Dermatology and Syphilology*, **65**, 334.

Korting G.W. (1967) Phthiriasis palpebrarum und ihre ersten historischen Erwährungen. *Hautarzt*, **18**, 73.

Nielsen A.O. & Secker L.S. (1980) Pediculosis pubis in a patient treated with topical corticosteroids. *Cutis*, **25**, 655.

Ronchese F. (1953) Treatment of pediculosis ciliorum in an infant. *New England Journal of Medicine*, **249**, 897.

Safdi S.A. & Farrington J. (1947) Constitutional reactions and maculae caeruleae attending phthiriasis pubis. *American Journal of Medical Science*, **214**, 308.

Sylvest B. (1951) Seasonal variation in the incidence of crab lice among loose women in Copenhagen. *Acta Dermato-venereologica*, **31**, 676.

Insect bites

The cutaneous reactions to the bites of most insects depend on an acquired allergic sensitivity to antigens in the insects' saliva. This allergic reaction may be of Type I manifest as an immediate weal of rapid onset, or of Type IV manifest as a firm and more persistent papule developing in 24–48 hours. The intensity of the reaction shows wide variation and in the most severe cases there may be bulla formation or necrosis.

Many biting insects occasionally bite in the scalp and the resulting inflammatory reaction may lead to some temporary shedding of hair from the site of the bites and from a narrow zone surrounding each of them. The minute gnats and midges of the family Ceratopogonidae particularly favour the scalp. On summer evenings they may be present in such vast swarms that they cause quite intolerable irritation. The reaction to the bites and secondary infection following the scratching may lead to patchy loss of hair but this normally regrows rapidly (Fig. 13.8).

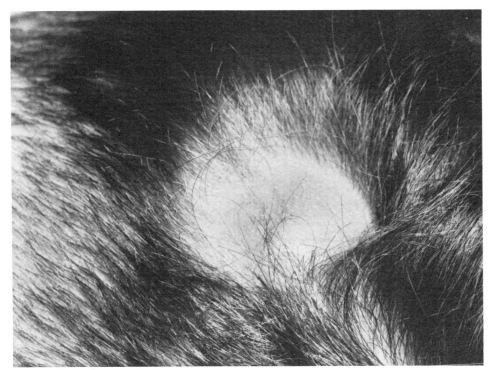

Fig. 13.8. An insect bite, heavily secondarily infected, was followed by temporary shedding of hair in the oedematous skin around the lesion. The hair regrew leaving a barely detectable central scar without hair (Addenbrooke's Hospital, Cambridge).

Tick bites
(References p. 396)

Ticks can carry a variety of infections by their bites and they can induce a wide range of allergic reactions (Marshall 1967), and also nodular reactions which can last for months or indefinitely.

The saliva of the tick contains numerous antigens and other substances, including anticoagulant. It seems possible that the anticoagulant is responsible for the alopecia which is associated with tick bites and which may be far more extensive than the narrow zone of temporary hair loss which may be associated with the inflammatory changes induced by other arthropods.

Seven to ten days after a tick bite in a child's scalp the hair may be shed in an area up to 4 cm in diameter. The bald patch resembles alopecia areata, except for the central area of crusting at the site of the bite (Saughar 1921; Marshall 1966). Complete regrowth of hair is usual except in a small central area of scarring. In two cases in which there were multiple tick bites (Ross & Friede 1955) multiple small areas of cicatricial alopecia up to 1.3 cm in diameter persisted.

References
Marshall J. (1966) Alopecia after tick bite. *South Africa Medical Journal*, **40**, 555.
Marshall J. (1967) Ticks and the human skin. *Dermatologica*, **135**, 60.
Ross M.S. & Friede H. (1955) Alopecia due to tick bite. *Archives of Dermatology*, **71**, 524.
Saughar L. (1921) Alopécie peladoide consecutive à une piqûre de tique. *Bulletin de la Sociétè Française de Dermatologie et Syphiligraphie*, **28**, 442.

Cutaneous myiasis

Myiasis is the infestation of the body by the larvae of certain species of Diptera—two-winged flies. Some species lay their eggs in existing wounds or ulcers but others deposit them on normal skin, and others such as *Dermatobia hominis*, important in Latin America, lay them on mosquitoes or house flies, which transfer them to the human body (Hubler *et al.* 1974).

The lesion of obligate and specific cutaneous myiasis in man are usually on exposed skin and sleeping babies are particularly at risk. The lesions present as furuncular nodules, single or multiple. There may be mild constitutional symptoms and eosinophilia. In one outbreak (Macias *et al.* 1973) the affected children were already suffering from pediculosis and pyoderma of the scalp. Around each nodule there may be temporary shedding of hair in a zone up to 3 cm in width. When the infection is controlled only the small central area at the site of the actual lesion remains bald. In a distinctive but uncommon clinical variant the larva migrates under the skin to produce one form of creeping eruption.

The lesions in myiasis are not uncommonly in the scalp, particularly where it is traditional to shave the scalp of babies and young children as in some parts of Africa.

Semispecific myiasis in which the eggs are laid in a wound, has complicated an infected ulcer of the scalp (Calero 1949).

Myiasis is more common in tropical than in temperate climates, but the species of fly (bot-fly or warble-fly) causing myiasis are widely distributed in temperate regions as well, and cases can occasionally occur there (Morgan *et al.* 1964).

In treating cutaneous myiasis the larvae should be evacuated from the nodules—they can sometimes be removed with fine forceps—and an antibiotic should be given systemically to control secondary infection.

References
Calero C. (1949) Cutaneous myiasis due to *Chryosostomomyia bergi*. *Journal of Parasitology*, **35**, 545.
Hubler W.R., Rudolph A.H. & Dougherty E.F. (1974) Dermal myiasis. *Archives of Dermatology*, **110**, 109.

Macies E.G., Graham A.J., Green M. & Pierce A.W. (1973) Cutaneous myiasis in South Texas. *New England Journal of Medicine*, **289**, 1239.

Morgan R.J., Moss H.B. & Hansker W.L. (1964) Myiasis. *Archives of Dermatology*, **90**, 180.

Piedra

Aetiology

The term piedra is applied to two distinct infections of the hair. Black piedra is caused by the ascomycete *Piedraia hortai* and the infection is endemic throughout the tropics and subtropics. Prevalence surveys show that in some areas, e.g. the Matto Grosso in Brazil, it is common at all ages, but particularly in young adults (Fischman 1973). The infection is endemic in a number of wild mammals, which may serve as reservoirs of infection (Kaplan 1959).

White piedra on the other hand is a relatively rare condition, usually encountered in temperate regions. It is caused by the imperfect yeast-like fungus, *Trichosporon cutaneum* (formerly known as *T. beigelii*).

Pathology

Piedraia hortai penetrates the hair cuticle, proliferates in the shaft and then breaks out to surround the shaft forming a hard brown to black nodular concretion, consisting of branched hyphae and containing asci and ascospores.

Trichosporon cutaneum also invades the hair shaft, damaging it so that breaking and splitting readily occur. The soft whitish nodules consist of hyphae which fragment into arthrospores.

Clinical features

In black piedra hard black nodules form on the scalp hairs. Other hairy regions, including the backs of the hands (Adams *et al.* 1977) may be affected.

In white piedra soft spongy white nodules develop on the pubic hair (Smith *et al.* 1973), but they too may appear in other hair regions including the beard and moustache, and to a limited extent, the scalp.

Treatment

Affected hairs may be cut short and the hair washed daily.

References

Adams B.A., Soo Hoo T.S. & Chung K.C. (1977) Black piedra in West Malaysia. *Australasian Journal of Dermatology*, **18**, 45.

Fischman O. (1973) Black piedra among Brazilian Indians. *Revista do Instituto de Medicina Tropical de Sao Paolo*, **15**, 103.

Kaplan W. (1959) Piedra in lower animals. *Journal of the American Veterinary Medical Association*, **134**, 113.

Smith J.D., Murtishaw W.A. & McBride M.E. (1973) White piedra (Trichsporosis). *Archives of Dermatology*, **107**, 439.

Trichomycosis axillaris

Aetiology and pathology

In trichomycosis axillaris nodules consisting of masses of bacteria develop in the axillary and sometimes in the pubic hairs. The condition is common in many populations. The cause is the diphtheroid *Corynebacterium tenuis*. It was found in 23 of 100 consecutive patients examined in the United States (Crissey *et al.* 1953). In an institution for the mentally retarded in England (Savin *et al.* 1976), trichomycosis was found in the axillae of 26%. About 2% had trichomycosis of scrotal hair, sometimes without axillary involvement. Axillary trichomycosis was present in about the same percentage of healthy male adults at physical education centres. Axillary sweating and low hygienic standards are said to favour the infection.

Microbiological studies have not reliably established whether *Corynebacterium tenuis* is a normal inhabitant of the axilla. Affected hairs have a larger number of diphtheroid species than control hairs (Savin *et al.* 1970). It has been suggested that different types give rise to the different colours. (Freeman *et al.* 1969). There are three colour varieties, yellow, black and red, but the black and red are unusual outside the tropics (Crissey & Murray 1954).

In the electronmicroscope colonies of bacteria can be seen invading and destroying cuticular and cortical keratin (Montes *et al.* 1963; Orfanos *et al.* 1971) (Fig. 13.9).

Clinical features

Commonly the patient is not aware of the presence of the infection, but sometimes yellow, red or black staining of the clothing brings it to his notice.

The affected hairs fluoresce under Wood's light, and the irregularly nodular granules can be seen with a hand lens.

Treatment

Regular washing usually suffices to clear the condition. Clindamycin 1% in alcohol has been found to be effective (White & Smith 1979).

References

Crissey J.T. & Murray P.F. (1954) Trichomycosis axillaris. *New York State Journal of Medicine*, **54**, 2841.

Crissey J.T., Rebell G.C. & Laskas J.J. (1953) Studies on the causative organism of trichomycosis axillaris. *Journal of Investigative Dermatology*, **19**, 187.

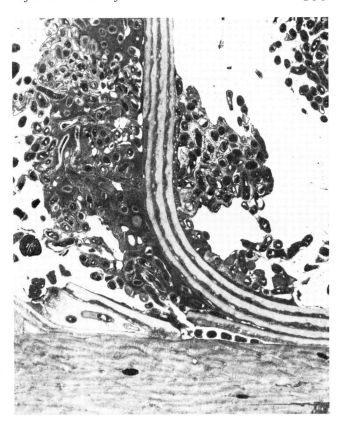

Fig. 13.9. *Corynebacteria* within the cuticle of an axillary hair. The cortex, seen at the bottom of the picture, is not affected (Slade Hospital, Oxford).

Freeman R.G., McBride M.E. & Knox J.M. (1969) Pathogenisis of trichomycosis axillaris. *Archives of Dermatology,* **100,** 96.

Montes L.F., Vasquez C. & Cataldi M.S. (1963) Electron microscopic study of infected hairs in trichomycosis axillaris. *Journal of Investigative Dermatology,* **40,** 273.

Orfanos C.E., Schloesser E. & Mahrle G. (1971) Hair-destroying growth of *Corynebacterium tenuis* in the so-called trichomycosis axillaris. *Archives of Dermatology,* **103,** 632.

Savin J.A., Sommerville D.A. & Noble W.C. (1970) The bacterial flora of trichomycosis axillaris. *Journal of Medical Microbiology,* **3,** 352.

White S.W. & Smith J. (1979) Trichomycosis pubis. *Archives of Dermatology,* **115,** 444.

Impetigo
(References p. 401)

Definition

Impetigo is a contagious superficial infection of the skin due to streptococci, staphylococci or both (Dillon 1972).

Normal skin is relatively resistant to invasion by bacteria; impetigo is very difficult to produce in laboratory animals (Johnson 1961).

Primary impetigo occurs as two types, impetigo contagiosum of Tilbury Fox, typically due to Group A streptococci, and bullous impetigo due to pyogenic staphylococci.

Secondary impetigo implies colonization and infection of already abnormal skin by streptococci or staphylococci.

Epidemiology and bacteriology (Marples 1965)
The relative importance of streptococci or staphylococci as the cause of impetigo varies from epidemic to epidemic and from country to country. Pure staphylococci impetigo is common in temperate climates, typically due to group II types 71 or 80/81. The streptococcal strains involved are usually of group A though rare cases may be due to groups B (impetigo neonatorum), C or G.

Primary impetigo is highly communicable and mainly affects pre-school children in late summer and early autumn. Staphylococci may infect the skin following initial nasal colonization whilst streptococci may directly infect the skin. Crowding, poor hygiene, and neglected minor trauma may contribute to the spread in epidemics. Localized outbreaks may occur in athletes taking part in contact sports.

Pathology
The inflammatory changes are superficial and commonly found near hair follicles. Vesiculation occurs in the epidermis at the level of the stratum granulosum. Epithelial cell debri, leucocytes and organisms are present in the vesicle. Smears for cytodiagnosis may show acantholytic cells. The skin heals without scarring.

Clinical findings
Primary impetigo. Streptococcal impetigo begins as a transient thin-roofed vesicle with a surrounding inflammatory halo; in this type, pustulation and crusting occur early. Removal of established crusts leads to rapid drying of serous exudate and further crust formation. The face, particularly around the nose and mouth, is the site of predilection; lesions may be multiple and become generalized. Staphylococcal impetigo is characterized by intact blisters often without any surrounding inflammatory reaction. Impetigo neonatorum is usually staphylococcal.

Secondary impetigo ('impetiginization') may occur in skin altered by minor trauma, insect bites, pediculosis capitas and eczema. Scalp infection associated with increasing serous matting of hair is usually associated with pediculosis capitis, atopic eczema, lichen simplex or insect bites.

Regional lymphadenitis and fever may both occur.

Laboratory findings include neutrophil leucocytosis and Gram smears showing positive staining cocci. Swab cultures readily yield colonies of staphylococci or streptococci.

Complications

The most severe complication of streptococcal impetigo is acute glomerulonephritis, less commonly acute guttate psoriasis and erythema multiforme may be precipitated. Toxic epidermal necrolysis ('scalded skin syndrome') may develop from staphylococcal impetigo (Lyall 1967).

Treatment

Very mild cases may respond simply to removal of crusts and bathing with saline or hydrogen peroxide. The use of topical antibiotics for treating impetigo is limited by the tendency of many to cause allergic sensitization. Sodium fucidate is active against most staphylococci.

   Impetigo remits most quickly when oral antibiotics are used. A single dose of intramuscular soluble penicillin G sodium followed by oral phenoxymethyl penicillin for one week is satisfactory for streptococcal infection; in childhood the dose will depend on the age of the patient. Most staphylococci respond to the same regime though penicillinase-producing strains may require flucloxicillin. Erythromycin is the treatment of choice for patients who are allergic to penicillins.

   In impetigo secondary to pediculosis capitis, eczema or lichen simplex, treatment of the infection is the first priority. Once bacterial inflammation has subsided, treatment appropriate to the primary disease must be started; if such treatment is inadequate, impetigo may recur. Since the normal bacterial flora may protect against virulent pathogens (Shinefield, 1965) in diseases such as eczema, only organisms causing inflammatory signs should be treated (Savin & Noble 1977).

References

Dillon H.C. (1972) Streptococcal infections of the skin and their complications: impetigo and nephritis. In *Streptococci and Streptococcal Diseases*, eds. L.W. Wannamaker & J.M. Matson. New York, Academic Press, p. 571.
Johnson J.E. (1961) Studies on the pathogenesis of staphylococcal infection. I. The effect of repeated skin infections. *Journal of Experimental Medicine*, 113, 235.
Lyall A. (1967) A review of toxic epidermal necrolysis. *British Journal of Dermatology*, 79, 662.
Marples M.J. (1965) *The Ecology of the Human Skin*, 1st edn. Springfield, Thomas.
Savin J.A. & Noble W.C. (1977) Opportunism and skin infections. In *Recent Advances in Dermatology*, vol. 4, ed. A. Rook. Edinburgh, Churchill Livingstone.

Furuncles and carbuncles
(Reference p. 403)

Aetiology

The furuncle is an acute, usually necrotic, infection of the hair follicle with *Staphylococcus aureus*, causing a perifollicular abscess. Furuncles occur most commonly in later childhood and in adolescence and reach a peak incidence in young adult life. They are more frequent in males than in females. Episodes of furunculosis may be short and acute but they may consist of crops at irregular intervals over a long period. Fatigue and stress are among many predisposing factors incriminated but without any statistical evidence that they are relevant. Malnutrition is however certainly a predisposing factor but otherwise most cases occur in apparently healthy young males.

A carbuncle is a deep infection with *Staphylococcus aureus* of a group of neighbouring hair follicles; the inflammatory changes involve the surrounding connecting tissue and subcutaneous fat. Carbuncles occur in the middle-aged and elderly, particulary in men, and systemic diseases, notably diabetes and cardiac failure, and corticosteroid therapy are among the important predisposing factors.

In both furuncles and carbuncles the patient may himself have been a chronic carrier of *Staphylococcus aureus* in the nose, axillae, perineum, toe-clefts or on the hair (Noble 1981). In other cases there is repeated reinfection from an asymptomatic carrier in the household or among nursing and medical attendants. The patient who has clinically recovered from these infections may remain a carrier.

Clinical features
Furuncles affect predominantly vellus hair follicles and are unusual in the scalp although they may frequently occur on the face and neck; they are also common around the axillae and in the anogenital region and on the hands and arms. They present single or multiple tender red follicular nodules which become pustules from which a necrotic core is discharged. They heal to leave small scars.

Carbuncles on the other hand are most often seen on the nape of the neck within the scalp margin; they may also occur on the shoulders, hips or thighs. An acutely tender smooth red nodule reaches a diameter of 8–10 cm within a few days. Focal necrosis is followed by the discharge of pus from multiple follicular orifaces. This is followed by more extensive necrosis and the separation of the whole central core, or such necrosis may occur rapidly without the preliminary follicular discharge. In either case a large ulcer results and heals to leave a permanent scar. Fever and other constitutional symptoms occur during the acute stage.

Diagnosis
Furunculosis in the scalp is sufficiently unusual for this diagnosis to be suspect. Superficial pustules complicating pediculosis must be excluded as must ringworm infection, and myiasis.

A carbuncle is simulated by anthrax but the haemorrhagic crust and vesicular margin of the latter infection are distinctive.

In all cases of furunculosis or of carbuncle a swab should be taken for bacteriological confirmation of the diagnosis and it is an advantage if phage typing can be carried out and antibiotic sensitivities established although treatment should not be postponed until this information is available.

The urine should be tested and underlying disease should be sought.

Treatment

Treatment of furunculosis and the careful search for the source of infection in the patient or his environment are described in general textbooks of dermatology. In chronic cases prolonged courses of antibiotics are not the ideal solution.

For carbuncles Penicillin G, the full dosage, should be given at the earliest opportunity.

Reference

Noble W.C. (1981) *Microbiology of the Human Skin*, 2nd ed. London, Lloyd Luke, p. 159.

Erysipelas
(Reference p. 402)

Aetiology

Erysipelas is an acute superficial cellulitis, caused by streptococci, usually of Group A. It occurs most frequently in infants and in the elderly, but can occur at any age. A wound or a non-infective skin lesion may provide an obvious point of entry for the infection, but in many cases no portal of entry is evident. Defective lymphatic drainage favours the development of erysipelas, and the infection tends to recur in such areas. Erysipelas most commonly affects the legs but the face is the next most frequent site (Schneider 1973). The scalp may be spared in erysipelas which may stop short at the scalp margin. However, the scalp may be involved by extension from the face or pinna or primarily in the presence of a scalp wound.

Clinical features

Fever and malaise often precede the development of visible cutaneous lesions and the patient may be severely ill; without effective treatment high fever may continue for several days and, particularly in the malnourished, the disease can be fatal.

Soon after the onset of the fever a sharply marginated plaque of erythema and oedema appears, sometimes with vesicles or bullae. The hair in affected areas of the scalp may be shed within a week to 10 days. Before antibacterial agents were available the early localized hair loss was followed after about 3 months by diffuse alopecia of the whole of the scalp, as a result of the prolonged high fever.

Diagnosis
Streptococci are not easily isolated from the skin lesions and are by no means
always present in the patient's throat. The clinical diagnosis is not difficult.

Treatment
A course of systemic penicillin or other appropriate antibiotic should be given at
the earliest possible stage.

Reference
Schneider I. (1973) Klinik und Pathogenese des rezidivierenden Erysipels. *Hautarzt*, **24**, 145.

Viral warts
(References p. 406)

Warts are benign tumours of the skin or adjacent mucous surfaces due to a DNA
virus, the human papilloma virus (HPV); most clinical types regress spontaneously (Rees 1979).

Viral spread is by direct inoculation into damaged skin. The incubation
period varies from 1 to 20 months with a mean value of approximately 4
months. Warts appear to have increased in incidence during the last 20 years.

Pathology
Individual lesions show irregular acanthosis and hyperkeratosis; the stratum
granulosum contains foci of virus-infected vacuolated cells whilst the horny
layer may be parakeratotic with basophilic nuclear inclusions. Lesions present
for more than 1 year may show little or no evidence of active viral presence.

Local immunity against the wart virus is cell-mediated, as with most viral
infections; during the phase of resolution complement-fixing (IgG) antibodies are
detectable. Until recently all the clinical manifestations of HPV infection were
considered to be due to a single strain of HPV. It is now evident that several
distinct sub-types exist (Gissmann *et al.* 1977; Coggin & Zur Hausen 1979). The
suggested types and their relationship to the clinical groups are as follows (Rees
1981):

Virus type	*Clinical type*
HPV 1 a, b, c	Plantar or common
HPV 2	Common
HPV 3	Plane, or epidermodysplasia verruciformis (EV)
HPV 4	Plantar, common or EV
HPV 5	EV (scaly lesions)
HPV 6	Genital (?); laryngeal (?)

Warts may occur at any age but their peak incidence is in childhood.

Recent work by Viac *et al.* (1977) suggests that once HPV virus can be harvested in culture, it will be possible to produce an effective anti-HPV vaccine.

Warts tend to involute spontaneously within months (Massing & Epstein 1963), but there is wide individual variation in their course. There is a suggestion that T lymphocytes may be reduced in patients with persistent warts (Chretien *et al.* 1978). The cell-mediated response and humoral complement-fixing IgG antibodies are both involved (Ivanyi & Morrison 1976; Pyrhönen & Johansson 1975). Very numerous warts may be present in patients with immune deficiencies especially Hodgkin's disease (Morrison 1975) and warts are particularly prevalent in elderly patients with systemic lupus erythematosus (Johansson *et al.* 1977).

Clinical types

Common warts (verruca vulgaris) are firm papules with a horny surface; sites of predilection are the hands and knees though any part of the body may be affected including the scalp.

Generalized verrucosis, which may be associated with impaired cell-mediated immunity, consists of common and sometimes plane warts disseminated widely over the body surface; individual lesions may coalesce to produce large verrucous plaques.

Plane warts are small (1–5 mm) smooth, flat or slightly elevated lesions. The colour varies from skin colour, to grey or brown. The face, shins and hands are commonly affected. Multiple plane or filiform warts of the beard area are due to seeding of the wart virus into sites of minor damage from shaving. Individual lesions may affect follicular openings. Plane warts often last for several years. The differential diagnosis depends on the site and number of lesions present but flat epidermal naevi and lichen planus may give a similar appearance.

Filiform or digitate warts occur more frequently in men than women; most lesions are found on the head or neck; hundreds of small filiform warts may develop in the beard area. Grouped filiform lesions on the scalp may mimic epidermal naevi.

Treatment

In carrying out treatment for warts one must constantly temper enthusiasm with the knowledge that most lesions will remit sponaneously within a few months of onset leaving no permanent scar (Rees 1981); warts that are causing little in the way of symptoms may therefore be left untreated or a placebo may be appropriate.

Plane warts may be treated with salicylic acid preparations. Therapy of common warts depends on their size and site; single large lesions can be removed by curettage or cryosurgery, preferably using liquid nitrogen spray. Filiform or digitate warts can be treated by electrocautery or cryosurgery; isolated large lesions on the scalp are best treated by curettage under local anaesthetic.

References

Chretien J.H., Esswin J.G. & Garagus P.F. (1978) Decreased T cell levels in patients with warts. *Archives of Dermatology*, **114**, 313.

Coggin J.R. & Zur Hausen H. (1979) Workshop on papilloma viruses and cancer. *Cancer Research*, **39**, 545.

Gissman L., Pfister H. & Zur Hausen H. (1977) Human papilloma viruses (HPV): characterization of four different isolates. *Virology*, **76**, 569.

Ivanyi L. & Morrison W.C. (1976) In vitro lymphocyte stimulation by wart antigen in man. *British Journal of Dermatology*, **94**, 523.

Johansson E., Pyrhönen S. & Rostili T. (1977) Warts and wart virus antibodies in patients with systemic lupus erythematosus. *British Medical Journal*, **i**, 74.

Massing A.M. & Epstein W.C. (1963) Natural history of warts. *Archives of Dermatology*, **87**, 306.

Morrison W.C. (1975) Viral warts, herpes simplex and herpes zoster in patients with secondary immune deficiencies or neoplasms. *British Journal of Dermatology*, **92**, 625.

Pyrhönen S. & Johansson E. (1975) Regression of warts: an immunological study. *Lancet*, **i**, 592.

Rees R.B. (1979) Warts. *Cutis*, **23**, 588.

Rees R.B. (1981) The characterization, immunopathology and treatment of viral warts. *International Journal of Dermatology*, **20**, 110.

Viac J., Thivolet J. & Chardonnet Y. (1977) Specific immunity in patients suffering from recurring wart before and after repetitive intra-dermal tests with human papilloma virus. *British Journal of Dermatology*, **91**, 365.

Molluscum contagiosum

Molluscum contagiosum is a common infection of skin and rarely of mucous membranes due to a large (200–300 nm) DNA poxvirus which usually affects children (Postlethwaite 1970). It is mainly a human infection but has been described in chimpanzees in captivity and in a kangaroo (Bagnall & Wilson 1974).

It occurs in all races and has a world-wide distribution. In Britain, school-age children up to 15 years of age are commonly affected; the recent increased incidence in the age group 20–30 years is mainly due to venereal spread. Transmission of the virus is by direct contact or via infected fomites. Communal living is associated with a high incidence of infection; however, multiple family cases are rare. In children under 14 years of age, boys are more frequently affected than girls.

The incubation period is from 14 to 50 days.

The earliest stage pathologically shows minute intracellular granules which coalesce into large eosinophilic hyaline bodies (molluscum, or Henderson–Paterson bodies); these infected cells associated with increased cell proliferation

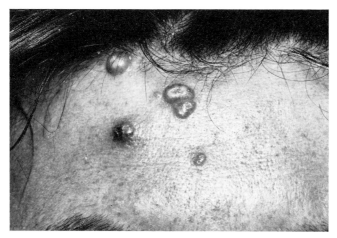

Fig. 13.10. Molluscum contagiosum of the forehead: smooth, pearly umbilicated lesions.

give the characteristic light microscopic appearance of scrapings or curettings (Fig. 13.10).

Clinical features

Individual lesions are shiny, pearly white, umbilicated papules varying in size from 1–10 mm. Cheesy white material can be expressed from the centre of any papule. In hairy areas, follicular lesions may mimic furunculosis though careful observation will always reveal associated pearly-white lesions.

The sites affected vary with factors such as climate, the mode of contact and the presence of an eczematous diathesis. Atopic subjects may develop hundreds of papules (Solomon & Telner 1966). In non-atopic subjects the infection is usually localized to one area, often on the trunk or axilla—apart from inpatients who are immunosuppressed or taking cytotoxic or steroid therapy (Rosenberg & Yusk 1970; Schorfinius 1972).

In temperate regions the neck and trunk are sites of predilection whilst in the tropics the limbs are more often involved; less commonly the face, scalp and mucous membranes are affected. Not infrequently, molluscum contagiosum causes conjunctivitis and an eczematous reaction in the affected area; these clear on resolution of the viral lesions.

In normal subjects, most cases clear within 3–4 months; a minority may persist for up to 3–4 years. However, occasionally a solitary lesion or more rarely a cluster of contiguous lesions may reach a diameter of 2 cm or more and persist for years. Such giant mollusca have been reported in the scalp (Fox 1902; Foelsche 1965).

Clinical diagnosis of the typical lesions presents no difficulty. The diagnosis of a giant molluscum is rarely suspected and is made histologically after the lesion has been curetted or excised.

Treatment is not necessary in most cases due to the good prognosis and absence of symptoms. Large, visible or irritating and sore lesions may require treatment. All the recommended therapeutic modalities involve irritating the papules, i.e. using trichloracetic acid or phenol applied on a pointed orange stick, or cryosurgery. Localized large lesions may be removed by curettage. Topical retinoic acid has been suggested by some authorities. Associated eczema may require treatment with topical anti-pruritic agents, or weak local corticosteroid creams; oral anti-histamines are helpful particularly if eczematous itching leads to sleeplessness.

References

Bagnall B.G. & Wilson G.R. (1974) Molluscum contagiosum in a red kangaroo. *Australasian Journal of Dermatology*, **15**, 115.

Foelsche W. (1965) Mollusca contagiosa seltener Extensität und Lokalisation. *Zeitschrift für Haut und Geschlechtkrankheiten*, **37**, 268.

Fox T.C. (1902) Case presentation, Dermatological Society of London. *British Journal of Dermatology*, **14**, 216.

Postlethwaite R. (1970) Molluscum contagiosum: a review. *Archives of Environmental Health*, **21**, 432.

Postlethwaite R., Watt J.A., Horley T.G., Simpson I. & Adam H. (1967) Features of molluscum contagiosum in the north east of Scotland and in Fijian settlements. *Journal of Hygiene (Cambridge)*, **65**, 281.

Rosenberg E.W. & Yusk J.W. (1970) Molluscum contagiosum: eruption following treatment with prednisolone and methotrexate. *Archives of Dermatology*, **101**, 439.

Schorfinius H.H. (1972) Molluscum Contagiosum als Symptom. *Hautarzt*, **23**, 34.

Solomon L.M. & Telner P. (1966) Eruptive molluscum contagiosum in atopic dermatitis. *Canadian Medical Association Journal*, **95**, 978.

Chapter 14
Psychological Factors and Disorders of the Hair

Introduction

The effective diagnosis, assessment and management of many disorders of the hair is impossible without some appreciation of the special psychological significance of the hair. Diseases which produce patterns of hair growth which deviate even slightly from that which the patient regards as normal may in extreme cases cause emotional stress of such a degree as may perpetuate the abnormality, whether or not stress played a role in initiating it.

The unconscious significance of hair
(References p. 414)

In a monograph with this title Charles Berg (1950) reviewed the anthropological and psychiatric literature. He emphasized the importance of the hair in many rituals in a variety of primitive peoples. He pointed out that hair has in modern man practically no other significance except as a sexual symbol and he claimed that there is no normal person without some degree of hair fetishism. He referred to a young woman with total alopecia who stated that she would rather have lost an arm or a leg, and he discussed the general overvaluation of hair. He mentioned that even minimal facial hair in a woman may cause great distress—'these affects are not based upon reality values, but like all the affects connected with hair have their source in those unconscious constellations which we are endeavouring to plumb'.

Charles Berg was a psychoanalyst of the Freudian school and he believed that the normal concern about the hair becoming thin, falling out or greying was a displacement of castration anxiety. Whether or not this explanation is acceptable we are not competent to decide but there can be no doubt that some disorders of the hair give rise to anxieties more profound than their objective severity would appear to justify.

Disturbance of the body image

In 1965 Meador introduced the concept of non-disease and pointed out that the absence of diagnostic signs and symptoms need not imply an absence of significant symptomatology. Of 28 such patients studied by Cotterill (1981) the symptoms were confined to the scalp in 9, the face in 8 and to the perineum in 8; there were 16 females and 12 males. The age ranged from 16 to 76 years with a mean age of 46. The scalp symptoms were loss of hair and some irritation and facial symptoms were burning, itching and hirsutism. We have seen similar patients whose principal scalp complaint apart from hair loss was extreme tenderness of the scalp. In all these patients the objective changes, if indeed there are any, are so slight as to seem trivial even to the most sympathetic observer, yet the patients insist that the symptoms are ruining their life.

From the psychiatric point of view these patients are not a uniform group. Most have a disturbed body image and the majority are depressed. They require most careful management and the more severely affected, who are potential suicide risks, should be referred to a psychiatrist.

Common causation of emotional and hair disorders

Depressive illness in young women may be accompanied by androgenetic cutaneous changes. Although the patient may herself tend to blame her alopecia, hirsutism or acne for her depression, a detailed history often establishes that the emotional and cutaneous changes developed in parallel. Possible mechanisms are discussed on p. 75.

Stress as a precipitating factor in diseases of the hair
(References p. 414)

Diffuse shedding of hair can occur in patients under very severe stress (p. 119) but diffuse alopecia should not be glibly attributed to the minor stresses which with perseverence can be elicited in the history of most individuals. Diffuse shedding of hair beginning some 3 or 4 months after a well-defined major stressful episode may, however, he accepted as provoked by that episode and to be potentially reversible in the same way as post-partum or post-febrile alopecia.

However, stress, acute and severe or chronic and prolonged, can induce the androgenetic syndrome (p. 75) and unless early investigation and treatment are undertaken, skin changes which are not easily reversed or are irreversible may be produced. The first symptom of androgenetic alopecia is profuse but predominantly frontovertical shedding of telogen hairs (p. 103). It can be seen that this symptom is very easily confused with true diffuse telogen shedding as mentioned above.

The role of stress in precipitating alopecia areata is well discussed by Whitlock (1976). The literature (p. 281) is conflicting. The time interval between the alleged precipitating stress and loss of hair has varied from a few days to 4 months. It follows that if stress can indeed precipitate an attack of alopecia areata, it must do so by more than one mechanism. Some writers suggest that alopecia may be an autoimmune disorder (p. 278). Should this prove to be the case it does not preclude the possible precipitation of an attack by stress. The evidence incriminating stress remains controversial, but it is probable that no dermatologist of experience would exclude its possible role in certain cases.

Stress as a perpetuating factor

In the cutaneous androgenetic syndromes the distress caused by the skin changes can contribute to their perpetuation. Acne and/or hirsutism can seriously impair the sensitive adolescent's capacity to establish normal social relationships with his contemporaries and if severe may retard his or her psychosocial development. The evidence that a self-perpetuating vicious circle can become established has not yet been proven biochemically, but clinical experience suggests that it may occur and that it may indeed be of common occurrence.

Alopecia areata can be extremely disfiguring. Whether or not stress plays a part in provoking it, it is certain that the alopecia is often itself a source of severe stress. It is not proven that this stress perpetuates the condition but the possibility should be borne in mind in the management of these patients.

Artefacts (Lyell 1972)

Artefacts are self-inflicted lesions, but the term as usually employed excludes such lesions produced accidentally through the abuse of mechanical or chemical cosmetic procedures. The most frequent form of deliberate artefact of the scalp consists of plucking the hair, so-called trichotillomania (p. 266). In children the partially bald patches so produced are seldom of serious psychiatric significance, but the plucking systematically of all the head hair in an adult usually indicates a very serious personality disorder as does extensive self-mutilation of the skin in any region of the body (Sneddon & Sneddon 1975).

Deliberate physical or chemical production of other injuries of the scalp is very unusual but it is possible that some such cases are undiagnosed.

Hair in the social sciences*
(References p. 414)

Hair cutting as punishment

Cutting off or shaving the hair as a punishment has been practised by many peoples. The Ainu of the island of Hokkaido, north of Japan, have a long-established reputation for hirsutism; they are in fact a proto-Caucasoid stock who are no more hirsute than many other Caucasoids, although very hairy by contrast with their Japanese neighbours (Harvey & Brothwell 1969). Among the Ainu great emphasis is placed on the possession of a very full beard and abundant head hair and the enforced cutting of hair was regarded as a severe punishment associated with loss of honour. Women's hair was cut as punishment for adultery. The same punishment was used in Europe after the Second World War on women who had associated with soldiers of occupying armies.

The importance placed on short hair by the armed forces of many countries reinforces the popular association between short hair and authority and discipline.

Hair style

The importance of hair as a component of the body image has been mentioned. The length, the colour and the style in which it is worn must conform to an accepted stereotype. Some knowledge of recent research on such stereotypes is helpful in increasing the dermatologist's understanding of some of his patients who appear to be perversely endeavouring to demand from their hair qualities with which nature failed to endow it.

Opler (1970) in discussing long hair in males in the United States, feels that hair style is a reflection of group attitudes culturally defined rather than of personal feelings of sexual identity. The findings of some investigators on male students classified as 'deviant' in hair length were not unexpected (Larsen &

* The remainder of this chapter is designed to introduce the clinician to the rapidly growing literature on the hair published in the journals of the social sciences. It is not cited in textbooks of dermatology and is largely unknown to dermatologists, but its relevance to clinical situations is evident.

White 1974). The deviants, with hair reaching below their shoulders, assigned more value to independence and less value to recognition and conformity than the non-deviant students. The stereotypes accepted among students have been found to vary from one university to another even during the same period, being influenced by the conservatism or liberalism of the community in which the university is situated. Long hair has been seen as a protest but, 'the increasing number of hair stylists for young men seem to indicate that many of them need an artificial aid to win or to retain a desired self-esteem' (Rom 1973).

Hair colour

As with other stereotypes those concerning hair colour apply only to the communities studied and to the period of the study. Nevertheless they throw considerable light on deeply rooted concepts and prejudices. Lawson (1971) found that 79 male psychology students, rating the females by hair colour, put brunettes first in 37 of 63 possible comparisons, blondes in 17, redheads in 5 and artificial blondes in 2. The 161 female students voted dark males superior to blond males in the proportion of 34 to 4 out of 42 possible comparisons.

Beards

Numerous psychological studies carried out during the '70s on the subject of beards show a generally positive correlation between the amount of hair on the subject's face and high ratings for masculinity, maturity, good looks, dominance, self confidence and other desirable traits (Pellegrini 1973). Similar findings have been reported from the University of Chicago (Freedman 1969). However, at the rural and more conservative University of Wyoming only 12.8% of females preferred men with a very full beard whereas 40% preferred no facial hair and 42% preferred a moustache but no beard (Feinman & Gill 1977).

Moustaches

Few investigations have been made of the correlation of moustaches with personality traits or of observer reactions to them. Peberdy (1961) studied candidates for commission in the British Army. He classified moustaches into four types: (1) Trimmed, flatly covering most of the lip; (2) Clipped—'toothbrush'; (3) Line; (4) Bushy. Those with trimmed moustaches did not differ in their assessments from clean-shaven candidates. All those with clipped moustaches failed to pass the selection board (but not of course on account of their moustaches). They were limited in imagination with little appreciation of the opinions of others and they tended to create rather than to decrease interpersonal tensions. Men with line moustaches passed the board at only half the normal rate; those that failed showed obsessive health consciousness. Men with bushy moustaches passed at the normal rate; those that failed tended to self-indulgence and self-display.

Parker's (1970) study carried out in Australia is sub-titled 'semi scientific'. He presents interesting facts and figures, tending to show an association between moustaches and sexual pathology, but not allowing any firm conclusions to be drawn.

References

Berg C. (1950) *The Unconscious Significance of Hair*. London, Allen & Unwin.

Cotterill J.A. (1981) Dermatological non-disease: a common and potentially fatal disturbance of cutaneous body image. *British Journal of Dermatology*, **104**, 661.

Feinman S. & Gill G.W. (1977) Females' response to males' beardedness. *Perceptual and Motor Skills*, **44**, 533.

Freedman D. (1969) The survival value of the beard. *Psychology Today*, **3**, 36.

Harvey R.G. & Brothwell D.R. (1969) Biosocial aspects of Ainu hirsuteness. *Journal of Biosocial Science*, **1**, 109.

Larsen J.P. & White B.A. (1974) Comparison of selected perceptual and personality variables among college men deviant and non-deviant in hair length. *Perceptual and Motor Skills*, **38**, 1315.

Lawson E.D. (1971) Hair color, personality and the observer. *Psychological Reports*, **28**, 311.

Lyell A. (1972) Dermatitis artefacta and self-inflicted disease. *Scottish Medical Journal*, **17**, 187.

Meador C.K. (1963) The art and science of non-disease. *New England Journal of Medicine*, **272**, 92.

Opler M. (1971) Long hair in contemporary males. *Medical Aspects of Human Sexuality*, 144.

Parker N. (1970) The moustache: a semi-scientific study. *Australia and New Zealand Journal of Psychology*, **4**, 49.

Peberdy G.R. (1961) Moustaches. *Journal of Mental Science*, **107**, 40.

Pellegreni R.J. (1973) Impressions of the male personality as a function of beardedness. *Psychology*, **10**, 29.

Rom P. (1973) Hair style and life style. *Individual Psychology*, **10**, 22.

Sneddon I. & Sneddon J. (1975) Self-inflicted injury: a follow-up of 43 patients. *British Medical Journal*, **iii**, 527.

Whitlock F.A. (1976) *Psychophysiological Aspects of Skin Disease*. London, Saunders, p. 181.

Chapter 15
Hair Cosmetics

Introduction
(References p. 426)

Twentieth-century woman has become increasingly concerned at modifying her appearance by cosmetic preparations and nowhere is this concern more strongly manifest than in connection with the hair, no doubt a measure of its psychological and sexual importance. The production of shampoos, dyes, waving and other hair applications has become big business in every 'Western' country. Science has benefited enormously from this industry since many of the advances in our knowledge of the structure of the hair follicle and hair have come from cosmetic science laboratories (Harry 1973; Schoen 1978).

Shampoos (Corbett 1976; Robbins 1979)
(References p. 426)

In modern terms a shampoo may be defined as a suitable detergent for washing hair that leaves the hair in good condition. Originally shampoos were used solely for cleansing hair but their range of function has extended in recent years to include conditioning, and the treatment of some hair and scalp diseases.

In principle, to wash hair a shampoo must remove grease since it is the latter which attracts dirt and other particulate matter. The polar group of a detergent achieves this by displacing oil from the hair surface. The evaluation of shampoo detergency is difficult and complicated. The consumer tends to equate detergency with foaming and this is scientifically incorrect; however, in Western society few shampoos sell unless they possess good foaming power. In the evaluation of detergents as shampoos no single criterion can be used though instrumental methods have been devised (Prall 1970). Efficacy can be based only on the subjective impression of the consumer. The factors taken into consideration include (a) ease of distribution of shampoo over the hair, (b) lathering power, (c) ease of rinsing and combing of wet hair, (d) lustre of hair, (e) speed of

415

drying, and (f) ease of combing and setting of dried hair. Safety is of paramount importance.

Shampoo formulations vary enormously but the basic ingredients can be resolved into a few groups—water, detergent and some fatty material. Soap shampoos are made from vegetable or animal fats and remove dirt and grease as efficiently as detergents; however, a scum forms with hard water and the trend has therefore been increasingly towards detergents as the principal washing ingredient. Detergents are synthetic petroleum products and form no hard water scum.

In essence shampoos contain (a) principal surfactants for detergency and foaming power, (b) secondary surfactants to improve and 'condition' hair, and (c) additives which both complete the formulation and add 'special' effects; whatever the claims of some manufacturers most special additives end up down the sink! (Spoor 1973).

Principal surfactants
The main ones are anionic substances e.g. alkyl sulphates made from alcohols obtained from fatty acids of coconut and palm kernel oil, the so-called lauryl sulphates. Other surfactants which may be the principal constituent are cationics—functionally good but in general too irritant, non-ionics—rather deficient in foaming power, and ampholytics—a low irritancy potential but rather expensive. Specific types include fatty acid soaps which are alkaline and cause 'rough' hair, paraffin sulphonates, alkyl benzene sulphonates that are in some low-cost liquid shampoos, and alkyl ether sulphates; the latter are relatively expensive but more soluble than lauryl sulphate. All have properties that can be utilized in combination with principal anionic substances.

Secondary (auxiliary) surfactants
These are added to improve the foaming and 'conditioning' characteristics of shampoos. In practice, most are ampholytic or anionic. Examples include secondary alkyl sulphates (teepols), monoglyceride sulphates (like lauryl sulphate), turkey red oil, alkyl phosphates, methyl taurides, fatty acid alkanolamides—often combined with lauryl sulphate for richness of lather and 'after condition', acyl aminoacids, sarcosines and peptides.

Additives
These include germicides, conditioners, pearlescents, sequestrants, colours, perfumes and preservatives.

Conditioners may be detergent in action, as already described under secondary surfactants, or non-detergent, for example natural polymers such as polyvinyl pyrrolidone (PVP), fatty materials (lanolin) or natural products such as herbs, peptides and egg fractions. Protein additives made from hydrolysed collagen have become popular (Karjala *et al.* 1966, 1967). As applied to shampoo formulations, the term conditioner can only be defined qualitatively. It must act to add body to 'thin' hair and improve the appearance and manageability, particularly of damaged hair, e.g. add gloss, lustre and minimize tangling and 'flyaway'. They should perhaps be called 'reconditioners', but any changes they induce are only temporary.

Shampoo formulations
In general cosmetic shampoos can be dry (powder and liquid types), liquid, solid cream, aerosol or oily. Anti-dandruff, 'medicated' and scalp treatment shampoos contain antiseptics and active agents such as coal and wood tar fractions. Clear liquid shampoos are the most popular, including 'cleansing' types, sold for treating greasy hair, and 'cosmetic' types having good conditioning action and popular among women with dry or 'normal' hair. For details of other specific formulations the reader is recommended to read larger texts (Harry, 1973).

Shampoo safety
Shampoos evidently must be non-toxic, and at concentrations used by the consumer irritate neither skin nor eyes. New shampoo formulations are tested exhaustively prior to marketing, particularly to assess their propensity to cause eye irritation, scarring and corneal opacities. Skin irritation is not usually encountered from shampoos that have low eye irritancy potential. Eye safety is assessed by the technique known as the Draize test; standard solutions of shampoo are instilled into the conjunctival sac of an albino rabbit. In general the eye irritancy of detergents is greatest with cationics, followed by anionics, and least with non-anionics. There are exceptions to this, suggesting that shampoo irritancy may be due to properties other than detergency including surface activity, pH, wetting power, foaming power (Ross–Miles Test), and wetting and foaming power together. Most shampoos are, in fact, irritant but not dangerously so.

Cosmetic hair colouring (Corbett & Menkart 1973; Burnett & Corbett 1977)
(References p. 426)

Since the days of the pharaohs, women in particular have used hair dyes both to hide grey hair and for reasons of fashion. The latter use has increased enormously during the past 40 years and now men are using them, mostly in the treatment of grey hair.

The penetration of dyes into hair depends on molecular size and the aqueous swelling of the hair at the time of application of the dye (Zviak 1966); basicity of the dye is also important. The most successful dyes are relatively small molecules.

Excluding bleaches, hair colouring materials can be divided into three groups; vegetable, metallic and synthetic organic dyes. In advanced countries vegetable and metallic hair colorants are almost obsolete because of the more 'natural' colours obtained with synthetic organic chemicals.

Vegetable dyes

Henna may be used to give reddish-auburn shades. It is obtained from shrubs found in North Africa and the Middle-East—*Lawsonia alba*, *L. spinosa* and *L. inermis*. The dye is produced from dried leaves which are removed before the plant flowers. The active principle is an acidic naphthoquinone (lawsone); it is still to be found in some hair rinses. Traditionally it is applied as a paste 'pack' which is left in situ for from 5 to 60 minutes. This process is non-toxic but messy, and fingernails may become stained. Henna rengs are mixtures of henna and powdered indigo leaves that produce blue-black shades. A wide range of colours can be obtained from henna combined with metallic salts or pyrogallol—compound henna. Ground flower heads or Roman or German chamomile yield a yellow dye, 1, 3, 4 trihydroxyflavone (apigenin). It stains only the cuticle and can be used to lighten or brighten hair. Other vegetable dyes include extracts from logwood and walnut shell.

Metallic dyes

Traditionally hair dyes for men have been of this type since the colour changes occur less rapidly and are not as immediately obvious as with the oxidative dyes. Inorganic salts are used which are altered by the hair and coat surface as either oxides from reduction of the metal salts by keratin, or sulphides from the action of the sulphur in keratin on the metal. They all give a rather dull (metallic) appearance and may cause brittle or damaged hair if used too often.

Lead acetate, with precipitated sulphur or sodium thiosulphate, gives brown to black shades; grey hair may be changed through yellow to brown or black. Silver nitrate used alone produces a greenish-black colour; pyrogallol is used as developer. Colours from ash blond to black are possible by mixing silver nitrate variously with copper, cobalt or nickel; brownish-black skin staining is the great disadvantage. Bismuth salts give shades of brown.

Newer metallic dyes, containing a metal plus an organic ligand, are used on textile fibres and in some hair dye patents.

Metallic dyes cannot be removed without hair damage and should be left to grow out.

Synthetic organic dyes

This group have now been in use for more than 40 years. They are the most important type because of the comprehensive range of 'natural' colours that can be obtained. Most penetrate the hair cuticle, i.e. they are potentially permanent, but in recent years less-permanent types have been introduced.

Synthetic organic colorants are of three types:

(1) *Temporary.* These wash out with one shampoo and last no longer than 1 week. Many temporary rinses belong to this group, including fashionable unnatural colours used by avant garde sects and groups! They are available in aerosol sprays by incorporation into transparent polymeric plastics such as PVP; the disadvantages of such vehicles is their tendency to flake off onto pillows and clothing.

(2) *Semi-permanent.* In Great Britain these have the widest appeal. They are of sufficiently small molecular size to penetrate into the cortex. They are intrinsically coloured, i.e. no developing is required, cf. the oxidative permanent group. They are relatively easy to wash out with shampoos containing ammonia; other shampoos must be used 6–10 times to remove them. The nitro group, for example the nitrophenylenediamine and nitroaminophenols, when mixed give colours from red or yellow to blond to chestnut; satisfactory brown colours can be obtained by including anthroquinones which are intrinsically blue. Some semi-permanent dyes have an affinity for thioglycollate—waved hair. Many are now used in colour shampoos.

(3) *Permanent* (syn. developed or oxidation dyes). These do not rely on the natural colour of a single chemical dye stuff, cf. semipermanents, but require an oxidative developer—H_2O_2—to produce the final colour i.e.:

Paraphenylenediamine (PPD)
and/or
Paratoluenediamine (PTD)
$\downarrow + H_2O_2$
Applied to hair
$\downarrow$
Quinone diimine (small molecule)
$\downarrow$
penetrates hair—to cortex
$\downarrow$
large molecules   (by diimine 'self' condensation and
produced   modifiers e.g. pyrogallol)

Other substances may be included in specific formulations to give greater intensity to the dye, for example resorcinol, and polyhidric phenols. For the range of formulations the reader is referred to more detailed texts (Zviak 1966).

Oxidative dyes are potentially hazardous. The need for hydrogen peroxide enables lighter shades to be obtained, but structural damage to hair may occur if care is not exercised. Additives such as pyrogallol and resorcinol are potential irritants. The greatest problem is the potential of PPD (less so with PTD) to cause allergic dermatitis. Up to 10% of users may develop type IV allergy (Blohm & Rajka 1970; Lubowe 1973). All dyes in this group are therefore sold with instructions to carry our preliminary patch testing 24–48 hours before the proposed dye, i.e. the dye system is applied to skin either behind one ear or on the forearm—any redness, swelling or blistering implies allergy and the dying should not therefore proceed. A negative patch test does not mean that subsequent allergy cannot develop, it simply shows the subject not to be allergic at the time the test was carried out. If allergy is shown, it is not sufficient merely to stop all future use of oxidative dyes—unfortunately cross sensitization occurs with other aromatic benzenes e.g. sulphonamides and some local anaesthetics, which must also be avoided for life. Hair dyes of this group have recently been incriminated as possible carcinogens (Burnett 1980). Chromosome breaks have occurred under experimental conditions (Kirkland *et al.* 1978) and an increased incidence of tumours has been found in regular users (Burnett & Menkart, 1978). It has also been intimated that aplastic anaemia could be produced by hair dyes (Burnett *et al.* 1978). None of these reports is sufficiently conclusive to warrant the withdrawal of such dyes.

Permanent dyes last for several months; they must not be applied more frequently than every 3–4 weeks, since hair damage will occur. Permanent waving or straightening too soon after dying may also induce hair damage. Permanent dyes must therefore be allowed to grow out. However, if a light shade has been produced and the subject wishes for a darker shade, then temporary rinses may safely be used since these only coat the hair surface and have no propensity to cause structural damage.

For less commonly used permanent dye formulations the reader is referred to larger texts (Harry 1973).

Bleaches (Wolfram *et al.* 1970; Wall 1972)
Whitening hair involves the use of hydrogen peroxide and ammonia mixtures. Melanin pigments are destroyed by this procedure, whilst combined cysteine is broken down to give cysteic acid residues which evidently damage hair—over-use may lead to disruption and fracture of hair (Selzle & Wolff 1976). Consequently bleaching, permanent waving and dyeing are never carried out together. The human eye perceives a more aesthetically acceptable blonde ('platinum' blonde) when the bleached hair is treated with a blue certified colour; methylene blue 1 : 100,00 is the most frequently used. The pigment destruction in bleached hair is chiefly localized in the surface portion of the cortex (Orfanos & Mahrle 1971).

Permanent waving (Corbett 1976)
(References p. 426)

Permanent waving has been defined as the process of changing the shape of the hair so that the new shape persists through several shampoos. Ancient Egyptian women used wet mud for this purpose and even as recently as 1910 the only methods available were heat, using a hot curling iron, or boiling water. During the last 70 years, increasing knowledge of keratin chemistry has enabled semi-permanent chemical methods to be developed. Whatever the process used, three stages are involved in hair waving (a) Physical or chemical softening of the hair, (b) Re-shaping, and (c) Hardening of fibres to retain the reshaped position.

Softening

Water can extend the hydrogen bonds between adjacent polypeptide in the keratin molecule, allowing temporary reshaping to be carried out—exposure to high humidity or re-wetting immediately reverses the process. To obtain a more durable effect from water, steam may be used which in a limited way disrupts disulphide bonds. Heat and steam alone are rarely acceptable to modern women because their effects are temporary and the treatment is uncomfortable. Heat can be more effectively utilized in conjunction with ammonium hydroxide and potassium bisulphite or triethanolamine as agents to reduce —S=S— bonds; great skill is involved in this process since failure to judge the time of application of chemicals and heat may cause severe damage. Chemical heat pads are still rarely used, for example utilizing heat produced from exothermic reactions, e.g. quicklime.

Since 1945, cold wave processes utilizing substituted thiosulphates, i.e. thioglycollates, have largely superseded hot waving. Thioglycollates are potent reducers of disulphide bonds in the keratin molecule:

$$-S{=}S{-} \longrightarrow 2{-}SH$$

A typical cold waving lotion contains thioglycollic acid plus ammonia ormonoethanolamine.

Reshaping

The type of rollers or curlers used to reshape the softened hair depends on the training of the hairdresser and the fashion desired. The diameter of curl is evidently related to curler size; 'curl tightness' depends on the effective curl diameter when the curl is completely hardened (neutralized); hardening is thus carried out with the rollers or curlers still in situ. Increasing the waving time up to 25 minutes gives increasing tightness of curl even to the extent of producing a frizzy appearance—still longer exposure times may cause decreasing tightness of curl. 'Tepid' shampooing involves using a weaker thioglycollate solution plus warm air. The reshaping stage is thus a great test of hairdressing skill and experience.

Hardening (neutralizing or setting)
In general this process involves a reversal of the softening (reduction) stages:

$$2\ SH \xrightarrow{\text{oxidation}} -S{=}S-$$

It is important to note that complete reversal to presoftened 'strength' cannot occur since many free —SH groups may not be in a position for oxidation to be effective.

$$2{-}SH \longrightarrow -S{-}C{-}S-$$

or

$$2{-}SH \longrightarrow -S{-}Ba{-}S-$$

Atmospheric oxidation may effectively neutralize the waving process. This method is slow and rollers must be left in position for several hours overnight. Chemical oxidation is now the rule. Hairdressers generally use hydrogen peroxide whilst most solutions for home contain sodium perborate or percarbonate (UK) or sodium or potassium bromate (USA). Some neutralizers contain shellac which may react with alcohol groups to cause hair discoloration.

Practical procedures
Hot waving involves the following sequence:
(a) Shampooing.
(b) The hair is divided and rollers or curlers applied under slight tension.
(c) Waving solution is applied.
(d) Heating. This varies according to the solution used or the type of wave required. Electric rollers or exothermic reactive chemicals may be used. The latter allow free head movement during the waving. The skill of this procedure lies in good hair sectioning, judging the right amount of solution, correct winding tension and appropriate steaming time.

Cold waving also involves initial shampooing, hair division into locks, moistening with waving lotion and application of croquignole curlers. Further solution may then be applied. The softening time is from 10 to 40 minutes. Rinsing then takes place, followed by neutralization with the oxidizing solution for up to 10 minutes. After removing the curlers further 'hardening' solution is usually applied. 'Loose' curl waves last for no more than a few weeks but 'tight' curl styles may persist for 4–6 months.

Evaluation of permanent waving
(1) *Fibre extension studies.* These are used to assess changes in mechanical properties of hair due to waving. Hair fibres show a hysteresis curve of extension and relaxation after the application of a load (stress). It has been shown that after

application of thioglycollates the total work of extending to 30% was lowered to 65% of its original value after reduction; oxidation reversed this.

(2) *Scanning electronmicroscopy.* This is used to study anatomical changes due to permanent waving. Along with bleaching, waving is potentially very damaging (Swift & Brown 1972; Robinson 1976) which is hardly surprising in view of the molecular disruption intrinsic to the procedure.

(3) *Human trials* are evidently important to test efficacy and potential toxicity. Factors to be assessed include (a) ambient temperature giving best results, (b) optimum duration of the mechanical process, for example curlers, the perming and hardening solutions.

(4) *Toxicity.* This depends on the process used. In view of the pH at which they are used, waving solutions must be kept away from the eyes and prolonged skin contact is to be avoided. Because of the unavoidable smell of thiols, some manufacturers put perfumes into the solution and these may cause dermatitis. Other toxicity is the result of poor technique, for example over-use of heat, overlong contact with softening agents. In general, the scalp resists irritants better than most sites on the body; any reactions from skin contact are therefore more liable to occur on the face or neck or elsewhere.

Hair straighteners (Gershen *et al.* 1972)
(References p. 426)

In principle the methods used to straighten hair are similar to those used in permanent waving. The practice is almost exclusively used to straighten Negroid hair.

(1) *Pomades.* These are mostly used by men with relatively short hair. They are greasy and act by 'plastering' hair into position.

(2) *Hot comb methods.* Shampooing is carried out and the hair is towelled dry; oil is then applied, e.g. petroleum jelly or liquid paraffin, which act as heat-transferring agents. Heat pressing with hot combing is then used ($148-260°F$) causing breakage and reforming of —S+S— bonds allowing the hair to be moulded straight. Structural damage (and breakage) of hair is common with this process and scarring alopecia may occur as a result of hot waxes entering the follicles. Sweating and rain reverse this procedure.

(3) *Cold methods.* The chemical methods employed utilize caustics, thioglycollates, ammonium carbonate or sodium bisulphite. Caustic soda preparations are usually creams and require the application of protective scalp oil or wax. These preparations are limited to salon use because of their potential to cause irritant dermatitis. Thioglycollate creams are the commonest agents used; the cream is applied liberally to the hair, which is then combed until it is straight. The cream is then washed off and a neutralizer (oxidizing agent) applied (Corbett 1976). Other straighteners ('relaxers') do not contain thioglycollates, e.g. sodium bisulphite

and ammonium carbonate, acidic ethylene glycol or 1.3-propylene glycol. Bisulphite straighteners are suitable for home use in combination with alkaline stabilizers.

Hair setting lotions and sprays
(References p. 426)

Setting lotions have changed considerably in recent years. The traditional semi-liquid gels based on water-soluble gums, for example tragacanth, karaya and acasia, have been replaced by various synthetic polymers in a bewildering array of forms—aerosol foams and sprays, liquids and gels. Most are based on PVP in a gelled aqueous solution and given an attractive glossy non-greasy appearance (Friefeld *et al.* 1962). Some preparations incorporate other ingredients to condition or to add antistatic action, lustre or sheen.

Setting lotion and spray formulations are considered safe, after early reports of foreign body granulomatous inflammation (Bergmann *et al.* 1958; Eddston 1959) had been questioned and not supported by further cases. Hair sprays were incriminated as a possible cause of peri-pilar keratin casts (Scott 1959) but this was not confirmed by later work (Dawber 1979).

Hair strengtheners

Many cosmetic preparations, by their action on the keratin molecule, irreversibly weaken the hair. The cosmetic scientist has produced chemicals that attempt to combat this problem. The formulations contain methylolated compounds of varying strength depending on the type of hair under treatment and the solubility of the compound. Early preparations were not satisfactory and released more than the legally permitted level of formaldehyde whilst in contact with the hair. Later preparations containing alkylated methylol compounds have greater stability and release very little formaldehyde.

Hair removers
(References p. 426)

The terms 'epilation' and 'depilation' have varied in their exact definition over the years. It is more convenient to define the exact process used, or the principle behind it, under the general term 'hair removers'. Superfluous hair may be masked by bleaching or removed by a variety of methods such as plucking, waxing, shaving, chemical processes and electrolysis—only the latter is permanent. No method is entirely satisfactory and the one adopted will depend on personal preference, and the character, area and amount of hair growth.

Bleaching is widely used for hair, particularly on the upper lip and the arms.

It is painless, and when repeated often inflicts sufficient damage to cause hair breakage. A simple method may be used such as 6% hydrogen peroxide (20 vol. peroxide) with 20 drops ammonia (household NH_3 or common NH_3 water) per 25 ml of peroxide. The bleach is added immediately on mixing and left for approximately 30 minutes. Some individuals develop an irritant reaction to bleach; it is therefore advisable to carry out a preliminary test—if irritation occurs within 30–60 minutes the peroxide strength and the duration of application should be reduced.

Shaving is unacceptable to some women as being too 'masculine'; however, the majority are happy to shave axillary and leg hair. There is no scientific basis for the belief that shaving stiffens hair or increases its pigmentation.

Waxing is one of the oldest methods known to man. Typically the wax is preheated, applied to the area to be treated, allowed to cool, then stripped off taking the embedded hair with it. Some 'cold' waxes are available that act in the same way. Glucose and ZnO waxing has the advantage of lasting up to several weeks before a repeat is required. Only relatively long hair can be treated in this way. Some women find it painful and irritating. It is more often used by beauticians than in the home (Rentoul & Aitken 1980).

Plucking is really satisfactory only for individual or small groups or scattered coarse hairs. It is usually done with tweezers. As with waxing, it requires to be repeated only every few weeks.

Chemical hair removers are now widely used for superfluous hair removal from most sites bar the face. The reason for not using them on the face is their irritancy potential. Sulphides and stannites, widely used in the past, have now been largely superseded by substituted mercaptans. Sulphides were unsatisfactory both because of skin irritancy and because of their odour—hydrogen sulphide—generated particularly when the preparation was washed off; strontium sulphide preparations are still available. Stannites, popularized some 30–40 years ago, had good hair-removing properties but were rather unstable. Substituted mercaptans form the basis of virtually all modern chemical depilatory preparations. They are slower in action than the sulphides but are safe enough for facial use if necessary. Thioglycollates are used in a concentration between 2–4% and typically act within 5–15 minutes (Turley & Windus 1937). Of the thioglycollates, the calcium salt is most favoured as it is the least irritant—the pH is maintained by an excess of calcium hydroxide which also acts to prevent the excess alkalinity known to irritate skin. Attempts to formulate products which accelerate the rather slow thioglycollate action have not been particularly successful. Modern preparations are available in foam, cream, liquid and aerosol forms, the one chosen depending on personal preference. Since thioglycollates attack keratin, not specifically hair, they may have adverse effects on the epidermis if manufacturers' recommendations are not adhered to; it is generally suggested that a small test site should first be treated in order to prevent more extensive irritant reactions in susceptible individuals. The ideal hair-removing chemical has still to be found—new substances are tested constantly for hair removal properties using in vitro methods such as the hair swelling test.

Electrolysis (Savill & Warren 1962)
All the above methods are temporary, the only practical permanent procedure being electrolysis. This involves passing a fine wire needle into the hair follicle and destroying the bulb with an electric current passed along it—the hair is loosened and plucked from each treated follicle. Either a galvanic, or modified high frequency electric current is used. Galvanic electrolysis is slower but destroys more follicles in one treatment. High-frequency current (electrocoagulation) is quicker but more regrowth is seen with this method. Relatively cheap, battery-operated machines have recently been developed for home use. These have all the disadvantages and potential hazards of those used by electrolysists with the added problem of an amateur operator.

The limitations of electrolysis in skilled hands are those of cost and time; even the best operators can only deal with 25–100 hairs per sitting and hair regrows in up to 40% of the follicles treated. In general, electrolysis is mostly used for localized coarse facial hair and alternative methods employed for excess hair on other body sites. Apart from regrowth of hair the problems that can occur with this mode of hair removal include discomfort during treatment, perifollicular inflammation and scarring, punctate hyperpigmentation and rarely bacterial infection.

A controlled investigation was carried out comparing the results of electrolysis with those of diathermy depilation. Permanent destruction of the hairs could be achieved by either method and the time required for the total destruction of all hair roots in a given area was the same, but the diameter of hairs regrowing after diathermy was greater than that of hairs regrowing after electrolysis (Peereboom-Wynia 1975). The results of depilation depend on the skill and dexterity of the operator (Blackwell 1973). In countries such as Britain, in which a Diploma in Medical Electrolysis exists, patients should wherever possible be referred to technicians who have obtained this certification of their proficiency. In the United States the American Electroysis Association regulates professional standards.

References
Bergmann M., Flance I.J. & Blumenthal A.T. (1958) Thesaurosis following inhalation of hair spray; a clinical and experimental study. *New England Journal of Medicine,* **258,** 471.
Blackwell G. (1973) Permanence in electrolysis epilation. *Cutis,* **11,** 753.
Blohme S.G. & Rajka G. (1970) The allergenicity of paraphenylene diamine. *Acta Dermato-venerologica,* **50,** 49.
Burnett C.M. & Corbett J.F. (1977) Chemistry and toxicology of hair dyes. In *Cutaneous Toxicity.*

Proceedings of the Third Conference on Cutaneous Toxicity, Washington, 1976, eds. V.A. Drill and P. Lazar. New York, Academic Press.

Burnett C.M. & Menkart T. (1978) Hair dyes and breast cancer. *New England Journal of Medicine*, **299**, 1253.

Burnett C.M., Corbett J.F. & Lanman B.M. (1978) Hair dyes and aplastic anaemia. *Drug and Chemical Toxicology*, **1**, 45.

Burnett C.M. (1980) Evaluation of toxicity and carcinogenicity of hair dyes. *Journal of Toxicology and Environmental Health*, **6**, 247.

Corbett J.F. & Menkart T. (1973) Hair colouring. *Cutis*, **12**, 190.

Corbett J.F. (1976) The chemistry of hair-care products. *Journal of the Society of Dyers and Colorists*, **92**, 285.

Dawber R.P.R. (1979) Hair casts. *British Journal of Dermatology*, **100**, 417.

Edelston B.G. (1959) Thesaurosis following inhalation of hair spray (Letter). *Lancet*, **ii**, 465.

Friefeld M., Lyons J. & Martinelli A.T. (1962) Polyvinylpyrrolidone in cosmetics. *American Perfumery*, **77**, 25.

Gershen J., Goldberg B. & Reiger A. (1972) Hair straighteners. In *Cosmetics, Science and Technology*, 2nd edn., eds. B. Balsam & E. Sagarin. New York, Wiley Interscience.

Harry R.G. (1973) *Harry's Cosmeticology*, 6th edn., revised J.B. Wilkinson. London, Leonard Hill Books.

Kirkland D.J., Lawler S.D. & Venitt, S. (1978) Chromosome damage and hair dyes. *Lancet*, **ii**, 124.

Lubow I. (1973) Allergic dermatitis and cosmetics. *Cutis*, **11**, 431.

Orfanos C.E. & Mahrle G. (1971) Human hair and its changes with cosmetic treatments in vivo. *Parfume Kosmet*, **52**, 203.

Peereboom-Wynia J.D.R. (1975) The effect of electrical epilation on the beard hair of women with idiopathic hirsutism. *Archives of Dermatological Research*, **254**, 15.

Prall J.K. (1970) *Proceedings of the Sixth Congress of the International Federation of Societies of Cosmetic Chemists*. Unpublished.

Rentoul J.R. & Aitken A.A. (1980) The cosmetic treatment of hirsutism. *Practitioner*, **24**, 1171.

Robbins C.R. (1979) *Chemical and Physical Behaviour of Human Hair*, 1st edn. New York, Van Nostrand Reinhold.

Savill A. & Warren C. (1962) *The Hair and Scalp*, 5th edn. London, Arnold, p. 304.

Schoen L.A. (1978) *Skin and Hair Care*. 1st English edn. Harmondsworth, England, Penguin Books.

Selzle D. & Wolff H.H. (1976) Exogener Haarschaden durch Bleichen und Kaltwelle. *Hautarzt*, **27**, 453.

Scot M.J. (1959) Peripilar keratin casts. *Archives of Dermatology*, **79**, 654.

Spoor H.J. (1973) Shampoos. *Cutis*, **12**, 671.

Swift J.A. & Brown A.C. (1972) The critical determination of fine changes in the surface architecture of human hair due to cosmetic treatment. *Journal of the Society of Cosmetic Chemists*, **23**, 695.

Turley H.G. & Windus W. (1937) In *Stiasny Festschrift*, 1st edn. Darmstadt, Edward Roether.

Wall C. (1972) In *Cosmetics Science and Technology*, eds. B. Balsam & E. Sagarin. New York, Wiley Interscience.

Wolfram L.J., Hall K. & Hui I. (1970) The mechanism of hair bleaching. *Journal of the Society of Cosmetic Chemists*, **21**, 875.

Zviak C. (1966) *Problemes Capillaires*, eds. E. Sidi & C. Zviak. Paris, Gauthier Villars.

Chapter 16
Hair and Scalp in
Systemic Diseases

Introduction

Throughout this book emphasis has been placed on the frequency with which abnormalities of hair growth are caused by, are related to, or are associated with systemic processes. The most important examples are the disturbances in the cyclical activity of hair follicles described in Chapter 5 and the disorders of hair patterns described in Chapter 4. In the present chapter we have grouped together a number of conditions in which the hair or scalp may be affected, and which are not readily classified in other chapters.

Infections

Syphilis (references p. 430)

Precise figures for the prevalence of syphilis are seldom obtainable because only a proportion of identified primary infections are notified and because unidentified primary infections are frequent, particularly in women and in male homosexuals. The widespread use of antibiotics in common diseases of adolescents and young adults, such as acne vulgaris, also distorts the natural history of syphilitic infections.

Syphilis may involve the scalp in the secondary stage of the infection. In its classical form the irregular 'moth-eaten' appearance is highly suggestive of the diagnosis, but a somewhat similar appearance may occasionally be seen in acute disseminated lupus erythematosus. The eyebrows may be shed, particularly in their lateral third, and there may be patchy alopecia of the beard. The pattern of hair loss is indeed very variable; in one patient, loss of the eyebrows was accompanied only by moderate alopecia of the pubic hair (Fig. 16.1) (Pirozzi *et al.* 1972).

Three to five months after infection, however, a diffuse shedding of telogen hairs may occur, differing in no way from the alopecia which may follow certain other infections. A very rarely reported phenomenon is the acceleration of hair loss in secondary syphilis as a feature of a febrile Jarisch–Herxheimer, a few hours after the initiation of treatment with penicillin (Pareek 1977). Serological tests for syphilis are advisable in unexplained acute diffuse alopecia.

The two principal forms of cutaneous syphilis in the tertiary stage also may involve the scalp. The serpiginous nodulosquamous syphilide can occur

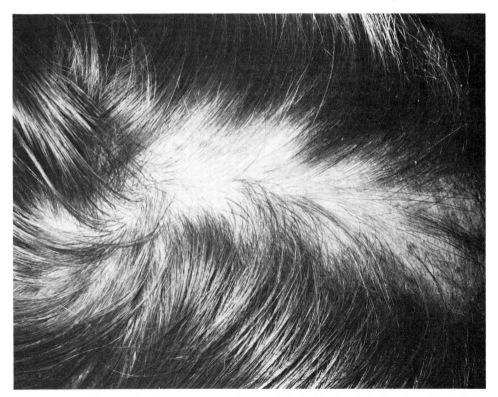

Fig. 16.1. Irregular, patchy alopecia in secondary syphilis (Addenbrooke's Hospital, Cambridge).

anywhere but it favours the face, the back and the extensor aspects of the limbs. The grouped reddish-brown indolent scaly papules may spread into the scalp from the forehead or from the nape of the neck. This eruption can be mistaken for psoriasis or for sarcoidosis. Later the nodules break down to form crusted ulcers. The syphilitic gumma may begin in the skin or in bone. It gradually forms a painless mass of rubbery consistency, breaking down to form a punched-out ulcer.

The confirmation of a suspected diagnosis depends on positive serological tests for syphilis. Full clinical evaluation and a properly planned course of treatment and careful follow-up are essential. Inadequate treatment which merely heals the cutaneous lesions exposes the patient to the serious risk of later cardiovascular or neurological involvement.

References

Pareek S.S. (1971) Syphilitic alopecia in Jarisch–Herxheimer reaction. *British Journal of Venereal Disease*, **53**, 389.

Pirozzi D.J., Lockshia N.A. & Rosenberg P.E. (1972) An unusual manifestation of cutaneous syphilis. *Cutis*, **20**, 451.

Tuberculosis

Apart from lupus vulgaris, which is itself uncommonly found in the scalp, tuberculosis in the scalp is excessively rare. At the end of his career Sabouraud (Boutelier 1953) had great difficulty in recalling a single case.

Where tuberculosis is prevalent lupus vulgaris is usually the most frequent cutaneous form. It occurs as a post-primary infection in patients with some degree of immunity to tuberculosis. The distribution of the lesions depends on the extent to which the body is covered by clothing. In temperate climates 80% of lesions are on the head and neck; in the tropics lesions on the trunk are relatively more frequent. The scalp is protected to some extent from inoculation of the infection, but lupus may extend into the scalp from contiguous non-hairy skin and it may at times begin in the scalp itself.

Soft reddish-brown nodules extend slowly but irregularly, leaving scarring in their wake. Without treatment the lesion tends to persist indefinitely and, particularly in the malnourished, may be very destructive. The diagnosis should be considered in the presence of soft granulomatous nodules and should be confirmed histologically. After full investigation to establish whether tuberculosis is present in other organs, treatment with antituberculous drugs may be initiated.

Reference

Boutelier A. (1953) *Tuberculose du cuir chevelu in affections de la chevelure et du cuir chevelu*, ed. A. Desaux. Paris, Masson, p. 606.

Leprosy (references p. 432)

Loss of scalp hair caused by leprosy is very unusual. Jeanselme, the French authority on tropical dermatology, wrote 'La lèpre ne fait pas de chauves' (Gaté & Rousset 1953). In lepromatous leprosy the eyebrows, particularly in their lateral third, may be shed, and body hair may be lost, but lesions in the scalp are exceptional (Fig. 16.2) (Parikh *et al.* 1974). In both the cases reported by these authors the lesions occurred in a scalp which was already bald. It has been suggested that the sparing of the scalp in leprosy may be due to the higher surface temperature in the skin in this site, resulting from the abundant blood supply and further increased by a normal covering of hair (Dutta *et al.* 1981). *Mycobacterium leprae* is known to favour the cooler parts of the body (Binford & Meyers 1978).

Jopling (1980, pers. comm.), who has had very extensive experience of leprosy, is impressed by the rarity with which the scalp is involved in leprosy. He

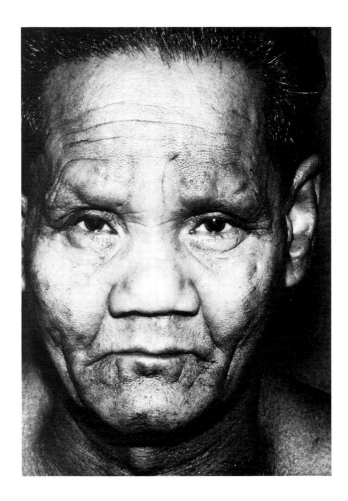

Fig. 16.2. Leprosy. Loss of eyebrows (Slade Hospital, Oxford).

is impressed also by the better than average scalp hair growth in male patients with lepromatous leprosy and he suggests (Jopling 1978) that the testicular atrophy which occurs in lepromatous leprosy reduces testosterone levels and thus retards the development of androgenetic alopecia.

References

Binford C.H. & Meyers W.M. (1978) Leprosy. In *A Window on Leprosy*, ed. B.R. Chatterjee. Calcutta, Statesman Commercial Press, p. 153.

Dutta A.K., Mandal S.B. & Jopling W.H. (1981) Surface temperature of bald and hairy scalp in reference to leprosy affection. *International Journal of Leprosy*.

Gaté J. & Rousset J. (1953) Le cuir chevelu dans la lèpre. In *Affections de la Chevelure et du Cuir Chevelu*, ed. A. Desaux. Paris, Masson, p. 292.

Jopling W.H. (1978) *Handbook of Leprosy*, 2nd edn. London, Heinemann, p. 20.

Parikh A.C., D'Souza N.G., Chaulawala R. & Ganapati R. (1974) Leprosy lesions in the scalp. *Leprosy in India*, **46**, 39.

Leishmaniasis (references p. 433)

The protozoan parasite *Leishmania* occurs in three forms: *L. tropica*, associated with dermal leishmaniasis, *L. donovani*, associated with kalaazar, and *L. braziliensis*, associated with South American (mucocutaneous) leishmaniasis. The three 'species' are morphologically identical by normal criteria, but show antigenic differences (Zuckerman 1975).

The natural reservoirs of infection are wild rodents, dogs and foxes, from which the parasites are conveyed to man by the bites of the sandfly *Phlebotomus*, and possibly sometimes by mosquitoes.

Dermal leishmaniasis (Haghighi *et al.* 1971)
This disease is widely distributed throughout the tropics and subtropics. In Europe it is endemic in the Mediterranean littoral, including some areas of the South of France (Rioux *et al.* 1968). The lesions are commonly on exposed skin, particularly the face and arms. Most infections occur in childhood and in the indigenous population of an endemic area, but may develop at any age in previously unexposed tourists and other visitors. We have seen lesions in the scalp margin and they can occur in bald areas of the scalp. Clinically the lesion, single or multiple, forms a granulomatous nodule, dry or ulcerated, which heals after months or years to leave an ugly or depressed scar.

Kala-azar
Skin lesions do not occur except in the 10% who, one or more years after apparent cure, develop post-Kala-azar dermal leishmaniasis with an extensive maculopapular eruption on the face, which later spreads to other parts of the body.

Mucocutaneous leishmaniasis (Azulay 1968)

The initial lesions are granulomatous ulcers which occur on exposed skin including that of the scalp. Progressive involvement of the mucous membranes occurs some 3 years later.

Diagnosis of leishmaniasis

The diagnosis is suggested when granulomatous skin lesions develop in an individual at an appropriate interval of weeks or months after the patient has visited an area in which either dermal or mucocutaneous leishmaniasis is endemic. The diagnosis is confirmed by the demonstration of *Leishmania* in a biopsy or in a smear taken from the edge of the lesion.

Treatment

Treatment is not entirely satisfactory and when this diagnosis has been reliably established advice should be sought from a physician with experience in the management of these diseases.

References

Azulay R.D. (1968) Leishmaniasis Americana. *Dermatologia Ibero Latino Americana*, **3**, 235.

Haghighi I., Kavoussi A. & Hayat-Davendi G.H. (1971) Some practical aspects of cutaneous leishmaniasis. *International Journal of Dermatology*, **10**, 129.

Rioux J.A., Golvan Y., Lauret H., Haim R. & Tour S. (1968) Enquete ecologique sur les leishmanioses dans le sud de la France. *Bulletin de l'I.N.S.E.R.M.*, **23**, 1125.

Zuckerman A. (1975) Parasitological review: current status of the immunology of blood and tissue parasites. I. *Leishmania*. *Experimental Parasitology*, **38**, 374.

Onchocerciasis (reference p. 434) (Convit 1975)

Onchocerciasis is caused by the filarial parasite *Onchocerca volvulus*, which is transmitted by the bites of small flies of the genus *Simulium*. The disease is endemic in much of equatorial Africa, and in the Yemen, and there are smaller foci in several Central American countries and in Venezuela and Colombia. The biting habits of the vector influence the clinical picture of the disease, notably the distribution of the nodules which are on the lower part of the body in Africa but tend to be on the upper trunk and in the scalp in Latin America.

About a year after infection a pruritic eruption develops with weals and oedema and sometimes with fever and joint pains. Gradually over the years the skin becomes thickened and lichenified from scratching and there are often patchy areas of decreased pigmentation.

Firm painless nodules develop over the bony prominences and in Latin America these nodules are often in the scalp, particularly in the occipital region. The serious manifestation of the late stage of the disease is eye involvement leading to blindness.

During the earlier stages the diagnosis is made by taking a skin 'snip' and examining a smear in saline for microfilariae. If nodules are present they may be excised to confirm the diagnosis and when this has been done the remainder should be excised as a stage in the therapeutic attack on the disease, which should include the administration of diethyl carbamazine.

The diagnosis should be suspected in a patient with scalp nodules who has the associated lichenified pruritic lesions on the trunk and who has visited, however briefly, an endemic area.

Reference

Convit J. (1975) In *Clinical Tropical Dermatology*, ed. O. Canizares. Oxford, Blackwell, p. 220.

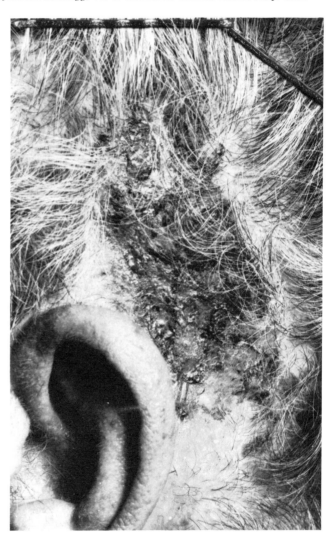

Fig. 16.3. Herpes zoster (Addenbrooke's Hospital, Cambridge).

Varicella–herpes zoster

Varicella is the usual response of the previousy unexposed subject to infection with the varicella–zoster virus, and zoster is commonly due to reactivation of the latent virus, but it is probable that zoster can also follow exogenous infection (Nally & Ross 1971; Luby 1973).

The eruption of varicella occurs in successive crops of small clear vesicles on the trunk, face and scalp. Scalp involvement may be extensive but there is little or no permanent scarring unless secondary infection has been severe or the normal immune response is depressed by disease or by drugs.

Herpes zoster is often preceded by localized pain and tenderness. The eruption consists of closely grouped vesicles in segmental distribution (Fig. 16.3). In the elderly or malnourished the lesions may be haemorrhagic, necrotic or even gangrenous (Fig. 16.4). The scalp is involved in zoster of the ophthalmic division of the trigeminal nerve or of the cervical segments 1–3. Zoster of C.2 3—Herpes occipito-collaris (Payten & Dawes 1972)—is associated with an eruption of the pre-auricular region of the cheek, the pinna, the side of the neck and the occipital scalp.

There is temporary hair loss from the affected areas of scalp and if the lesions have been necrotic or secondary infection has been severe, there may be persistent scars.

References

Luby J.P. (1973) Varicella–zoster virus. *Journal of Investigative Dermatology*, **61**, 212.
Nally F.F. & Ross I.H. (1971) Herpes zoster of the oral and facial structures. *Oral Surgery, Oral Medicine, Oral Pathology*, **32**, 221.
Payten R.J. & Dawes J.D.K. (1972) Herpes zoster of the head and neck. *Journal of Laryngology & Otology*, **86**, 1031.

Other diseases

Sarcoidosis (references p. 437)

Sarcoidosis rarely involves the scalp. In some of the few cases reported the patients have been Negroid women (Golitz *et al.* 1968; Rudolph *et al.* 1975), but elderly Europeans, male and female, have also been affected (Fazio *et al.* 1979).

The lesions may be initially nodular or papular, coalescing to form plaques, which flatten to leave an area of cicatricial alopecia.

The clinical presentation, as diffuse and sometimes extensive cicatricial alopecia, will not suggest the correct diagnosis, although this may be suspected if other more typical cutaneous or systemic lesions of sarcoidosis are present.

The diagnosis is made on the histological appearances and a positive Kveim test.

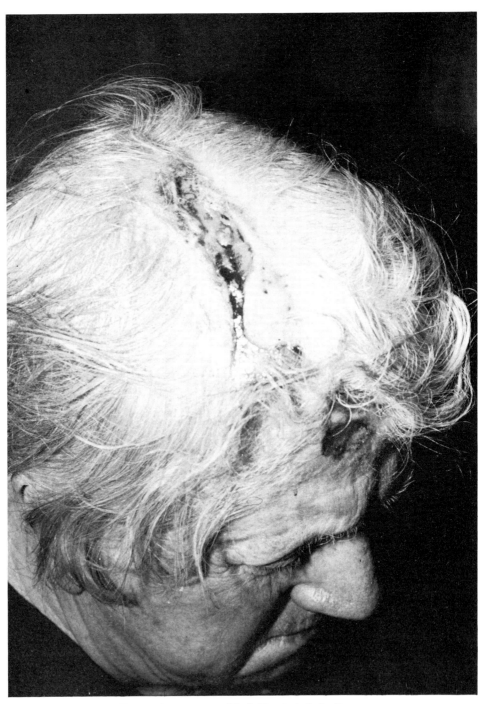

Fig. 16.4. Ulceration following herpes zoster (Slade Hospital, Oxford).

References

Bluefarb S.M., Szymanski F.J. & Rostenberg A. (1955) Sarcoidosis as a cause of patchy alopecia. *Archives of Dermatology*, **71**, 602.

Fazio M., Bassetti F., Santucci B., Argentieri R. & Gentili G. (1979) Sarcoidosi anulare cicatriziale e necrobiosi lipoidica atipica del cuoio capelluto. *Bollettino dell'Istituto Dermatologico San Gallicano*, **10**, 85.

Golitz L.E., Shapiro L., Hurwitz E. & Stritzler R. (1968) Cicatricial alopecia of sarcoidosis. *Archives of Dermatology*, **107**, 758.

Rudolph R.I., Holzwanger J.M. & Heaton C.L. (1975) Diffuse cicatricial alopecia of the scalp caused by sarcoidosis. *Cutis*, **15**, 524.

Histiocytic reticuloendotheliosis

This term groups together the conditions known as Letterer–Siwe disease, eosinophilic granuloma of bone, Hand–Schüller–Christian, and xanthoma disseminatum. Each condition is usually encountered as a distinctive clinico-pathological entity, but intermediate cases also occur.

Letterer–Siwe disease

Skin lesions are a characteristic and almost constant feature of this rare disease of infancy and very early childhood. Discrete yellow-brown scaly papules appear in crops on the scalp, neck and face, trunk and buttocks. They may become haemorrhagic, particularly on the trunk. Larger nodules are occasionally seen, mainly in the flexures, and both scalp and flexures may develop crusting and secondary infection (Nyholm *et al.* 1967).

Apparent seborrhoeic dermatitis in an obviously ill child, especially if the spleen is enlarged, is an indication for urgent biopsy, as early diagnosis is important. In some cases the disease is apparently confined to the skin (Esterly & Sevick 1969) but the skin lesions may precede other evidence of the disease by weeks or months (Jones *et al.* 1967).

Scalp involvement of 'seborrhoeic' type is much rarer in other forms of histiocytic reticuloendotheliosis, but does occur in children (Graciansky *et al.* 1953) and in adults (Bender & Holtzman 1958).

References

Bender B. & Holtzman I.N. (1958) Histiocytosis X (granulomatous reticuloendotheliosis. *Archives of Dermatology*, **78**, 692.

Esterly N.B. & Sevick H.M. (1969) Cutaneous Letterer–Siwe disease. *American Journal of Diseases of Children*, **117**, 236.

de Graciansky P., Leclerq R. & Janet (1953) A propos d'un cas de reticulose histiomonocytaire subaiguë chez un nourrisson. *Semaine des Hôpitaux*, **29**, 1643.

Jones B., Welton W.A. & Gilbert E.F. (1967) Congenital Letterer–Siwe Disease. *Cutis*, **3**, 750.

Nyholm K., Reed G. & Sjalin K.-E. (1967) Letterer–Siwe disease. *Acta pathologica et microbiologica Scandinavica*, **70**, 481.

Amyloidosis

In primary systemic amyloidosis the most characteristic skin lesions are yellowish, waxy papules, which may be haemorrhagic, most commonly on the face, particularly the eyelids, and in the scalp, on the neck and in the anogenital region. There may also be nodules and plaques but usually not in the scalp.

Alopecia may be conspicuous (Brownstein & Helwig 1970). There may be diffuse or patchy loss of scalp hair, and body hair may be completely or partially lost. The pilosebaceous units are destroyed by the pressure of amyloid deposits. The diagnosis must be confirmed histologically.

The tumefactive form of cutaneous amyloidosis is very rare. Waxy nodules have been reported in the scalp (Ratz & Bailin 1981).

References
Brownstein M.H. & Helwig E.B. (1970) The cutaneous amyloidoses. II. Systemic form. *Archives of Dermatology*, **102**, 20.
Ratz J.L. & Bailin P.L. (1981) Cutaneous amyloidosis. *Journal of the American Academy of Dermatology*, **4**, 21.

Lupus erythematosus

Scalp changes are not uncommon in both systemic and the chronic discoid forms of lupus erythematosus.

During the acute phase of systemic lupus erythematosus alopecia is present in at least 50% of cases (Armas-Cruz *et al.* 1958). There is diffuse shedding of hair and there may be some erythema of the scalp. The hair is dry, fragile and broken, and short hairs are often seen, particularly at the frontal margin—so-called 'lupus hair' (Alarcon-Segovia & Citina 1974). Much less frequently cicatricial alopecia may be present in systemic lupus erythematosus, usually in cases in which the systemic phase has been preceded by chronic discoid lupus erythematosus.

Alopecia closely simulating alopecia areata, but with the histological features of lupus erythematosus, has been reported (Borda *et al.* 1963).

Chronic discoid alopecia may involve the scalp. In its typical form an area of erythema and scaling with horny follicular plugs extends irregularly, leaving scarring. At this stage a tentative diagnosis is possible; follicular plugging, erythema and telangiectasia in association with scarring and alopecia are highly suggestive. Later, only the scarring remains and a confident diagnosis may not be possible. Lupus erythematosus of the scalp affects women more than men. When the disease begins on the face, as is usually the case, scalp lesions ultimately develop in 20% of men but 50% of women.

Squamous carcinoma has been reported in chronic cicatricial lupus erythematosis of the scalp (Vidal-Lliteras & Cabré 1971).

References

Alarcon-Segovia D. & Cetina J.A. (1974) Lupus hair. *American Journal of Medical Science*, **267**, 241.

Armas-Cruz R., Harmaker J., Ducaun G., Jebil J. & Gonzales F. (1958) Clinical diagnosis of systemic lupus erythematosus. *American Journal of Medicine*, **25**, 409.

Borda J.M., Abulafia J. & Buchsbaum, E. (1965) Lupus eritematosa peladoide de cuero cabelludo. *Archivos Argentinos de Dermatologia*, **15**, 129.

Vidal-Lliteras J. & Cabré J. (1971) Carcinoma espinocelular sobre alopecia cicatricial eritematodica. *Actas Dermosifiligraficas*, **62**, 63.

Dermatomyositis

Dermatomyositis is a rare disorder affecting predominantly the skin and the muscles. Its cause is unknown but immunological mechanisms are probably involved. Over 50% of patients over the age of 40 have malignant disease.

Clinical features

The onset is usually insidious, with fatigue, malaise, pain and stiffness of the limbs and loss of weight. Muscle weakness is more marked in the shoulder and pelvic girdles and in the proximal muscles of the limbs.

There is no correlation between the severity of the myositis and the extent of the skin lesions. Periorbital oedema is the most frequent. It may be accompanied by bluish-pink discoloration of the eyelids with telangiectasia, which is pathognomonic of the disease. Also frequent and distinctive are scaly bluish-red plaques over the elbows, knees, ankles and knuckles. Many cases show less specific changes, spreading erythema of face and neck, or of the limbs, and fleeting or more persistent oedema of face or limbs. A wide variety of other skin lesions has been reported in occasional cases.

Diffuse alopecia is present in 15–20% of cases (O'Leary & Waisman 1940; Roberts & Brunsting 1954). Complete or almost complete regrowth is possible. Also during the acute stage hypertrichosis may be conspicuous, especially on the face and limbs (Reich & Reinhardt 1948) (see p. 252).

In the chronic stage poikilodermatous changes with marked atrophy may replace the acute inflammatory lesions, and when such lesions involve the scalp or other hairy regions cicatricial alopecia results. In some unusual cases reported in Hong Kong, (Wong 1969) cicactricial alopecia was associated with horny follicular papules.

References

O'Leary P.R. & Waisman M. (1940) Dermatomyositis. *Archives of Dermatology and Syphilology*, **41**, 1001.

Reich M.E. & Reinhardt J.B. (1948) Dermatomyositis associated with hypertrichosis. *Archives of Dermatology and Syphilology*, **57**, 725.

Roberts H.M. & Brunsting L.A. (1954) Dermatomyositis in childhood. *Postgraduate Medicine*, 16, 393.

Wong K.O. (1969) Dermatomyositis: a clinical investigation of twenty-three cases in Hong Kong. *British Journal of Dermatology*, 81, 544.

Giant-cell arteritis (syn. temporal arteritis, Horton's disease)

This granulomatous arteritis affects the larger and medium-sized arteries in the elderly. It forms part of the polymyalgia rheumatica complex (Fritsch *et al.* 1980). The acute phase of temporal arteritis may be precipitated by over-exposure to sunlight (Kinmont & McCallum 1965). Giant-cell arteritis is probably an autoimmune disorder.

Histologically the intima is thickened and the lumen partially obstructed. There is fibrinoid necrosis of the intimal elastic lamina, with histiocytic and giant-cell infiltration. Fibrosis becomes progressively more extensive.

During the early stages the symptoms are often indefinite and vague; weakness, fatigue, malaise, loss of appetite and aching pain in the limbs are common complaints. There may also be unexplained light sensitivity. The development of temporal arteritis is associated with unilateral or bilateral headache. There may also be unilateral loss of vision, and pain and ulceration of one side of the tongue.

The skin over the scalp arteries may be red and tender or pigmented: there may be loss of hair. Bullae, ulceration and necrosis may occur (Kinmont & McCallum 1964). Necrosis of the scalp may be unilateral or bilateral and can be very extensive (Tirschek 1957; Poppy 1959; Schucke & Kaul 1967).

The diagnosis is made on the clinical features and a high ESR, and may be confirmed by biopsy. Treatment with systemic corticosteroids is necessary; a maintenance dose may be required for many months.

References

Fritsch P., Gschnait F. & Wolff K. (1980) *Temporal Arteritis in Vasculitis*, eds. K. Wolff & R.K. Winkelmann. London, Lloyd-Luke, p. 285.

Kinmont P.D.C. & McCallum D.I. (1964) Skin manifestations of giant-cell arteritis. *British Journal of Dermatology*, 76, 299.

Kinmont P.D.C. & McCallum D.I. (1965) Aetiology, pathology and course of giant-cell arteritis. *British Journal of Dermatology*, 77, 193.

Poppy F. (1959) Gangränöses Ulkus des Capillitiums als Folge einer sogenannten Arteriitis temporalis. *Wiener klinische Wochenschrift*, 71, 783.

Schucke G. & Kaul A. (1967) Doppelseitige Kopfschwentennekrosis an Pareitalberion bei Riesenzellarteritis. *Dermatologische Wochenschrift*, 153, 825.

Tirschek H. (1957) Gangraena regionis temporo-parietalis durch Arteriitis temporalis. *Winer klinische Wochenschrift*, 69, 610.

Sjögren's syndrome

In this syndrome, which occurs mainly in women between the ages of 30 and 70, but occasionally in younger women and in men, the hair may be dry, sparse and brittle, and diffuse alopecia may involve the pubic and axillary hair as well as the scalp.

The syndrome is one in which autoimmune mechanisms are involved and other such diseases, for example rheumatoid arthritis, Hashimoto's thyroiditis, lupus erythematosus and alopecia areata may be associated (Bunim 1961).

There is lymphocytic and plasma cell infiltration of the exocrine glands, such as the salivary glands, sweat glands, the lacrymal glands and the submucous glands of the respiratory tract, the upper alimentary tract and the vagina. These glands become atrophic. Degenerative changes have been reported also in the external root sheaths of hair follicles (Ferreira-Marques 1960).

The clinical picture is very variable. In the patient presenting with fine, dry sparse hair the diagnosis will be suggested by the general dryness of the skin, by the presence of red, sore dry eyes, a dry mouth or dry and sore anogenital mucous membranes.

To confirm the diagnosis an ophthalmologist's opinion is helpful. Screening for autoantibodies may be informative. Biopsy of the labial salivary glands is advisable if the diagnosis is in doubt (Greenspan 1974).

Only symptomatic treatment is possible.

References

Bunim J.J. (1961) A broader spectrum of Sjögren's syndrome and its pathogenic implications. *Annals of Rheumatic Diseases*, **20**, 1.

Ferreira-Marques J. (1960) A contribution to the study of Sjögren's syndrome. *Acta Dermatovenereologica*, **40**, 485.

Greenspan J.S. (1974) The histopathology of Sjögren's syndrome in labial salivary gland tissue. *Oral Surgery*, **37**, 217.

Benign and malignant lymphoproliferative disorders
(References p. 449)

Classification of both benign and malignant lymphoreticular proliferative disorders is difficult because of the fact that cells of this type have a degree of biological versatility that is first expressed in their change from the stem cell to lymphoblasts and histiocytes or to reticulum cells and histiocytic cells. This position is further complicated by the fact that many factors in both health and diseases such as neoplasia may modify this versatility and give rise to changes in the morphological stability of the cell.

At present, the benign lymphoreticular proliferative disorders are classified according to clinical, pathological and cytological characteristics. The malignant lymphomas are typed by their degree of differentiation and also according to the relative presence of lymphocytes and histiocytic cells together with the identification of lymphoid cells as either thymus-dependent (T cell) or bone-marrow dependent (B cell) in type. Electronmicroscopic and light microscopic examination of epon-embedded $1\ \mu$ sections have considerably improved the morphological identification of cells (Lutzner 1975).

Benign lymphoplasias

Benign lymphoreticular proliferation may be caused by external influences such as insect bites (Gross 1971; Horen 1972) or mechanical trauma, and inflammatory diseases such as lupus erythematosus. Excluding these specific factors, there remains a number of cryptogenic conditions which have been described under many titles and have distinct clinical and morphological characteristics (Clark 1974; Stiegleder 1976). They are classified according to clinical differences and the type of cellular infiltrate (From 1979).

Lymphocytic infiltrate of skin (Jessner-Kanof 1953)
This is a superficial benign skin disease characterized by erythematous plaques which became annular. It typically waxes and wanes, often for several years before spontaneous resolution occurs with no residual scarring; it mainly affects men below 50 (Calnan 1957).

Histology. There is a dense lymphocytic infiltrate in the dermis without germinal centre formation; the cells are often predominantly around hair follicles, sweat pores and blood vessels. Elastic tissue shows basophilic degeneration, and hyaluronic acid can be demonstrated using toluidine blue or colloidal iron stains. The histological changes may be difficult to differentiate from lupus erythematosus (LE) and polymorphic light eruption. IgG and C3 are usually found at the dermo-epidermal junction in LE by immunofluorescence, which is universally negative in lymphocytic infiltration.

Clinical features. Individual lesions consist of infiltrated erythematous papules which spread peripherally with central clearing; follicular hyperkeratosis is not a feature. Any part of the body may be affected, but typical cases affect the face, temples, ears and the interscapular region of the upper back. The bald scalp may be affected. Sunlight may be a provoking factor in some cases.

Treatment. No curative therapy is known but oral antimalarials give the best results. Other treatments that have been suggested include sunscreens, topical steroids, gold and X-irradiation.

Lymphocytoma cutis (syn. Spiegler–Fendt pseudo-lymphoma or sarcoid; miliary lymphocytoma; benign lymphocytomatoid granuloma)

Many authors have attempted to define specific sub-types of lymphocytoma cutis but clinical overlap is so frequent that they are considered here as a single condition.

Lymphocytoma cutis is a benign lymphoproliferative condition in which single or multiple papules or plaques develop around the face and ears (Gross 1971). No cause has been found but infection, rudimentary lymphoid hyperplasia and other factors have been suggested as possibly important.

The dense dermal lymphocytic infiltrate usually spares a small band below the epidermis but is most dense in the upper and mid dermis (Caro & Helwig 1969). Hair follicles are not often affected. In some cases lymphocytes are organized into lymphoid germinal follicles.

Women are more frequently affected than men; onset may be from childhood to old age. Unlike lymphocytic infiltration of Jessner–Kanof, lesions do not become annular. Differential diagnosis includes granuloma faciale, angiolymphoid hyperplasia, insect bite reactions; the latter two conditions show a greater predominance of eosinophils in the dermal infiltrate and may affect the scalp and other sites. Diffuse and disseminated forms may resemble polymorphic light eruption and adenoma sebaceum.

No uniformly successful treatment is known. Localized lesions with a mainly lymphoid follicular infiltrate may respond to X-irradiation. Some cases improve with sun-screens. Unlike lymphocytic infiltration of Jessner-Kanof, anti-malarials are not useful.

Prognosis is poor, particularly in the diffuse and disseminate types, most cases lasting many years or even decades. The condition requires careful observation since malignant features have been demonstrated histologically in typical cases.

Malignant lymphomas

Mycosis fungoides

Mycosis fungoides is an uncommon, slowly neoplastic disease of the reticulo-endothelial system in which the first and often the only expression of the disease may be in the skin. It is now considered to be a tumour of the thymus-dependent lymphocyte (T-cells). The early ill-defined pre-mycotic phase may show no clear evidence of neoplasia in the pathological sense but the later stages of infiltration and tumour formation have all the hallmarks of a malignant lymphoma. This three-phase description of mycosis fungoides is attributable to Bazin (1876) though the earliest description of the disease was by Alibert (1835); he first used the name mycosis fungoides because of the mushroom-like tumours. Until recently the condition was considered to be a pure skin lymphoma but extra-cutaneous changes are now known to occur (Long & Mihm 1974; Rappaport & Thomas 1974). Erythrodermic mycosis fungoides (Hallopeau & Besnier 1892) and the Sézary syndrome (Sézary 1949) can now be classified pathologically with the commoner Alibert type, but the exact status of the tumeur d'emblée variety (Vidal & Brocq 1885) remains unclear.

Epidemiology. All races are affected equally; it is twice as common in men. The peak age of onset of the pre-tumour phase is in the fourth decade. There are no more than 200 deaths per year directly attributable to mycosis fungoides.

Pathogenesis. Electronmicroscopic techniques have shown that the T-lympho-cyte is the cell undergoing malignant transformation in mycosis fungoides but the cause of this is still not known; in particular, no infective agent has ever been found. In both the classical and leukaemic (Sézary) forms, T cells have been noted to have 'helper' cell function in that such cells will promote B-cell transformation into immunoglobulin-producing cells (Broder 1976).

The immunological reactivity of patients with mycosis fungoides to antigens provoking either type IV allergy or circulating antibody, usually stays normal until the late stage of plaques, tumours or the leukaemic phase (Nordqvist & Kinney 1976).

Histology (Rappaport & Thomas 1974). Even in the earliest stage, some histological change consistent with mycosis fungoides will be evident, particu-larly if several biopsies are taken.

Characteristic changes include: (a) a band-like infiltrate in the upper dermis 'hugging' the epidermis; the main cell type is an atypical lymphoid cell with an irregular infolded nucleus. (Other cells in the infiltrate include normal lympho-cytes, plasma cells, histiocytes and eosinophils). Some spread of the infiltrate may occur into the mid and lower dermis along adnexal structures and blood vessels; (b) epidermal Pautrier micro-abscesses consisting of local clusters of atypical lymphoid cells; (c) mycosis, or Lutzner cells which are larger than atypical lymphocytes and possess hyperchromatic, irregular indented nuclei, the so-called cerebriform nuclei.

Follicular mucinosis (p. 493) may be seen at any stage of the disease but most typically when the disease is well advanced.

Autopsy sections of tissue from many internal organs may reveal mycosis cells and occult changes consistent with mycosis fungoides.

Clinical features. The course of the disease may be divided into the pre-tumour and tumour stages; transformation into the latter may occur within months, or only several decades after the onset of the pre-tumour stage. The eruption of the pre-tumour phase may be highly characteristic; several well-defined types are known:

(i) Chronic superficial scaly dermatitis, alternatively called parapsoriasis in plaque or digitate dermatosis. It consists of non-itchy brownish-red scaly plaques occurring mainly on the trunk and limbs. Lesions on the upper trunk may be digitate in appearance, particularly on the lateral chest wall. It has been suggested that this pattern never progresses to the tumour stage; this opinion is strengthened if the histology reveals only mild eczematous changes. Those cases in this group which are pre-mycotic usually develop itching and some poikilodermatous areas early in the course of the disease.

(ii) The poikilodermatous pre-mycotic eruption (syn. poikiloderma atrophicans vasculare; parapsoriasis lichenoides; atrophic parapsoriasis). The eruption consists of macular patches showing reticulate pigmentation, atrophy and telangiectasia within them; these changes are similar to the atrophy following X-irradiation.

Acquired poikiloderma of this type is unequivocally pre-mycotic (pre-tumour).

Mycosis cells may be present in the monocytic dermal infiltrate and occasionally also in the epidermis which is atrophic and shows degenerative changes in the basal layer. Upper dermal capilaries are often dilated.

(iii) Parakeratosis variegata (Stevenson 1974) is a very rare red scaly striped eruption (zebra-like) which is considered pre-reticulotic.

(iv) Lymphomatoid papulosis (Macauley 1968) is a papular variant of pityriasis lichenoides. Histologically, individual lesions show a dense dermal infiltrate of malignant-looking cells of T-cell type which may invade the epidermis (Valentino & Helwig 1973). Most cases wax and wane for many years and eventually remit spontaneously, but typical cases may change into mycosis fungoides or other types of lymphoma.

Tumour phase. This phase may supervene within months or as late as 20–30 years after the onset of the pre-tumour phase, consisting most commonly of the poikilodermatous form. During transformation asymptomatic plaques may begin to itch and become palpable, scaly and often inflamed (Fig. 16.5). Rarely typical infiltrated tumours may develop without a preceding pre-tumour phase, the so-called tumeur d'emblée variety.

Infiltrated lesions increase in number, become larger and more indurated and many eventually ulcerate. With the advent of modern suppressive treatment this phase is now rare. Any part of the body may be affected.

Variants from the above may occur. Follicular mucinosis may be manifest as widespread follicular accentuation of the eruption with hair loss. Erythroderma is usually a late stage which may be associated with diffuse hair loss. The Sézary syndrome (Sézary 1949; Winkelmann 1974) is an acute 'leukaemic' form of

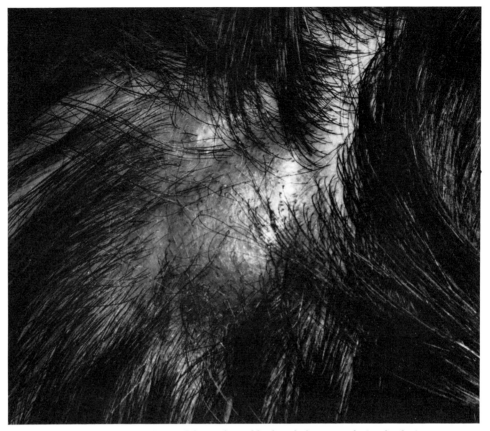

Fig. 16.5. Lymphomatous nodules of the scalp (Addenbrooke's Hospital, Cambridge).

mycosis fungoides (T-cell erythroderma); generalized erythroderma is associated with skin histology consistent with mycosis fungoides and mycosis (or Lutzner cells) in the blood and bone marrow. Considerable generalized hair loss occurs in this type without follicular mucinosis. The nails are usually all dystrophic and are like severe psoriasis. The variant has a high mortality. Death often occurs suddenly after several years of activity of the eruption and minimal systemic findings.

Prognosis. Apart from cases starting in childhood, life expectancy is not usually modified by mycosis fungoides though the late tumour stage may considerably interfere with the quality of life; few recorded cases exist of death before 60. The development of lymphadenopathy is suggested as a sign that death may occur from disease spread within 3 years (Clendenning 1964).

Treatment. No specific treatment is available. Most authorities recommend a conservative approach, though in view of the neoplastic nature of the condition it has been suggested that an aggressive 'anti-tumour' regime should be instituted from the earliest stage. Early asymptomatic pre-tumour eruptions are usually left untreated. Parapsoriatic morphology may be suppressed by topical corticosteroids and natural or artificial ultraviolet radiation (UVB). Poikilodermatous lesions may completely remit with methoxsalen photochemotherapy (PUVA). Indeed, recent studies with PUVA have suggested that this line of treatment may also prove to be the best and least toxic therapy for the early tumour stage also (Roenigk 1977). Topical cytotoxic therapy (Zackheim & Epstein 1975) and systemic anti-cancer drugs are often used but cannot offer more than temporary suppression. Individual lesions may best be treated by local X-irradiation (60–120 kV). Whole body electron beam therapy may cause complete remission; this can be repeated if required, unlike large doses of conventional X-irradiation. It seems likely that radiotherapeutic methods will be used much less as experience with PUVA increases and it becomes more widely available. PUVA and X-irradiation may cause complete remission of the clinical signs of follicular mucinosis but unfortunately satisfactory regrowth of hair is rare.

B-cell lymphomas
These were formerly classified as sarcomata of lymphocytic or histiocytic types but it is now evident that the majority are tumours of the B lymphocyte. They are seen much less by dermatologists than T-cell lymphomas (Braylan 1975). Those derived from lymphocytes in various stages of blast transformation (large cell, immunoblastic type) carry a poor prognosis; in practice, the majority of B-cell lymphomas are small cell types and are derived from plasma cell precursors which have a good prognosis for life.

Histology. Skin lesions show a dense monocytic infiltrate composed almost entirely of lymphocytes; differential diagnosis is from lymphocytoma cutis and Jessner's lymphocytic infiltration of skin.

Clinical features. Specific skin lesions are rare. They are usually firm, pink or skin-coloured papules or plaques up to several centimetres in diameter. Grouped lesions usually develop on the trunk or limbs; they may expand or coalesce to produce bizarre gyrate shapes. Cases have been described with nodules affecting only the scalp (Samman 1979).

Individual nodules or plaques in the skin are sensitive to X-irradiation; fractionated doses (60–120 kV) up to 2000 rad may eradicate the disease though recurrences are common.

Hodgkin's disease
Hodgkin's disease is a malignant lymphoma of the reticuloendothelial system characterized histologically by the presence of abnormal reticulum (Sternberg–Reed) cells in the cellular infiltrate of affected organs (Berard 1975). It has still not been clearly shown whether it is the Sternberg–Reed cell or the abundant T lymphocytes that are truly malignant. Many authorities believe that Hodgkin's disease can be divided into several distinct diseases based on clinical and pathological differences.

Histologically four sub-types are recognized: lymphocytic predominance, nodular sclerosing, mixed cellularity and lymphocytic depletion (Berard 1975). The first two have a relatively good prognosis.

Hodgkin's disease is a multi-system disease; based on accurate staging using clinical, lymphangiographic and laparotomy findings (including splenectomy), four stages (each sub-divided into A and B sub-types—presence or absence of systemic symptoms—can be defined:

Stage 1—Limited to one or two adjacent anatomical sites on one side of the diaphragm.
Stage 2—As for 1, but more than two regions affected.
Stage 3—Disease on both sides of the diaphragm; only lymph nodes, spleen and Waldeyer's rings, involved.
Stage 4—Involvement of many organs throughout the reticuloendothelial system, including the skin.

This classification suggests that specific skin lesions imply a bad prognosis which is generally but not universally true.

Clinical features. The skin may rarely be specifically infiltrated with Hodgkin's disease tissue as with most organs. There are usually firm erythematous nodules which may ulcerate; the scalp may be the first site of involvement (Samman 1979).

Non-specific skin symptoms and signs occur in up to 50% of cases (Bluefarb 1959). These may predate evidence of active Hodgkin's disease by months or years. Included are pruritus or prurigo, pigmentation mimicking Addison's disease, acquired ichthyosis, generalized exfoliative dermatitis, herpes zoster and erythema nodosum. Hair loss may occur because of rubbing and scratching due to irritable dry skin, or because of pituitary or adrenal destruction by the disease process. Less commonly alopecia may be due to diffuse infiltration of the skin.

Treatment. Specific skin infiltrates are usually treated together with other sites of involvement using X-irradiation or chemotherapy or both. Pruritus and dry skin are best treated by regular oiling of the skin and oral antihistamines.

Histiocytic medullary reticulosis (syn. malignant histiocytosis)

This rare malignant proliferation of hystiocytes (and their precursors) is a rapidly fatal tumour in all the cases so far described (Scott & Robb-Smith 1939; Berard 1975).

Men are more frequently affected than women in this condition which presents with asthenia, weight loss and pyrexia; the lymph nodes, spleen and liver are enlarged and pancytopenia may develop. Rarely leucocytosis occurs. Jaundice and purpura are common.

The skin may be specifically infiltrated. Lesions are tender bluish/purple nodules which may coalesce to form plaques on the scalp, forehead, extremities and back.

The condition is progressive and death occurs within one year; no successful treatment is known.

References

Alibert J.L.M. (1835) *Monographie des Dermatoses*. Paris, Bellière.

Bazin P.A.E. (1876) *Maladies de la Peau Observeés à l'Hôpital*. Paris, St. Louis.

Berard C.W. (1975) Reticuloendothelial system. An overview of neoplasia. In *The Reticuloendothelial System. International Academy of Pathology Monographs*, 16, ed. J.W. Rebuck. Baltimore, Williams & Wilkins.

Bluefarb S.M. (1959) *Cutaneous Manifestations of the Malignant Lymphomas*. Springfield, Thomas.

Braylan R.C. (1975) Malignant lymphomas: current classification and new observations. In *Pathology Annual*, ed. S.C. Summers. New York, Appleton-Century-Croft.

Broder S. (1976) The Sézary syndrome. A malignant proliferation of helper T cells. *Journal of Clinical Investigation*, **58**, 1297.

Calnan C.D. (1957) Lymphocytic infiltrate of skin. *British Journal of Dermatology*, **69**, 169.

Caro W.A. & Helwig E.B. (1969) Lymphocytoma cutis. *Cancer*, **24**, 487.

Clark W.H. (1974) The lymphocytic infiltrates of the skin. *Human Pathology*, **5**, 25.

Clendenning, W.E. (1964) Mycosis fungoides. Relationship to malignant and cutaneous reticulosis and the Sézary syndrome. *Archives of Dermatology*, **89**, 785.

Gross P.R. (1971) Benign lymphoid hyperplasia. *Archives of Dermatology*, **103**, 347.

Hallopeau H. & Besnier F. (1892) On the erythroderma of mycosis fungoides. *Journal of Cutaneous Genetic Diseases*, **10**, 453.

Horen W.P. (1972) Insect and scorpion sting. *Journal of the American Medical Association*, **221**, 894.

Jessner M. & Kanof N.B. (1953) Lymphocytic infiltration of skin. *Archives of Dermatology*, **68**, 447.

Long J.C. & Mihm M.C. (1974) Mycosis fungoides with extracutaneous entity. *Cancer*, **34**, 1745.

Lukes R.J. & Collins R.D. (1974) Immunologic characteristics of human malignant lymphomas. *Cancer*, **34**, 1488.

Lutzner M. (1975) The Sézary syndrome, mycosis fungoides and related disorders. *Annals of Internal Medicine*, **83**, 534.

Nordqvist B.C. & Kinney J.P. (1976) T and B cell and cell-mediated immunity in mycosis fungoides. *Cancer*, **37**, 714.

Pinkus H. (1957) Lymphocytic infiltrate of skin. *British Journal of Dermatology*, **69**, 169.

Rappaport H. & Thomas L.B. (1974) Mycosis fungoides; the pathology of extracutaneous involvement. *Cancer*, **34**, 1198.

Roenigk H.H. Jr (1977) Photochemotherapy for mycosis fungoides. *Archives of Dermatology*, **113**, 1047.

Samman P.D. (1979) Lymphomata of B cells. In: *Textbook of Dermatology*, 3rd edn., eds. A.J. Rook, D.S. Wilkinson & F.J.G. Ebling. Oxford, Blackwell Scientific Publications, p. 1555.

Scott R.B. & Robb-Smith A.H.T. (1939) Histiocytic medullary reticulosis. *Lancet*, **ii**, 194.

Sézary A. (1949) Une nouvelle réticulose cutanée, la réticulose maligne leucémique à histio-mono-cytes monstrueuses et à forme d'érythrodermie oedemateuse et pigmentée. *Annales de Dermatologie et Syphilologie (Paris)*, **9**, 5.

Stevenson C.J. (1974) Parakeratosis variegata. *Proceedings of the Royal Society of Medicine*, **57**, 316.

Stiegleder G.K. (1976) Benign and malignant proliferative response. *Acta Dermato-venerologica (Stockholm)*, **56**, 33.

Vidal E. & Brocq L. (1885) Etude sur le mycosis fungoides. *France Médicale*, **2**, 946.

Winkelmann R.K. (1974) Symposium on the Sézary cell. *Mayo Clinic Proceedings*, **49**, 513.

Zackheim H.S. & Epstein E.H. (1975) Treatment of mycosis fungoides with topical nitrosurea compounds. *Archives of Dermatology*, **111**, 1564.

Common non-infective diseases of the scalp

Pityriasis capitis (references p. 455)

History and nomenclature

In 1842 John Erichsen, later to become an eminent surgeon, published a monograph on *Diseases of the Scalp*. Of pityriasis he wrote 'The diagnosis of pityriasis from the other scaling affections is sufficiently simple, indeed it is impossible to confound the small, thin white or greyish loose scales . . . It never causes the permanent loss of hair.' He regarded pityriasis as a simple cosmetic defect and not a precursor of baldness. The microbiological discoveries of the next

* Skin diseases causing cicatricial alopecia are considered in Chapter 11.

hundred years provided fuel for imaginative speculation on the relationship of pityriasis to seborrhoea, and of both to baldness. This cautionary tale is summarized on p. 90. It now seems reasonable to accept pityriasis as near-physiological scaling of the scalp or other hairy regions, which may or may not be fortuitously associated with 'seborrhoea' or with baldness. Pityriasis simplex or furfuracea is popularly known as dandruff.

Aetiology
Pityriasis is a cosmetic affliction of adolescence and adult life and is relatively rare and mild in children. Its peak incidence and severity are reached at the age of about 20 and it becomes less frequent after 50. At 20 some 50% of Caucasoids are affected in some degree. Figures for other races appear not to have been published.

The age incidence suggests that an androgenic influence is important and the level of sebacious activity may be a factor. However, gross seborrhoea may occur without pityriasis and commonly severe pityriasis may be present without clinically apparent excessive sebaceous activity. Quantitative studies have not been reported.

The microbial origin of pityriasis was accepted by Sabouraud (p. 92) but a number of later authors (e.g. Whitlock 1953) could establish no correlation between the degree of pityriasis and the population of *Pityrosporon ovale*. However, the role of *P. ovale* is still disputed. This yeast increases in number at puberty, and it elaborates substances which inhibit the growth of dermatophytes (Weary 1968). The large numbers of *P. ovale* in scalps with pityriasis has been regarded as secondary to the increased scaling (Ackermann & Kligman 1969). In another investigation of yeasts in subjects with and without pityriasis (Roia & Vanderwyk 1969) it was concluded that although no specific organism was significantly related to pityriasis, an increase in the total microbial flora was a factor in the increase of pityriasis. It had previously been demonstrated that the application of yeast inhibitors to one half of the scalp produced a greater reduction in pityriasis than did the application of a bacteria-inhibitor to the other half of the same scalp (Vanderwyk & Hechemey 1967). When the scalp flora of 11 subjects was almost completely eliminated by the application of nystatin and neomycin, the production of pityriasis was reduced by over 60%; and when a nystatin-resistant strain of *P. ovale* was then introduced the severity of the pityriasis increased by over 80% (Gosse & Vanderwyk 1969). However, some antimicrobial agents will decrease the flora without affecting the severity of pityriasis (Ackermann & Kligman 1969). Further quantitative studies of the microflora have not finally resolved the problem of their precise role in the production of pityriasis; *P. ovale* is more abundant in pityriasis than in the normal scalp, and still more so in seborrhoeic dermatitis, while *Corynebacterium acnes* is less abundant in pityriasis than in normal scalps, and almost disappears in seborrhoeic dermatitis (McGinley *et al.* 1975); these changes could be influenced by increased blood flow since *C. acnes* is strictly anaerobic.

Some of the investigations mentioned above, tending to attribute a pathogenic role to micro-organisms, were not well controlled (Priestly & Savin 1976) and the balance of evidence at present supports the considered judgement of Klingman's team (Leyden *et al.* 1976) that scalp organisms play no role in causing pityriasis capitis but are present in abundance because of the increased availability of scalp nutrients.

The antigenicity of *Pityrosporon* has been much investigated, but the clinical significance of allergic sensitivity to components of pityriasis scale has not been firmly established. It has been suggested that it may be of importance in some patients with atopic dermatitis. Over 75% of defatted human dandruff is non-allergenic mucopolysaccharide; the allergen is probably a glycoprotein (Berrens & Young 1964).

Similarly the significance of sensitivity to *P. ovale* is difficult to evaluate. Antibody to *P. ovale* is often present in high titre in patients with or without hair loss. However, Alexander (1967) found that patients with common baldness had more pityriasis than control subjects and that they had higher titres of antibody to *P. ovale* than had patients with alopecia areata.

Investigation on pityriasis requires a technique for the quantitative assessment of scaling, such as was described by Van Abbé (1964).

Pathology

Although their cause may be disputed the nature of the epidermal changes resulting in pityriasis is not. In the normal scalp the horny layer consists of 25–35 fully keratinized and closely coherent cells; in pityriasis there are usually fewer than ten layers of cells, and these are often parakeratotic and irregularly arranged, with deep crevices resulting in the formation of the flakes visible clinically (Ackermann & Kligman 1969). The permeability of such a horny layer is of course greater than normal. Autoradiographic studies (Plewig & Kligman 1969, 1970) showed a high labelling index and stratum corneum transit time of 3–4 days. Application of selenium sulphide reduced the labelling index and slowed down the transit time.

Clinical features

Small white or grey scales accumulate on the surface of the scalp in localized, more or less segmental, patches, or more diffusely. After removal with an effective shampoo the scales form again within 4–7 days. The condition first becomes a cosmetic problem during the second and third decades, but there are long- and short-term variations in its severity, without obvious cause (Van Abbé 1964). There are also variations in the ease with which the scales become detached and drift unaesthetically among the hair shafts or fall on the collar and shoulders. Although pityriasis usually clears spontaneously during the fifth or sixth decade, it may persist in old age.

In those subjects whose scalps become greasy at or after puberty, the seborrhoea binds the scale in a greasy paste and it is no longer shed, but accumulates in small adherent mounds—as so-called pityriasis steatoides. The development of clinically evident inflammatory changes in such individuals leads to seborrhoeic dermatitis. Pruritus is not a feature of simple pityriasis. It is very much more common when inflammatory changes develop in seborrhoeic scalps, and such recurrent episodes may be clearly related to periods of stress. Acne necrotica (p. 475), which may be intensely irritable, also can complicate pityriasis.

Diagnosis

The presence of more than very mild pityriasis in a young child throws doubt on the diagnosis. Extreme and persistent scaling, even though it lacks the characteristic features of psoriasis, is always suspect, particularly if there is a family history of this disease. Widespread scaling, sometimes with scarring, may occur in some forms of ichthyosis (p. 489). At any age, if pruritus is troublesome, pediculosis must be carefully excluded.

Small areas of scaling with dull broken hair shafts are typical of *Microsporon* ringworm. Localized scaling in children is therefore an indication for examination of the scalp under Wood's light, and of the broken hairs under the microscope. A nervous hair-pulling tic may result in twisted and broken hairs of normal texture in a patch of post-inflammatory scaling.

Profuse sticky silvery scale should suggest pityriasis amiantacea (p. 455).

Treatment

Pityriasis in its milder forms is a physiological process. The object of treatment is to control it at the lowest possible cost and inconvenience to the patient, appreciating that any procedure found to be effective will need to be repeated at regular intervals.

In some cases, particularly if seborrhoea is associated, a tar preparation such as Oil of Cade ointment (see p. 466) or a proprietary preparation such as Pragmatar, may be rubbed into the scalp and washed out after a few hours with a detergent shampoo. This treatment may need to be repeated at intervals, but after two or three applications it can often be replaced by a tar shampoo, which has been shown to be more effective than the vehicle alone (Alexander 1967a, b).

In the average case one of the many proprietary shampoos may be found effective. Selenium sulphide, which has been shown to reduce epidermal turnover (Plewig & Kligman 1970) is very useful for many patients but fails inexplicably in others. The same may be said of preparations containing zinc pyrithione of zinc omadine, which are said to reduce the yeast populations (Brauer *et al.* 1966).

References

Ackermann A.B. & Kligman A.M. (1969) Some observations on dandruff. *Journal of the Society of Cosmetic Chemists*, **20**, 81.

Alexander S. (1967a) Do shampoos affect dandruff? *British Journal of Dermatology*, **79**, 92.

Alexander S. (1967b) Loss of hair and dandruff. *British Journal of Dermatology*, **79**, 549.

Berrens L. & Young E. (1964) Studies on the human dandruff allergen. *Dermatologica*, **128**, 3.

Brauer E.W., Opdyke D.L. & Burnett C.M. (1966) The anti-seborrhoeic qualities of zinc pyrithione in a cream vehicle. *Journal of Investigative Dermatology*, **47**, 174.

Erichsen J.E. (1842) *A Practical Treatise on the Diseases of the Scalp*. London, Churchill, p. 180.

Gosse R.M. & Vanderwyk R.W. (1969) The relationship of a nystatin-resistant strain of *Pityrosporon ovale* to dandruff. *Journal of the Society of Cosmetic Chemists*, **20**, 603.

Leyden J.J., McGinlay K.J. & Kligman A.M. (1976) Role of micoorganisms in dandruff. *Archives of Dermatology*, **112**, 333.

McGinley K.J., Leyden J.J., Marples R.R. & Kligman A.M. (1975) Quantitative microbiology of the scalp in non-dandruff, dandruff and seborrhoeic dermatitis. *Journal of Investigative Dermatology*, **64**, 401.

Plewig G. & Kligman A.M. (1969) The effect of selenium sulphide on epidermal tumours of normal and dandruff scalps. *Journal of the Society of Cosmetic Chemists*, **20**, 767.

Plewig G. & Kligman A.M. (1970) Zellkinetische Untersuchungen bei Kopfschuppenerkrankung. *Archiv für klinische und experimentelle Dermatologie*, **236**, 406.

Priestly G.L. & Savin J.A. (1976) The microbiology of dandruff. *British Journal of Dermatology*, **94**, 469.

Roia F.C. & Vanderwyk R.W. (1969) Residual microbial flora of the human scalp and its relationship to dandruff. *Journal of the Society of Cosmetic Chemists*, **20**, 113.

Van Abbé N.J. (1964) The investigation of dandruff. *Journal of the Society of Cosmetic Chemists*, **15**, 609.

Vanderwyk R.W. & Hechemey K.E. (1967) A comparison of the bacterial and yeast flora of the human scalp and their effect upon dandruff production. *Journal of the Society of Cosmetic Chemists*, **18**, 629.

Weary P.E. (1968) *Pityrosporon ovale*. *Archives of Dermatology*, **98**, 408.

Whitlock F.A. (1953) *Pityrosporon ovale* and some scaly conditions of the scalp. *British Medical Journal*, **i**, 484.

Pityriasis amiantacea (references p. 457)

History and nomenclature

The clinical features of this poorly documented but not uncommon syndrome were known before Alibert (1832) named it 'fausse teigne amiantaćee', which may be translated as asbestos-like pseudo-ringworm. Since then it has often been referred to as tinea amiantacea, but as the term 'tinea' ordinarily implies a ringworm infection many others have preferred the non-committal 'pityriasis amiantacea', as we do. Gschwandtner (1974) has given his etymological reasons for using the old term 'porrigo', but this term proved such a source of confusion throughout the nineteenth century that it seems better to let it die.

Aetiology (Becker & Muir 1929; Brown 1948)

Pityriasis amiantacea is a pattern of eczematous reaction of the scalp to trauma or to infection, or without evident cause. It may complicate seborrhoeic dermatitis, psoriasis or lichen simplex. Its association with these and other conditions is difficult to evaluate. It depends on the initial clinical diagnosis. Cases which some dermatologists would accept as early psoriasis are labelled pityriasis amiantacea by others. If such cases are excluded then there is no definite association between pityriasis amiantacea and psoriasis (Hersle *et al.* 1979). In Knight's (1977) study of 71 patients, 2 had associated psoriasis and 9 had eczema. Pityriasis amiantacea may occur at any age but in Knight's (1977) series, the average age was 25, and the range 5–40 years.

Pathology

Biopsies from eighteen patients were examined by Knight (1977). The most consistent findings were spongiosis, parakeratosis, migration of lymphocytes into the epidermis, and a variable degree of acanthosis. The essential features responsible for the asbestos-like scaling are diffuse hyperkeratosis and parakeratosis together with follicular keratosis, which surrounds each hair by a sheath of horn (Kiess 1925; Jossel 1932; Gschwandtner 1974).

Clinical features (Dunbreuilh 1930; Jordan & Nolting 1971; Gschwandtner 1974)

Masses of sticky silvery scales, overlapping like the tiles on a roof, adhere to the scalp and are attached in layers to the shafts of the hairs which they surround. The underlying scalp may be red and moist or may show simple erythema and scaling, or the features of psoriasis of seborrhoeic dermatitis or of lichen simplex (Fig. 17.1).

A relatively common form seen mainly in young girls complicates recurrent or chronic fissuring behind one or both ears. The scales extend some distance into the neighbouring scalp. Another form extends upwards from medical patches of lichen simplex and is seen in middle-aged women. The disease is usually confined to small areas of the scalp, but may be very extensive, either involving a large area diffusely, or affecting a number of small patches. The latter form in children often proves by its subsequent course to be psoriasis. The majority of patients notice some hair loss in areas of severe scaling (Knight 1977). The hair regrows when the scaling is effectively treated.

Diagnosis

The distinctive clinical appearance makes the diagnosis but the identification of the underlying disease may not be easy; indeed none may be found.

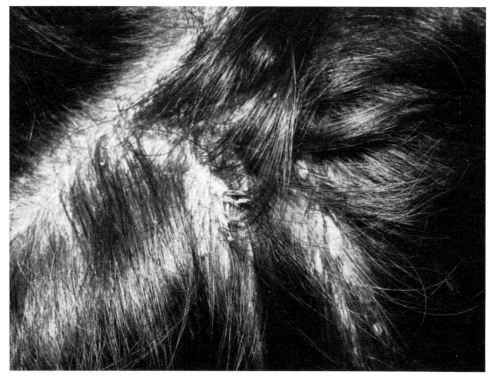

Fig. 17.1. Pityriasis amiantacea (Addenbrooke's Hospital, Cambridge).

Treatment

Where the pityriasis complicates lichen simplex or psoriasis the underlying condition must be treated, but it may be useful initially to eliminate the abundant scale by the use of Oil of Cade ointment of Pragmatar which is effective also in many cases in which no preceding disease of the scalp is discovered. Either preparation should be washed out of the scalp after 4 or 5 hours with a detergent shampoo. Even then the condition tends sometimes to recur.

References

Alibert J.L. (1832) *La Porrigine Amiantacée. Monographie des Dermatoses*, vol. 1. Paris, Imprimerie de Ridgnoux, p. 293.

Becker S.W. & Muir K.B. (1929) Tinea amiantacea. *Archives of Dermatology and Syphilology*, **20**, 45.

Brown W.H. (1948) Some observations on neurodermatitis of the scalp with particular reference to tinea amiantacea. *British Journal of Dermatology*, **60**, 81.

Dubreuilh W. (1930) De la forme teigne amiantacée d'Alibert. *Annales de Dermatologie et de Syphiligraphie*, **1**, 61.

Gschwandtner W.R. (1974) Porrigo amiantacea (pityriasis amiantacea). *Hautarzt*, **25**, 134.

Hersle K., Lindholm A., Mobaeken H. & Sandberg L. (1979) Relationship of pityriasis amiantacea to psoriasis. *Dermatologica*, **159**, 245.

Jordan P. & Nolting S. (1971) Tinea amiantacea. *Schriften der Alfred-Marchionini-Stiftung,* **2,** 55.

Jossel B. (1932) Zur Kenntnis der sogennaten Alibertischen tinea amiantacea. *Dermatologische Wochenschrift,* **94,** 677.

Kiess O. (1925) Die Porrigo amiantacea. *Dermatologische Wochenschrift,* **81,** 1355.

Knight A.G. (1977) Pityriasis amiantacea: a clinical and histopathologic investigation. *Clinical and Experimental Dermatology,* **2,** 137.

Seborrhoea (references p. 460)

Definition

Seborrhoea has been defined as the production of a quantity of sebum which is excessive for the age and sex of the individual, but this definition is inadequate in clinical practice, since many patients in whom the level of sebum excretion is not abnormal nevertheless seek advice because they find the greasiness of their hair cosmetically unacceptable. Seborrhoea in practice is that level of sebum production which the patient considers to be excessive.

Aetiology

Sebaceous glands are present over the entire skin surface except the palms and the soles and the dorsa of the feet. The largest glands are on the face and scalp and on the scrotum. The glands in the central areas of the chest and back are larger than those elsewhere in the trunk. Sebaceous glands in the skin all open into hair follicles, but the pilary component of the pilosebaceous unit may be only a very small vellus hair.

The sebaceous glands are functional at birth, and in early infancy under the influence of maternal androgens, but throughout childhood they remain tiny and inactive. With the approach of puberty, at which androgen levels begin to rise, usually at about the age of 9 or 10, the sebaceous glands enlarge and the production of sebum begins. Between 13 and 16 the production of sebum is equal between males and females but the level increases in males to reach a peak at the age of about 20. From about 16 onwards the production of sebum is significantly greater in males than females. In males it remains high to extreme old age; in females there is a marked decrease after the menopause (Strauss & Pochi 1968). Sebaceous gland activity in males is dependent mainly on testicular androgen. In females it depends on adrenal and ovarian androgen.

Oestrogen decreases the size of sebaceous glands and thus the production of sebum (Pochi & Strauss 1973), but in pregnancy there is no reduction in sebum production and there is a decrease post partum (Burton *et al.* 1970).

There is considerable variation in the normal level of sebum production in sexually normal males and those with abundant sebum may complain about it. In those genetically predisposed to acne this may accompany the seborrhoea. Men with common baldness may complain of the conspicuous greasiness of the scalp, but in such patients greasiness is merely more evident and the level of sebum production is no greater than in non-bald control subjects (Maibach *et al.* 1968). During the course of development of baldness the total number of sebaceous glands does in fact decrease significantly (Rampini *et al.* 1968).

In women seborrhoea may have far greater significance. Seborrhoea (and acne in those so predisposed), together with hirsutism and baldness, is one of the triad of cutaneous parameters of androgenic activity.

Increased sebaceous activity, quite apart from the levels of androgenic stimulation may occur in Parkinson's disease and in epilepsy (Grasset & Brun 1959).

There are satisfactory quantitative techniques available for the measurement of the rate of sebum excretion (Ebling 1974) and the rate of replacement sebum on the hair (Eberhardt & Kuhn-Bussiers 1975). Sebum replacement curves show wide variations and four types of curve are identified.

Clinical features
The patient complains that his, or more often her, hair is excessively greasy and therefore unmanageable and may insist that the frequent removal of the grease by shampooing tends to increase the rate of its production (Goldsmidt & Kligman 1968).

Management
Symptomatic treatment without any attempt to evaluate the significance of the symptom is hard to justify. Admittedly the seborrhoea may be a physiological variant and the patient be otherwise entirely normal. However, in a significant proportion of women the seborrhoea is a manifestation of increased androgenic activity which has other consequences than purely cosmetic.

The association of hirsutism or of androgenetic alopecia should be noted. The menstrual history should be recorded. If the association of hirsutism, or of alopecia of androgenetic pattern, or of menstrual irregularity, suggests the possibility of an abnormality in systemic androgen metabolism this should be investigated and treated (see Chapter 4). If the seborrhoea is an isolated symptom topical means to control it are recommended. Gloor (1979) outlined the aims of topical treatment as (a) inhibition of depletion of sebaceous glands, (b) inhibition of lipid synthesis in the glands and (c) inhibition of microbial lipolysis of triglycerides. He states that the use of isopropyl alcohol as a vehicle reduces sebum depletion, tar or oestrogens reduce lipid synthesis, and lipolysis is reduced by isopropyl alcohol, colloidal sulphur or selenium disulphide. The use of lotions containing oestrogens is often advocated in some European countries and its thorough investigation and evaluation is clearly desirable. In Britain it is usual in cases in which there is no indication for systemic treatment, to prescribe Unguentum Cadimi Co. (see p. 468) or Pragmatar and a detergent shampoo, and to establish empirically the choice of preparation and the frequency of application to provide the greatest symptomatic relief.

References
Burton J.L., Cunliffe W.J., Millar D.G. & Shuster S. (1970) Effect of pregnancy on sebum excretion. *British Medical Journal*, ii, 769.
Eberhardt H. & Kuhn-Bussius H. (1975) Bestimmung der Ruckfettungskinetik der Haare. *Archiv fur Dermatologische Forschung*, **252**, 139.
Ebling F.J. (1974) Hormonal control and methods of measuring sebaceous gland activity. *Journal of Investigative Dermatology*, **62**, 161.
Gloor M. (1979) Aspekte zur Therapie der Seborrhoea Oleosa und des Pityriasis simplex capillitii. *Hautarzt*, **30**, 236.
Goldschmidt H. & Kligman A.M. (1968) Increased sebum secretion following selenium sulphide shampoo. *Acta Dermatologica et Venerealogica*, **48**, 489.
Grasset N. & Brun R. (1959) Etude de fonction sebacée de sujets sains et de patients atteints d'epilepsie ou de maladie de Parkinson. *Dermatologica*, **119**, 132.
Maibach H.I., Feldmann R., Payne B. & Hutshell T. (1968) Scalp and forehead sebum production in male pattern alopecia. In *Biopathology of Pattern Alopecia*, eds. A. Baccareda-Boy, G. Moretti & J.R. Frey. Basel, Karger, p. 171.
Pochi P.E. & Strauss J.S. (1973) Sebaceous gland suppression with ethinyl oestradiol and diethinylstilbestrol. *Archives of Dermatology*, **108**, 210.
Rampini E., Bertamino R. & Moretti G. (1968) Size and shape of sebaceous gland in male pattern alopecia. In *Biopathology of Pattern Alopecia*, eds. A. Baccareda-Boy, G. Moretti & J.R. Frey. Basel, Karger, p. 155.
Strauss J.S. & Pochi P.E. (1968) The change in human sebaceous gland activity with age. In *Biopathology of Pattern Alopecia*, eds. A. Baccareda-Boy, G. Moretti & J.R. Frey. Basel, Karger, p. 166.

Seborrhoeic dermatitis (references p. 463)

History and nomenclature (Colcott Fox 1911)
Willan introduced the concept of pityriasis, consisting of irregular patches of small thin scales. He included both pityriasis capitis and pityriasis versicolor in this group. Hebra in 1870 introduced the term and the concept of seborrhoea oleosa, with increased sebaceous gland activity as its essential feature, and he included Willan's pityriasis capitis as seborrhoea sicca which he claimed was due to sebaceous gland dysfunction. In 1887 Unna used the term seborrhoeic eczema and emphasized the inflammatory component. Subsequent work of Sabouraud and others incriminating various micro-organisms has been discussed elsewhere (p. 92).

The prevalence of seborrhoeic dermatitis shows wide geographical variation, but the extent to which this is climatic or racial is still uncertain. In Britain seborrhoeic dermatitis appears to be significantly more frequent among the Celts than in other ethnic groups. International comparisons are still more difficult to make as differences in diagnostic criteria and in nomenclature are so frequent.

Aetiology

The cause of seborrhoeic dermatitis is unknown but a genetic factor is almost certainly implicated. Clinically different syndromes with some features in common occur in the infant with sebaceous activity induced by maternal androgens and in the adolescent and adult in whom sebaceous activity has been re-established by endogenous androgen production. The sebum excretion rate, however, is not increased in seborrhoeic dermatitis but the sebum contains less than the normal proportion of free fatty acids, squalene and wax esters, and relatively increased quantities of triglycerides and cholesterol (Gloor *et al.* 1972). The incidence of seborrhoeic dermatitis is increased in Parkinsonism and the dermatitis in such patients is improved by l-dopa which reduces the abnormally high sebum excretion rate (Parish 1970).

Attempts to relate seborrhoeic dermatitis to the activities of yeasts or bacteria have been unconvincing, but secondary bacterial infection is common. Claims that autoimmune mechanisms are involved (Hashimoto 1966) are also unproven. Stress seems at times to be a precipitating factor.

Pathology

The histological changes combine features of chronic eczema with features of psoriasis. The histological differential diagnosis of seborrhoeic dermatitis from psoriasis is discussed on p. 464. The ultra-microscopic appearance (Metz & Metz 1975) is not specific and resembles that seen in nummular eczema.

Clinical features (Rook 1954; Borda & Abulafia 1967)

Pityriasis simplex capitis is widely regarded as the precursor or the mildest form of seborrhoeic dermatitis of the scalp but until much more knowledge of the conditions becomes available the nature of this possible relationship must remain a matter for speculation.

Pityriasis steatoides is regarded as a slightly more severe form of seborrhoeic dermatitis of the scalp. Large greasy scales of dirty yellow colour, combine with exudate to form crusts, beneath which the scalp is red and moist (Fig. 17.2). The eyebrows and the nasolabial folds are often also involved. As the condition deteriorates perifollicular erythema and scaling gradually extends to form sharply marginated patches, dull red in colour and covered by greasy scales. There may be only a few discrete patches or the scalp may be diffusely affected with extension of the dermatitis beyond the frontal margin to give the 'corona seborrhoeica'. Scratching and secondary infection may produce eczematization with much exudation and crusting, and secondary infection may cause an increase of these inflammatory changes or the development of pustulation.

Often associated with seborrhoeic dermatitis of the scalp is a characteristic blepharitis. Small crusts form along the eyelid margins and separate to leave scars. Some eyelashes may be destroyed.

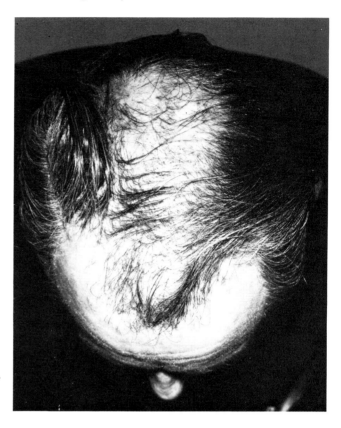

Fig. 17.2. Seborrhoeic dermatitis (Addenbrooke's Hospital,
Cambridge).

The retro-auricular region is commonly affected by seborrhoeic dermatitis
either alone or in association with scalp lesions. There may be a crusted
retro-auricular fissure from which dull red scaling extends into the scalp and to
the back of the pinna. The concha and the external auditory canal may be
similarly affected.

The renewed popularity of beards in some countries has led to an increase of
seborrhoeic dermatitis at this site (Parish & Arndt 1972). Erythema and greasy
scaling are most severe on the cheeks. On the shaven chin a superficial folliculitis
of the beard (barbers' rash) is common. Less often a deep follicular infection gives
rise to sycosis which may leave scars.

Seborrhoeic dermatitis of other hairy regions of the body may accompany
dermatitis of the scalp.

Seborrhoeic dermatitis of infancy
The relationship of this distinctive syndrome to seborrhoeic dermatitis of adults is
problematical. During the early days or weeks of life grey greasy crusts form on

the scalp, particularly on the frontal and parietal regions. A pink scaly erythema may develop in the neck folds and in other skin flexures (Fig. 3.4).

Diagnosis

There is a tendency to diagnose seborrhoeic dermatitis too freely. Many other skin conditions may occur in grossly seborrhoeic subjects and the diagnostic criteria should therefore be strict.

The heavy palpable scales of psoriasis are usually easy to differentiate, particularly if psoriatic lesions can be found in the skin and on the nails. Occasionally the existence of a hybrid condition may be suspected. In cases of doubt a biopsy may be helpful (p. 464).

Tinea capitis may readily be confused with seborrhoeic dermatitis, particularly those forms of tinea caused by anthropophilic *Trichophyton* species (p. 377).

Lichen simplex of the nape, a relatively common condition in women, can be confused with seborrhoeic dermatitis but the characteristic site and the severity and persistence of the itching suggests the correct diagnosis. Less commonly lichen simplex may occur at the side of the scalp above the ear.

Treatment

The treatment of pityriasis capitis is considered on p. 454. Seborrhoeic dermatitis of the scalp may respond to the same measures but if it is extensive or severe daily application of a corticosteroid lotion is helpful. The scalp should be shampooed twice or more each week until the dermatitis is under control. A preparation containing tar and sulphur such as Pragmatar or Oil of Cade ointment should be rubbed gently into the scalp at least 2 hours before the hair is shampooed.

If secondary infection is present a topical antibiotic/corticosteroid combination should be prescribed; if the secondary infection is severe and extensive systemic antibiotics are to be preferred.

Seborrhoeic dermatitis of the beard may be kept under control by regular washing (Parish & Arndt 1972).

Severe and extensive seborrhoeic dermatitis may tend to relapse. The patient's way of life should be discussed and efforts made to provide relief from physical and emotional stress.

References

Borda J.M. & Abulafia J. (1967) Sindrom Eccematoid. *Archives Argentins de Dermatologic*, **17**, 203.

Colcott Fox T. (1911) Pityriasis *in a System of Medicine*, vol. 4, eds. C. Allbutt & H.D. Rolleston. London, Macmillan, p. 202.

Gloor M. (1972) Uber Menge und Zusammensetzung der Hautoberflachenlipide beim sogennanten Seborrhoischer Ekzem. *Dermatologische Monatschrift*, **158**, 759.

Hashimoto I. (1946) Autoimmune phenomena in eczema seborrhoeicum. *Tohoku Journal of Experimental Medicine*, **89**, 45.

Metz J. & Metz G. (1975) Zur Ultrastruktur der Epidermis bei Seborrhoeischer Ekzem. *Archiv für Dermatologische Forschung*, **252**, 285.

Parrish J.A. & Arndt K.A. (1972) Seborrhoeic dermatitis of the beard. *British Journal of Dermatology*, **87**, 201.

Parish L. (1970) L-dopa for seborrhoeic dermatitis. *New England Journal of Medicine*, **283**, 879.

Rook A. (1954) Seborrhoeic dermatitis. *Practitioner*, **172**, 522.

Psoriasis of the scalp (references p. 467)

Aetiology

Psoriasis is a genetically determined disorder of the skin. There is some racial variation in its prevalence but few large-scale and reliable surveys have been reported. The prevalence in adults in north-west Europe is about 1.5–2%. The mode of inheritance of psoriasis is not known and there may indeed be more than one genotype.

In the genetically predisposed individual the first attack may develop at any age, but the mean age of onset is in the third decade and psoriasis is uncommon in the first 2 or 3 years of life. The initial attack and subsequent recurrences may be provoked by streptococcal infection, and perhaps by stress but may also occur for no discoverable reason.

The pathogenesis of psoriasis is being extensively studied and good reviews are available (Baker & Wilkinson 1979; Farber & Cox 1977). A long account of this work would be out of place in this book and a brief summary could be misleading.

Pathology

The distinctive histological features of psoriasis are acanthosis with elongation of the reti ridges and absence or reduction of the granular layer. The horny layer is parakeratotic and there are collections of polymorphonuclear lymphocytes—Monro abscesses—in the upper epidermis. The dermal papillae are oedematous. Braun-Falco *et al.* (1979) defined the criteria for the histological differential diagnosis of psoriasis from seborrhoeic dermatitis of the scalp. Features favouring psoriasis were condensed hyperkeratosis with focal parakeratosis, PAS-positive serum inclusions, Monro abscesses within the horny layer, and spongiform pustules and polymorphonuclear leucocytes within the epidermis. The criteria for seborrhoeic dermatitis were irregular acanthosis with a relatively thin ortho- or parakeratotic horny layer, spongiosis and spongiotic vesicles, and exocytosis of lymphocytes.

The rate of hair growth is not increased in psoriasis (Comaish 1969). The calibre of the shafts of hairs growing in plaques of psoriasis is significantly reduced (Wyatt & Riggott 1981). Electronmicroscopic studies (Braun-Falco & Rassner 1966; Orfanos *et al.* 1970; Wyatt *et al.* 1972) showed changes in the hair shafts in psoriasis; the cuticular cells were irregular and dystrophic.

Using a labelling technique Shahrad & Marks (1976) found an increased index only in the upper part of the external root sheath.

Clinical features

The scalp is frequently involved in psoriasis. In children and young adults it is sometimes the first site to be affected and in some patients it remains the only one. In the majority of cases, however, other sites are sooner or later involved. Sometimes the scalp remains constantly affected to some degree over many years, whilst lesions elsewhere may come and go.

The classical feature of psoriasis is a palpable bright pink plaque covered in silvery scale, and such lesions occur in the scalp (Fig. 17.3). However, the earliest changes, particularly in children, may be less distinctive. There may be patchy or a diffuse scaling without any special features, or there may be asbestos-like scale in layers (pityriasis amiantacea, see p. 455). The correct diagnosis may be suspected if there is a family history of psoriasis or if the patient has lesions elsewhere.

Although extensive loss of hair occurs only in the erythrodermic forms of psoriasis, some increased shedding of telogen hairs and some reduction in hair density is common in plaques of psoriasis.

In severe psoriasis of the scalp masses of heaped up scale form a solid cap which may extend just beyond the hair margin.

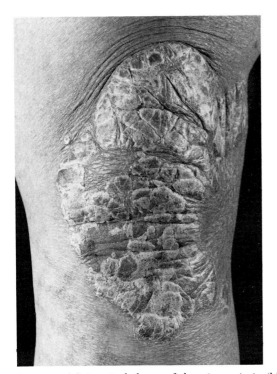
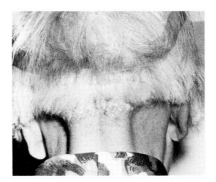

Fig. 17.3. (a) A typical plaque of chronic psoriasis. (b) Extensive psoriasis of the scalp extending below the scalp margin on the nape of the neck (Slade Hospital, Oxford).

Psoriasis is traditionally seldom irritable but irritation is sometimes severe in the scalp as elsewhere.

Seborrhoeic dermatitis (see p. 460) is a common condition in some populations and it frequently involves the scalp, extending further beyond the scalp margins than does psoriasis, spreading behind the ears, to the forehead and into any bald areas of the scalp. In the patient predisposed to psoriasis the lesions of seborrhoeic dermatitis may become increasingly psoriasiform, showing clinical and histological features of both conditions.

Lichen simplex of the nape may be confused with psoriasis, but as with seborrhoeic dermatitis hybrid lesions occur, showing features of both conditions.

Diagnosis

The diagnosis of typical psoriasis is rarely difficult. Atypical lesions suggestive of psoriasis should lead to a thorough examination of the commonly affected sites, including the nails, for traces of psoriasis, even if the patient denies their presence. Small patches on knees or elbows are easily overlooked by the patient.

A very persistent scaly plaque on the bald scalp should be histologically examined to exclude Bowen's disease. Small psoriasiform plaques (even in the hairy scalp) remaining unchanged over many years except perhaps for some slow increase in size, should also be suspected of being Bowen's disease (see p. 517).

Treatment

A detailed explanation of the problems of psoriasis should always be given, and the patient should be reassured that although the tendency to psoriasis cannot be eradicated, the attacks can be controlled and very long complete remissions may occur.

The commonest cause of treatment failure, particularly in scalp lesions, is the patient's inability to carry out the treatment thoroughly, and the lack of anyone else to help him. In mild cases a tar shampoo may suffice, or a proprietary preparation such as Pragmatar may be rubbed into the patches 3 or more hours before the scalp is shampooed once or twice a week.

In more severe cases Oil of Cade ointment is helpful

Oil of Cade	6
Precipitated sulphur	2
Salicylic acid	2
Emulsifying ointment to	100

Other preparations which may be effective when chronic lesions are present are the proprietary Alphosyl H.C. or Dithrocream 0.1%. Either preparation should be rubbed into the patches and washed out after a few hours.

In conjunction with such measures a corticosteroid lotion or gel may be applied daily.

Patients with psoriasis require careful supervision. The disease itself can be a cause of severe stress and full discussion of the problems arising as a result, forms an important part of treatment.

References

Baker H. & Wilkinson D.S. (1979) Psoriasis. In *Textbook of Dermatology*, 3rd edn., eds. A. Rook, D.S. Wilkinson & F.J. Ebling, Oxford, Blackwell Scientific Publications, p. 1315.

Braun-Falco O., Heilgemeir G.P. & Lincke-Plewig H. (1979) Histologische Differentialdiagnose von Psoriasis vulgaris und seborrhoischem Ekzem des Kapillitium. *Hautarzt*, **30**, 478.

Braun-Falco O. & Rassner B. (1966) Haarwurzelmuster bei Psoriasis vulgaris der Kopfhaut. *Archiv. für Klinische und Experimentelle Dermatologie*, **225**, 42.

Comaish S. (1969) Autoradiographic Studies of Hair Growth in various dermatoses: Investigation of a possible circadian rhythm in normal hair growth. *British Journal of Dermatology*, **81**, 283.

Farber E.M. & Cox A.J. (1977) *Psoriasis. Proceedings of the Second International Symposium.* New York, Yorke Medical Books.

Orfanos C., Mahler G. & Christenhurz R. (1970) Verhornungstörungen am Haar bei Psoriasis: Eine Studie im Raster-Elektronmikroscop. *Archiv für Klinische und Experimentelle Dermatologie*, **236**, 107.

Sharad, P. & Marks R. (1976) Hair follicle kinetics in psoriasis. *British Journal of Dermatology*, **94**, 7.

Wyatt E., Bottoms E. & Comaish S. (1972) Abnormal hair shafts in psoriasis in scanning electron microscopy. *British Journal of Dermatology*, **87**, 368.

Wyatt E. & Riggott J.M. (1981) The influence of psoriasis on hair diameter.

Lichenification and lichen simplex (references p. 469)

Lichenification is a 'leathery' thickening of skin resulting from repeated rubbing and scratching. The surface skin lines and creases are exaggerated within the abnormal area. Lichenification may occur secondary to many pruritic dermatoses or develop as a localized abnormality without any predisposing diseases, the so-called lichen simplex or primary lichenification.

The pathological changes vary from site to site. Typical findings include hyperkeratosis and acanthosis; localized areas of spongiosis and parakeratosis may be present. All components of the epidermis are hyperplastic; though labelling indices are usually 25–30% greater than normal, the transit time of the thickened epidermis is longer than that of psoriasis (Marks & Wells 1973a, b). The dermal changes vary according to the primary cause and the duration of the lesion. A mixed chronic inflammatory cell infiltrate is usually present in the upper dermis sometimes associated with fibrosis and Schwann cell proliferation.

Emotional tensions play an important part in favouring the development and persistence of lichenification which may indeed persist long after the primary disease has remitted. This fact is the basis of the often-used synonym

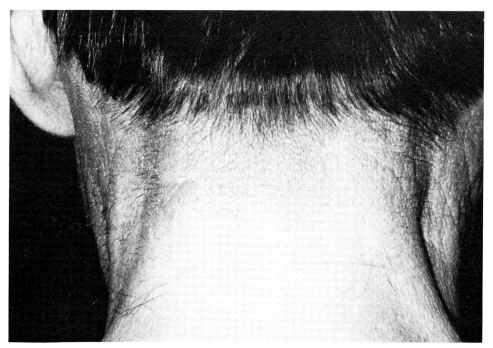

Fig. 17.4. Lichen simplex of the nape: confluent lichenoid papules (Slade Hospital, Oxford).

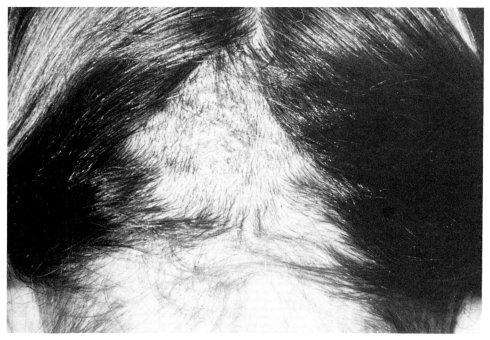

Fig. 17.5. Lichen simplex of the nape: hair loss from rubbing (Slade Hospital, Oxford).

neurodermatitis. Not all individuals produce lichenified skin on rubbing and scratching; atopic subjects are particularly prone, as are the Mongoloid race. In many subjects, the same disease and chronic rubbing and scratching produce nodules—nodular prurigo or nodular lichenification. Negroid subjects frequently produce papular and follicular lichenification.

The main symptom is pruritus which may be very severe despite minimal signs. The most common diseases predisposing to secondary lichenification are atopic dermatitis, nummular eczema, pruritus ani and vulvae, lichen planus, seborrhoeic dermatitis, stasis dermatitis, asteototic eczema and, rarely, psoriasis. In the condition termed actinic reticuloid (Ive *et al.* 1969) chronic photodermatoses and psoriasis may cause a lichenified appearance in areas where little scratching and rubbing occur. Lichenified patches may occur on any pruritic area that is amenable to rubbing and scratching.

Lichen simplex is defined as localized lichenification due to rubbing and scratching of skin previously apparently normal i.e. primary lichenification (Schaffer & Beerman 1951; Cleveland 1936). In general, the local physical signs and histopathological changes are the same as in secondary lichenification.

Lichen simplex is rare before puberty, the peak incidence being between 30 and 50; women are more frequently affected than men. In lichen simplex only a few lesions are present, in 50% of cases only one lesion occurs. The commonest areas affected are the nape of the neck, the shin and the calves, the upper thigh, the extensor surface of the forearms and various sites on the external genitalia (Figs. 17.4, 17.5).

Lichen nuchae occurs as a single plaque on the nape of the neck; it may be very scaly and mimic psoriasis; attacks of secondary bacterial infection are common. On other parts of the scalp the presenting sign may be localized breaking of hair associated with underlying pruritus and scaling. This pattern is particularly likely to affect the temporal and parietal areas of the scalp. Allergic or irritant reactions to hair cosmetics must be carefully excluded.

Treatment

Primary lichenification requires careful psychological assessment and treatment; the patient should be given insight into the underlying stresses and an understanding of the need to break the scratching habit. Topical treatment needs to be anti-inflammatory, occlusive in sites where this is possible such as the limbs, and antibacterial if secondary infection is present; topical steroid creams are most commonly used whilst intralesional triamcinolone may be effective in recalcitrant cases.

References

Cleveland D.E.H. (1936) Lichen simplex chronicus. *Archives of Dermatology and Syphilology,* **33,** 316.

Ive F.A., Magnus I.A., Warin R.P. & Wilson-Jones E. (1969) 'Actinic reticuloid', a chronic
    dermatosis associated with severe photosensitivity and the histological resemblance to
    lymphoma. *British Journal of Dermatology,* **81,** 469.
Marks R. & Wells G.C. (1973a) Lichen simplex; morphodynamic correlates. *British Journal of
    Dermatology,* **88,** 249.
Marks R. & Wells G.C. (1973b) A histochemical profile of lichen simplex. *British Journal of
    Dermatology,* **88,** 557.
Shaffer B. & Beerman H. (1951) Lichen simplex chronicus and its variants. *Archives of Dermatology
    and Syphilology,* **64,** 340.

Contact dermatitis (references p. 474)

Contact dermatitis (syn. contact eczema) may be conveniently defined, for
present purposes, as an inflammatory condition of the skin caused by an external
agent. If photodermatitis is excluded, two broad divisions are recognized, irritant
and allergic dermatitis.

Irritant dermatitis

A skin irritant is defined as a substance that is capable of causing cell damage in
most people if it is applied for a sufficient length of time, frequently enough and in
great enough concentration. The scalp is generally considered to be resistant to
irritant damage, possibly because of a relatively thick epidermis and horny layer;
also, the scalp has a rapid epidermal 'turn-over time' i.e. it replaces its natural
barrier layer relatively quickly after any cell damage. It should be noted,
however, that substances which are recognized as highly irritant on other sites
are rarely applied to the scalp frequently enough, for long enough or in
high-enough concentrations. For example, hairdressers frequently develop
irritant contact dermatitis of the hands from contact with shampoos, but the
dilute shampoo solution applied to the scalp does not cause dermatitis.
Shampoos may rarely irritate the skin of the forehead and scalp margins in
susceptible individuals, such as atopic eczema subjects, and inflame the
conjunctival surface of the eye.

   In practice, the misuse of thioglycollates, bleaching preparations and heat
are the commonest causes of irritant dermatitis of the scalp. It is important to
remember that irritant dermatitis affects only skin that has been in direct contact
with the offending agent.

Allergic dermatitis

Allergic dermatitis implies dermatitis due to the development of allergy to a
substance previously applied to the skin. Most substances causing dermatitis of
this type are of small molecular weight—less than 10,000—and act only as
partial antigens or haptens. To form complete antigens they must combine with
epidermal protein. The immunological response requires the presence of

epidermal langerhans cells to recognize the allergen and normal regional lymph glands for the cell-mediated antibody response to occur in the epidermis. The dermatitis developing in this way may spread away from the site of contact, particularly if the allergen is applied repeatedly. The scalp is relatively resistant to allergens; as with irritants, this resistance may be due to the thick horny layer but this cannot be the only factor since eczematous contact allergy is not entirely dose related.

Less well defined is the occurrence of immediate-type hypersensitivity with or without concurrent eczematous allergy (Calnan & Shuster 1963; Cronin 1979).

Clinical appearance
Irritant dermatitis affecting the scalp may commence with burning, or soreness and tightness of the scalp, within a short time of contact with the irritant. Liquid irritants most typically cause these symptoms at the scalp margins. The signs vary from slight erythema to marked oedema and exudation. Complete resolution usually takes no more than a few days. Hair breakage may occur from certain substances e.g. thioglycollates; if the scalp inflammation is severe enough diffuse hair loss may occur days to weeks after the insult, due to local inflammatory telogen effluvium.

Allergic dermatitis; the clinical picture varies considerably. Irritation of the scalp or scalp margins with little visible change, and occipital lichenification due to chronic scratching may be the only signs. More severe cases present with acute, sub-acute or chronic eczema either localized to the scalp and adjacent areas or spreading to affect other parts of the head and neck. Acute signs may mimic angio-oedema, bilateral erysipelas or dermatomyositis if periorbital oedema occurs. Many weeks, rarely months, may elapse between the onset and the spontaneous cure of allergic dermatitis.

Agents causing contact dermatitis
In a report of 70 cases of cosmetic allergy, Schorr (1974) found that 6 were due to hair dyes and rinses and that 2 were caused by shampoos.

Hair dyes. Approximately 40% of women in the USA use some form of hair dye (Corbett & Menkart 1973).

Vegetable dyes are still used though less commonly than in the past. Henna does not cause eczematous allergy but may precipitate allergic rhinitis and asthma (Cronin 1979). Chamomile is still present in some shampoos and rinses; the dye-stuff is apigenin (trihydroxyflavone). It is a potent sensitizer in those handling the plant but not when used cosmetically.

Metallic dyes are now only rarely used. Some contain nickel and chromium which are, however, securely chelated into complex molecules.

Temporary dyes (colour rinses) and semi-permanent dyes are generally safe products though the latter are often marketed as shampoos and may give an irritant reaction in susceptible individuals, or allergic dermatitis due to o-nitroparaphenylenediamine (ONPPD).

Permanent dyes are more prone to cause allergic sensitization than any other hair cosmetic preparation (Fig. 17.6). Paraphenylenediamine (PPD) may cause very acute eczematous dermatitis of the head and neck though hand dermatitis in those handling PPD is the commonest pattern. PPD is a potent sensitizer; Kligman (1966) using the maximization test and 10% PPD was able to sensitize all 24 subjects tested. Such is the notoriety of PPD that it has been banned as a hair dye in many countries; this stringent abolition may soon be relaxed since the European Economic Community has decreed that hair dyes may contain up to 6% PPD. Cases of PPD allergy are now less common, partly from better education of hairdressers and users, and also because the chemical reaction during the dyeing process is more accurately controlled and completed, leaving

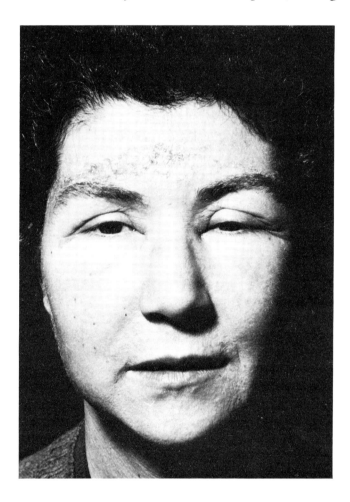

Fig. 17.6. Allergic contact dermatitis from hair dye (Slade Hospital, Oxford).

little or no free PPD. Fully polymerized PPD is harmless and inert; reactions to dyed wig hair do not therefore occur. In practice, hair dyed by individuals at home is more likely to produce allergy in the user or in those afterwards in contact with the hair, due to residual free dye remaining on the hair if adequate care is not exercised during the dying process. Paratoluenediamine (PTD) is 50% less likely to cause allergy than PPD.

If allergy to a hair dye is suspected, patch testing should be carried out to 1% ONPPD, 1% PPD and 1% PTD. Cross-reactivity may be a problem in such cases; thus para-dye dermatitis may be potentiated by certain antihistamines (MacKie & MacKie 1964) and rubber antioxidants (Schønning & Hjorth, 1969).

Hair bleaches. These are commonly sold as twin packs containing hydrogen peroxide and ammonium persulphate. The latter is potentially both an irritant and a sensitizer; Calnan & Shuster (1963) showed it to be a histamine releaser causing facial swelling and scalp itching—this is more likely in dermographic subjects. The propensity of persulphate to liberate histamine was confirmed by Mahzoon *et al.* (1977). If too-high concentrations are applied for too long, an acute irritant reaction may occur with hair breakage (Fisher & Dooms-Goosens 1976). For patch testing, 1% aqueous ammonium persulphate should be used.

Permanent wave solutions. Sensitivity reactions to thioglycollates are extremely rare though mild transient irritant dermatitis is not uncommon. Necrosis of the scalp has been described from incorrect use of a thioglycollate solution, compounded by attempted reversal of the reaction with a borate neutralizer (Ippen & Seubert 1975); the necrosis may have been due to the heat generated.

Hair straighteners and depilatories. These often contain thioglycollates but are less likely to cause significant reactions than permanent wave solutions (Foussereau & Benezra 1970).

Setting lotions. The main ingredient is usually polyvinylpyrrolidone which seems to have no allergic potential. If a reaction to such lotions occurs it is more likely to be due to added dyes.

Hair tonics, stimulants and restorers. Such preparations are generally innocuous. Kerner *et al.* (1973) described burning and exudation of the scalp due to a stimulant containing century plant extract which was used on the scalp in common baldness.

Shampoos. Since they are applied in dilute solution for a short time irritant reactions are rare though shampoos are the commonest cause of hand dermatitis in hairdressers.

Men's hair creams. Allergy to perfume, lanolin or preservatives may occur.

Shaving preparations. The recorded cases of irritant and allergic reactions have been to perfumes found mostly in after-shave lotions.

Hair nets. These are no longer popular but may still be worn by some older women. Calnan *et al.* (1958) described 27 cases of nylon hair net dermatitis; 23 of the patients were over 40 years of age. The eruption affected the neck, ears and frontal hairline, simulating seborrhoeic dermatitis and lichen simplex. All the cases showed positive patch tests either to the net or to its marginal elastic. Azo- and anthroquinone dyes, PPD and certain disperse dyes are the commonest specific allergens: several of the cases had noted skin reactions to nylon

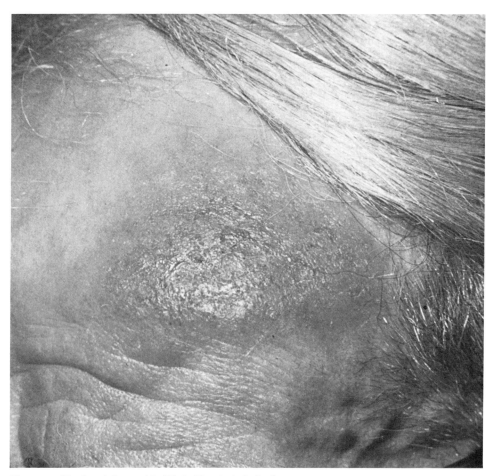

Fig. 17.7. Hat-band dermatitis (Slade Hospital, Oxford).

stockings, clothing or gloves. Six other cases of hairnet dermatitis were documented by Cronin (1980).

Hat-band dermatitis. The site affected by the dermatitis varies, though most cases involve the forehead (Fig. 17.7). Leather used to be the most frequent allergen (Bett 1958) but fabric or plastic are now the more likely offenders. Dermatitis has been described from laurel oil used to add lustre to felt hats (Foussereau *et al.* 1967). Some hat bands have a varnish finish containing colophony.

Wig reactions. Ill-fitting wigs frequently cause friction and irritant damage to localized parts of the scalp, typically under the adhesion band. Allergic dermatitis may occur to adhesive substances; allergy cannot develop against completely polymerized hair dye in wigs.

References
Bett D.C.G. (1958) The potassium dichromate patch test. *Transactions of St. John's Hospital Dermatological Society*, **40**, 41.
Calnan C.D., Marten R.H. & Wilson H.T.H. (1958) Nylon hairnet dermatitis. *British Medical Journal*, **ii**, 544.
Calnan C.D. & Shuster S. (1963) Reactions to ammonium persulphate. *Archives of Dermatology*, **88**, 812.
Corbett J.F. & Menkart J. (1973) Hair colouring. *Cutis*, **12**, 190.
Cronin E. (1979) Immediate type hypersensitivity to henna. *Contact Dermatitis*, **5**, 198.
Cronin E. (1980) *Contact Dermatitis*, 1st edn. Edinburgh, Churchill Livingstone.
Fisher A.A. & Dooms-Goosens A. (1976) Persulphate hair bleach reactions. *Archives of Dermatology*, **112**, 1407.
Foussereau J., Benezra C.I. & Durisson G. (1967) Contact dermatitis from laurel. I. Clinical aspects. *Transactions of St. John's Hospital Dermatological Society*, **53**, 141.
Foussereau J. & Benezra C.I. (1970) *Les Eczemas Allergiques Professionals*. Paris, Masson, p. 385.
Ippen H. & Scubert A. (1975) Kopfhautnekrosen durch Haarbehandlung—eine Erklarurgsmoglichkeit. *Hautarzt*, **26**, 598.
Kerner J., Mitchell J. & Maibach H.I. (1973) Irritant contact dermatitis from *Agave Americana* L. *Archives of Dermatology*, **108**, 102.
Kligman A. (1966) The identification of contact allergens by human assay. *Journal of Investigative Dermatology*, **47**, 393.
MacKie B.S. & MacKie L.S. (1964) Cross-sensitivity in dermatitis due to hair dyes. *Australian Journal of Dermatology*, **7**, 189.
Mahzoon S., Yamamoto S. & Greaves M.W. (1977) Response of the skin to ammonium persulphate. *Acta Dermato-venerologica*, **57**, 125.
Schønning L. & Hjorth N. (1969) Gross-sensitivity between hair dyes and rubber chemicals. *Berufsdermatosen*, **17**, 100.
Schorr W.F. (1974) Cosmetic allergy: diagnosis, incidence and management. *Cutis*, **14**, 844.

Acne necrotica (references p. 477)

History and nomenclature
The variability of this clinical syndrome no doubt accounts for the multiplicity of

terms applied to it. In current use for two clinical variants are acne frontalis, suggested by Hebra, and acne necrotica, suggested by Boeck. The acne pilaris of Bazin and the acne varioliformis of Hebra are commonly regarded as redundant synonyms (Pignot 1953).

Acne miliaris necrotica of Sabouraud is a third clinical variant, with some distinctive features.

Aetiology

These syndromes have been regarded as a folliculitis, probably of staphylococcal origin, occurring in seborrhoeic subjects with an allergic hypersensitivity to this organism (Pignot 1953). There appears to be no recent work substantiating this hypothesis and it is perhaps wisest to consider these syndromes as being of unknown origin, with stress often incriminated in precipitating recurrences (Calnan & O'Neill 1952). Men are affected more often than women; most patients are aged 30–50 but cases occur at any age past puberty.

Pathology

The histological changes are not pathognomonic. There is a folliculitis, complicated in the more severe lesions by necrosis destroying the follicle and the neighbouring dermis. Some lesions submitted to biopsy show only infected excoriations.

Clinical features (Müller 1964)

Acne necrotica and its variant acne frontalis present as indolent papulopustules with central necrosis, healing slowly to leave varioliform scars. They may be slightly painful and are sometimes pruritic. They occur most characteristically along the frontal hairs, but also involve the scalp where they may leave small patches of cicatricial alopecia; less often they occur on the cheeks and neck or on the chest and back (Stritzler *et al.* 1951). Untreated the condition runs a long course, although there may be only a small number of active lesions present at any one time.

Acne necrotica miliaris (Montgomery 1937) may coexist with the forms just described, but much more commonly occurs alone. Pruritus, which may be distressingly severe, takes the patient to his doctor. The primary lesions are minute follicular vesicles but these are rapidly excoriated. There may be a few or many. New lesions continue to develop at irregular intervals, but the pruritus seems often to be disproportionately severe in relation to the objective change.

Diagnosis

In acne necrotica the distribution of the lesions and their morphology serve to differentiate such diseases, now uncommon in temperate regions, as papulonecrotic tuberculides and tertiary syphilis.

The pruritic miliary form should never be diagnosed unless pediculosis and dermatitis herpetiformis have been excluded, the former by searching for the lice, and the latter by the presence of lesions elsewhere.

Treatment

All forms show a temporary response to a broad spectrum antibiotic and such treatment is useful in severe cases. Many patients find it necessary to take a small maintenance dose, e.g. oxytetracycline 250 mg daily, as in acne vulgaris. Topical corticosteroid/antibiotic preparations are of limited value. If it is practicable attempts should be made to reduce stress.

References

Calnan C.D. & O'Neill D. (1952) Some observations on acne necrotica. *Transactions of the St. John's Hospital Dermatological Society*, **31**, 12.

Miller H. (1964) Beitrag zur Therapie der Akne nekroticans. *Dermatologische Wochenschrift* **149**, 495.

Montgomery H. (1937) Acne necrotica miliaris of the scalp. *Acta Dermo-Sifiliograficas*, **36**, 10.

Pignot M. (1953) L'Acné nécrotique du cuir chevelu. In *Affections de la Chevelure et du Cuir Chevelu*, ed. A. Desex. Paris, Masson, p. 132.

Stritzler C., Friedman R. & Loveman A.B. (1951) Acne necrotica. Relation to acne necrotica miliaris and response to penicillin and other antibiotics. *A.M.A. Archives of Dermatology and Syphilology*, **64**, 464.

Folliculitis cheloidalis nuchae (syn. acne cheloidalis)

This chronic inflammatory folliculitis of the nape of the neck occurs exclusively in males and is certainly more severe and probably also more frequent in Negroids than in Caucasoids. It may begin at any time after puberty, usually between 14 and 25. Many of those affected suffer or have suffered from acne vulgaris, many more have no other skin lesions. The cause of the condition is unknown; a genetic factor is probably implicated. Histologically chronic folliculitis and foreign body granulomata surrounding fragments of hair are the main features.

Follicular papules and pustules develop in irregularly linear clusters on the nape just below the hair line and extend in further crops at long or short intervals towards the occiput. Firm cheloid papules follow the folliculitis and become confluent to form horizontal bands or plaques. These may co-exist with new follicular papules and discharging sinuses.

Treatment with topical antibacterial agents and with systemic antibiotics may possibly restrain the progress of the inflammatory changes but not reliably or completely. The cheloids may be successfully excised by plastic surgery (Cosman & Wolff 1972).

Reference
Cosman B. & Wolff M. (1972) Acne keloidasis. *Plastic and Reconstructive Surgery,* **50,** 25.

Pseudofolliculitis

Pseudofolliculitis is a common inflammatory disorder of the follicles, most commonly occurring when tightly coiled or very curly hair is closely shaved, and the tips of shaved hairs either penetrate the follicular wall or grow back to re-enter the skin near the follicle. Pseudofolliculitis may occur also if the hairs are plucked (Dilaimy 1976) and in such cases is caused by the abnormal regrowth of the hairs in injured follicles. Cocci can sometimes be grown from the lesions, but the condition is primarily mechanical in origin (Straus & Kligman 1956).

Pseudofolliculitis of the beard is extremely common in Negroid men, amongst whom it is almost universal in some degree (Brauner & Flandermeyer 1977) but it occurs in other races and may be seen also in hirsute women (Fig. 17.8). The importance of genetic predisposition has been emphasized (Alexander 1974). It was present extensively in the scalps of four Negroid boys whose heads had been shaved, and regressed spontaneously as the hair regrew (Smith & Odom 1977).

Pseudofolliculitis presents clinically as an eruption of follicular papules or pustules on the sides of the neck and over the angles of the jaw. In some cases unsightly nodules may form and may leave conspicuous scars (Fig. 17.9).

The logical and effective treatment is to stop shaving and there are cases in which this provides the only solution. If wearing a beard is not acceptable to the patient a corticosteroid/antibiotic cream may be helpful in mild cases. In severe

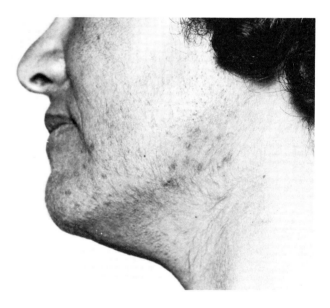

Fig. 17.8. Pseudofolliculitis in a hirsute woman aged 35 (Addenbrooke's Hospital, Cambridge).

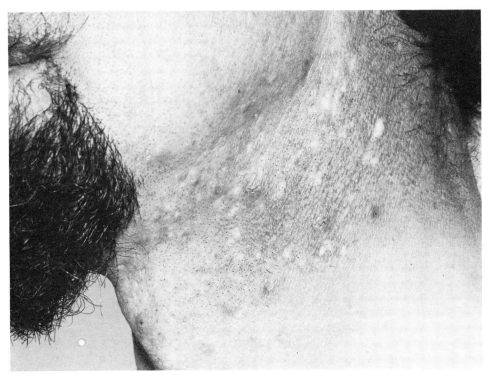

Fig. 17.9. Pseudofolliculitis leaving unsightly scars (Addenbrooke's Hospital, Cambridge).

cases the use of a chemical depilatory every 3 days may be recommended (Straus & Kligman 1956).

References

Alexander A.M. (1974) Pseudofolliculitis diathesis. *Archives of Dermatology*, **109**, 729.
Brauner C.J. & Flandermeyer L.K. (1977) Pseudofolliculitis barbae. *International Journal of Dermatology*, **16**, 520.
Dilaimy M. (1976) Pseudofolliculitis of the legs. *Archives of Dermatology*, **112**, 507.
Smith J.D. & Odom R.B. (1977) Pseudofolliculitis capitis. *Archives of Dermatology*, **113**, 328.
Straus J.S. & Kligman A.M. (1956) Pseudofolliculitis of the beard. *Archives of Dermatology*, **74**, 533.

Pruritus of the scalp

Many inflammatory diseases of the scalp may be associated with itching. It may both precede and accompany the development of allergic reactions to hair dyes and other chemicals and it may accompany urticaria.

Itching of the scalp may be troublesome in psoriasis (p. 465) especially in patients who are under stress or who are depressed. Pityriasis capitis may cause some irritation but in this condition too the irritation is rarely severe except under stress. The scalp may be involved, but seldom sufficiently severely to be a specific cause of complaint in generalized pruritus, the causes of which will not be discussed here. More frequently, in generalized pruritus without visible skin changes, the scalp is spared.

Irritation of the scalp may occur in dermatitis herpetiformis in which the lesions in other parts of the body may suggest the diagnosis.

Persistent irritation of the scalp, particularly in children but also at any age and at all levels of social respectability, may be caused by pediculosis, and in all circumstances lice and their eggs should be carefully sought.

Intense pruritus, temporarily localized to small focal sites is characteristic of acne necrotica (p. 475) which is seen mainly in men working under continuous tension. More diffuse irritation of the scalp, without visible lesions, may occur in either sex.

Itching or tenderness or sometimes other uncomfortable sensations may occur as a prominent symptom of mild androgenetic alopecia in a depressed patient (p. 77).

The treatment of pruritus of the scalp is the treatment of its cause.

Hair casts

Definition

Hair casts (syn. peripilar keratin casts) are firm, yellowish-white accretions ensheathing but not attached to scalp hairs and freely movable up and down the affected shafts (Kligman 1957).

Such lesions found in scaly and seborrhoeic disorders of the scalp had previously been termed 'hair eaters' (Crocker 1932).

Pathology

In cross-section casts are composed of a central layer of retained internal root sheath and an outer thick keratinous layer. Scalp histology shows the follicular openings to be packed with parakeratotic squames which break off at intervals to form hair casts.

Casts are found quite commonly in scaly, mainly parakeratotic conditions of the scalp such as psoriasis, pityriasis capitas, seborrhoeic dermatitis and pityriasis amiantacea (Dawber 1979). Cases have been described in association with traction hair styles (Rollins 1961; Crovato *et al.* 1980) and hair sprays (Scott 1959).

Clinical findings

Hair casts may occur as an isolated abnormality unrelated to any overt scalp disease (Figs. 17.10, 17.11); such cases may mimic pediculosis capitis (Brunner & Facq 1957) and have been termed pseudonits (Keipert 1974; Kohn 1977). Girls and young women are most commonly affected; hundreds of casts may

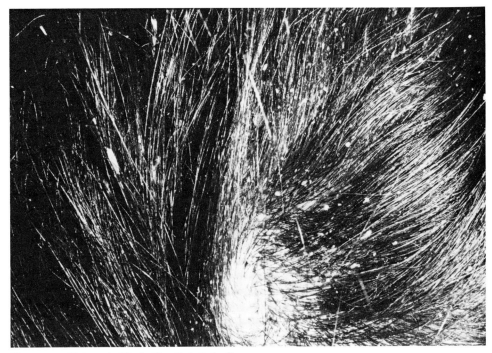

Fig. 17.10. Hair casts (Slade Hospital, Oxford).

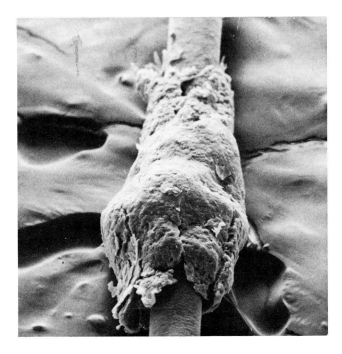

Fig. 17.11. Hair cast in the scanning electronmicroscope (Slade Hospital, Oxford).

develop within a few days. No cause is known but sex-linked inheritance has been suggested (Kligman 1957). It is possible that this type may represent an unusual manifestation of psoriasis.

If patients with scaly parakeratotic diseases of the scalp complain of persistent dandruff which resists apparently adequate treatment this is likely to be due to multiple hair casts.

Diagnosis

In the absence of associated scalp disease, casts may be mistaken for pediculosis capitas, trichorrhexis nodosa or hair knots (Dawber 1974). Of these nodal shaft abnormalities, only hair casts are freely movable along the hair.

Treatment

Any causative scalp disease must be treated. Keratolytic preparations and shampoos that readily improve scalp scaling frequently fail to remove casts; prolonged brushing and combing is necessary to slide casts off the affected hairs (Bowyer 1974; Dawber 1977).

References

Bowyer A. (1974) Peripilar keratin casts. *British Journal of Dermatology*, **90**, 231.
Brunner M.J. & Facq J.M. (1957) A pseudoparasite of scalp hair. *Archives of Dermatology*, **75**, 583.
Crocker R. (1932) In *Jadassohn's Handbuch der Haut und Geschlechtskrankheiten*, vol. 13. Berlin, Springer-Verlag.
Crovato F., Rebora A. & Crosti C. (1980) Hair casts. *Dermatologica*, **160**, 281.
Dawber R.P.R. (1974) Knotting of scalp hair. *British Journal of Dermatology*, **91**, 169.
Dawber R.P.R. (1977) The scalp and hair care in psoriasis. *Journal of the Psoriasis Association*, **16**, 5.
Keipert J.A. (1974) Peripilar keratin casts (pseudonits) and psoriasis. *Medical Journal of Australia*, **1**, 218.
Kligman A.M. (1957) Hair casts. *Archives of Dermatology*, **75**, 509.
Kohn S.R. (1977) Hair casts or pseudonits. *Journal of the American Medical Association*, **2–8**, 2058.
Rollins T.G. (1961) Traction folliculitis with hair casts and alopecia. *American Journal of Diseases of Children*, **101**, 131.
Scott M.J. (1959) Peripilar keratin casts. *Archives of Dermatology*, **79**, 654.

Rosacea (references p. 484)

Aetiology

Rosacea is a common disorder affecting principally the facial skin. Episodes of flushing are followed by persistent telangiectasia, and the development of papules and pustules. The cause of the condition is unknown. The traditionally accepted association between rosacea and gastrointestinal disease has not been confirmed (Søbye 1950; Marks *et al.* 1977). Psychological factors are widely believed to play some part in rosacea but there is no reliable evidence that they cause it (Marks 1968) although some secondary anxiety and depression are common.

Females are affected more frequently than males and usually between the ages of 30 and 50 but earlier and later onset are not unusual.

Exposure to light appears to play some part in the pathogenesis of rosacea as suggested by the predominant involvement of light-exposed skin, by the peak hospital attendance during the spring and early summer and by the histological changes. On the other hand rosacea is not confined to exposed skin.

Pathology
The papules consist of a pleomorphic lymphohistiocytic infiltrate. Granulomatous changes may be present. The dermis shows a higher degree of elastotic change than is seen in the facial skin of control subjects (Marks & Harcourt Webster 1969).

Clinical features
Telangiectasia, papules and pustules occur in very variable proportions. There may be extensive and conspicuous telangiectasia as the only change, or this may be associated with dull red papules or the papules may predominate and the telangiectasia be relatively mild. The cheeks and the forehead are most commonly affected. Papules in area other than the face—the limbs, shoulders and the chest—are more frequent when the facial rosacea is severe, but can also occur in the presence of only mild facial changes (Marks & Wilson-Jones 1969; Röckl *et al.* 1969).

Involvement of the bald scalp (Gajewska 1975) by papules, pustules or telangiectasia is not uncommon, and may accompany severe or mild facial rosacea (Fig. 17.12).

Untreated rosacea may run a very long course and be a source of intense embarrassment to the patient. Moreover in a proportion of cases, and not necessarily in the more severe cases, occular involvement may lead to keratitis.

Diagnosis (Steigleder 1971)
Diagnostic difficulties are likely only when rosacea of the scalp accompanies minimal facial lesions.

Treatment
The use of fluorinated topical steroids should be avoided for they intend to increase the telangiectasia and to give rise to a troublesome folliculitis. In very mild cases the regular application of 2% precipitated sulphur in emulsifying ointment may suffice. In other cases oral tetracycline is the treatment of choice, unless contraindicated by pregnancy or the possibility of pregnancy. Most cases will respond to oxytetracycline 250 mg twice daily for 3–6 months. About 20% relapse rapidly when the antibiotic is discontinued, and some others do so within

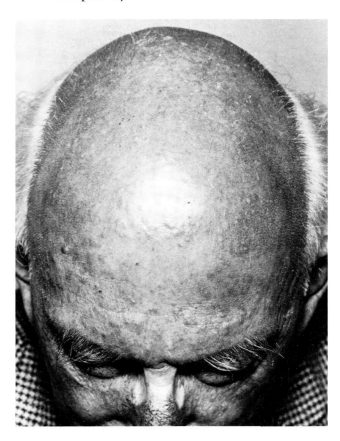

Fig. 17.12. Rosacea of the
bald scalp in an elderly man
(Addenbrooke's Hospital,
Cambridge).

a few months, but some remain symptom-free for long periods (Knight & Vickers
1975).

References
Gajewska M. (1975) Rosacea of common male baldness. *British Journal of Dermatology*, **93**, 65.
Knight A.G. & Vickers C.F.H. (1975) A follow-up of tetracycline treated rosacea. *British Journal of
    Dermatology*, **93**, 577.
Marks R. (1968) Concepts in the pathogenesis of rosacea. *British Journal of Dermatology*, **80**, 170.
Marks R., Beard R.J., Clark M.L., Kwok M. & Robertson W.B. (1967) Gastrointestinal observations
    in rosacea. *Lancet*, **i**, 739.
Marks R. & Harcourt-Webster J.N. (1969) Histopathology of rosacea. *Archives of Dermatology*, **160**,
    683.
Marks R. & Wilson-Jones, E. (1969) Disseminated rosacea. *British Journal of Dermatology*, **81**, 16.
Röckl H., Schropl F. & Scheren M. (1969) Rosacea mit extrafacialer Localisation. *Hautarzt*, **20**,
    349.
Søbye P. (1950) Aetiology and pathogenesis of rosacea. *Acta Dermato-venereologica (Stockholm)*,
    30, 117.
Steigleder G.K. (1971) Differentiale diagnose der Rosacea. *Hautarzt*, **22**, 91.

Rare diseases which characteristically affect the scalp

Dissecting cellulitis of the scalp

History and nomenclature
This rare disease was first described by Nobl of Vienna in 1905. Three years later Hoffmann (1908) gave it the name perifolliculitis capitis abscedens et suffodiens, by which it is still sometimes known. In English-speaking countries the term 'dissecting cellulitis of the scalp' (Barney 1931) is usually preferred.

Aetiology
Dissecting cellulitis occurs predominantly in males between 18 and 40 and more often in Negroids than in Caucasoids. Its cause is unknown. No specific organism has been isolated from the lesions, and although the process has much in common with acne conglobata, with which it may coexist, the latter too is of unknown origin. The description of the pathological process as a 'keratinous granuloma' (Moyer & Williams 1962) throws no light on the source of the follicular disruption.

Pathology
The follicles are destroyed by an intense folliculitis, which is succeeded by a chronic granulomatous infiltrate containing foreign-body giant cells.

Clinical features (Hoffmann 1908; Carmie 1962)
Firm skin-coloured nodules develop near the vertex, and later become softer and fluctuant. By confluence the nodules form tubular ridges in an irregularly cerebriform pattern, on a red and oedematous background. Thin blood-stained pus exudes from crusted sinuses, and pressure on one region of the scalp may cause the discharge of pus from a sinus in a neighbouring intercommunicating ridge. There is patchy loss of hair. In some cases cervical adenitis may develop, but it is usually absent even when the disease is acute (Moyer & Williams 1962).

The extent of the disease is variable but its course is prolonged with partial remission and acute exacerbations. Depressed scars at the sites of healed nodules may be seen in areas still active. Spontaneous recovery can occur, when the scarring determines the cosmetic prognosis; hair shed from temporarily oedematous skin regrows. Squamous carcinoma is a rare late complication of dissecting cellulitis (Curry *et al.* 1981).

Diagnosis
The follicular pustules of a ringworm infection should not cause confusion. In cutis verticis gyrata inflammatory changes are usually absent, and if present are follicular and only a minor and inconsistent feature of the disease.

Treatment
This is most unsatisfactory. Some authors have found no response to antibiotics (Moyer & Williams 1962) and this is certainly to be expected in the later stages of the disease. At an early stage oxytetracycline or clindamycin reduces the inflammatory reaction, and may in severe cases be combined with systemic corticosteroids. 'Scalping' and grafting have been recommended in intractable chronic cases (Moschella *et al.* 1967).

References
Barney R.E. (1931) Dissecting cellulitis of the scalp. *Archives of Dermatology and Syphilology*, **23**, 503.
Carmine R.L. (1962) Perifolliculitis capitis abscedens et suffodiens. *Scottish Medical Journal*, **7**, 488.
Curry S.S., Gaither D.H. & King L.E. (1981) Squamous carcinoma arising in dissecting perifolliculitis of the scalp. *Journal of the American Academy of Dermatology*, **4**, 673.
Hoffmann E. (1908) Sitzungsberichte. *Dermatologische Zeitschrift*, **15**, 122.
Moschella C.L., Klein M.H. & Miller R.J. (1967) Perifolliculitis capitis abscedens et suffodiens. *Archives of Dermatology*, **96**, 195.
Moyer D.G. & Williams R.M. (1962) Perifolliculitis capitis abscedens et suffodiens. *Archives of Dermatology*, **85**, 378.
Nobl G. (1905) Verhandlungen der Wiener Dermatologischen Gesellschaft. *Archiv für Dermatologie und Syphilologie*, **74**, 80.

Cutis verticis gyrata

History and nomenclature
The term 'cutis verticis gyrata' describes the hypertrophy and folding of the skin of the scalp, to present a gyrate or cerebriform appearance. The term was proposed by Unna in 1907, but many cases had previously been reported under other diagnostic labels (see Polan & Butterworth (1953) for historical review). Cutis verticis gyrata (CVG) is now used by authorities on mental deficiency to describe the distinctive disorder of which the scalp changes are one feature, and which in dermatological texts has been often referred to as 'Primary' or 'Idiopathic' CVG. Dermatologists on the other hand use the term to describe a morphological syndrome with many causes. The French term pachydermie plicaturée invites further confusion with pachydermoperiostosis, of which CVG is a feature (Touraine & Golé 1938; Touraine 1955).

Pathology
The essential abnormality appears to be overgrowth of the scalp in relation to the underlying skull. Some predisposing factor must be postulated since it occurs in only a small proportion of cases of each of the conditions with which it is associated. The histological findings depend on the essential disease. The naevoid forms usually prove to be melanocytic. Biopsies in the primary form of CVG (Paulson & Dudley 1966) showed possible sebacous hyperplasia, but no obvious excess of collagen.

Aetiology and clinical features

Primary CVG. This syndrome, which occurs almost exclusively in males, is probably genetically determined, but its mode of inheritance is uncertain (Åkesson 1965a). In one pedigree sex-linked recessive inheritance seemed possible (Åkesson 1965b) but most cases appear to be sporadic. It has been reported in association with Darier's disease and with tuberous sclerosis. It accounts for 0.5% of the retarded population in Sweden (Åkesson 1964), Scotland (MacGillivray 1967) and the United States (Paulson 1974), and for 1–2% of institutionalized severely retarded males. The prevalence of the condition may be still higher since there is evidence that at least some patients with the Lennox–Gastart syndrome—retardation with an electroencephalograph showing slow and irregular spate and wave complexes—later develop CVG (Paulson 1974).

The longitudinal and irregularly parallel folds of the scalp may appear in late childhood or at puberty and slowly become more accentuated. The IQ is rarely over 35 and cerebral palsy (spastic diplegia) and epilepsy are present (Kratter 1958; Berg & Windrath-Scott 1962; Åkesson 1964).

Pachydermoperiostosis. This genetically determined syndrome also occurs mainly in men and has often been confused with CVG. It differs from it in several particulars. The scalp is folded but the skin of the face is affected, as is that of the hands and feet. The cutaneous changes, which are accompanied by thickening of the phalanges and of the long bones of the limbs, progress for 10 to 15 years, then become static.

Acromegaly. Mild degrees of CVG are not uncommon in acromegaly, but more severe forms have been reported (Zeisler & Wieder 1940; Hung-Chiung 1955; Serfling & Foelsche 1959).

Other endocrine disorders. Rarely CVG has been associated with cretinism or myxoedema, but the significance of these case reports is uncertain (Polan & Butterworth 1953).

Naevi. Naevi may assume a folded or cerebriform structure and thus simulate CVG. The naevus is present at birth and usually covers only a relatively small area (Hammond & Ransome 1937) but may slowly increase in size to cover most of the scalp (e.g. Lenormant 1920). Most of the reported cases have been naevi of melanocytic type, but neurofibromas and fibromas can assume this form (McConnell & Davies 1943).

Treatment
In the majority of cases only symptomatic measures are practicable. Plastic

surgery was helpful in CVG in acromegaly (Abu-Jamra & Dinsich 1966) and may of course be indicated in cerebriform naevi.

References

Abu-Jamra F. & Dinsich D.F. (1966) Cutis verticis gyrata. *American Journal of Surgery,* 111, 274.

Åkesson H.O. (1964) Cutis verticis gyrata and mental deficiency in Sweden. *Acta medica Scandinavica,* 175, 115.

Åkesson H.O. (1965a) Cutis verticis gyrata and mental deficiency in Sweden. II. Genetic aspects. *Acta medica Scandinavica,* 177, 459.

Åkesson H.O. (1965b) Cutis verticis gyrata, thyroid aplasia and mental deficiency. *Acta Geneticae Medicae et Gemellologiae,* 14, 200.

Berg J.M. & Windrath-Scott A. (1962) Cutis verticis gyrata with particular reference to its association with mental subnormality. *Journal of Mental Deficiency Research,* 6, 75.

Hammond G. & Ransome H.K. (1937) Cerebriform nevus resembling cutis verticis gyrata. *Archives of Surgery,* 35, 309.

Hung-Chiung L. (1955) Cutis verticis gyrata associated with acromegaly. *Chinese Medical Journal,* 73, 320.

Kratten F.I. (1958) The incidence of cutis verticis gyrata in three low-grade mental defectives. *Journal of Medical Science,* 104, 850.

Lenormant C.H. (1920) La pachydermie vorticellée du cuir chevelu. *Annales de Dermatologie et de Syphiligraphie,* 1, 225.

MacGillivray R.C. (1967) Cutis verticis gyrata and mental retardation. *Scottish Medical Journal,* 12, 450.

McConnell L.H. & Davies A.J.M. (1943) Massive fibroma of the scalp. *Annals of Surgery,* 118, 154.

Paulson G.W. (1974) Cutis verticis gyrata and the Lennox syndrome. *Developmental Medicine and Child Neurology,* 16, 196.

Paulson G. & Dudley A.W. (1966) Cutis verticis gyrata. *Confinia Neurologica,* 28, 432.

Polan S. & Butterworth T. (1953) Cutis verticis gyrata. *Americana Journal of Mental Deficiency,* 57, 613.

Serfling H.J. & Foelsche W. (1959) Extensive Form einer *Cutis verticis gyrata* bei Hypophysenadenome. *Zentralblatt für Chirurgie,* 84, 473.

Touraine A. & Golé L. (1938) La pachydermie plicaturée avec pachypériostose des extremités. (Etat actuel de la question). *Progrès Médical,* 65, 263.

Touraine A. (1955) *L'Hérédité en Médecine.* Paris, Masson, p. 486.

Zeisler E.P. & Wieder L.J. (1940) Cutis verticis gyrata and acromegaly. *Archives of Dermatology and Syphilology,* 42, 1092.

Lipedematous alopecia

This rare condition has so far been reported only in Negroid women, was first described by Cornbleet in 1935, and was named lipedematous alopecia by Coskey *et al.* (1961). The cause is unknown. Hyperextensible joints were present in one case (Curtis & Heising 1964).

The epidermis shows some atrophy and some follicles are replaced by scar tissue. The subcutaneous fat was increased in thickness at the expense of the dermis. The latter showed some lymphocytic infiltration.

The patients, aged 28–75, complained of itching, soreness or tenderness of the scalp. The hair was sparse and short. The scalp was palpably thickened and was of spongy or boggy consistency.

References

Cornbleet T. (1935) Cutis verticis gyrata? lipoma? *Archives of Dermatology and Syphilology*, **32**, 688.

Coskey R.J., Fosnough R.P. & Finn G. (1961) Lipedematous alopecia. *Archives of Dermatology*, **84**, 619.

Curtis J.W. & Heising R.A. (1964) Lipedematous alopecia associated with skin hyperelasticity. *Archives of Dermatology*, **89**, 819.

Skin diseases in which lesions may occur in the scalp

Ichthyosis

The term ichthyosis is traditionally applied to a heterogeneous group of mainly hereditary disorders characterized in some degree by dryness and scaling of the skin. Ichthyosis vulgaris comprises two different diseases (Wells & Kerr 1965).

Autosomal dominant ichthyosis

In this, the commonest form of ichthyosis, dryness and scaling of the skin become apparent during the second year or later. The changes are most marked on the back and on the exterior aspects of the limbs, and the flexures are spread. The scales are small and white. Keratosis pilaris is frequent, and is often conspicuous. There may be some fine scaling of the scalp but there is no hair loss.

Sex-linked recessive ichthyosis

From early infancy large dark scales are present on the trunk and the side of the face, and tend to encroach on the flexures. The scalp is scaly and the hair is sometimes coarse and dry; there may be patches of cicatricial alopecia (Harris 1947).

References

Harris H. (1947) A pedigree of sex-linked ichthyosis vulgaris. *Annals of Eugenics*, **14**, 10.

Wells R.S. & Kerr C.B. (1965) Genetic classification of ichthyosis. *Archives of Dermatology*, **92**, 1.

Darier's disease (references p. 491)

History and nomenclature

Jean Darier (1856–1938) of the Hôpital St Louis, Paris, described in 1889 the disease which now bears his name. Misinterpretation of the histological findings was responsible for the misleading term 'psorospermosis', which was soon abandoned. 'Keratosis follicularis', the term commonly applied, invites confusion with other forms of follicular keratosis, and the eponymous Darier's disease is therefore preferred.

Aetiology

Darier's disease is a hereditary defect of keratinization determined by an autosomal dominant gene (Getzler & Flint 1966). Its prevalence in Denmark has been estimated as 1:100,000 (Svendsen & Albuchtron 1959); it has been reported from most countries.

The essential abnormality is a defect in the tonofilament–desmosome complex.

Pathology

Several lacunae appear above the basal cells and thence extend irregularly through the malpighian layer. Cells around the lucunae undergo premature keratinization and become enlarged and separated from their neighbours; a dark nucleus is surrounded by clear cytoplasm. These cells are the so-called 'corps ronds', which give rise to the 'grains', shrunken cells seen in the upper layer of the epidermis.

Clinical features

The appearance of the first lesion is commonly in childhood, but may be developed until the fourth decade or later. The characteristic lesion is a brown, warty, rather greasy papule. These papules may coalesce to form warty, malodorous plaques (Fig. 17.13).

The sites most commonly affected are the face, the flexures and the mid-chest and back. Some involvement of the scalp is frequent and may simulate seborrhoea. Less commonly, there are hypertrophic lesions of the scalp and behind the ears (Elsbach and Nater 1960). In such cases there may be some hair loss; exceptionally there may be extensive cicatricial alopecia (Kuske & Krebs 1965).

Whilst physical development may be normal, some affected individuals are of short stature, and in many intellectual development also is retarded. Distinct changes in the nails—longitudinal white and red bands associated with terminal V-shaped splits—may support the diagnosis, which can usually be made with confidence on clinical grounds, and is readily confirmed histologically.

Treatment

Treatment is on the whole disappointing, but the topical application of retinoic acid (Hesbacher 1970) causes temporary regression of the lesions, and can be repeated as necessary.

Encouraging results are being obtained by oral treatment with the aromatic retinoid 10-9359, Tigasone.

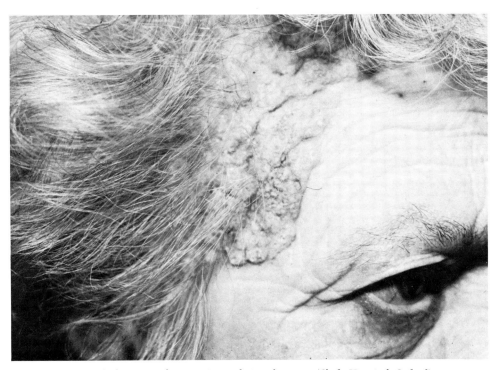

Fig. 17.13. Darier's disease with extensive scalp involvement (Slade Hospital, Oxford).

References

Darier J. (1889) De la psorospermie folliculaire végétante. *Annales de Dermatologie et de Syphiligraphie*, **10**, 597.

Elsbach E.M. & Nater J.P. (1960) La forme hypertrophique de la maladie de Darier. *Dermatologica*, **120**, 93.

Getzler N.A. & Flint A. (1966) Keratosis follicularis. *Archives of Dermatology*, **93**, 545.

Hesbacher E.N. (1970) Zosteriform keratosis follicularis treated topically with Tretinoin. *Archives of Dermatology*, **102**, 209.

Kuske H. & Krebs A. (1965) Morbus Darier mit subtotaler Alopecie. *Dermatologica*, **131**, 108.

Svendsen I.B. & Albuchtron B. (1959) The prevalence of dyskeratosis follicularis (Darier's disease) in Denmark. *Acta Dermato-venereologica*, **39**, 256.

Dermatitis herpetiformis (references p. 493)

History and nomenclature

The bullous erythemas have suffered to an unusual extent from international confusion in nomenclature. Dermatitis herpetiformis is now increasingly accepted. Duhring-Brocq disease is the only synonym in current use. The history of the disease was reviewed by Alexander in 1975.

Aetiology

The disease affects all ages, but onset between 10 and 50 is usual. The pathogenesis is not fully understood; a gluten-sensitive enteropathy is commonly associated and immunofluorescence studies of the apparently normal skin show granular deposits of IgA in the tips of dermal papillae, or sometimes a band-like deposit of the same immunoglobulin (Seah & Fry 1975).

Pathology

The bullae are subepidermal. The initial lesion is a small collection of polymorphonuclear and eosinophil leucocytes which invade a papilla, accumulate at its summit, and separate epidermis from dermis (Piérard and Whimster 1961). These lesions are the site of IgA deposition.

Clinical features

A chronic, more or less symmetrical, papulovesicular eruption is present in variable severity for many years (Fig. 17.14). The sites of predilection are the elbows, buttocks, shoulders, knees, scalp and forearms. The neck, thigh, sacral area, temples and face are not uncommonly involved. In the early stages the scalp, or the scalp and face, may be the only sites affected (Björnberg & Hellgren

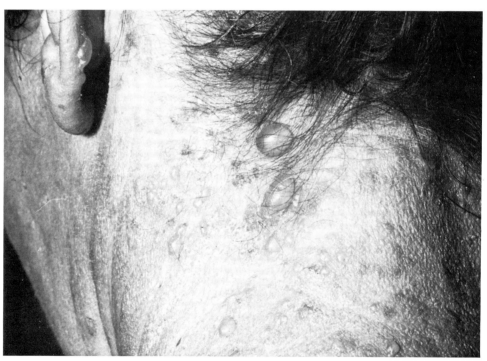

Fig. 17.14. Dermatitis herpetiformis with unusually florid lesions of the neck and scalp (Slade Hospital, Oxford).

1962) and the scalp is involved at some stage in some 30% of cases (Alexander 1975).

The presence of unexplained intensely irritable papules in the scalp should lead to a search for similar lesions elsewhere. Only in the rarer cases in which the scalp alone is involved initially or at some stage, will differentiation arise, and this can be resolved by biopsy.

Treatment

Thorough examination, investigation and evaluation should precede treatment with dapsone and perhaps a gluten-free diet.

References

Alexander J. O'D. (1975) *Dermatitis Herpetiformis*. London, Saunders, p. 22.
Björnberg A. & Hellgren L. (1962) Dermatitis herpetiformis. *Dermatologica*, **125**, 205.
Piérard J. & Whimster I. (1961) The histological diagnosis of dermatitis herpetiformis, bullous pemphigoid and erythema multiforme. *British Journal of Dermatology*, **73**, 253.
Seah P.P. & Fry L. (1975) Immunoglobulins in the skin in dermatitis herpetiformis and their relevance in diagnosis. *British Journal of Dermatology*, **92**, 157.

Follicular mucinosis (references p. 496)

History and nomenclature

Descriptions of this distinctive clinico-pathological entity were published by Kreibich in 1926 and by Gougerot and Blum in 1932 (Degos *et al.* 1962). The clinical and histological features were clearly defined by Pinkus in 1957. He proposed the term alopecia mucinosa, but most subsequent authors have preferred 'follicular mucinosis', since alopecia is clinically evident only when sites bearing terminal hairs are involved.

Aetiology

The cause of follicular mucinosis is unknown. Most of the reported cases of this uncommon, but far from rare, disorder fall into one of three groups (Coskey & Mehregan 1970; Emmerson 1969). The largest group consists of patients with solitary or few lesions, often on the face and scalp, clearing spontaneously in 2 months to 2 years. In a second group, also benign, the lesions are more extensive and persistent, or continue to develop at intervals for years without any evidence of associated disease. These benign forms occur at any age from early childhood onwards, but are most frequent between 10 and 40. In a third group of patients, somewhat older on average, the mucinosis is associated with a reticulosis, histological evidence of which is present from the onset.

Pathology

The outer root sheath and sebaceous gland become oedematous and develop cystic spaces in which mucin accumulates. These changes may extend to the full depth of the follicle, which may then be converted into a cystic cavity containing mucin and degenerate root sheath cells. Variable inflammatory changes in the dermis range from a sparse lymphocytic infiltrate to a granulomatous reaction. Unless the follicle is destroyed complete or almost complete reversion to normal usually occurs. Any cellular infiltrate should be carefully studied for evidence of a reticulosis.

With the electronmicroscope (Orfanos & Gahlen 1964) the epidermis has been shown to be involved. Mainly in the stratum malpighii and the granular layer organelles in the perinuclear cytoplasm disappear and the nucleus shrinks.

Clinical features (Kim & Winkelmann 1962; Emmerson 1969)
The acute benign form commonly affects the face, scalp, neck and shoulders. Skin-coloured papules or plaques of erythema show some fine scaling and patulous prominent follicles. If the scalp or eyebrows or male beard are involved the patient seeks advice on account of the loss of hair from the affected follicles. In sites covered by vellus hair the loss is less conspicuous. The plaques tend to be 2–5 cm in diameter and change little until they resolve, usually without trace after a few months, or sometimes rather longer. There may be a single plaque, or multiple plaques developing more or less simultaneously or at intervals.

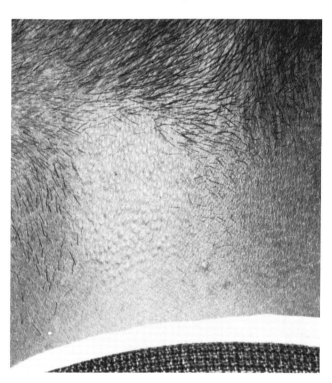

Fig. 17.15. Follicular mucinosis of the nape: typical appearance (Addenbrooke's Hospital, Cambridge).

Variations in the clinical picture have been reported, and may not be as rare as the paucity of recorded cases suggests, for they are easily misdiagnosed. A generalized eruption of papules with horny plugs, not grouped into plaques, was associated with redness and scaling of the scalp and small patches of alopecia in the eyebrows (Fig. 17.15) (Bazex *et al.* 1962). In a boy aged 11, groups of papuls on the neck, popliteal flexures, one knee and one buttock were followed by the appearance of a single patch of alopecia of the scalp (Fig. 17.16) (Zackheim 1958). The hairs remaining in this patch were distorted telogen hairs. A man aged 36 had suffered for 3 months from an eruption of pink papules of the face and scalp, with branny scaling and patchy alopecia. The dilated follicles contained horny plugs (Goldschlag & Jablonska 1960).

In the chronic benign form lesions are more numerous, more widely ditributed and more diverse in their morphology. There may be red scaly patches or soft gelatinous plaques or nodules. The lesions may persist unchanged for

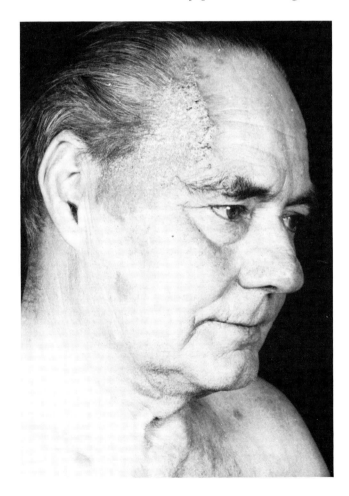

Fig. 17.16. Follicular mucinosis; more extensive erythema and scaling (Addenbrooke's Hospital, Cambridge).

years and the destruction of some follicles may lead to patches of permanent alopecia, sometimes studded with horny plugs. A characteristic case of this form of follicular mucinosis was a man aged 38 in whom multiple plaques of the scalp, arms and buttocks were unchanged after 3 years (Stevanovic 1964).

In some 15–20% of all chronic cases a reticulosis is associated (Plotnich & Abrecht 1965). The skin lesions, which do not differ from those of the chronic benign form, may develop when the reticulosis is well advanced, or the latter may first be diagnosed in a biopsy of the mucinosis (Emmerson 1969; Pinkus 1964).

In all forms pruritus is an inconstant symptom. Occasionally it may be troublesome in the chronic forms.

Differential diagnosis

Problems in diagnosis occur when only the scalp is involved or when the lesions elsewhere are disseminated or otherwise atypical. A circumscribed plaque of erythema and scaling with total or partial loss of hair, especially in a child, may easily be confused with tinea: if examination under Wood's light is negative, and so is microscopy of epilated hairs, the diagnosis of follicular mucinosis should be considered. In all cases of unexplained patchy hair loss the whole skin surface should be examined. The diagnosis is confirmed by biopsy. Biopsy is advisable even in clinically obvious cases in adults, to exclude a reticulosis.

Treatment

None has been proved to be effective.

References

Bazex A., Dupré A., Parant M. & Christol B. (1962) Mucinose folliculaire; forme spinulosique généralisée. *Bulletin de la Societé française de Dermatologie et de Syphiligraphie*, **67**, 484.

Coskey R.J. & Mehregan A.H. (1970) Alopecia mucinosa. *Archives of Dermatology*, **102**, 193.

Degos R., Civatte J. & Baptista A.P. (1962) Mucinose folliculaire: La 'dermatose innominée alopéciante' de H. Gougerot et P. Blum (1932) en est-elle le premier cas? *Bulletin de la Societé française de Dermatologie et de Syphiligraphie*, **69**, 228.

Emmerson R.W. (1969) Follicular mucinosis. *British Journal of Dermatology*, **81**, 35.

Goldschlag F. & Jablonska S. (1960) Mucinosis follicularis. *Australian Journal of Dermatology*, **5**, 173.

Kim R. & Winkelmann R.K. (1962) Follicular mucinosis (alopecia mucinosa). *Archives of Dermatology*, **85**, 490.

Kreibich, C. (1926) Mucin bei Hauterkrankung. *Archiv für Dermatologie und Syphilologie*, **150**, 243.

Orfanos C. & Gahlen W. (1964) Elektronmikroskopische Befunde bei der Mucinosis follicularis. *Archiv für klinische und experimentelle Dermatologie*, **218**, 435.

Pinkus H. (1957) Alopecia mucinosa. *A.M.A. Archives of Dermatology*, **76**, 419.

Pinkus H. (1964) The relationship of alopecia mucinosa to malignant lymphomas. *Dermatologica*, **129**, 266.

Plotnich H. & Abrecht M. (1965) Alopecia mucinosa and lymphoma. *Archives of Dermatology*, **92**, 137.

Stevanovic D.V. (1964) Mucinosis follicularis diffusa idiopathica. *Dermatologische Wochenschrift*, 149, 352.
Zackheim H. (1958) Alopecia mucinosa. *A.M.A. Archives of Dermatology*, 78, 715.

Granuloma annulare

Granuloma annulare rarely affects the scalp, but subcutaneous nodules in the scalp have accompanied typical lesions in other parts of the body (Grauer 1934).

Reference
Grauer F.H. (1934) Granuloma annulare. *Archiv für Dermatologie und Syphilologie*, 30, 785.

Elastosis perforans serpiginosa

This unusual condition occurs particularly in persons with inherited abnormalities of connective tissue, but also in Down's syndrome, in patients receiving penicillamine, and in some apparently normal subjects.

The lesions occur most often on the face and neck, and in the latter site they extend some distance into the scalp (see Fig. 17.17).

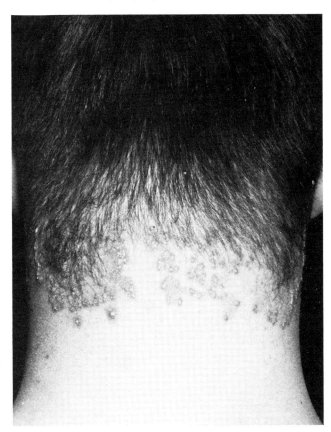

Fig. 17.17. Elastosis perforens serpiginosa in an 18-year-old male with Down's syndrome (Addenbrooke's Hospital, Cambridge).

The papules, which appear to be hyperkeratotic, are classically but not invariably grouped in circles or segments of circles.

The diagnosis is confirmed by the histological appearance of a focal increase of large elastic fibres, which, in a necrotic state, are seen to be extruded through the overlying epidermis.

Reference

Uitto J., Santa Cruz D.J. & Eisen A.Z. (1980) Connective tissue naevi of the skin. *Journal of the American Academy of Dermatology*, **3**, 441.

Eosinophilic cellulitis

History and nomenclature

Wells (1971) described as recurring granulomatous dermatitis with oesinophilia a distinct clinical entity, the cause of which remains unknown. Subsequently several similar cases have been recorded, the majority in adults but three in boys aged 11 and 12 (Wells & Smith 1979). In one of the children scalp lesions were present (Nielsen *et al.* 1981).

Pathology

During the acute stage there is dermal oedema with eosinophilic infiltration. This is followed by granulomatous changes with focal masses of disintegrating eosinophils and necrobiotic collagen fibres. These 'flame figures' are surrounded by histocytes and foreign body giant cells.

Clinical features

Large infiltrated erythematous, oedematous, pruritic plaques develop with fever and marked peripheral eosinophilia. They resolve after a few weeks to leave slight atrophy. They may be associated with bullae which are sometimes haemorrhagic. Recurrences at irregular intervals are usual but not invariable.

In the only case in which the scalp has been involved by indurated plaques (Nielson *et al.* 1981), these left large patches of permanent cicatricial alopecia.

Treatment

Systemic treatment with corticosteroids may shorten the course of the individual attack although these are eventually self limiting without treatment. There may be only a single attack but more often the condition ends after one or more recurrences.

References

Nielsen T., Schmidt H. & Søgaard H. (1981) Eosinophilic cellulitis (Wells' syndrome) in a child. *Archives of Dermatology*, **117**, 427.

Wells G.C. (1971) Recurring granulomatous dermatitis with eosinophilia. *Transactions of St John's Hospital Dermatological Society*, **57**, 44.

Wells G.C. & Smith N.P. (1979) Eosinophilic cellulitis. *British Journal of Dermatology*, **100**, 101.

Chapter 18
Naevi, Tumours and Cysts
of the Scalp

Superficial benign epidermal tumours
    Epidermal naevi
    Seborrhoeic keratoses
    Solar keratosis
    Cutaneous horn
Hair follicle tumours
    Keratoacanthoma
    Multiple self-healing epithelioma
    Pilomatrixioma
Sebaceous gland tumours
    Naevus sebaceus (see Epidermal naevi)
    Sebaceous adenoma
    Sebaceous carcinoma
Sweat gland tumours
    Syringocystadenoma papilliferum (see Epidermal naevi)
    Dermal eccrine cylindroma
    Syringoma
Basal cell carcinoma
Bowen's disease
Squamous cell carcinoma
Melanocytic tumours
    Melanocytic naevi
    Congenital pigmented naevi
    Juvenile melanova
    Blue naevus
    Naevus of Ota
    Malignant melanoma
Tumours of dermis and subcutis
    Dermatofibrosarcoma protuberans
    Gingival fibromatosis and multiple hyaline fibromas
    Neurofibromatosis
    Encephalocraniocutaneous lipomatosis
    Mastocytosis
Tumours of vessels
    Granuloma telangiectaticum
    Angiolymphoid hyperplasia with eosinophilia
    Vascular naevi
    Malignant angioendothelioma
Cutaneous meningioma
Carcinoma metastatic to the scalp
Cysts of the scalp
    Trichilemmal cysts
    Episdermoid cysts
    Congenital inclusion dermoid cysts

Superficial benign epidermal tumours

Of the very large number of different tumours of the skin now recognized as distinct entities, the majority have at some time or another been reported as occurring in the scalp. The role of light exposure is such an important factor in increasing the incidence of many common tumours that they are rarely found in the scalp of those who retain a good protective covering of hair in old age. In the many who develop frontovertical baldness in early adult life however, the scalp, so conspicuously exposed to light, becomes very vulnerable.

The dense population of large pilosebaceous follicles in the scalp results in a relatively higher incidence of tumours derived from that source than the surface area would lead one to expect. The special anatomical peculiarities of the scalp modify the morphology and course of other tumours or demand special procedures in treating them.

In this account of tumours of the scalp only a brief description is given of tumours which are uncommon in this site, with no mention of those that have rarely if ever been reported in the scalp. Tumours which are common in the scalp and elsewhere receive greater attention, with emphasis on differential diagnosis. For more detailed information on skin tumours and on the general problem of carcinogenesis the reader is referred to standard textbooks of dermatology and oncology. A relatively longer account is given in this chapter of tumours which are particularly characteristic of the scalp, such as the dermal eccrine cylindroma.

Epidermal naevi (references p. 504)

The epidermal naevi are circumscribed developmental defects. They are classified according to their predominant component. Although many naevi contain other epidermal structures, this classification remains useful for the different types show differences in distribution, morphology and course.

Verrucous naevi

These naevi, warty and often linear, are not common in the scalp. In two patients with extensive verrucous naevi the scalp appeared normal but there were patches of hair abnormal in colour and texture (Bassas Grau *et al.* 1969).

Sebaceous naevi (Robinson 1932; Conner & Bryan 1967)

Sebaceous naevi are present at birth or in early infancy but may first appear later in childhood (Fig. 18.1). The majority are in the scalp or on the face (Wilson Jones & Heyl 1970). In infancy the naevus, which may be 1 or 2 cm in diameter, or may cover a large area, is a flat or slightly elevated plaque with a velvet-like surface composed of numerous small elevations. It may be yellow or yellow-

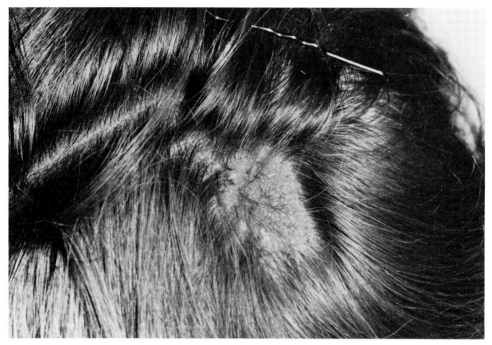

Fig. 18.1. Naevus sebaceus in the scalp of a man aged 19. It had enlarged during the previous 3 or 4 years. The granular texture of the surface can be seen (Addenbrooke's Hospital, Cambridge).

brown in colour. It is often more evident in infancy than in childhood for the sebaceous gland component regresses (Mehregan & Pinkus 1965; Steigleder & Cortes 1971). However, sebaceous naevi enlarge again with the approach of puberty. It is this enlargement which frequently induces the child's parents to seek medical advice.

Basal-cell carcinoma may develop in these naevi (Zugerman 1961; Castellain & Spitalier 1962) and enlargement, induration or ulceration in one part of the naevus is an indication for biopsy.

Plastic excision of sebaceous naevi is the treatment of choice.

Naevus syringocystadenomatosus papilliferus (Helwig & Hackney 1955)
In this clumsily named naevus the apocrine sweat gland component predominates. The essential histological changes are villous papillary projections into the lumen of dilated sweat ducts, and cystic dilatation of the associated gland. The epidermis may be normal but may be grossly acanthotic and hyperkeratotic.

The typical lesion is a pink, domed, umbilicated nodule 2–10 mm in diameter. There may be a cluster of discrete nodules or they may be grouped to form a plaque with a warty surface (Fig. 18.2). Some 50% occur in the scalp. In about 30% of cases a sebaceous naevus is associated.

This naevus is present at birth or develops in infancy. It may enlarge at puberty and become more verrucous (Pinkus 1954). Malignant change may eventually develop in about 10%.

Treatment is by excision.

Comedo naevus

The comedo naevus is perhaps not a single entity but a group of conditions characterized by dilated and plugged follicles (Leppard & Marks 1973). This naevus may be present at birth or may appear during childhood; exceptionally it may develop in old age (Nabai & Mehregan 1973). It may occur in any part of the body but in most cases on the neck, face or trunk. It is rare in the scalp but this was involved in a patient with extensive bilateral lesions (Page & Mendelson 1967). In two cases (Leppard & Marks 1973; Peyri *et al.* 1978) lesions of the scalp were associated with palmoplantar lesions.

Histologically there are large horny plugs in dilated follicles with small atrophic sebaceous glands (Beerman & Homan 1959). Clinically the naevus

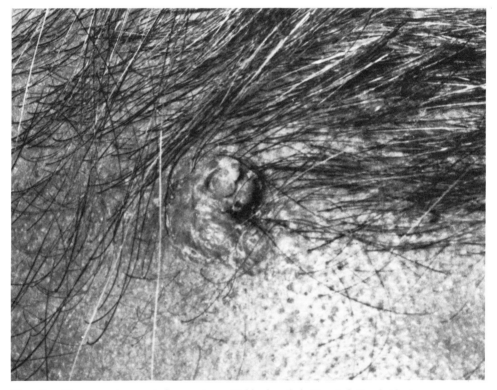

Fig. 18.2. Naevus syringocystadenomatosus (Addenbrooke's Hospital, Cambridge).

presents as a circumscribed, often irregularly linear area in which dilated follicles contain large horny plugs. The intervening surface epidermis may appear normal or may be thickened.

Treatment is not entirely satisfactory. If the naevus is small excision may be considered but this is not appropriate in most cases. Retinoic acid 0.1% has been reported to be 'very effective' (Dechard *et al.* 1972) but we have not found it always to be so.

Epidermal naevus syndrome

An epidermal naevus of any of the four types described may be associated with other defects, skeletal and ocular, epilepsy and mental retardation. The syndrome was formerly linked principally to naevus sebaceous (Feuerstein & Mims 1962) but naevus syringocystoadenoma papilliferus (Jancar 1970) and naevus comedonicus (Rook 1953) may also form part of this somewhat variable syndrome. In the presence of such naevi the other defects should be sought, though in many cases the epidermal naevus is an apparently isolated defect, but according to Solomon *et al.* (1968) some other developmental defects, although not the full syndrome, were found in some 60% of cases of epidermal naevus.

References

Bassas Grau E., Capdevela J., Castells A., Pinol Aguade J. (1969) Naevus sistematizado con heterocromia areata del cabello. *Medicina Cutanea,* **3,** 1.

Beerman H. & Harman J.B. (1959) Naevus comedonicus. *Archiv für klinische und experimentelle Dermatologie,* **208,** 325.

Castellain P.Y. & Spitalier J.M. (1962) Epiteliome basocellulaire pigmentée sur naevus sebacée de Jadassohn. *Annales de Dermatologie et Siphilagraphie,* **69,** 956.

Conner A.E. & Bryan H. (1967) Nevus sebaceus of Jadassohn. *American Journal of Diseases of Children,* **114,** 626.

Dechard J.C., Mills O. & Leyden J.J. (1972) Naevus comedonicus—treatment with retinoic acid. *British Journal of Dermatology,* **86,** 528.

Feuerstein R.C. & Mims L.C. (1962) Linear Nevus Sebaceus with convulsions and mental retardation. *American Journal of Diseases of Children,* **104,** 605.

Helwig E.B. & Hackney V.C. (1955) Syringadenoma papilliferum. Lesions with and without naevus sebaceus and basal cell carcinoma. *Archives of Dermatology and Syphilology (Chicago),* **71,** 361.

Jancar J. (1970) Naevus syringocystadenomatosus papilliferus. *British Journal of Dermatology,* **82,** 402.

Leppard B. & Marks R. (1973) Comedone naevus. *Transactions of the St. John's Hospital Dermatological Society,* **59,** 45.

Mehregan H. & Pinkus H. (1965) Life history of organoid nevi. *Archives of Dermatology,* **91,** 574.

Nabai H. & Mehregan H. (1973) Naevus comedonicus. *Acta Dermatovenilogica (Stockholm),* **53,** 71.

Paige T.M. & Mendelson C.G. (1967) Bilateral nevus comedonicus. *Archives of Dermatology,* **96,** 172.

Peri J., Ferrandiz C., Palou J. & Mascaro J.M. (1978) Naevus comedonicus palmoplantar y de cuero caballudo. *Medicina Cutanea I.L.A.* **6,** 227.

Pinkus H. (1954) Life history of naevus Syringocystadenomatosus papilliferus. *Archives of Dermatology and Syphilology,* **69**, 305.

Robinson S.S. (1932) Nevus sebaceus (Jadasson). *Archives of Dermatology and Syphilology,* **26**, 663.

Rook A.J. (1953) Naevus comedonicus unilateralis with partial Sturge-Weber syndrome and extensive vascular naevi with haemangiomatous hypertrophy of leg. *Proceedings of Tenth International Congress of Dermatology.* London, 421.

Solomon L.M., Fretzin D.F. & De Wald R.I. (1968) The epidermal nevus syndrome. *Archives of Dermatology,* **97**, 273.

Steigleder G.K. & Cortes A.C. (1971) Verhalten der Talgdrusen in Talgdrussenaevus während des Kindersalters. *Archiv für klinische und Experimentelle Dermatologie,* **239**, 323.

Wilson Jones E. & Heyl T. (1970) Naevus sebaceus. *British Journal of Dermatology,* **82**, 97.

Zugerman I. (1961) Basal-cell epithelioma in nevus Syringocystadenomatosus papilliferus. *Archives of Dermatology* (Chicago), **84**, 672.

Seborrhoeic keratoses (references p. 505)

Nomenclature

Numerous terms have been applied to these common lesions, Unna called them seborrhoeic verrucas: they are also known as senile warts and as basal-cell papillomas.

Aetiology

Seborrhoeic keratoses are benign neoplasms. They are so frequent that it is difficult to assess the role of genetic factors, but autosomal dominant inheritance seems probable in some families (Reiches 1953). They are extremely rare in childhood but have been reported as early as the age of 5 (Becker 1951). They become more frequent from the age of 30 onwards and are common in middle and old age.

Pathology (Becker 1951)

The epidermis is thickened and cells resembling basal cells form a solid epithelial mass, flat or irregularly serrated, or a retiform pattern with horn cysts or pseudocysts.

Clinical features

Typical seborrhoeic keratoses are sharply marginated flat papule, bright or dark brown in colour, with a velvety surface, greasy to the touch. They may become pedunculated with a smooth dull cerebriform surface. They can occur anywhere except on the palms and soles, but are most frequently seen on the face and scalp and on the trunk. There may be only one or two keratoses or very large numbers.

The rapid development of very numerous keratoses may be a manifestation of systemic malignant disease.

Differential diagnosis

The most important problem in differential diagnosis presented by seborrhoeic keratoses in the hairy scalp is that of distinguishing them from a melanocytic naevus or a malignant melanoma. The smooth dome-shaped seborrhoeic keratoses may be very deeply pigmented. If the diagnosis is in doubt the lesion should be excised if small, or submitted to biopsy if large.

The typical flat seborrhoeic keratosis seen more often on the bald scalp must be differentiated from a solar keratosis and from a basal cell carcinoma. If the diagnosis is uncertain a biopsy is essential.

Treatment

These keratoses are not premalignant and their removal is undertaken solely on cosmetic grounds. They are very easily curetted to leave less scarring than would follow excision.

References

Becker S.W. (1951) Seborrheic keratosis and verruca, with special reference to the melanotic variety. *Archives of Dermatology and Syphilology,* **63,** 358.

Reiches A.J. (1953) Seborrheic keratoses. *Archives of Dermatology and Syphilology,* **65,** 600.

Solar keratosis

Nomenclature

The synonym senile keratosis is not appropriate, for the incidence of these keratoses is related to age only in so far as the latter is a measure of cumulative exposure to solar radiation. Actinic keratosis is an acceptable synonym.

Aetiology

Solar keratoses are very common lesions of all exposed skin, including the bald or balding scalp. Their age of onset depends on the amount of light exposure in relation to the individual skin's capacity to tan. Given the same exposure to light, the fairer the skin, the earlier the onset of the keratoses.

Pathology (Pinkus 1958)

The parakeratotic epidermis has lost its granular layer. The prickle-cells are oedematous and vary in size and shape, and have lost their normal orderly stratified arrangement. The dermo-epidermal junction may be flat and the epidermis thin, or there may be acanthosis, but in either case the normal regular pattern of ridges and papillae is no longer apparent. The keratosis has sharp margins which slope upwards and inwards. The dermal collagen shows solar degenerative changes.

Clinical features

The patient complains initially of dry patches. Later, well-circumscribed, rough, adherent crusts develop. They are removed with difficulty and soon recur. In a simple keratosis the lesion feels superficial, and there is no underlying induration. If such is present the possibility of early squamous carcinoma must be considered.

Diagnosis

The sharply marginated rough patch on evidently light-damaged skin is not readily confused with seborrhoeic keratosis or with the red, often crusted appearance of Bowen's disease.

Treatment

If a single lesion is present it may be curetted under local anaesthesia, or destroyed with liquid nitrogen or trichloracetic acid. If there are numerous lesions, as if often the case, 5 fluorouracil cream may be used (Almeida Gonçalves & de Noronia 1970).

If the lesions are indurated, biopsy or excision-biopsy is essential.

References

Almeida Gonçalves J.C. & de Noronia T. (1970) 5 Fluorouracil (5 FU) ointment in the treatment of skin tumors and keratoses. *Dermatologica,* **140** (Suppl.) 1, 97.
Pinkus H. (1958) Keratosis senilis. *American Journal of Clinical Pathology,* **29,** 193.

Cutaneous horn

A cutaneous horn is a horny projection, a few millimetres or several centimetres in length, forming when conditions, such as protection from trauma, favour the accumulation of horn. It may arise on a wide variety of different lesions including virus warts, epidermal naevi, solar or seborrhoeic keratoses and squamous carcinoma.

When this purely clinical diagnosis is made, it must be regarded as the first stage of a two-stage diagnosis and the nature of the underlying lesion must be established clinically or, preferably, histologically.

Hair follicle tumours

Keratoacanthoma (references p. 507)

Aetiology

The keratoacanthoma (Fig. 18.3) is a common tumour of the skin occurring in the same populations as squamous carcinoma and in response to such carcinogenic environmental hazards as actinic radiation and tar, but at a significantly lower age than squamous carcinoma. In one large series of cases (Rook & Champion 1963) 24% of keratoacanthomas but only 6% of squamous carcinomas occurred in patients under 50 years of age, and only 9% of keratoacanthomas, but 18% of squamous carcinomas occurred in patients over 80 years of age. In this same series of cases of keratoacanthoma only 1% occurred on the scalp, 4% on the forehead, 5% on the thighs, 7% on the eyelids, 20% on the nose and 26% on the cheeks. Most of the remainder were on other areas of the face and neck or on the exposed skin of the back and forearms.

Pathology (Kopf 1976)

The keratoacanthoma is compact, circumscribed and superficial. A central mass of horn is surrounded by columns of hyperplastic epithelium, orderly and symmetrical; mitoses are numerous. The general architecture of the lesion (Fig. 18.4) is usually characteristic.

Clinical features

A firm hemispherical papule enlarges rapidly to reach a diameter of 1–2 cm in 4 or 5 weeks, though further enlargement is unusual. The lesion is now a crateriform nodule of rubbery consistency, the central crater of which is filled by horn. After 6 or 8 weeks the lesion becomes softer and flatter and the plug of horn is shed. The rim slowly flattens and only a puckered scar remains.

Recurrence after removal is not unusual (Rook *et al.* 1967) but the recurrent lesion runs essentially the same course if left untreated.

Malignant change is possible and should be suspected in atypical lesions, particularly those on the lip or ear, and in elderly patients (Rook & Whimster 1979).

Diagnosis

The short history and the clinical appearance suggest the diagnosis which may be confirmed histologically from an adequate biopsy specimen. If the diagnosis is still in doubt, the lesion must be treated as a carcinoma.

Treatment

In the high proportion of cases in which the diagnosis is not in doubt the lesion can be curetted under local anaesthesia.

References

Kopf A.W. (1976) Keratoacanthoma. In *Carcinoma of the Skin*, eds. R. Andrade, S.L. Gumport, G.L. Popkin & T.D. Rees. Saunders, Philadelphia, p. 755.
Rook A. & Champion R.H. (1963) Keratoacanthoma. *National Cancer Institute Monograph*, **10**, 257.
Rook A. & Whimster, I. (1979) Keratoacanthoma—a thirty year retrospect. *British Journal of Dermatology*, **100**, 41.

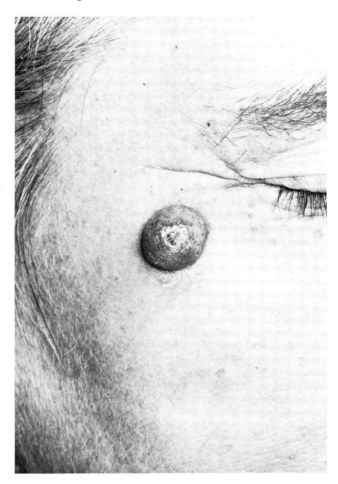

Fig. 18.3. Keratoacanthoma
(Slade Hospital, Oxford).

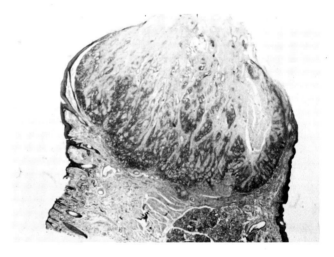

Fig. 18.4. Keratoacanthoma,
showing the characteristic
architecture (Slade Hospital,
Oxford).

Rook A., Kerdel-Vegas F. & Young J.A. (1967) Las recidivas en el queratoacantoma. *Medicina cutanea*, **2**, 17.

Multiple self-healing epithelioma (references p. 510)

In this uncommon syndrome, characterized by Ferguson Smith in 1934, the development of self-healing epitheliomas begins in the third or fourth decade, sometimes earlier (Sommerville & Milne 1950). There may be a family history of the disorder.

The tumours may be very widely distributed, but in most cases they have occurred predominantly in the scalp, on the face and ears, on the hands and in the anogenital region (Epstein *et al.* 1957). The presence of tumours in the scalp is a feature of almost all reported cases.

Clinically the tumours do not show the almost consistently crateriform structure of the keratoacanthoma. They are more deeply set irregular nodules.

Histologically the columns of squamous cells extend into the dermis and differentiation from an ordinary squamous cell carcinoma may be difficult. The history and presence of other lesions will suggest the diagnosis.

References
Epstein N.M, Biskind G.R. & Pollack R.S. (1957) Multiple benign self-healing 'epitheliomas' of the skin. *Archives of Dermatology and Syphilology*, **75**, 210.

Ferguson Smith J. (1934) A case of multiple primary squamous celled carcinoma of the skin in a young man, with spontaneous healing. *British Journal of Dermatology*, **46**, 267.

Sommerville J. & Milne J.A. (1950) Familial primary self-healing epithelioma of the skin (Ferguson Smith type). *British Journal of Dermatology*, **62**, 485.

Pilomatrixioma (syn. benign calcifying epithelioma of Malherbe)

History and nomenclature

This distinctive tumour was named by Malherbe in 1880 (Malherbe and Chénartins 1880), 'calcified epithelioma of the sebaceous glands'. It had first been described in 1858 by Wilckens in his thesis at the University of Göttingen (Geiser 1959). The origin of the tumour was disputed for many years, but it is now accepted that it arises from the primitive epidermal germ cells differentiating towards hair matrix cells (Forbès & Helwig 1961) and the term pilomatrixioma is generally favoured.

Pathology Forbès & Helwig 1961)

Pilomatrixioma is a circumscribed tumour situated in the lower dermis, and consisting of lobulated masses of cells. The small outer cells have large round basophilic nuclei. The central cells are large with eosinophilic cytoplasm, but no nuclear staining—the so-called shadow cells. Calcification may be seen in these cells and also sometimes in the abnormal connective tissue stroma. There is no reliable evidence that the tumour is inherited, but more than one case in a family has been reported on several occasions (Geiser 1960).

Clinical features

The tumours, which are usually solitary, though rarely up to four may be present, are often first observed in childhood and have been observed in early infancy: some 40% have been found in patients under 40. The majority are on the upper half of the body—scalp 6%, face 21%, neck 13%, arms 35% in one series of cases (Forbès & Helwig 1961); scalp 12%, face 36.5%, arms 24.2% in another (Martins 1956).

The lesion presents as a slowly enlarging dermal or subcutaneous lobular nodule up to 3 cm in diameter and of firm or hard consistency.

Treatment

Excision is the only effective treatment. Malignant change does not occur, but recurrences have followed incomplete excision.

References

Forbès R. & Helwig E.B. (1961) Pilomatrixioma. *Archives of Dermatology,* **83,** 601.
Geiser J.D. (1959) L'Epithéliome calcifié de Malherbe. *Annales de Dermatologie et de Syphiligraphie,* **86,** 259 and 583.
Geiser J.D. (1960) Forme familiale de l'epithéliome (calcifié) de Malherbe. *Dermatologica,* **130,** 361.
Martins A.G. (1956) Tumor mumificado de Malherbe. *Arquivo de Patalogia,* **28,** 123.

Sebaceous gland tumours

Sebaceous adenoma

These benign tumours are uncommon. They occur most frequently in men, usually over the age of 40. Histologically the tumours have a well-defined sebacous structure. The peripheral cells of the lobules are small and eosinophilic; the more central cells contain lipid globules.

Clinically sebaceous adenomas are small nodules, skin coloured or yellow, and may have a keratotic surface. They are most common on the nose, cheeks or scalp. Multiple sebaceous adenomas should suggest the possibility of Torre's syndrome and a search for associated visceral cancer (Rulon & Helwig 1973).

The adenomas should be excised.

Reference

Rulon D.B. & Helwig E.B. (1973) Multiple sebaceous adenomas of the skin. *American Journal of Clinical Pathology,* **60,** 745.

Sebaceous carcinoma (references p. 511)

History and nomenclature
Lever (1948) distinguished between the sebaceous carcinoma derived from the
cells of the sebaceous gland and the basal cell or squamous epithelioma with
sebaceous differentiation. Relatively few cases of sebaceous carcinoma of the skin
have been reported; these tumours arise rather more frequently in the
Meibomian glands. The confusion of these sebaceous carcinomas with epithelioma with sebaceous differentiation (Urban & Winkelmann 1961) accounts for
the conflicting opinions as to its degree of malignancy.

Pathology (Civatte & Tsoitis 1976)
The tumour consists of lobules of sebaceous cells in various stages of
differentiation. Atypical cells and mitoses are frequent. The eosinophylic
cytoplasm is foamy or finely granular. Lipid may be demonstrable, particularly in
the better differentiated cells. The stroma which may be dense and fibrous
contains lymphocytes and plasma cells. Histological distinction from basal cell
epithelioma or squamous cell epithelioma with sebaceous differentiation must be
made.

Clinical features (Warren & Warvi 1943)
The tumour occurs most often on the face or scalp mainly over the age of 50. The
clinical appearance is not diagnostic; there is a solid or ulcerated nodule which
enlarges slowly. It may be yellow in colour but is not invariably so. Local
invasion and metastasis may occur. The diagnosis must be confirmed histologically.

Treatment
Wide excision is advisable in an attempt to reduce the risk of recurrence (Beach &
Serurann 1942).

References
Beach A. & Serurann A.D. (1942) Sebaceous gland carcinoma. *Annals of Surgery*, **115**, 258.
Civatte J. & Tsoitis G. (1976) Adenaxal skin carcinomas. In *Cancer of the Skin*, vol. 2, eds. R.
    Andrade, S.L. Gumporte, G.L. Popkin & T.D. Rees. Philadelphia, Saunders, p. 1045.
Lever W.F. (1948) Pathogenesis of benign tumours and cutaneous appendages and basal cell
    epithelioma. *Archiv für Dermatologie und Syphilogie* (Berlin), **57**, 679.
Urban F.H. & Winkelmann R.K. (1961) Sebaceous malignancy. *Archives of Dermatology*, **84**, 63.
Warren S. & Warvi W.N. (1943) Tumors of Sebaceous Glands. *American Journal of Pathology*, **19**,
    441.

Sweat gland tumours

Dermal eccrine cylindroma (syn. turban tumour; Spiegler's tumour)

History and nomenclature
The earliest account of the scalp tumours that later acquired the name of cylindromas was given by Ancell in 1842. Many accounts were published, under almost as many different names, but the terms most widely adopted have been cylindroma, turban tumours and Spiegler's tumours. The term dermal eccrine cylindroma is preferred; it is more precise. Not all 'turban tumours' are eccrine cylindromas (Parker 1958) and the latter tumour does not always present in 'turban' distribution.

Trichoepitheliomas of the face may be present in association with cylindromas of the scalp and the two tumours form part of a single genetic entity (Welch *et al.* 1968). Inheritance is determined by an autosomal dominant gene with variable expression: either tumour may predominate. Penetrance probably approaches 100% in adult life.

Pathology (Sutherland 1956; Crain and Helwig 1961; Nödl 1965)
The cylindroma is of eccrine sweat gland origin. Closely packed masses of darkly staining cells are invested by condensed hyaline strands in variable mucinoid infiltration. Histological changes transitional between cylindroma and trichoepithelioma may occur.

Clinical features
The cylindroma is a firm or hard raised nodule, pink or bluish-red in colour, domed or mushroom-shaped, and enlarging very slowly (Fig. 18.5). It may ultimately reach a diameter of several centimetres, or remain no more than pea-sized for several years. The first tumours have appeared in childhood, but the greatest number begin between the ages of 10 and 40.

Solitary lesions may occur in any part of the body, but both solitary and multiple lesions favour the forehead and scalp where, if present in great numbers, they may justify the clinical diagnosis 'turban tumour'. They normally run an entirely benign course, but as they increase in number and size, may constitute a serious cosmetic disability.

Rarely local invasion and malignant degeneration with fatal metastasis may overtake in middle life lesions present since childhood (Luger 1949). In one woman in whom dedifferentiation and metastasis occurred at the age of 67 in an epithelioma present for 3 years, brachydactyly and rachet nails were also present (Greither & Rehrmann 1980). The authors suggest that this may represent an unrecognized syndrome.

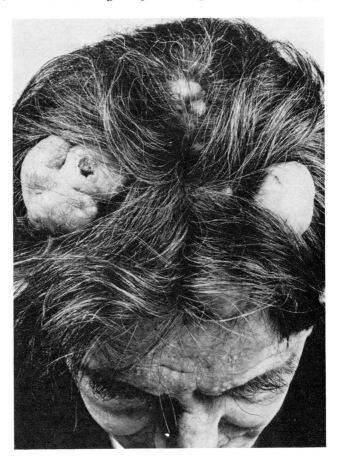

Fig. 18.5. Cylindromata (turban tumours) of the scalp (Dr C. Darley, London Hospital).

Cylindromas formed part of a syndrome with milia in addition to trichoepitheliomas (Rasmussen 1975). The milia developed in the fourth decade.

Diagnosis
The confident clinical diagnosis of the solitary cylindroma may be impossible and biopsy is always advisable. Where multiple cylindromas of the scalp are present, epidermoid cysts must be excluded. Very rarely familial turban tumours have proved to have a modified squamous structure (Parker 1958).

Treatment
Excision, followed if necessary by grafting, is usually the treatment of choice, but local recurrence is frequent (Crain & Helwig 1961). Radiosensitivity is low, but the skilled application of contact therapy in high dosage can give excellent results (Graul 1954).

References

Ancell H. (1842) History of a remarkable case of tumour development on the head and face. *Medicochirurgical Transactions,* **25,** 227.

Crain R.C. & Helwig E.B. (1961) Dermal cylindroma (dermal eccrine cylindroma). *American Journal of Clinical Pathology,* **35,** 504.

Graul E.H. (1954) Strahlenbiologische und strahlentherapeutische Untersuchungen an Spieglerschen Zylindromen. *Strahlentherapie,* **93,** 549.

Greither A. & Rehrmann A. (1980) *Spiegler-Karzinone mit associerten Symptome. Dermatologica,* **160,** 361.

Luger A. (1949) Das Cylindrom der Haut und seine maligne Degeneration. *Archiv für Dermatologie und Syphilologie,* **188,** 155.

Nödl, F. (1965) Zur Histogenese der dermaler ekkriner Cylindroma. *Archiv für klinische und experimentelle Dermatologie,* **222,** 171.

Parker R.A. (1958) Familial multiple cutaneous tumours of the head with a modified squamous structure. *Journal of Pathology and Bacteriology,* **75,** 435.

Rasmussen J.E. (1975) A syndrome of trichoepitheliomas milia and cylindromas. *Archives of Dermatology,* **111,** 610.

Sutherland T.W. (1956) Non-papillary hyalinising hidradenoma, sometimes forming turban tumours. *Journal of Pathology and Bacteriology,* **72,** 663.

Welch J.P., Wells R.S. & Kerr C.B. (1968) Ancell–Spiegler cylindromas (turban tumours) and Brooke–Fordyce trichoepitheliomas: evidence for a single genetic entity. *Journal of Medical Genetics,* **5,** 29.

Syringoma

Aetiology

This benign tumour, apparently not hereditary, is a malformation of the ecrine sweat ducts.

Pathology

In the upper part of the dermis are convoluted and cystic sweat ducts. On one side of the lesion a tail-like projection extends into the fibrous stroma, like the tail of a tadpole.

Clinical features

Syringomas, which are usually but not invariably multiple, develop from adolescence in crops or singly on the eyelids and the orbital skin, on the chest and on the abdomen. They are small, skin-coloured papules.

One patient, a man aged 47, had a plaque of cicatricial alopecia with a papular surface. He also had syringomas of the eyelids and cutis laxa (Dupré *et al.* 1981). The bald cicatricial area showed the pathological changes of syringoma.

A woman aged 57 with progressive, irregular cicatricial alopecia of twenty years' duration, with no other skin changes was found histologically to have multiple syringomas of the scalp, replacing the hair follicles (Shelley & Wood 1970).

Diagnosis

In retrospect, knowing that syringoma can give rise to cicatricial alopecia, the diagnosis could have been suspected in the first case. The second case merely underlines the importance of taking a biopsy in unexplained cicatricial alopecia for there were no clinical grounds on which a diagnosis of syringoma could have been considered.

References

Dupré A., Bonafe J.L. & Christoe B. (1951) Syringoma as a causative factor for cicatricial alopecia. *Archives of Dermatology*, **117**, 315.
Shelley W.B., Wood M.G. (1980) Occult syringoma of the scalp associated with progressive hair loss. *Archives of Dermatology*, **116.** 843.

Basal cell carcinoma
(syn. basal cell epithelioma; rodent ulcer)
(References p. 517)

Aetiology

Basal cell carcinoma is not a rare tumour in the scalp; this was the site in some 5% of tumours in one series (Battle & Patterson 1960).

Tumours on the bald scalp do not differ from those in other light-exposed areas. Those in the hairy scalp may develop in scars, but many arise in previously normal skin for no known reason. X-ray overdosage for epilation in childhood ringworm may leave persistent radiodermatitis and cicatricial alopecia, but a somewhat smaller dose may be followed by a reasonable regrowth of hair, and atropy and the progressive reduction in follicle density may not be clinically apparent until age changes have added to those induced by the X-rays. The development of one or more basal cell carcinomas in the scalp in middle age should lead to a careful enquiry concerning ringworm in childhood.

Pathology

The pathology of these lesions in the scalp shows no features which distinguish it from that of basal cell carcinomas in other sites, other than those imposed by the anatomy of the scalp and by the greater tendency of patients to neglect lesions concealed by hair. Thus lesions tend to be larger and more advanced with destructive invasion of the periosteum, and even of bone (Howell & Riddell 1954). The depth of invasion may not be the same in all parts of a large tumour, and extension may occur along nerve sheaths as well as blood vessels and lymphatics.

Clinical features (Geiser 1980)

The typical smooth, translucent, fire nodule, very slowly enlarging, with a few telangiectatic vessels crossing its surface occurs in the scalp as elsewhere. The nodule may be slightly or even deeply pigmented. Ulceration is frequent. The duration of the lesion when the patient seeks advice is measured in months or years: if a lesion of more than trivial size is reliably known to have been present only a few weeks, serious doubt should be thrown on the diagnosis.

The multicentric basal cell carcinoma is particularly characteristic of the scalp. It presents a rolled mother-of-pearl margin; its surface is moist and crusted and atrophic or ulcerated. Throughout the lesion some hair follicles are present in patches. Such lesions can be alarmingly destructive, involving even the meninges if they are neglected (James *et al.* 1950).

The uncommon morphoeic type of basal cell carcinoma also occurs in the scalp (Howell and Riddell 1954). The indurated, thickened plaque is not readily recognised as a tumour.

Diagnosis
A biopsy should be taken as soon as the diagnosis is suspected. If the lesion is

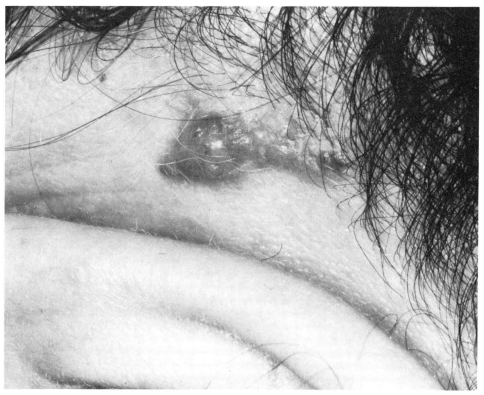

Fig. 18.6. Basal cell epithelioma arising at the age of 66 in a congenital epidermal naevus of the scalp (Addenbrooke's Hospital, Cambridge).

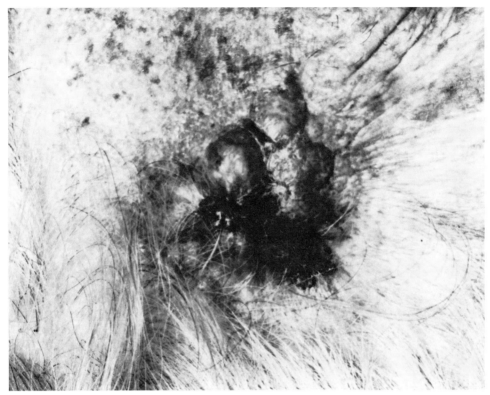

Fig. 18.7. Basal cell epithelioma of the scalp in a man aged 82 (Addenbrooke's Hospital, Cambridge).

large biopsies should be taken from two or more sites, to give some indication of the depth of invasion of dermis or periosteum.

Treatment
Very small carcinomas may be effectively treated by curettage, provided the patient can be kept under supervision, but wide excision is advisable. Whether excision or radiotherapy is preferred it is of the greatest importance to ensure that the initial treatment is adequate, for the treatment of recurrences presents even greater difficulties than in other parts of the body.

References
Battle R.J.V. & Patterson T.J.S. (1960) The surgical treatment of basal-celled carcinoma. *British Journal of Plastic Surgery,* **12,** 118.
Geiser T.D. (1980) Les tumeurs cutanées malignes du cuir chevelu. *Revue de Therapeutique* **37,** 578.
Howell J.B. & Riddell J.M. (1954) Cancer of forehead and scalp. *Journal of the American Medical Association,* **154,** 13.

James A.G., Anderson R.G., Scholl J.A. & Martin B.C. (1950) Cancer of the scalp. *American Journal of Surgery*, **80**, 441.

Bowen's disease

This intra-epidermal carcinoma may occur in any part of the skin. In the scalp it occurs most frequently in areas long exposed to solar damage by balding but multicentric Bowen's disease has occurred in the hairy scalp (Mora *et al.* 1980).

The lesion is a crusted, sharply marginated plaque which has been mistaken for psoriasis. It enlarges very slowly. An invasive squamous carcinoma may eventually develop.

The diagnosis should be confirmed histologically and the lesions should be excised.

Reference
Mora R.G., Jolly H.W. & Vaughn G.E. (1980) Localised multicentric Bowen's disease of the scalp. *Archives of Dermatology*, **116**, 841.

Squamous cell carcinoma

Aetiology
Squamous cell carcinoma in the scalp is uncommon, but early diagnosis is of such importance in prognosis that a knowledge of its precursors is essential.

The most frequent precursor of squamous carcinoma of the scalp is a solar keratosis (p. 505). Such lesions occur in scalp which has long been bald and the lack of hair ensures that changes in the appearance of the keratosis should be rapidly detected.

The scalp is not infrequently the site of burns or scalds in childhood. Squamous carcinoma may develop after an interval of many years in long-forgotten scar tissue (Lawrence 1952; Cruickshank *et al.* 1963).

Skin damaged by X-ray epilation in the treatment of ringworm (p. 331) may later be the site of squamous carcinoma. Lupus vulgaris was at one time treated with X-rays and such lesions too may develop squamous carcinoma as may also chronic lupus erythematosus (Ratzer & Strong 1967).

Clinical features
The development of induration around the base of a solar keratosis should raise the suspicion of malignant change. Ulceration of a long-standing scar does not necessarily imply a diagnosis of squamous carcinoma but it too is an indication for urgent biopsy. Any change in size or any ulceration of a chronic skin lesion of the scalp should be submitted to biopsy with the minimum of delay.

Treatment
If histological examination establishes the diagnosis of squamous carcinoma the management of the patient should be entrusted to a plastic surgeon.

References

Cruickshank A.H., McConnell E.M. & Miller D.G. (1963) Malignancy in scars, chronic ulcers and sinuses. *Journal of Clinical Pathology*, **16**, 573.

Lawrence E.A. (1952) Carcinoma arising in the scars of thermal burns. *Surgery, Gynaecology and Obstetrics*, **95**, 579.

Ratzer E.R. & Strong E.W. (1967) Squamous cell carcinoma of the scalp. *American Journal of Surgery*, **114**, 570.

Melanocytic tumours

Melanocytic naevi

Melanocytic (syn. pigmented naevi) are formed by the proliferation of melano-cytes at the dermo-epidermal junction. Some naevi are present at birth but the majority appear during childhood or adult life. Relatively few new naevi develop after middle age and fewer are present in old age. If the activity at the dermo-epidermal junction ceases the naevus gradually becomes intradermal. If junctional activity persists after the intradermal naevus has formed then this is said to be of the compound type (Fig. 18.8).

Junctional naevi are flat brown macules. At a rate which varies with the site and with the individual, junctional naevi form compound naevi and become raised to a variable degree. At puberty the enlargement of some naevi and the growth of coarse hair in some, often brings them to the notice of parents. Each naevus may reach its maximum size in childhood or during adult life. Pigmented naevi may ultimately become pedunculated and be shed. It is important to think of the pigmented naevi in any individual as a changing population. Some new ones appear from time to time; the existing naevi mature at varying rates.

Pigmented naevi of the ordinary types are not uncommon in the scalp. Medical advice is often sought because of enlargement or because the comb catches in the naevus or because of a change in the appearance of the naevus.

An increase in size or in the depth of pigmentation, ulceration, bleeding or pain are indications for immediate excision and histological examination. The risk of melanoma developing in any individual naevus is slight, but this tumour is of such importance that early diagnosis is essential.

A naevus, usually on the neck in women, or in male adolescents may suddenly become swollen and tender. On careful examination it is often evident that the inflammatory swelling is situated beneath rather than within the naevus. The lesion is in fact a foreign body granuloma which will resolve or may

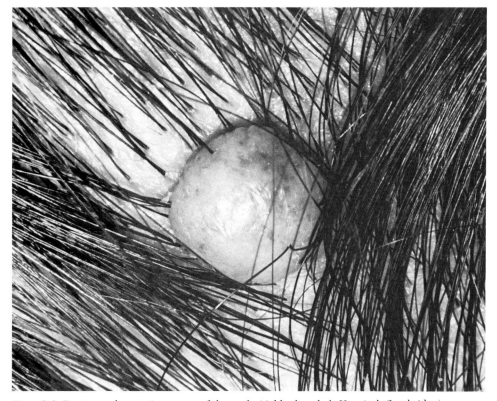

Fig. 18.8. Benign melanocytic naevus of the scalp (Addenbrooke's Hospital, Cambridge).

recur. Excision is desirable both for this reason and because it allows histological confirmation of the diagnosis. We have seen these granulomas on the nape of the neck but not in other regions of the scalp.

The patient's attention may first be drawn to a previously unnoticed naevus of the scalp by the development of a mesh of white hairs which on closer examination can be shown to arise in a halo of leucoderma surrounding the naevus.

Treatment
In almost every case in which treatment is considered necessary or desirable, excision is to be preferred; if malignancy cannot be excluded or if the diagnosis is in any doubt, excision is mandatory. If malignancy is thought probable, plans must be made for further surgery to be undertaken without delay, should malignancy be proven. If the naevus is certainly benign the probable cosmetic benefits of excision should be carefully evaluated and unnecessary surgery should be avoided.

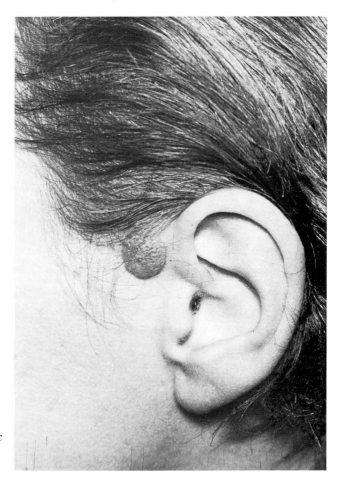

Fig. 18.9. Benign melanocytic naevus (Slade Hospital, Oxford).

Congenital pigmented naevi

Pigmented naevi present at birth differ in their morphology and natural history from the commoner pigmented naevi appearing during childhood or during adult life.

Histologically they are similar to compound naevi but the naevus cells extend more deeply.

Clinically they may be quite small with a surface which is warty or hairy, or both, but they may be very extensive, with a dermatomal distribution. If on the lower back they tend to involve the buttocks and thighs in a 'bathing trunk' pattern, if on the upper back they invest the shoulders and arms and if in the cervical region, the scalp. There may be associated melanocytic infiltration of the meninges; this is associated particularly with cranial and cervical naevi but may occur with giant congenital naevi in any site (Read *et al.* 1965).

Congenital naevi are dark brown with an irregularly thickened, sometimes verrucous surface. The naevus becomes thicker and darker and the coarse hairs which are usually present, become more conspicuous with the approach of puberty. Dark brown or black nodules may also be present.

Malignant melanoma develops in infancy, childhood, or less commonly in adult life in at least 10% of cases. In one series of giant naevi the incidence of malignancy was 17.5% (Pack & Davis 1961). Neurocutaneous melanosis is frequently fatal (Netherton 1936).

Another still rarer form of congenital naevus of the scalp is the cerebriform naevus (Gibson 1960). This irregularly convoluted naevus is melanocytic but is not clinically pigmented. Malignant change is rare in such naevi but does occur (Gross & Carter 1967).

Treatment

The high incidence of malignant melanoma even in infancy in congenital naevi, together with the serious cosmetic disfigurement they inflict, make excision the treatment of choice. A plastic surgeon should be consulted as soon as possible and excision in stages should be planned as soon as the child is old enough. Sometimes with very large naevi only very limited surgery can safely be undertaken in infancy. In such cases priority should be given to excising those areas in which the naevus appears to be most active. Techniques of excision which preserve the follicles may be applicable in some cases (Cronin 1953).

References

Cronin T.D. (1953) Extensive pigmented naevi in the hair-bearing areas: resection of pigmented layer whilst preserving the follicles. *Plastic and Reconstructive Surgery*, **11**, 94.

Gibson A.A.M. (1960) A giant benign naevus of the scalp. *Journal of Pathology and Bacteriology*, **80**, 185.

Gross P.R. & Carter D.M. (1967) Malignant melanoma arising in a giant cerebreform naevus. *Archives of Dermatology*, **96**, 536.

Netherton E.W. (1936) Extensive pigmented nevus associated with primary melanoblastosis of leptomeninges of brain and spinal cord. *Archives of Dermatology and Syphilology (Chicago)*, **33**, 238.

Pack G.T. & Davis J. (1961) Naevus giganticus pigmentosus with malignant transformation. *Surgery (St. Louis)*, **89**, 347.

Reed W.B., Beck S.Q. & Nickel W.R. (1965) Giant pigmented nevi, melanoma and leptomeningeal melanocytosis. *Archives of Dermatology*, **91**, 100.

Juvenile melanoma (references p. 523)

This tumour is generally considered to be a special form of benign compound naevus. Before it was characterized by Spitz in 1948 many such tumours were misdiagnosed as melanomas and unnecessarily radical treatment was carried out (Kernen & Ackerman 1960).

Aetiology
The peak incidence of juvenile melanoma is between 3 and 15, but onset in infancy or adult life may occur and persistence of lesions into adult life is not unusual. They are most frequently seen on the face, particularly the cheeks, or on the arms or legs. They are less common on the trunk. They have been reported in the scalp (Gartmann 1959).

Pathology
The cells of the juvenile melanoma are larger than ordinary naevus cells, polygonal or spindle-shaped, with abundant eosinophilic cytoplasm, and are arranged in nests or cords in the upper or mid dermis. There are few or no mitoses. Characteristic but inconstant are large giant cells, usually with three or four nuclei. Pigment is absent or scanty. There may be an abundant lymphocytic infiltrate. Telangiectases may be conspicuous in the oedematous subepidermal zone.

Clinical features
The juvenile melanoma commonly presents as a firm elevated nodule, pink, red, or red brown, with a smooth or slightly warty surface. It is commonly said to have developed very slowly. Bleeding with slight trauma is often noted, and the vascularity may suggest the diagnosis. The lesion persists but remains benign.

Differential diagnosis
Pyogenic granuloma, melanocytic naevus, malignant melanoma and lupus vulgaris are the main diagnostic problems.

Treatment
Simple excision is adequate.

References
Gartmann H. (1959) Probleme des sogenannten Juvenilen Melanom. *Medizinische Kosmetik*, **8**, 301.
Kernen J.A. & Ackerman L.V. (1960) Spindle cell nevi and epithelioid cell nevi (so-called juvenile melanomas) in children and adults. *Cancer*, **13**, 612.

Blue naevus

Aetiology
Blue naevi are circumscribed developmental defects in which persisting melanocytes are situated in the dermis.

Pathology
The common type of blue naevus consists of groups of melanocytes in the lower

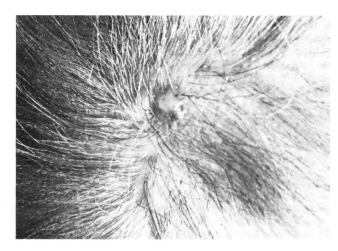

Fig. 18.10. Blue naevus. This patient also has ringed hair (Slade Hospital, Oxford).

dermis. In the so-called cellular type there are also larger cells arranged in a neuroid pattern.

Clinical features
The common type of blue naevus is a flat or slightly elevated blue-black papule, usually small (Fig. 18.10). The cellular type is sometimes larger and more raised. The lesions occur most frequently on the face and the extremities but have occurred in most sites, including the scalp (Gartmann & Lischka 1972; Dawber 1972). They may be present at birth or may first appear at any age. Malignant change is uncommon.

Treatment
If the naevus is over 1 cm in diameter, or if it is enlarging, it should be excised with an adequate margin of normal tissue.

   If it is small, flat and unchanging it may be removed on cosmetic grounds if the patient so wishes.

References
Dawber R. (1972) Investigation of a family with pili annulati associated with blue naevus. *Transactions of St. Johns' Hospital Dermatological Society*, **58**, 51.
Gartmann, H. and Lischka, G. (1972) Maligner blauer Naevus. Hautarzt, **23**, 175.

Naevus of Ota

The naevus of Ota is a developmental defect, not proved to be of hereditary origin, which consists of dermal melanocytosis in the distribution of the first two divisions of the trigeminal nerve. It is apparently considerably more frequent among the Japanese than in other races, but it is not confined to Mongoloids. About 80% of patients have been females. Bluish black pigmentation may be present at birth and it appears before the end of the first year in about 50%; onset after the third decade has not been reported (Fig. 18.13) (Kopf & Weidman 1962; Hidano *et al.* 1967).

At its maximum the pigmentation extends, particularly during early life, to orbital and zygomatic skin but it may cover a wide area and exceptionally may be bilateral (Hidano *et al.* 1967). The pigmentation may spread from the forehead some 2 cm or more into the scalp margin (Pariser & Beerman 1949; Findlay 1951).

Melanocytosis may affect ocular structures such as the sclera, cornea, iris and fundus, and also the oropharyngeal mucous membrane.

Ota's naevus is essentially a cosmetic disability, and no more can be done to relieve it than to obtain for the patient expert advice on the use of covering

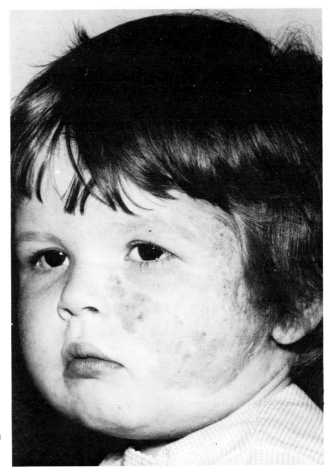

Fig. 18.11. Naevus of Ota in a girl aged 2 (Addenbrooke's Hospital, Cambridge).

creams. Malignant change is exceedingly rare but a fatal orbital melanoma has been reported in a woman age 64 (Jay 1965).

References

Findlay G.H. (1951) Mesodermal abnormalities of the face and sclera. *South African Journal of Clinical Science*, **2**, 281.

Hidano A., Kajima H., Ikeda S., Mizutani H., Miyasata H., Miimura M. (1967) Natural history of Nevus of Ota. *Archives of Dermatology*, **95**, 157.

Jay B. (1965) Malignant melanoma of the orbit in a case of oculodermal melanosis. *British Journal of Ophthalmology*, **49**, 359.

Kopf A.W. & Weidman A.I. (1962) Nevus of Ota. *Archives of Dermatology*, **85**, 195.

Pariser H. & Beerman H. (1949) Extensive blue patch-like pigmentation. *Archives of Dermatology and Syphilology*, **59**, 396.

Malignant melanoma (references p. 527)

Aetiology

In most countries for which adequate statistics are available the incidence of malignant melanoma is increasing, as is the mortality from it. This increase may be due in part to increased exposure to sunlight of those who are susceptible by virtue of their fair skins. The capacity to form protective pigment is of course itself genetically determined, but there is also a more specific hereditary tendency to develop melanoma; in such families the age of onset of the melanoma is early, multiple primary tumours are not unusual, and the survival rate is higher than in patients with non-familial melanomas (Anderson 1971).

Some 30–50% of melanomas arise in benign pigmented naevi; the remainder develop in apparently normal skin. Melanomas in the scalp are largely of the nodular type arising in congenital naevi and occurring mainly in children and young adults, or of the lentigo malignant melanoma type, in sun-damaged bald scalp in the elderly.

In most series of cases all tumours of the head and neck are grouped together. When the scalp is separately classified the incidence of tumours in this site varies from less than 1% (Daland & Holmes 1939) to 3% (Farrell 1932). The latter series, like many from the Mayo Clinic, may include an unduly high proportion of cases which presented special treatment problems. A series of 48 cutaneous melanomas in Algeria (Merssini-Montpellier & Striet 1952) included 7 in the scalp, of which 5 were in Europeans, one in a Negroid and one in an Asiatic. In 3 of 15 consecutive cases of disseminated melanomatosis, the primary tumour had been in the scalp (Tullis 1958). The early metastasis and poor prognosis of melanoma of the scalp is emphasized by a number of case reports (Russo 1947; Dionisi *et al.* 1951). In a French series of 623 melanomas (Maillard 1971) the 5-year survival rate for tumours of the forearm (70%) and face (50%) contrasted grimly with the 0% 5-year survival rate of melanomas of the scalp.

Pathology
The neoplastic melanocytes may invade the dermis laterally or vertically and the extent and direction of this invasion determines the indications for treatment and the prognosis (McGovern 1976).

Clinical features
Any change in a congenital naevus should be regarded with suspicion. In particular a localized increase in pigmentation, or bleeding from an area of erosion, or a complaint of itching or discomfort in the lesion.

The nodular form of melanoma, usually in middle-aged or elderly men, presents as a rather vascular reddish-brown nodule, raised or even pedunculated.

The melanomas in congenital naevi and the nodular melanoma may develop in hairy scalp and this delays their diagnosis, which in part accounts for their poor prognosis.

In contrast the lentigo maligna, melanoma usually develops in bald scalp as a flat brown patch; as this slowly extends the pigmentation becomes more intensely black in some areas and redder in others. Eventually a nodule may form at a point within the pigmented area and may first present as localized crusting and ulceration.

Diagnosis
This involves a high level of suspicion of any pigmented lesion in the scalp or of any reddish-brown vascular nodule. If melanoma is considered to be a possible diagnosis excisional biopsy is desirable. If, however, the lesion is very large and excision would be a mutilating procedure incisional biopsy may be justifiable.

Treatment
This should be entrusted to an experienced plastic surgeon. The result of the surgical procedure will be determined by careful assessment of the clinical and histological features.

References

Anderson D.E. (1971) Clinical characteristics of the genetic variety of cutaneous melanoma in man. *Cancer*, **28**, 721.

Daland E.M. & Holmes J.A. (1939) Malignant melanomas. *New England Journal of Medicine*, **220**, 651.

Dionisi P., Orcel L. & Kahn J. (1951) Evolution aigue d'un melanocarcinome du cuir chevelu. *Bulletin de L'Association française de Cancer*, **38**, 449.

Farrell H.J. (1932) Cutaneous melanomas. *Archives of Dermatology and Syphilology*, **26**, 110.

Maillard G.-F. (1971) Etude statistique de 623 mélanomes malins cutanés. *Annales de Dermatologie et de Syphiligraphie*, **98**, 5.

McGovern V.J. (1976) *Malignant Melanomas. Clinical and Histological Diagnosis*. Sydney, Wiley Medical.

Merssini-Montpellier J. & Striet R. (1952) Le mélanoblastome malin. Quelques aspects Algériens. *Bulletin Algérien de Carcinologie*, **5**, 19.

Russo P.E. (1947) Malignant melanoma in infancy. *Pediology*, **48**, 15.

Tullis J.L. (1958) Triethylenephosphoramide in the treatment of disseminated melanoma. *Journal of the American Medical Association*, **166**, 37.

Tumours of dermis and subcutis

Dermatofibrosarcoma protuberans (syn. Darier and Ferrand's tumour)

This rare tumour usually begins in early adult life, but the diagnosis is often made only after a considerable delay. It occurs most frequently on the trunk but is on the head or neck in over 10% of cases (Shapiro & Brownstein 1976) and has been reported in the scalp (Micoli *et al.* 1968).

Histologically the tumour consists of spindle-shaped cells in a closely woven pattern.

Clinically there are protuberant firm nodules arising on a diffusely thickened dermal plaque.

Excision must be wide as the risk of recurrence is considerable.

References

Micoli G., Leofreddi L. & Italia F. (1968) Dermatofibroma di Darier e Ferrand: Discuzione di un caso a localizzazione al Cuoio Cappelluto. *Gazzetta Istituto Medicinale Cuoio*, **73**, 2154.

Shapiro L. & Brownstein M.H. (1976) Dermatofibrosarcoma protuberans. In *Cancer of the Skin*, vol. 2, eds. R. Andrade, S.L. Gumport, G.L. Popkin & T.D. Rees. Philadelphia, Saunders, p. 1069.

Gingival fibromatosis and multiple hyaline fibromas

Aetiology

The inheritance of this very rare disease is determined by an autosomal recessive gene.

Clinical features

Gingival fibromatosis begins in infancy or early childhood. Soon numerous subcutaneous nodules appear on the scalp, face, shoulders and digits. Later they appear on the trunk and limbs. In the scalp they resemble cylindromas. Histologically they consist of amorphous, PAS-positive ground substance in which are embedded blood vessels and spindle-shaped cells.

There is no hypertrichosis.

Reference

Kitano W. (1976) Juvenile hyaline fibromatosis. *Archives of Dermatology*, **112**, 86.

Neurofibromatosis (syn. Von Recklinghausen's disease) (references p. 530)

Aetiology
Neurofibromatosis is a neuro-ectodermal disorder, the inheritance of which is determined by an autosomal dominant gene. It is relatively common and occurs in 1 in 2500–3000 births (Crowe *et al.* 1956).

Pathology
Neurofibromas are derived from peripheral nerves and their supporting structures and consist of Schwann cells in collagenous interstitial tissue. Pigmented macules may contain macromelanosomes (Jimbow *et al.* 1974).

Clinical features
Neurofibromata can occur anywhere in the skin including the scalp where they are not uncommon. They are seen in several distinct clinical forms. The small, soft, lilac-pink molluscum fibrosum—resembling a grape pip—contrasts with the diffuse elongated plexiform neuroma along the course of a nerve, and the diffuse overgrowth of skin and subcutaneous tissue producing the severely disfiguring pendulous folds of elephantiasis neuromatosa. Two types of pigmented lesion are characteristic of the disease: small freckles in the axillae and perineum are present in about 20% of cases and are pathognomonic (Crowe 1964): light-brown, more or less oval, café-au-lait spots are present in over 90% of cases: one or more such spots are present in 10% of normal subjects but the presence of six or more is highly suggestive of neurofibromatosis (Crowe *et al.* 1956).

The scalp may be involved with the face in neurofibromatous elephantiasis as in Treves' 'Elephant Man' (Howell & Ford 1980) but the commonest scalp lesions are single or multiple soft nodules, often appearing during the second or the third decade and sometimes becoming quite large. The soft consistency suggests the diagnosis and should lead to an investigation of the entire skin for other evidence of the disease. If this is found the patient should be kept under long-term supervision so that the involvement of other organ systems by the disease, should it occur, may be diagnosed early (Canale & Bebin 1972; Brasfield & Das Gupta 1972). The severity of neurofibromatosis is extremely variable and ranges from pigmentary changes with a few small mollusca to a grossly disfiguring and disabling disease with involvement of multiple systems.

Treatment
Excision is the only possible treatment and should be carried out if the scalp lesion is enlarging or is otherwise troublesome. Malignant change occurs in a significant proportion of lesions in deeper structures but is very unusual in superficial lesions.

References

Brasfield R.D. & Das Gupta T.K. (1972) Von Recklinghausen's disease—a clinicopathological study. *Annals of Surgery*, **175**, 86.

Canale D.J. & Bebin J. (1972) Von Recklinghausen's disease of the nervous system. In *Handbuch of Clinical Neurology*, vol. 14, eds. P.J. Vinken & G.W. Bruyn. Amsterdam, North-Holland, p. 132.

Crowe F.W. (1964) Axillary freckling as physical sign of neurofibromatosis. *Annals of Internal Medicine*, **66**, 1142.

Crowe F.W., Schull W.J. & Neel J.V. (1956) *A Clinical, Pathological and Genetic Study of Multiple Neurofibromatosis*. Springfield, Thomas.

Howell M. & Ford P. (1980) *The True History of the Elephant Man*. London, Allison & Busby.

Jimbow K., Szabo G. & Fitzpatrick T.B. (1974) Ultrastructure of giant pigment granules (macromelansomes) in the cutaneous pigmented macules of neurofibromatosis. *Journal of Investigative Dermatology*, **61**, 300.

Encephalocraniocutaneous lipomatosis

This syndrome, of which only four examples have been reported, cannot yet be too rigidly defined, as further cases may lead to some broadening of the clinical spectrum.

From birth soft papules and nodules are present in the scalp and on the face and neck; they have been unilateral in three cases and bilateral in one. Over the larger lesions in the scalp are patches of alopecia. Histologically the lesions are fibrolipomata or angiofibromata.

Intracranial lipomata may result in convulsions and mental retardation.

Reference

Sanchez N.P., Rhodes A.R., Mandell F. & Mihm M.C. (1981) Encephalocraniocutaneous lipomatosis: a new neurocutaneous syndrome. *British Journal of Dermatology*, **104**, 89.

Mastocytosis

The term mastocytosis is applied to a group of disorders in which mast cells are present in the tissues in excessive numbers.

In localized cutaneous mastocytosis one or sometimes two or three pigmented nodules are present at birth or appear in the first month of life. They may occur in any part of the body, including the scalp. The urtication of the nodules when they are rubbed is a diagnostic feature. Sometimes blisters form on the nodules. Spontaneous resolution occurs during childhood.

Generalized cutaneous mastocytosis beginning in early childhood consists of light brown macules or nodular lesions, which urticate when rubbed. If the lesions are numerous the quantity of histamine released by rubbing them may be sufficient to cause flushing. One boy aged 9 developed an attack of flushing when he visited his hairdresser (Marten 1957). Bullae may form on the lesions in early childhood; they have been sufficiently numerous to give rise to crusting of the

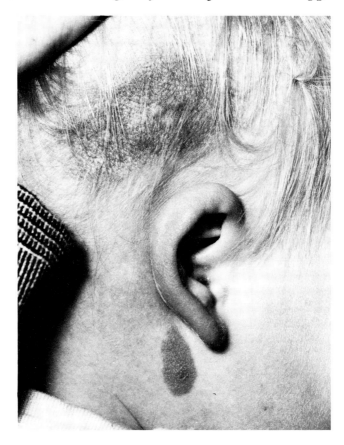

Fig. 18.12. Mast cell naevus in a child's scalp (Addenbrooke's Hospital, Cambridge).

scalp (Tavs 1947). This childhood form of the disease usually regresses before puberty.

Involvement of the scalp is not a feature of the other forms of mastocytosis.

References

Marten R.H. (1957) Urticaria pigmentosa. *British Journal of Dermatology*, **69**, 151.

Tavs L.E. (1947) Urticaria pigmentosa with bullae. *Archives of Dermatology and Syphilology*, **55**, 558.

Tumours of vessels

Granuloma telangiectaticum (syn. granuloma pyogenicum; pseudobotryomycoma) (references p. 532)

Aetiology

The granuloma telangiectaticum, as the commonly employed synonym implies, was believed to be an abnormal tissue response to pyogenic infection of a minor abrasion but infection is probably secondary (Kerr 1951). The role of a virus has not been excluded. The lesion is seen in both sexes and at all ages, but is more common in childhood. The sexes are equally affected.

Pathology (Martens & McPherson 1956)
The granuloma consists of a mass of thin-walled newly formed capillaries in a connective tissue stroma, mucoid or fibrous, with an inconstant mixed cellular infiltrate.

Clinical features
It is a bright red, soft and highly vascular papule or nodule ranging in size from 2–3 mm to several centimetres in diameter, globular and pedunculated, mushroom-shaped or sessile. It enlarges for several weeks and then persists more or less indefinitely. It may be eroded or covered with a dried crust of foul-smelling seropurulent exudate. The base may be surrounded by a collar of thickened epidermis. Haemorrhage is often troublesome. The majority occur on the exposed parts, usually on the face in infancy and the face, hands, arms and upper trunk in older children and in adults. About 3% of those on the skin occur in the scalp (Kerr 1951). The mucous membranes of the oral cavity and nares are frequently affected. Lymphangitis is an occasional complication.

Diagnosis
Juvenile melanoma, malignant melanoma, and angiomatous naevi are most commonly confused. The history and the extreme friability of the lesion should serve to differentiate it from the angiomatous naevi. The juvenile melanoma may not be clinically distinguishable.

Treatment
Curettage followed by cauterization usually is satisfactory, but since the clinical diagnosis may be incorrect in about one case in three (McGeoch 1961), excision should be performed if there is any doubt in the clinician's mind. The lesion should always be examined histologically to exclude a serious diagnostic error. Recurrences are occasionally seen, and excision is then advisable.

References
Kerr D.A. (1951) Granuloma pyogenicum. *Oral Surgery*, **4**, 153.
McGeoch A.H. (1961) Pyogenic granuloma. *Australian Journal of Dermatology*, **6**, 33.
Martens V.E. & McPherson D.J. (1956) Fibroangioma. *Archives of Pathology*, **61**, 120.

Angiolymphoid hyperplasia with eosinophilia

This recently characterized angiomatous disorder occurs usually between the years of 25 and 45, in women more often than in men, and affects the scalp, the

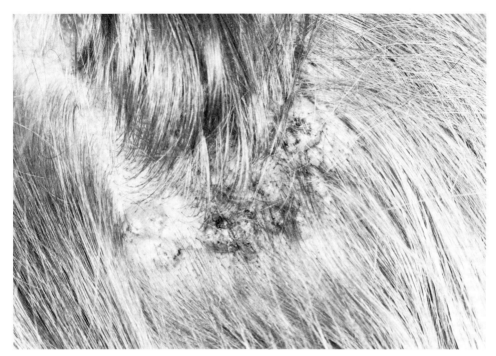

Fig. 18.13. Angiolymphoid hyperplasia (Dr P.W. Bowers).

ears and occasionally the face. The lesions, which may be multiple, present as dome-shaped vascular nodules which may bleed easily.

Histologically the lesions show abnormal hypertrophic capillaries with swollen endothelial cells and an infiltrate of lymphocytes, histiocytes and eosinophils (Fig. 18.13).

The condition is benign, although recurrence may follow excision, which is the treatment of choice.

References
Berretty P.J.M. & Faber W.R. (1980) Angiolymphoid hyperplasia with eosinophils. *British Journal of Dermatology*, **103**, 578.
Vasques Botet M. & Sanchez J.L. (1978) Angiolymphoid hyperplasia with eosinophilia: report of a case and review of the literature. *Journal of Dermatologic Surgery and Oncology*, **4**, 931.
Wilson Jones E. & Bleehen S.S. (1969) Inflammatory angiomatous nodules with abnormal blood vessels occurring about the ears and scalp (pseudo or atypical pyogenic granuloma). *British Journal of Dermatology*, **81**, 804.

Vascular naevi (references p. 537)

The vascular naevi of the skin are circumscribed developmental defects of the dermal or subcutaneous vasculature. A simple classification of these naevi is:

1. Flat vascular naevi—telangiectatic naevi
       naevus flammeus—port-wine naevus
       (may also form part of complex syndromes)
2. Raised vascular naevi—cavernous
       superficial—strawberry mark
       deep

Flat vascular naevi

Nuchal naevus. The commonest flat naevus occurs on the nape of the neck and is known as Unna's naevus. It was found in 20–30% of newborn babies in Malaya (Tan 1972). A study of 2171 Danish schoolchildren aged 6–17 showed a nuchal naevus in 46.2% of girls and 35.1% of boys (Oster & Nielsen 1970). The reported incidence of the naevus in other population groups has ranged from 12 to 57%. The incidence in any population is the same in infancy and in middle age. The naevus shows no tendency to disappear (Zumkeller 1957).

 The nuchal naevus is not a cosmetic problem, and is usually no more than an incidental finding when the scalp is being examined.

Sturge–Weber syndrome. In this syndrome a port-wine naevus involves part or the whole of the trigeminal distribution on the face and the front of the scalp. The cutaneous naevus is associated with ocular and intracranial angiomatosis. There is no constant relationship between the extent of skin involved and the extent of intracranial lesions (Fig. 18.14).

Raised vascular naevi
Superficial raised naevi—strawberry mark—are present at birth or develop during the first month after birth in some 90–95% of cases; in 5–10% they develop from the 2nd to the 5th month (Schnyder 1957; Simpson 1959). Subcutaneous cavernous naevi are essentially similar in their natural history. Both superficial and subcutaneous types are about twice as common in girls as in boys, and, although they may occur anywhere, are found predominantly on the head and trunk (Fig 18.15). In many reports the distribution of the naevi on the head is not recorded in great detail, but 14% of Simpson's cases involved the scalp.

 For the first 6–12 months the naevi continue to enlarge: indeed in a few cases enlargement, but at a decreasing rate, may continue for 3 or 4 years. After a year, but sometimes much earlier, greyish-blue patches mottle the previously bright red surface, and the naevus begins to flatten. About 50% have involuted without trace by the age of 5 and the process of involution continues in the remainder. The residual changes when spontaneous involution has ceased depend on the original size of the lesion and range from a few telangiectases to

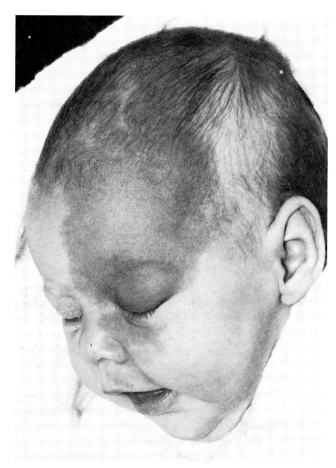

Fig. 18.14. Capillary naevus in the first two divisions of the left trigeminal nerve. This patient had Sturge–Weber syndrome (Addenbrooke's Hospital, Cambridge).

redundant folds of atrophic skin. Superficial ulceration of naevi is not unusual in infancy; it is not a serious complication and does not result in significant haemorrhage, but it may lead to some increase in scar formation. However, even in the scalp at least 50% of normal hair growth was preserved at the site of such a naevus (Simpson 1959).

Wallace (1953) had reported similar findings. Of 290 strawberry naevi, 120 disappeared without trace and a further 157 left slight atrophy which was no cosmetic disability. Of 121 deeper cavernous naevi 93 gave equally satisfactory results, though a slightly higher proportion had detectable atrophy. Bowers *et al.* (1960) made similar observations; they showed that spontaneous involution left only 6% with any ultimate cosmetic handicap.

Treatment. It is evident that in the majority of raised vascular naevi any form of treatment is unnecessary. Many potentially harmful measures, such as radio-

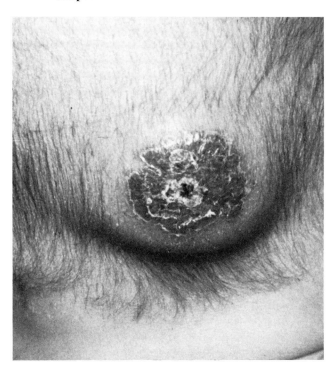

Fig. 18.15. Cavernous vascular naevus (Slade Hospital, Oxford).

therapy, have been used in the past, and the reluctance of the medical profession to accept the self-evident fact that most of the naevi involute spontaneously is now difficult to understand. Radiotherapy, even when it produced no local cutaneous damage, was associated with an increased incidence of thyroid carcinoma in childhood or adolescence (Brunner 1961).

A child's parents apprehensively watching the enlargement of a naevus on the face or scalp may put considerable pressure on their physician to provide some active treatment. Since such treatment is not in the best interests of the child it should never be given. If the parents can be shown serial photographs of the spontaneous involution of similar naevi, they will accept the advice that patience gives the best cosmetic results.

Where there are residual changes which require plastic surgery, this should be postponed until the comparison with photographs shows no further improvement over a year. Unnecessary surgery can then be avoided.

There are cases, however, in which active treatment is desirable or even essential. Treatment with systemic corticosteroids will hasten involution (Edgerton 1976) and is indicated when the naevus is obstructing orifices, or involves a vital organ or is causing cardiovascular decompensation (Lasser & Stein 1973).

References

Bowers R.E., Graham E.A. & Tomlinson K.M. (1960) The natural history of the strawberry nevus. *Archives of Dermatology*, **82**, 167.

Brunner K. (1961) Schilddrüsenkarzinon in Kinderalter nach Röntgenbestrahlen einer Nevus vascularis cutaneus von 12 Jahren. *Schweiz medizinische Wochenschrift*, **91**, 389.

Edgerton M.T. (1976) The treatment of haemangioma. *Annals of Surgery*, **183**, 517.

Lasser A.E. & Stein A.F. (1973) Steroid treatment of hemangiomas in children. *Archives of Dermatology*, **108**, 565.

Oster J. & Nielsen A. (1970) Nuchal naevi and interscapular telangiectases. *Acta paediatrica scandinavica*, **59**, 416.

Schnyder U.W. (1957) Zur Klinik und Histologie der Angiome. IV. Die plano-tuberösen und tuberonodösen Angiome des Kleinkindes. *Archiv für klinische und experimentelle Dermatologie*, **204**, 457.

Simpson J.R. (1959) *Natural history of cavernous haemangiomata. Lancet*, **ii**, 1057.

Tan K.L. (1972) Nevus flammeus of the nape, glabella and eyelids. A clinical study of frequency, racial distribution, and association with congenital anomalies. *Clinical Pediatrics*, **11**, 112.

Wallace H.J. (1953) The conservative treatment of haemangiomatous naevi. *British Journal of Plastic Surgery*, **6**, 78.

Zumkeller R. (1957) A Propos de la fréquence et de l'hérédité du 'Naevus vascularis nuchae—Unna'. *Journal de Génétique Humaine*, **6**, 1.

Malignant angioendothelioma (references p. 538).

Aetiology

Malignant angioendothelioma of the face and scalp has been characterized as a distinct clinicopathological entity (Wilson Jones 1964). Very rarely it may occur as early as the fourth decade but the average age of onset is between 70 and 80 and men are more frequently affected than women (Knight *et al.* 1980).

Pathology

The tumour consists of anastamosing irregular vascular channels and spaces which infiltrate but do not destroy the dermis. The channels are lined by atypical swollen endothelial cells which show a tendency to intraluminal budding to form cords and islands of cells in syncytial arrangement.

Clinical features

The commonest presentation is with single or grouped bluish red nodules of the face and scalp. There may be come thinning of the hair over the tumours (Suurmond 1958) but alopecia is not a conspicuous feature of this form of disease. Less well differentiated tumours appear as diffuse indurated plaques over which much hair is lost. Exceptionally there may be an extensive cicatricial alopecia (Knight *et al.* 1980).

Eventually a large area of face, neck and scalp may be involved, with gross oedema of the eyelids. The skin may ulcerate. Involvement of the cranial bones may occur and distant metastases are frequent. The average duration of survival after onset is under 2 years.

Treatment
Palliative radiotherapy is the best that can be offered.

References
Knight T.E., Robinson H.M. & Sina B. (1980) Angiosarcoma (angioendothelioma) of the scalp. *Archives of Dermatology*, **116**, 183.
Suurmond D. (1958) Haemangioendothelioma (Angioplastic sarcoma). *British Journal of Dermatology*, **70**, 132.
Wilson Jones E. (1964) Malignant angioendothelioma of the skin. *British Journal of Dermatology*, **76**, 21.

Cutaneous meningioma

This is an extremely rare tumour which may occur in the scalp. A solitary nodule, usually in the mid line of the occiput, is present from birth. The consistency of the tumour has been soft or rubbery. The overlying skin may be atrophic but has more often been thickened and sometimes hypertrophic. Some have enlarged slowly but others have remained unchanged. The ultimate size has ranged from 2 to 10 cm in diameter.

The diagnosis is suggested by the site and must be confirmed histologically.
Treatment is by surgical excision.

Reference
Bain G.O. & Schnitka T.A. (1956) Cutaneous meningioma (psammoma). *Archives of Dermatology*, **74**, 590.

Carcinoma metastatic to the scalp
(References p. 540)

Aetiology and nomenclature
Carcinoma of an internal organ may involve the skin directly from an underlying organ or by extension through lymphatics, by lymphatic or blood-stream embolic dissemination, or by accidental implantation of tumour cells during the course of a surgical procedure (Mehregan 1961).

The incidence of metastatic carcinoma in the skin in any population reflects to some extent the efficiency with which malignant disease is sought, detected and treated. However, a cutaneous metastasis may be the presenting manifestation of an otherwise asymptomatic carcinoma; and indeed, even when the patient is fully investigated, the primary growth may not be discovered. In some cases, notably of carcinoma of the breast, a metastasis has appeared as long as 30 years after surgical removal of the original tumour (Michel *et al.* 1971).

In reported series the total incidence of cutaneous metastasis in patients with internal carcinoma has ranged from 2% to over 4%. The scalp is the site of such metastasis, particularly in hypernephroma (Rosenthal & Lever 1957), and carcinoma of the breast (Michel *et al.* 1971), but scalp metastasis also occurs from primary growths in bronchus, stomach, colon, rectum, ovary and prostate, and, more uncommonly, pancreas, liver, uterus and bone (Gómez Orbaneja *et al.* 1967; Cueto *et al.* 1970; Hernanez *et al.* 1979). Meningiomas may reach the scalp by direct extension, through operative defects in the skull or by metastasis (Waterson & Shapiro 1970).

Pathology (Montgomery & Kierland 1940)
The cells in metastatic malignant deposits may retain recognizable character-istics of the primary tumour but may be too anaplastic for identification. Their metastatic origin is betrayed by their lack of any connection with cutaneous epithelial structures, but occasionally involvement of the epidermis by the cells of the metastasis may make diagnosis more difficult (Miescher 1955). Columns of cells may be seen within dilated lymphatics. Vascular dilatation is a variable feature.

The presence of mucin suggests that the primary tumour is in the digestive tract (Mehregan 1961). In metastasis from hypernephroma (Rosenthal & Lever 1957) the acinose arrangement of the cells of the original tumour may not be obvious, but vascular proliferation is often conspicuous.

Clinical features
Single or multiple firm non-tender nodules enlarging quite rapidly are the most frequent manifestation of metastatic carcinoma in the scalp. Sometimes when the patient's tissue reaction to the metastasis has been more effective there may be some oedema and inflammatory changes. In other changes dermal sclerosis around the deposit leads to destruction of hair follicles and the metastasis presents clinically as single or multiple areas of cicatricial alopecia (Fig. 18.16)—scleroderma-like plaques of a few weeks' or months' duration (Delacré-taz & Chapuis 1958; Baran 1969; Baum *et al.* 1981).

Multiple modules may simulate turban tumours (Ronchese 1940), but the latter develop slowly over many years.

Treatment
A biopsy should always be taken, and every attempt should be made to detect and treat the primary tumour. Usually the prognosis is very poor but, particularly in hypernephroma in which a solitary metastasis to the scalp may be the first evidence of the presence of the tumour, excision of both the affected kidney and the secondary may give a permanent cure.

Excision of the metastasis is always advisable unless of course it proves to be

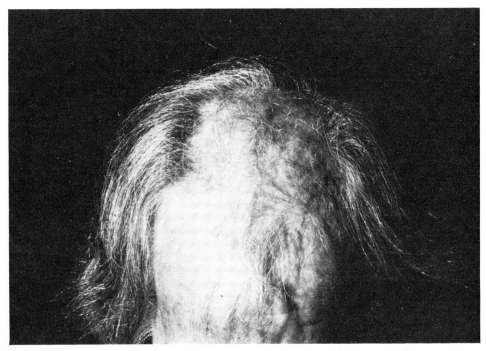

Fig. 18.16. Cicatricial alopecia caused by metastatic carcinoma of the breast (Slade Hospital, Oxford).

only one manifestation of generalized carcinomatosis. Even the long-delayed metastasis developing years after mastectomy should be excised (Michel *et al.* 1971) and the practicability of chemotherapy should be discussed. The patient's response to skin tests of delayed hypersensitivity may be of assistance in planning treatment (Anthony *et al.* 1974).

References

Anthony H.M., Templeman G.H., Madren K.E. & Mason M.K. (1974) The prognostic significance of DHS skin tests in patients with carcinoma of the bronchus. *Cancer*, **34**, 1901.

Baran R. (1969) Les métastases alopéciantes scleroatrophiques des cancers mammaires. *Dermatologica*, **138**, 169.

Baum E.M., Omura E.F., Payne P.P. & Little W.P. (1981) Alopecia neoplastica—a rare form of cutaneous metastasis. *Journal of the American Academy of Dermatology*, **4**, 688.

Cueto J.J., Rotman J.-C., Castellato R.H. & Veron C.W. (1970) Metastasis alopeciante escleruoatrofica. *Archivos Argentinos de Dermatologia*, **20**, 167.

Delacrétaz J. & Chapuis H. (1958) Métastases cutanées alopéciantes. *Dermatologica*, **116**, 372.

Gómez Orbaneja J., Ledo Pozueta A. & de Castro Torres A. (1967) Metastatic carcinomas to the skin. *Dermatologia Ibero Latino-Americana (English edn.)*, **2**, 13.

Hernanez J.M., Vives P., Garcia Almazno D. & Jacqueti G. (1981) Alopecia neoplàsica. *Actas dermosifilograficas*, **20**, 507.

Mehregan A.H. (1961) Metastatic carcinoma to the skin. *Dermatologica*, **123**, 311.

Michel P.-J., Cretin J. & Grimaud P.-S. (1971) A propos de certaines métastases cutanées isolées et tardives des Cancers du Sein. *Annales de Dermatologie et de Syphiligraphie*, **98**, 73.

Miescher G. (1955) Uber metastatische Invasar der Epidermis durch Tumorzellen (Melanom, Mammacarcinom). *Oncologia*, **8**, 203.

Ronchese F. (1940) Metastasis of the scalp simulating turban tumours. *Archives of Dermatology and Syphilology*, **41**, 439.

Rosenthal A.L. & Lever W.F. (1957) Involvement of the skin in renal carcinoma. *A.M.A. Archives of Dermatology*, **76**, 96.

Waterson K.W. & Shapiro L. (1970) Meningioma cutis. Report of a case. *International Journal of Dermatology*, **9**, 125.

Cysts of the scalp

The term sebacious cyst is still widely used and is applied indiscriminately to epidermal cysts or trichilemmal cysts. It is best abandoned (Leppard & Sanderson 1976).

Trichilemmal cysts

Aetiology

This relatively common cyst occurs mainly in middle age, and more frequently in women than in men. The tendency to form such cysts is inherited, and it is determined by an autosomal dominant gene (Ingram & Oldfield 1937; Stephens 1959).

Pathology

The cysts are derived from the external root sheath, the trichilemma (Pinkus 1969). The wall consists of epidermis and the cyst contains keratin, but no granular layer is formed.

Clinical features

The cysts occur most frequently in the scalp, as single, or more often multiple, firm rounded nodules. If the cysts are large hair growth in the overlying scalp may be impaired.

Treatment

Treatment may be required on cosmetic grounds. The cysts can usually be dissected out without difficulty; occasionally excision may be necessary.

References

Ingram J.T. & Oldfield M.C. (1937) Hereditary sebaceous cysts. *British Medical Journal*, **i**, 960.

Leppard B.J. & Sanderson K.V. (1976) The natural history of trichilemmal cysts. *British Journal of Dermatology*, **94**, 379.

Pinkus H. (1969) 'Sebaceous cysts' are trichilemmal cysts. *Archives of Dermatology*, **99**, 544.

Stephens F.E. (1959) Hereditary multiple sebaceous cysts. *Journal of Heredity*, **50**, 299.

Epidermoid cysts

Aetiology
Epidermoid cysts are common in adolescence and in adult life. They may occur as a complication of acne vulgaris.

They occur also in Gardner's syndrome.

Pathology
The wall of the cyst shows the normal layering of epidermis, but may be flattened by pressure. It contains lamellated keratin in which there may be cholesterol clefts.

Clinical features
Epidermoid cysts are firm and rounded nodules situated in the dermis and attached to the epidermis; there may be a central punctum.

They vary greatly in size, the largest cysts sometimes exceeding 50 mm in diameter. Recurrent episodes of inflammation are common, particularly in cysts associated with acne. The cysts occur most frequently on the face, neck and trunk, but are not uncommon in the scalp. They first appear in later childhood, and are frequently multiple.

Epidermoid cysts beginning in adolescence are a feature, often the earliest, of Gardner's syndrome, in which they are associated with fibromas, desmomas and lipomata of the skin and polyposis of the colon.

Treatment
Many cysts can be dissected out but cysts which have been inflamed may require excision, although some may be drained and pulverized.

Congenital inclusion dermoid cysts

Aetiology
Most dermoid cysts develop from sequestrated epithelial cells along lines of embryonic fusion. In the scalp groups of epidermal cells are cut off from the surface epithelium at the suture lines as the cranial bones grow together (Colcock *et al.* 1955).

Pathology
The cysts are lined by stratified squamous epithelium and contain greasy material, keratinized debris and hair.

Clinical features
About 40% are present at birth and 60% by the 5th year. They slowly enlarge to

reach a diameter of up to 5 cm. The skin is freely movable over them and they usually give rise to no symptoms.

Whilst the majority of cutaneous dermoids occur on the head and neck only a small proportion of them are in the scalp. In one series of cases the three cysts in the scalp were situated over the right parieto-occipital suture lines, the bregma and the anterior fontanelle respectively.

Treatment
Simple excision is usually adequate.

Reference
Colcock B.P., Sass R.D. & Standinger L. (1955) Dermoid cysts. *New England Journal of Medicine*, **252**, 373.

Chapter 19
Investigation of Hair and
Hair Follicle Diseases

On being presented with a patient complaining for example of pruritus or a blistering eruption, most clinicians are fully competent to carry out a careful clinical examination and to use appropriate histological, biochemical and other laboratory investigations if required. The details of specific techniques for studying the pathogenesis of hair diseases seem for many clinicians and pathologists to be shrouded in mystery, mainly because the methods concerned are not within the province of any one speciality.

Many of the techniques required for studying hair and hair follicle abnormalities will be found in the chapter relating to the disease in question. In this section are considered the clinical methods required for studying hair growth and also critical microscopic methods for detailed examination of hair shafts and hair follicles.

Hair growth and hair loss
(References p. 552)

History taking is of fundamental importance in assessing hair loss. A patient complaining of balding or hair loss may in fact have an increased shedding rate or a decrease in hairs per unit area. The complaint of thinning of hair may be due to a decrease in the number of hairs per unit area or a decrease in hair diameter; sometimes this may be worsened by a decrease in hair pigmentation. By careful questioning it is possible to assess these factors which guide one into particular lines of investigation and differential diagnosis. Table 19.1 shows categories of hair disorders based on the clinical presentation and mechanism of hair loss. It is important that these should be quantified in order accurately to assess the progress (and prognosis) of hair disease and also to assess the changes induced by treatment. For example, in androgenetic alopecia and hirsutism, changes in the telogen count, linear growth rate, diameter of hair and pigmentation are detectable before the affected individual is able subjectively to observe the changes.

Linear hair growth

Several simple methods are available for clinical or experimental use.

One method involves bleaching or dying hair in the affected area and observing the rate of growth of the normally pigmented hair that follows; using this method one can also crudely assess the number of hairs in anagen and telogen since only anagen hairs will show linear growth.

Hair may be shaved short or plane to the skin and standardized serial photography carried out. This has the advantage that measurements can be made at leisure from the photographic prints; its reliability depends entirely on careful photographic standardization. Saitoh *et al.* (1970) have modified this method to assess the hair cycle status in a more accurate way than the bleaching method. All the hair in the area to be studied is cut to approximately 1 mm long and photographed under standard conditions; after 1 week the photography is repeated and the hair is again cut to 0.5–1 mm. This process is repeated until enough pictures are available to compare individual hairs. The 'growth phase' is the period from the appearance of new hair in a given area to the end of its growth in length; the resting phase is from the time a hair attains its maximum length to when it is lost. By this method catagen is included in the growth phase.

Hair growth measurements can be made over very short periods of time using a capillary tube method (Saitoh *et al.* 1969). A glass capillary tube graduated every 0.2 mm is fitted around a growing hair and gently pressed to the surface of the skin. The image of the hair in the tube is magnified 16–25 times using a Zeiss Dermascope. This method allows growth to be measured at daily or even shorter intervals. The maximum error of the method is ±0.82% between 0 and 40°C and 0 and 100% humidity. The technique can of course be used without magnifying equipment if a larger margin of error is acceptable and growth measurement is only required every few days or longer.

To show that hair growth is constant during anagen, Saitoh *et al.* (1969) used time-lapse photography. Hair was shaved close to the skin in three regions, the vertex, the temple and the chin. To minimize blurring, a plaster mask was prepared to fix the head in the correct position; the photographic apparatus was also rigidly fastened. One exposure was taken every 15 minutes for 48 hours. By this method, all the hairs not in telogen were found to grow at a fairly constant rate.

A very accurate experimental method for the assessment of hair growth involves the use of radioactively labelled compounds (Downes & Syne 1959; Sims 1964). Intradermal injections of 35 S-cystine has been used in humans to assess growth in health and disease (Munro 1966; Comaish 1969 a, b).

Following the injection of the labelled cystine, hairs are plucked at specific intervals and subjected to autoradiography.

As already stated hair 'growth' abnormalities in clinical practice are not commonly associated with changes in linear growth but with other factors (Table 19.1). In order to quantify hair 'growth', Barman *et al.* (1964) devised the concept of the trichogram involving the measurement of growth rate, the state of the hair cycle, hair density, and hair thickness. Hair density and growth are measured using a microscope adapted for examining the skin surface; two eyepieces are used, one with a micrometer scale calibrated down to 1/40 mm

Table 19.1. Types of hair disorders in relation to clinical presentation

1. *Increased rate of shedding*
   Loss of telogen hairs (telogen effluvium)
   Loss of broken hairs (anagen effluvium)
   Loss of whole anagen hairs (anagen effluvium proper)

2. *Diffuse thinning of hair*
   Decrease in shaft diameter in all, or a proportion of hairs
   Decrease in hair pigmentation

3. *Patchy alopecia*
   Non-Scarring
      Loss of telogen hairs
      Loss of broken hairs
      Loss of whole anagen hairs
      Decrease in shaft diameter
   Scarring
      Loss of whole hairs
      Loss of follicular openings
      Hair twisting and kinking at edge of active areas

4. *Failure to grow long*
   Increased weathering of hair
   Loss of broken hairs
   Loss of telogen hairs

and the other containing a reticulum allowed measurements to be carried out on an area of 1/25 cm². As one parameter to assess hair follicle status they measured the 'regeneration period 90' which is the time lag for the reappearance of 90% of plucked hairs in a specific area. Using the trichogram method, hair 'growth' has been measured in prepubertal children (Pecoraro *et al.* 1964), adults (Barman *et al.* 1965) and pregnant women (Pecoraro 1967).

In attempting to grade hair growth on various body sites, Ferriman (1971) used a semi-quantitative hair scoring system in which hair growth was graded from 0 (absence of hair growth) through to 6 (very profuse hair growth); this method has been used for studying endocrine factors varying hair patterns.

Hair plucking and root analysis

To assess the status of hair in various body sites in relation to the hair cycle, and to study the changes in disease, hair root examination has long been used.

The simplest method used by clinicians is to grasp approximately ten hairs near to the scalp between the thumb and index finger and pull them firmly out of the scalp; under normal circumstances no more than two telogen roots (Fig. 1.9) will be present in the sample. This method may be repeated at several different sites. It is useful in observing the severity of androgenetic alopecitia, in which one can compare roots from the vertex with samples from the unaffected occipital area. This method is crude and is far inferior to more formal and standardized telogen counts. Approximately 50 plucked hairs are taken in this test; the group of hairs to be sampled is first held in a clamp such as needle holding or artery forceps, with elastoplast binding the jaws to give satisfactory grip. The hairs are then plucked with a quick action; the 40–50 hairs in the forceps can usually be plucked in groups of 8 or 10 but all the clamped hairs must be extracted and not simply those hairs which come out easily since most of the latter will be telogen roots. With experience the proportion of telogen (club) roots can be assessed macroscopically with the aid of a ×4 magnifying lens. For studying subjects with diffuse alopecia, telogen counts of this type, converted to a percentage of the total number plucked, are satisfactory. If accurate studies of anagen roots are required, for example, to assess the root changes induced by factors such as cytotoxic drugs or X-irradiation then the hairs must be mounted for microscopic examination (Van Scott *et al.* 1957). For anagen root examination it is essential that the hairs are plucked firmly and rapidly (Maguire & Kligman 1964) or many dysplastic roots will be obtained as in the studies of Archer & Luell (1960). Dysplastic roots are growing hairs with a constriction of the bulb or shaft, growing hairs with a constriction of the keratogenous zone, shafts broken at a constriction or hairs with a hook or bend in the bulb or keratogenous zone which is greater than 90°. Many of these changes may be seen from normal roots if plucking is not rapid—Van Scott *et al.* (1957) recommend floating the hairs in water prior to mounting for microscopy since hair roots can be more accurately staged when hydrated. If the roots are to be preserved, they should be mounted in balsam or a synthetic resin-mounting medium.

Hair and hair follicle microscopy

Hair shaft microscopy is essential for the diagnosis of many abnormalities, particularly fungal disease, congenital and hereditary hair shaft disorders and to assess hair weathering.

In the diagnosis of fungal diseases of hair (Rebell & Taplin 1976) plucked hairs are mounted in 20% potassium hydroxide solution; if the microscopy is to be carried out within 30 minutes then dimethylsulphoxide (DMSO) may speed the clearing time; DMSO may cause false negative results beyond this time since hyphal destruction occurs. The kerion type of infection may show only arthrospores on the proximal part of the plucked hair shaft despite massive inflammatory changes in the skin.

Optical microscopy

Routine light microscopy of hair shafts is essential for the diagnosis of diseases such as hereditary and congenital shaft abnormalities. To assess intrinsic shaft changes only the proximal 1–2 cm of plucked hairs should be examined since more distal changes may be extrinsic and due to weathering (Dawber 1980). Hairs may be mounted dry if they are required for further studies; however, in routine transmitted light microscopic examination the surface of dry-mounted hairs will scatter light. More detail is seen and higher magnification will be possible if a standard mounting medium is used; potassium hydroxide and water are not satisfactory. 'Colour' changes seen by routine light microscopy may be due to pigment alterations, or structural changes not transmitting light and thus giving dark areas. If reflected light is used then the dark areas in structural diseases such as pili annulati (Chapter 7) become light (Dawber 1972); pigmentation changes are not altered by this technique. Careful examination using routine light microscopy provides most of the information required in clinical practice. Polarization microscopy may provide extra information regarding the biochemical make-up of the hair and fine structural changes may become more obvious. Using this method it is possible to determine refractive index and the birefringence of fibres—the numerical difference between the refractive indexes parallel and perpendicular to the hair axis—a physical phenomenon that reflects the orientation of internal structures in the hair. In the examination of hair from patients with a neuroectodermal symptom complex (Price *et al.* 1980), polarizing microscopy revealed striking bright and dark regions on viewing the hair between cross polarizers. Turning the microscopic stage approximately 10° (5° on each side of the position of maximum extinction) reversed the bright and dark areas; between cross polarizers with the hair axis parallel to the vibration direction of the polarizer (maximum extinction or 0°), the hair revealed transverse lines. This abnormality was associated with sulphur, and high sulphur (matrix) protein deficiency. Brown *et al.* (1970) noted alternating birefringence in a congenital hair defect showing trichoschisis and low sulphur content. Dupré & Bonafe (1978) and Price (1979) have used polarization microscopy in many structural abnormalities of hair and have shown that the colour changes of polarization show up the abnormalities seen under transmitted light with greater clarity. The subtlety of optical microscopic methods can be enhanced by various specialized techniques (Swift 1977). The scale pattern can be examined in detail by examining a hair cast or impression of the hair in a suitable plastic material; an impression made by rolling the hair in the medium enables the whole circumference to be viewed. Interference microscopy, using monochromatic sodium light, greatly facilitates the examination of minute surface changes (Tolansky 1948).

Electron microscopy

Optical microscopy is limited in resolution to approximately 0.2 μm and has a narrow depth of focus. Transmission electron microscopy is capable of very high resolution (down to 2 nm for biological materials) and has a depth-of-image focus that is greater than the normal specimen thickness (approximately 100 nm). Routine electron microscopic preparation may be suitable for examination of hair follicles, but the presence of keratinized hair within the follicle and the nature of hair structure, make it necessary to modify routine procedure to get the best resolution and meaningful results. Glass knives give poor sectioning; a diamond knife is necessary for cutting ultra-thin sections of hair without distortion. Needless to say this is a very skilful procedure not always available in electron microscope laboratories. Hair is a rather amorphous structure and must be stained with a heavy metal to show anatomical detail. Uranyl acetate and lead citrate enable the overall structure to be seen; dodecatungstophoric acid gives added detail of cortex matrix proteins and cortical cell membranes. For transverse sections of hair fibres, ammoniacal silver, or the silver methenamine stain (Swift 1968) which specifically stain cystine, give more contrast to cuticular and cortical structure (Fig. 19.1) by highlighting the cystine-rich exocuticle and cortical matrix protein (Leonard *et al.* 1980). Other electron histochemical techniques already usefully applied to tissue from many other organs have not get been fully exploited in hair follicle disease; these include the identification and localization of enzyme systems and antigen–antibody reactions (Swift 1977).

Scanning electron microscopy is very diverse in its modes of operation and gives a wealth of information about surface architecture (Dawber & Comaish 1970; Brown & Swift 1975), elemental composition (if an X-ray microanalytical attachment is available), crystalline make-up and electrical and magnetic properties of specimens. It is a research tool and it cannot be stressed too greatly that all the detail needed by the clinician regarding hair microstructure can be obtained by optical microscopic methods.

Follicular microscopy

Biopsy technique must be considered carefully if useful histological results are to

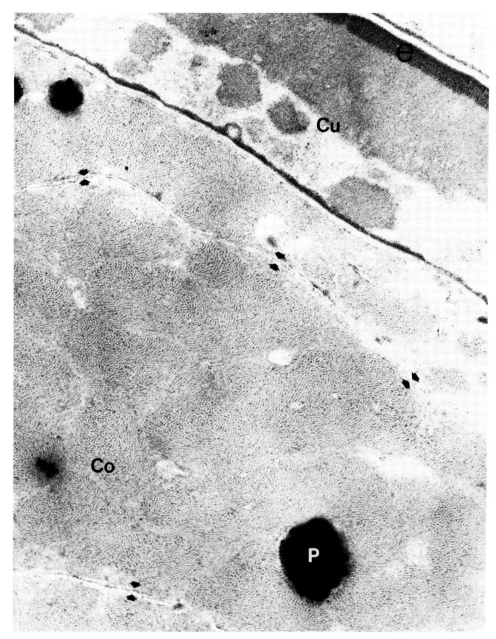

Fig. 19.1. Silver methenamine stain, showing the cystine-rich exocuticle A-layer (e); and matrix protein in the cortex (Cu) (Slade Hospital, Oxford).

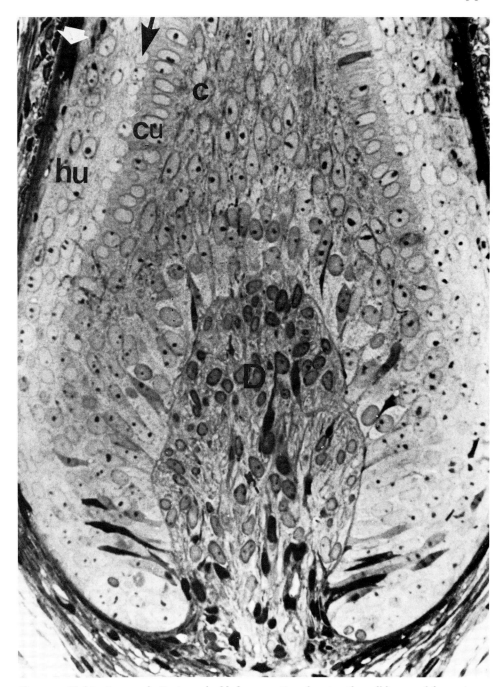

Fig. 19.2. Light micrograph. Resin-embedded 1 m section showing the cell layers of the cortex (C), cuticle of hair (Cu), the internal root sheath cuticle (black arrow), Huxley layer (white arrow) and the dermal papilla (D) (Slade Hospital, Oxford).

be obtained. The level of the biopsy must extend deep into subcutaneous fat to avoid cutting off hair bulbs. The epidermal surface of the excised tissue should be opposed to a rigid piece of paper, to avoid curling of the tissue, and immediately placed in fixative, if necessary it can be glued or pinned to the paper if longitudinal follicular cutting is desired (Fig. 19.2), since follicles have a great propensity for bending prior to hardening, leading to cross-cutting in the dermis. After processing, the embedded tissue requires careful orientation prior to cutting to maximize the chance of obtaining longitudinal follicular sections. Routine paraffin-embedded tissue has never been entirely satisfactory for visualizing cytological detail within the follicle; where possible, tissue should be fixed and embedded as for routine electronmicroscopy and 1μ sections cut (Fig. 19.2), this gives greater cytological clarity. Haematoxylin and eosin staining reveals the general detail of the various cell layers in the follicle. Other histochemical stains may specifically enhance the appearance of various cell layers (Pinkus 1968, 1980). The lower border of the internal root sheath takes up the Giemsa stain; this stains the keratinized internal root sheath specifically dark blue. The intra-follicular hair cuticle stains with toluidine blue and rhodamine B, first becoming visible as a thin blue layer surrounding the presumptive hair. The Van Gieson stain gives a yellow colour to the hair and the club in telogen roots; the tissue surrounding the club is brownish-red with PASHPA stain whilst rhodamine B stains the cuticle a faint blue colour and the surrounding tricholemmal layer brilliant red. Useful screening techniques for abnormal hair keratins are the fluorescence methods using either acridine orange or thioflavine T; normal hair keratin fluoresces blue with dilute acridine orange, whereas altered keratins such as the tip of hairs in trichorrhexis nodosa, dystrophic hairs in kwashiorkor, or weathered fibres, fluoresce red or orange. The peracetic oxidation and thioflavine T fluorescent method (Jarrett 1958) stain the disulphide bonds in cystine, enabling sites of mature keratin to be detected in the exocuticle or cortex. —SH bonds can be specifically stained by a fluorogenic meleimide, N(7-dimethyl-amino-methyl coumarinyl) maleimide (DACM). This substance only fluoresces on combining with —SH bonds (Taneda *et al.* 1980); this method requires frozen tissue; it has the advantage that the emission maximum of DACM does not overlap with any of the aromatic residues of proteins such as tryptophan.

References

Archer V.E. & Luell E. (1960) Effect of selenium sulphide suspension on hair roots. *Journal of Investigative Dermatology*, **35**, 65.

Barman J.M., Pecoraro V. & Astore I. (1964) Method, technique and computations in the study of the trophic state of human scalp hair. *Journal of Investigative Dermatology*, **42**, 421.

Barman J.M., Astore I. & Pecoraro V. (1965) The normal trichogram of the adult. *Journal of Investigative Dermatology*, **44**, 233.

Brown A.C. & Swift J.A. (1975) Hair breakage: the scanning electron microscope as a diagnostic tool. *Journal of the Society of Cosmetic Chemists*, **26**, 289.

Comaish S. (1969a) Autoradiographic studies of hair growth in various dermatoses: investigations of a possible circadian rhythm in human hair growth. *British Journal of Dermatology*, **81**, 283.

Comaish S. (1969b) Autoradiographic studies of hair growth and rhythm in monilethrix. *British Journal of Dermatology*, **81**, 443.

Dawber R.P.R. & Comaish S. (1970) Scanning electron microscopy of normal and abnormal hair shafts. *Archives of Dermatology*, **101**, 316.

Dawber R.P.R. (1972) Investigations of a family with pili annulati associated with blue naevi. *Transactions of St. John's Hospital Dermatological Society*, **58**, 51.

Dawber R.P.R. (1980) Weathering of hair in some genetic hair dystrophies. In *Hair, Trace Elements and Human Illness*, eds. A.C. Brown & R.G. Crounse. New York, Praeger.

Downes A.M. & Syne A.G. (1959) Measurement of the rate of growth of wool using cystine labelled with sulphur 35. *Nature*, **184**, 1884.

Dupré A. & Bonafe J.L. (1978) Pilar dystrophies studied by polarised light. *Annales de Dermatologie et de Venerologie*, **105**, 921.

Ferriman (1971) *Human Hair Growth in Health and Disease*, 1st edn. Springfield, Thomas, USA.

Jarrett A. (1958) Chemistry of inner root sheath and hair keratins. *British Journal of Dermatology*, **70**, 271.

Leonard J.N., Gummer C.L. & Dawber R.P.R. (1980) Generalised trichorrhexis nodosa. *British Journal of Dermatology*, **103**, 85.

Maguire H.C. & Kligman A.M. (1964) Hair plucking as a diagnostic tool. *Journal of Investigative Dermatology*, **43**, 73.

Munro D.D. (1966) Hair growth measurement using intradermal sulphur 35-cystine. *Archives of Dermatology*, **93**, 119.

Pecoraro V., Astore I., Barman J.M. & Araujo C.I. (1964) The normal trichogram in the child before the age of puberty. *Journal of Investigative Dermatology*, **42**, 427.

Pecoraro V., Barman J.M. & Astore I. (1967) The normal trichogram of pregnant women. In *Advances in Biology of Skin*, vol. IX, *Hair Growth*, eds. W. Montagna & R.L. Dobson. Oxford, Pergamon Press.

Pinkus H. (1980) Factors in the formation of club hairs. In *Hair, Trace Elements and Human Illness'*, eds. A.C. Brown & R.G. Crounse. New York, Praeder.

Price V.H. (1979) Strukturanomalien des Haarschaftes. In *Haar und Haarkrankheiten*, ed. C.E. Orfanos. Stuttgart, Fischer Verlag.

Price V.H., Odom R.B., Ward W.H. & Jones F.T. (1980) Trichothiodystrophy. *Archives of Dermatology*, **116**, 1375.

Rebell G. & Taplin D. (1976) *Dermatophytes: Their Recognition and Identification*, 2nd edn. Florida, University of Miami Press.

Saitoh M., Uzaka M. & Sakamoto M. (1969) Rate of hair growth. In *Advances in Biology of Skin*, vol. IX, *Hair Growth*, eds. W. Montagna & R.L. Dobson. Oxford, Pergamon Press.

Saitoh M., Uzaka M. & Sakamoto M. (1970) Human hair cycle. *Journal of Investigative Dermatology*, **54**, 65.

Sims R.T. (1964) The incorporation and fate of H_3 tyrosine in the hair cortex of rats observed by autoradiography. *Journal of Cell Biology*, **23**, 403.

Swift J.A. (1968) The electron histochemistry of cystine containing proteins in thin transverse sections of human hair. *Journal of the Royal Microscopical Society*, **88**, 449.

Swift J.A. (1977) The Histology of Keratin Fibres. In *The Chemistry of Natural Protein Fibres*, ed. R.S. Asquith. London, Wiley.

Taneda A., Ogawa H. & Hashimoto K. (1980) The histochemical demonstration of protein-bound sulphidryl groups and disulphide bonds in human hair by a new staining method (DACM staining). *Journal of Investigative Dermatology*, **75**, 365.

Tolansky S (1948) *Multiple Beam Interferometry*, Oxford, Clarendon Press.

Van Scott E.J., Reinertson R.P. & Steinmuller R. (1957) The growing hair roots of human scalp and morphological changes therein following amethopterin therapy. *Journal of Investigative Dermatology*, **29**, 197.

Index